The SAGES Manual of Hernia Repair

The SAGES Manual of Hernia Repair

Brian P. Jacob, MD, FACS
Mount Sinai School of Medicine, NY, USA

Bruce Ramshaw, MD, FACS
Transformative Care Institute, Daytona Beach, FL, USA

Editors

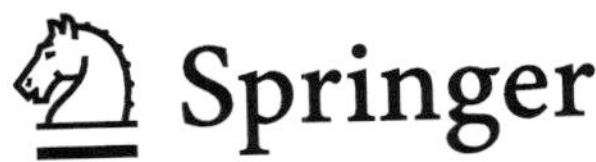

Editors
Brian P. Jacob, MD, FACS
Mount Sinai School of Medicine
Mount Sinai Medical Center
New York, NY, USA

Bruce Ramshaw, MD, FACS
Transformative Care Institute
Advanced Hernia Solutions
Department of General Surgery
Daytona Beach, FL, USA

ISBN 978-1-4614-4823-5 ISBN 978-1-4614-4824-2 (eBook)
DOI 10.1007/978-1-4614-4824-2
Springer New York Heidelberg Dordrecht London

Library of Congress Control Number: 2012948968

Printed on acid-free paper

Springer is part of Springer Science+Business Media (www.springer.com)

Preface

The evolution of abdominal wall hernia repair, both inguinal and ventral, continues as we begin the second decade of the twenty-first century. There is an ongoing influx of new techniques, new prosthetics and devices, and new hernia programs, each designed to optimize outcomes for our patients. Tomorrow's techniques and workflows will certainly be different than those we are utilizing today. With patient outcomes paramount, it is important to capture and summarize the current trends and debates into one manual that is easily accessible for all hernia surgeons. This new *SAGES Manual of Hernia Repair* provides practicing surgeons with immediate access in one handbook to many acceptable current ideas and strategies regarding hernia repair.

Each time we repair a hernia, the technique we choose and the mesh we implant will vary, based not just on surgeon experience but also on the individual patient we are trying to help. As surgeons lead the effort to implement evidence-based algorithms to define and improve patient care and outcomes, this manual can be used as a reference when considering a particular management strategy for hernia patients. We have added a unique section called Current Debates where readers can capture current opinions on many of the ongoing debates of this time period.

We want to genuinely thank all of the contributors for their hard work in preparing these manuscripts for this book, which we dedicate to all of the family members and colleagues who unconditionally support each of us.

New York, NY, USA — Brian P. Jacob
Daytona Beach, FL, USA — Bruce Ramshaw

Contents

Part IX Other Hernias

Contributors

Gina L. Adrales, MD, MPH
Department of Surgery, Dartmouth-Hitchcock Medical Center, Lebanon, NH, USA

Emily L. Albright, MD
Division of General Surgery, Department of Surgery, University of Kentucky College of Medicine, Lexington, KY, USA

A. Mariah Alexander, MD
Department of Surgery, University of Tennessee Graduate School of Medicine, Knoxville, TN, USA

Richard Alexander, MD
Department of Minimally Invasive Surgery, Texas Endosurgery Institute, San Antonia, TX, USA

Parviz K. Amid, MD
Department of General Surgery, Lichtenstein Hernia Institute, David Geffen School of Medicine at UCLA, Santa Monica, CA, USA

Maurice E. Arregui, MD, FACS
Department of General Surgery, St Vincent Hospital, Indianapolis, IN, USA

Charles Ascher-Walsh, MD
Department of Obstetrics, Gynecology and Reproductive Science, The Mount Sinai Hospital, New York, NY, USA

Gerardo Lozano Balderas, MD
Department of General Surgery, Hospital San José–Tec de Monterrey, Monterrey, Nuevo Leon, Mexico

Igor Belyansky, MD
Department of General Surgery, General Surgery Faculty, Anne Arundel Medical Center, Annapolis, MD, USA

Steven P. Bowers, MD
Department of General Surgery, Mayo Clinic Florida, Jacksonville, FL, USA

L. Michael Brunt, MD
Department of Surgery, Barnes-Jewish Hospital, St. Louis, MO, USA

Alfredo M. Carbonell II, DO
Division of Minimal Access and Bariatric Surgery, Department of Surgery, Greenville Hospital System University Medical Center, University of South Carolina School of Medicine–Greenville, Greenville, SC, USA

Jaime A. Cavallo, MD, MPHS
Section of Minimally Invasive Surgery, Department of Surgery, Washington University School of Medicine, St. Louis, MO, USA

David C. Chen, MD
Department of General Surgery, Lichtenstein Hernia Institute, David Geffen School of Medicine at UCLA, Santa Monica, CA, USA

Jenny J. Choi, MD
Department of Surgery, Montefiore Medical Center, Bronx, NY, USA

Andrei Churyla, MD
Department of Surgery, Berkshire Medical Center, Pittsfield, MA, USA

William S. Cobb IV, MD
Department of Surgery, Greenville Hospital System University Medical Center, Greenville, SC, USA

Gregory F. Dakin, MD
Department of Surgery, Weill Cornell Medical College, New York Presbyterian Hospital, New York, NY, USA

Corey R. Deeken, PhD
Department of Surgery, Washington University School of Medicine, St. Louis, MO, USA

Jose J. Diaz Jr., MD, FACS, FCCM
Department of Surgery, University of Maryland Medical Center, Baltimore, MD, USA

Juan J. Diaz-Hernandez, MD
Department of General Surgery, Florida Hospital Celebration Health, Celebration, FL, USA

Carl Doerhoff, MD, FACS
Department of Surgery, Capital Region Medical Center,
Jefferson City, MO, USA

David Earle, MD, FACS
Minimally Invasive Surgery and Esophageal Physiology Laboratory,
Baystate Medical Center, Tufts University School of Medicine,
Springfield, MA, USA

Chris Edwards, MD
Mission Bariatrics, Mission Hospitals, Asheville, NC, USA

Kevin El-Hayek, MD
Bariatric and Metabolic Institute, Cleveland Clinic, Cleveland, OH, USA

Jose E. Espinel, MD, FACS
Department of Surgery, Baystate Medical Center, Springfield, MA, USA

Nicole Fearing, MD
Malley Surgical, Mission, KS, USA

Edward L. Felix, MD, FACS
Department of Surgery, Central California Institute of Minimally
Invasive Surgery, Fresno, CA, USA

Abe Fingerhut, MD, FACS, FRCPS, FRCS Ed
European Association for Endoscopic Surgery, Eindhoven,
The Netherlands

Department of Surgery, Hippokration Hospital, University of Athens,
Athens, Greece

Robert J. Fitzgibbons Jr., MD, FACS
Department of General Surgery, Creighton University Medical Center,
Omaha, NE, USA

Dennis L. Fowler, MD, MPH
Department of Surgery, Reemtsma Center for Innovation
and Outcomes Research, College of Physicians and Surgeons,
Columbia University, New York, NY, USA

Morris Franklin Jr., MD, FACS
Department of Minimally Invasive Surgery, Texas Endosurgery
Institute, San Antonio, TX, USA

Matthew Goede, MD
Department of Surgery, University of Nebraska Medical Center,
Omaha, NE, USA

Rajat Goel, MBBS, MS, DNB
Mimimal Access and Bariatric Surgery, Columbia Asia Hospital, Palam Vihar, Gurgaon, India

Ross F. Goldberg, MD
Department of Surgery, Mayo Clinic Florida, Jacksonville, FL, USA

Dinakar Golla, MD
Department of Plastic Surgery, University of Pittsburgh Medical Center, Pittsburgh, PA, USA

Sheila A. Grant, PhD
Department of Biological Engineering, University of Missouri, Columbia, MO, USA

Kristi L. Harold, MD
Division of General Surgery, Mayo Clinic Arizona, Phoenix, AZ, USA

B. Todd Heniford, MD, FACS
Department of Surgery, University of North Carolina at Chapel Hill, Charlotte, NC, USA

Elizabeth Honigsberg, MD
Department of Surgery, Dartmouth-Hitchcock Medical Center, Lebanon, NH, USA

Brian P. Jacob, MD, FACS
Department of Surgery, Mount Sinai Medical Center, Mount Sinai School of Medicine, New York, NY, USA

L. Brian Katz, MD
Department of Surgery, The Mount Sinai Hospital, New York, NY, USA

Stephen M. Kavic, MD, FACS
Department of Surgery, University of Maryland School of Medicine, Baltimore, MD, USA

Michael L. Kendrick, MD
Department of Surgery, Mayo Clinic, Rochester, MN, USA

Kent W. Kercher, MD, FACS
Division of GI and Minimally Invasive Surgery, Carolinas Medical Center, Charlotte, NC, USA

Mousa Khoursheed, MD, FRCPS
Department of Surgery, Mubarak Al-Kabeer Hospital,
University of Kuwait, Safat, Kuwait

David A. Klima, BS, MD
Department of General Surgery, Carolinas Medical Center,
Charlotte, NC, USA

Matthew Kroh, MD
Department of General Surgery, Digestive Disease Institute,
Cleveland Clinic Lerner College of Medicine, Cleveland, OH, USA

David M. Krpata, MD
Division of Pediatric Surgery, Rainbow Babies and Children's Hospital,
Cleveland, OH, USA

Andrew B. Lederman, MD, FACS
Department of Surgery, Berkshire Medical Center, Pittsfield, MA, USA

John G. Linn, MD
Department of Surgery, Ohio State University Medical Center,
Columbus, OH, USA

Aaron M. Lipskar, MD
Department of General Surgery, The Mount Sinai School of Medicine,
New York, NY, USA

Davide Lomanto, MD, PhD
Minimally Invasive Surgical Centre, National University Health System,
Singapore, Singapore

Gregory J. Mancini, MD
Department of Surgery, University of Tennessee Graduate
School of Medicine, Knoxville, TN, USA

Daniel Marcus, MD
Department of Surgery, Marina del Rey Hospital,
Marina del Rey, CA, USA

St. Johns Health Center, Santa Monica, CA, USA

Roxbury Hernia Center, Beverly Hills, CA, USA

Viney K. Mathavan, MD
Department of General Surgery, St Vincent Hospital, Indianapolis,
IN, USA

Brent D. Matthews, MD, FACS
Section of Minimally Invasive Surgery, Department of Surgery, Washington University School of Medicine, St. Louis, MO, USA

David A. McClusky III, MD
Department of Surgery, Atlanta VAMC and Emory University School of Medicine, Decatur, GA, USA

Dean J. Mikami, MD
Department of Gastrointestinal Surgery, The Ohio State University Medical Center, Columbus, OH, USA

Marc Miserez, MD, PhD
Department of Abdominal Surgery, University Hospital Gasthuisberg, Leuven, Belgium

Yuri W. Novitsky, MD
Department of Surgery, Case Comprehensive Hernia Center, University Hospitals Case Medical Center, Cleveland, OH, USA

Dmitry Oleynikov, MD, FACS
Department of Surgery, University of Nebraska Medical Center, Omaha, NE, USA

Carlos M. Ortiz-Ortiz, MD
Department of General Surgery, Florida Hospital Celebration Health, Celebration, FL, USA

Mickey M. Ott, MD
Division of Trauma and Surgical Critical Care, Department of Surgery, Vanderbilt University Medical Center, Nashville, TN, USA

Pradeep Pallati, MD
Department of General Surgery, Creighton University Medical Center, Omaha, NE, USA

Adrian Park, MD, FRCSC, FACS, FCS(ECSA)
Department of Surgery, Anne Arundel Health System, Annapolis, MD, USA

Eduardo Parra-Davila, MD, FACS, FASCRS
Department of General Surgery, Florida Hospital Celebration Health, Celebration, FL, USA

Jonathan P. Pearl, MD
Norman M. Rich Department of Surgery, Uniformed Services University/Walter Reed National Military Medical Center, Bethesda, MD, USA

Scott Philipp, MD, FACS
Department of Surgery, The Permanente Medical Group, Inc, Vallejo, CA, USA

Lisa C. Pickett, MD
Departments of Surgery/Critical Care and Medicine, Duke University Hospital, Durham, NC, USA

Alfons Pomp, MD, FACS, FRCSC
Department of Surgery, New York Presbyterian Hospital/Weill Medical College of Cornell University, New York, NY, USA

Kimberly Ponnuru, MD, FACS
Department of General Surgery, Providence Medical Center, General Surgery Associates, Kansas City, KS, USA

Todd A. Ponsky, MD
Division of Pediatric Surgery, Akron Childrens Hospital, One Perkins Square Akron, OH, USA

Benjamin S. Powell, MD
Department of Surgery, University of Tennessee Health Science Center, Memphis, TN, USA

Archana Ramaswamy, MD
Department of General Surgery, University of Missouri Healthcare, Columbia, MO, USA

Bruce Ramshaw, MD, FACS
Department of General Surgery, Transformative Care Institute, Advanced Hernia Solutions, Daytona Beach, FL, USA

Lauren Rascoff, MD
Department of Obstetrics, Gynecology and Reproductive Science, Mount Sinai Hospital, New York, NY, USA

Mark A. Reiner, MD
Department of Surgery, The Mount Sinai Hospital, New York, NY, USA

E. Matthew Ritter, MD
Division of Academic Surgery, Norman M. Rich Department of Surgery, Uniformed Services University/Walter Reed National Military Medical Center, Bethesda, MD, USA

John R. Romanelli, MD
Department of Surgery, Baystate Medical Center, Tufts University School of Medicine, Springfield, MA, USA

Michael J. Rosen, MD
Division of GI and General Surgery, Department of Surgery, Case Comprehensive Hernia Center, Case Medical Center, Case Western Reserve University, Cleveland, OH, USA

J. Scott Roth, MD
Department of Surgery, University of Kentucky College of Medicine, Lexington, KY, USA

Karla Russek, MD
Department of Minimally Invasive Surgery, Texas Endosurgery Institute, San Antonio, TX, USA

Marc H.F. Schreinemacher, MD
Department of General Surgery, Maastricht University Medical Center, Maastricht, The Netherlands

C. Daniel Smith, MD, FACS
Department of Surgery, Mayo Clinic Florida, Jacksonville, FL, USA

Nathaniel Stoikes, MD
Department of Surgery, University of Tennessee Health Sciences Center, Memphis, TN, USA

Chee-Chee H. Stucky, MD
Department of General Surgery, Mayo Clinic Arizona, Phoenix, AZ, USA

Malini D. Sur, MD
Department of Surgery, Mount Sinai Medical Center, New York, NY, USA

Daniel E. Swartz, MD, FACS, FRCSC
Department of Surgery, Central California Institute of Minimally Invasive Surgery, Fresno, CA, USA

Victor B. Tsirline, MD, MS
Department of Surgery, Northwestern Lake Forest Hospital, Lake Forest, IL, USA

Jignesh V. Unadkat, MD, MRCS
Department of Plastic Surgery, University of Pittsburgh Medical Center, Pittsburgh, PA, USA

Guy Voeller, MD
Department of General Surgery, University of Tennessee Health Science Center, Memphis, TN, USA

Part I
Essentials of Inguinal Hernia

1. Establishing a Hernia Program and Follow-Up Regimen: A Complex Systems Design for Care and Improvement

Bruce Ramshaw

It is tempting to write a chapter describing the development of a hernia program in the traditional "center of excellence" model. In that model, there would be criteria developed for certification, documented protocols, and standardized process and outcome measures reported to a national regulatory group. This has been the model for bariatric surgery programs for the past decade. However, there is growing awareness that this "center of excellence" model, while helping to prevent extremely poor care, actually fosters mediocrity and inhibits positive innovation. By implementing standards and static criteria as well as requiring resources focused upon reporting, attention is often placed on maintaining the status quo rather than on continuous learning and improving. The transformation to a sustainable health care system will require us to design programs around patient problems in a way that allows for continuous learning and improving, facilitated by a diverse community that includes the patient and family.

The "center of excellence" model is also designed either around a limited portion of a patient's cycle of care and/or based on a particular physician specialty, rather than the entire cycle of care from the perspective of the patient. To understand why we need to evolve beyond the "center of excellence" model, it might be helpful to understand how our global health care system has become unsustainable in its current form. Our health care system has become what it is today through a complex history involving the evolution of hospitals, physicians, nurses, and other specialties, combined with insurance policies and other health

B.P. Jacob and B. Ramshaw (eds.), *The SAGES Manual of Hernia Repair*, DOI 10.1007/978-1-4614-4824-2_1,

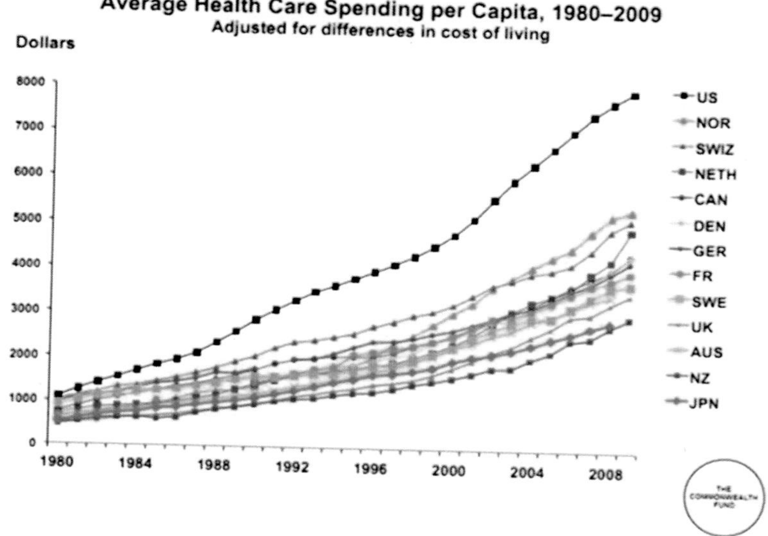

Fig. 1.1. Average health care spending per capita in many developed countries over a period of almost 30 years. Although the total spending per capita varies country to country, the overall spending trend over time (the *slope*) is similar for every country. This result reflects the predictable output of a complex system (our global health care system) where each part of the fragmented system is focused on revenue growth and profit margin (or bond rating for nonprofits). The system is producing the result (unsustainable costs) that it is designed to produce.

care laws, enacted in an attempt to help people be able to afford and have access to health care. Over time, the health care system has grown to become almost 18% of the US GDP. A look at other developed countries' spending on health care shows that, although they do not spend as much on total health care costs, the trends of increasing costs are essentially the same (Fig. 1.1). This represents a global health care system designed for the revenue growth of each part rather than for optimizing the value of the health of a population, including the entire patient cycle of care and the health care system itself. In addition to care givers and hospitals, a variety of industries within health care, led by the pharmaceutical industry, have grown to serve patients by providing diagnostic and therapeutic intervention and have also been successful in creating a large amount of wealth for a relatively small group of shareholders and top corporate executives. It is this fragmentation, with each part focused primarily on its own optimization, which has led to the current unsustainable situation in health care. [1, 2]

There are many other parts in the system that extract profit and resources which I will not describe (medical publishers, general purchasing organizations, etc.), but even with the few components mentioned, it is evident that the system inherently functions by attempting to optimize and protect its parts. Hospitals work to optimize hospital performance and maintain profit margin and growth targets; physicians focus on the financial needs of their individual and group practices as well as the portion of care they provide for the patient based on each physician's specialty. In addition to these providers of care, pharmaceutical and other health care companies have a fiduciary responsibility to maximize shareholder profit while they are producing products to be used in patient care. An understanding of complex systems science makes it clear that when each part is attempting to optimize itself, then the whole process (in this case, the hernia patient's entire cycle of care) WILL NOT be optimized [3].

Complex systems science also helps to explain why one type of treatment or device (such as hernia mesh) can be beneficial to one group of patients but cause harm to another. During the past decade, with the help of a dedicated hernia team and in collaboration with many hernia experts worldwide, we have discovered the complexity of mesh used to repair hernias, and just this one example is a reflection of the increasing complexity of the world, in general, and health care in particular. When I started residency (1989), there were basically a few meshes available, and today there are hundreds. Most importantly, the same mesh used with the same technique in two different patients can have significantly different outcomes. This variability is due to the fact that we are all (caregivers, patients, and the health care systems we function in) complex adaptive systems. The concept of complex systems means that outcomes are variable and dependent upon many variables, as well as the interactions between them. The design for organizations attempting to optimize the value of a complex system is very different from one that is designed to optimize the value of a simple system (in which the cause and effect are directly related and predictable—mass producing one type of hernia mesh, for example). For a simple system, the parts may be optimized to improve the entire process for a predictable, repeatable output. For a complex system, many parts may need to be suboptimized and all the interactions between the parts need to be managed, measured, and continuously improved. This allows for optimization of the whole process and output (providing care for a group of hernia patients, for example) [4].

Developing an Academic Hernia Program

The core concept behind the development of a hernia program using a complex systems approach is the design of the program with a new organizational structure. This must be one which provides person-centered care coordination with the implementation of continuous clinical quality improvement (CCQI) cycles. If these are developed as the essence of care delivery, it will drive increased value for both the patient and the system itself.

A core component of care coordination is the development of person-centered patient care managers. By facilitating patient and family member engagement and responsibility, the patient care managers ensure that an outcomes-based relationship is developed among the patient, their family, and the care team. With patient and family engagement, better decisions, better outcomes, and lower costs are more likely [5]. This patient and family relationship continues throughout the entire cycle of care for the patient, and of course, accountability is built into this important process.

The principles of care coordination and CCQI implementation include:

1. Identify a diverse group of people to address the needs of a definable group of patients with hernia disease and hernia-related complications and problems. This will make up the core hernia team. Figure 1.2 represents the concept of a diverse team designed around the needs of a defined group of patients with hernia disease and related complications.
2. Engagement and participation of patient and family in the care process, as a part of the hernia team and a part of the extended care community development (shared decision process for all elective care decisions).
3. Continuous access to all information (patient record, dynamic care processes, outcomes, etc.) for the patient and family.
4. Care coordination led by patient care managers who are considered and treated as equal members of the care team. This requires time to develop genuine relationships and trust between all core team members.
5. Development of transparent, dynamic care processes based upon best available evidence and which are continuously improved, based on evolving evidence.
6. Development of outcome measures that identify value of care for both the patient and the system: quality, satisfaction, safety, financial, etc.

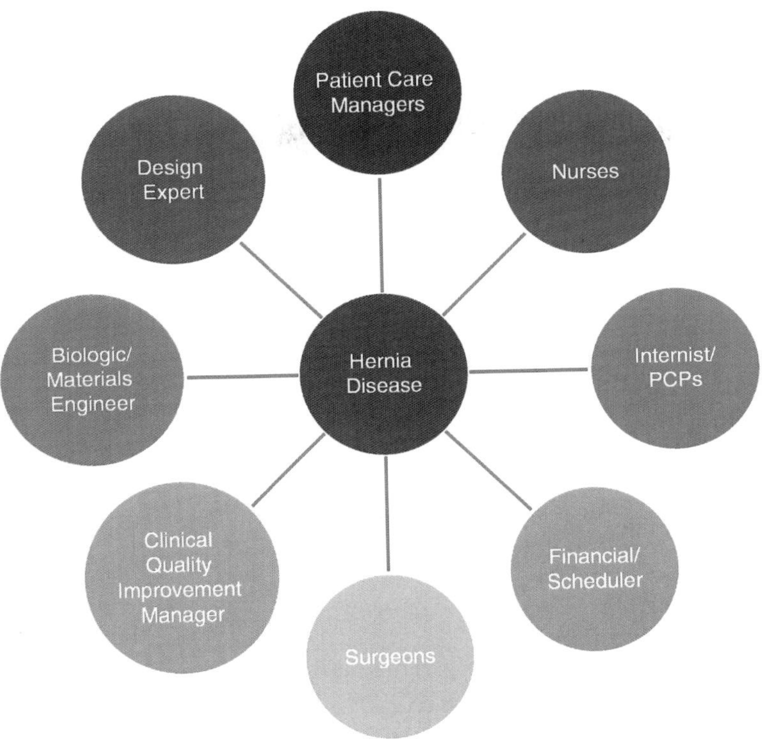

Fig. 1.2. An example of a diverse team built around a group of patients with hernia disease and hernia-related problems.

7. Care processes and outcome measures are developed and adapted to local environments and are continuously measured and improved through the CCQI process locally.
8. The hernia team has the authority and resources to function within this complex systems structure and is accountable to make outcome measures transparent to governing boards made up of leadership and the community.

This plan addresses the system structural problem of why our health care system has not been able to evolve into a sustainable model, namely, the vertical department and hierarchical structure of most health care organizations in addition to the individual physician practice model. These system structures have led to fragmentation of care, and as complexity has increased, this fragmentation has led to poorer outcomes, less efficiency, and more waste within the entire health care industry. Recent attempts to improve quality, such as surgical site marking and timing of antibiotic dose in suspected pneumonia patients in the emergency room, have not led to significant improvement and, in some cases, have caused unintended harm [6–12]. Because these attempts are simple solutions applied to complex problems and complex systems, they do not provide significant or sustainable improvement. Addressing complex problems within complex systems requires a different approach.

In person-centered care, the focus is based upon defined patient groups and problems rather than upon the physicians' specialties. The care is provided by diverse team members (including patients and family members) with the different skill sets necessary to effectively meet the needs of each patient group. For a person whose primary current problem is related to hernia disease, the hernia team provides integrated management for all care needs of the patient cutting across the traditional vertical department model. Integrated management of multiple comorbidities has been shown to improve outcomes [13, 14]. In CCQI, the cost of all steps of the health care process for patient groups are documented and analyzed, and the value is determined. This, in turn, is used to decrease the cost and waste as well as to improve the outcomes of care.

To effectively implement the CCQI process, an understanding of the patient processes associated with the entire cycle of care is necessary. These workflows document the patient steps, resources, data, and personnel associated with the care of the patient through the entire cycle of care. The care process begins with first contact with the patient and continues through the return to maximum quality of life, which may encompass the entire life span of the patient in some cases. One example of a dynamic patient care process is represented in Fig. 1.3.

One challenge in determining the value for these processes is to determine the real costs for each step in each care process, termed activity-based accounting. In "How to Solve the Cost Crisis in Health Care" (Harvard Business Review, September 2011), Robert Kaplan and Michael Porter outline a process by which the value of health care is documented [15]. This involves determination of the true cost of care through a seven-step process: (1) determine patient population to be examined, (2) define the delivery care chain, (3) develop process maps of care delivery, (4) obtain time estimates for each step, (5) estimate the cost of supplying each patient care resource, (6) estimate capacity of each resource provider, and (7) compute the total costs over the entire cycle of care for a patient [15]. True costs of each step in the patient care

a Types of Hernia Dynamic Care Processes

Elective Dynamic Care Processes

Pre-Clinic	Clinic	Pre-Op	Procedure	Post-Op	Discharge / Follow-up

- Inguinal hernia (uncomplicated and complicated)
- Ventral hernia (uncomplicated and complicated)
- Complex abdominal wall reconstruction
- Sports hernia (chronic groin pain without hernia)
- Chronic pain after prior hernia repair
- Chronic pelvic pain in females

b

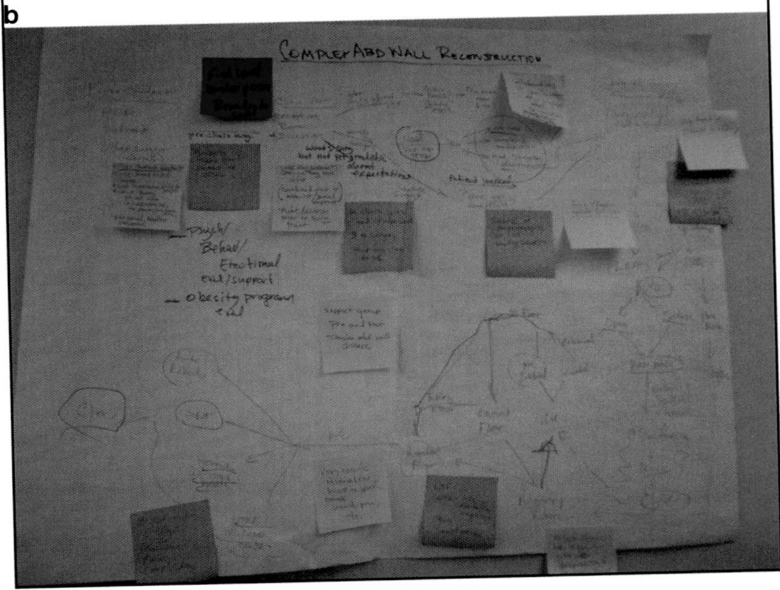

Fig. 1.3. (**a**) The list and basic diagram for hernia program dynamic care processes representing all groups of patients cared for by our hernia program and the design of the care processes to define the patient's entire cycle of care. (**b**) The early stages of developing a dynamic care process for a complex abdominal wall patient group. (**c**–**f**) A more complete example of the dynamic care process for a patient group with uncomplicated ventral hernia disease. Within many of these steps, there are data collection forms that will travel with the patient and team through the entire cycle of care and outcome measures that will be used to determine value and help to improve the process over time.

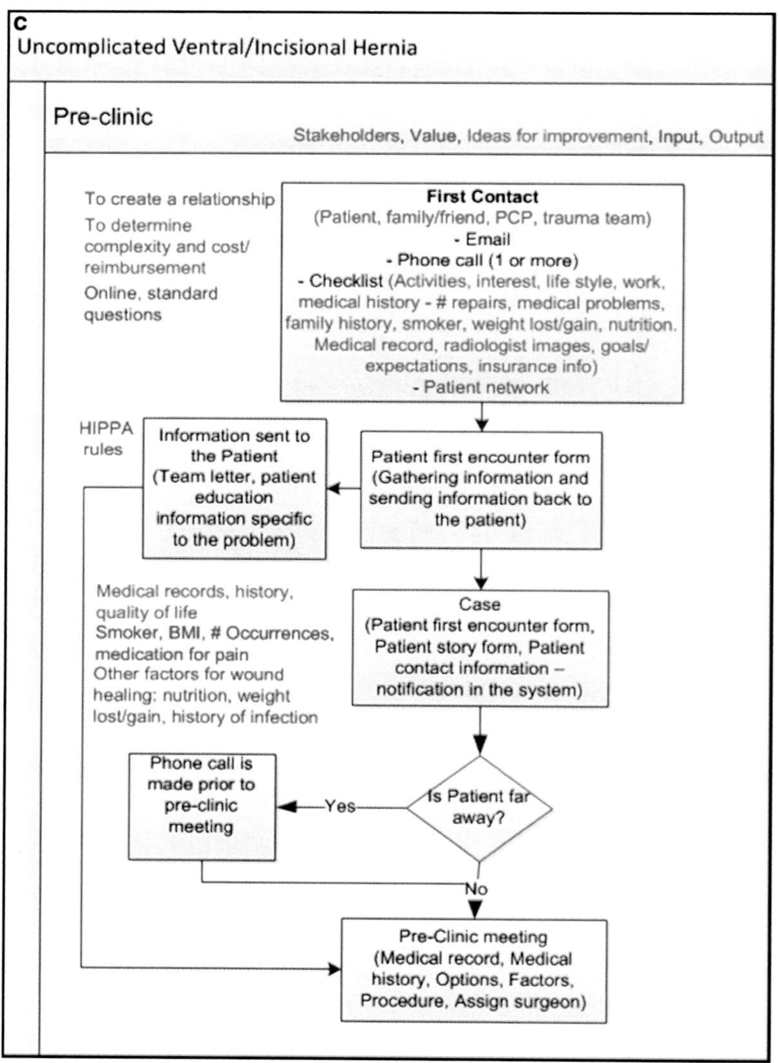

Fig. 1.3. (continued).

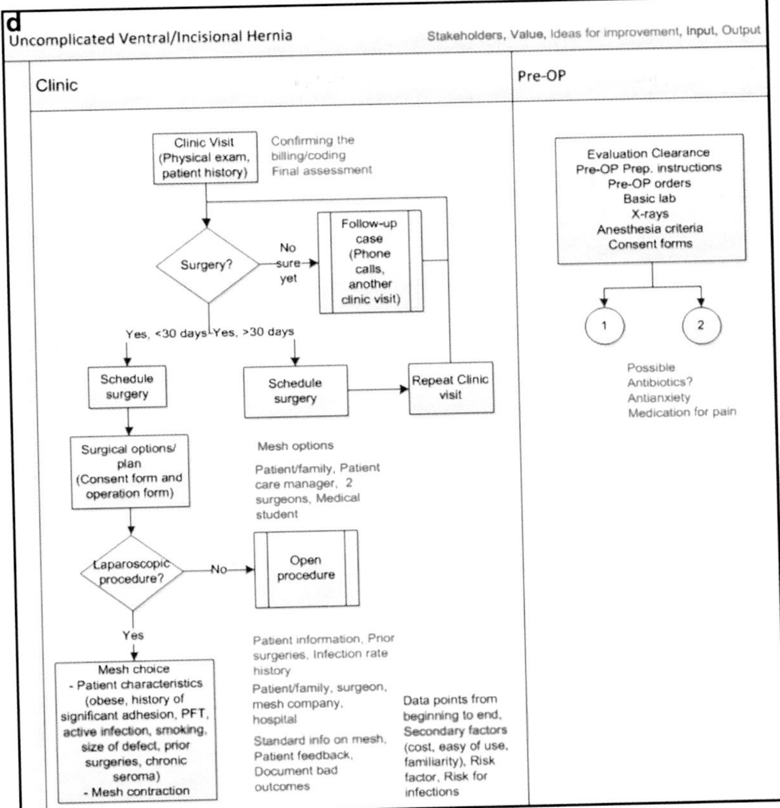

Fig. 1.3. (continued).

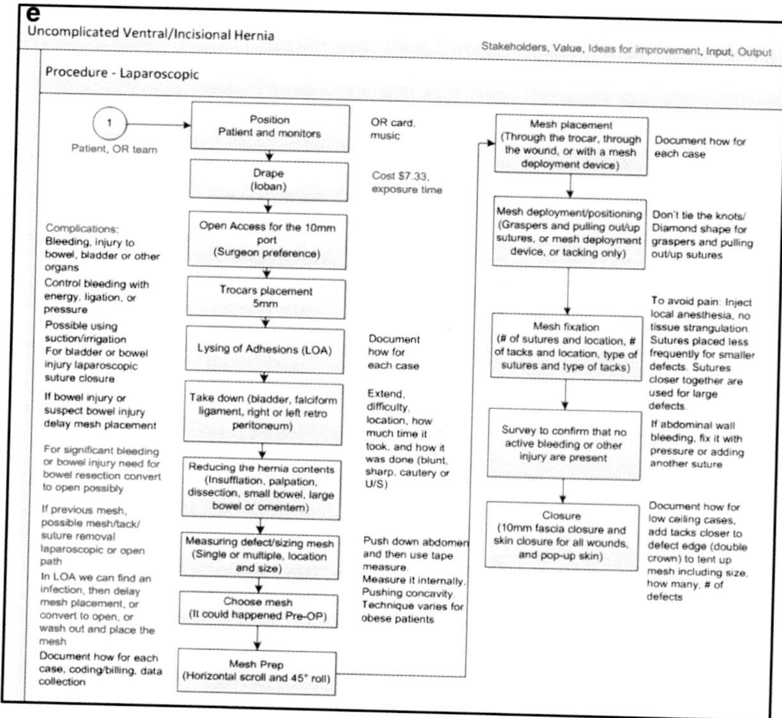

Fig. 1.3. (continued).

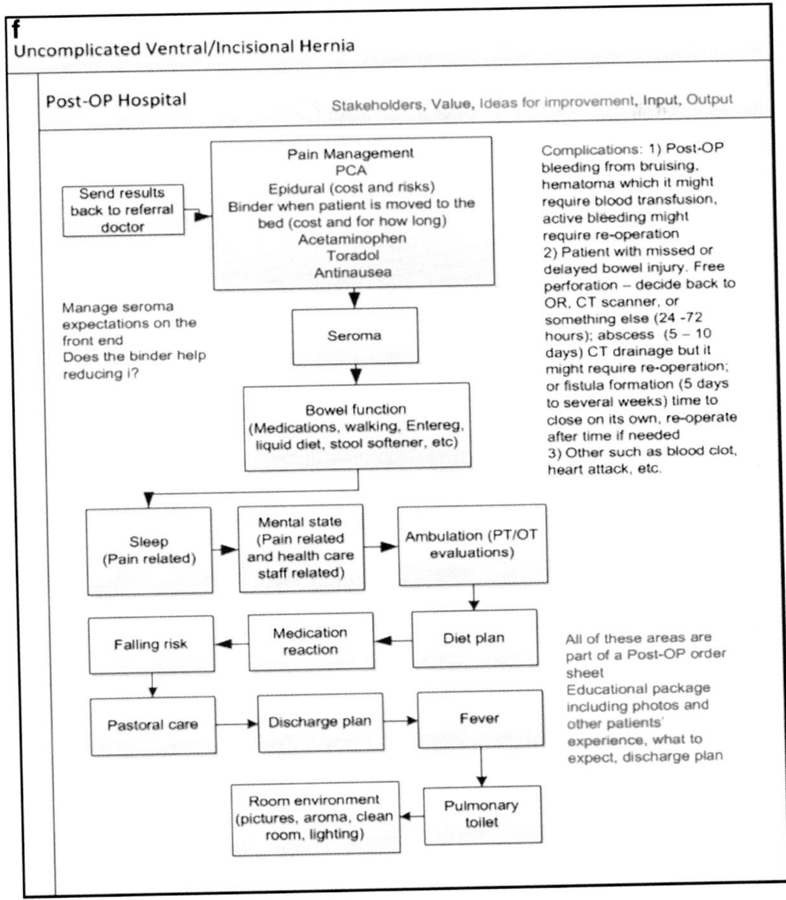

Fig. 1.3. (continued).

cycle are determined, and value is also determined as part of the analysis. This data is critical for the analysis of the true value as measured by outcomes, satisfaction, and cost.

A critical aspect of all care is the technology involved in providing the care, including the medical records software (electronic medical records or EMR). The majority of medical and health record software used by hospitals is proprietary and expensive. This makes having different software systems and software systems that might be implemented in different areas of care difficult to integrate. Software users are locked into the interfaces and capabilities of the software and do not have the ability to customize the software to their specific needs. This makes it difficult to track the patient in a person-centered model and can contribute to medical error and increased costs [16]. As part of the Transformative Care Institute (our academic medical center designed in a complex system model), the Advanced Hernia Solutions team will design software around the care processes and outcome measurements in collaboration with the larger hernia care community. This software will be open source and freely available. It will be capable of interfacing with software that is currently in use within hospitals and health care systems using the protocols being developed as part of the health information exchange (HIE) effort.

In summary, the care team outlined in this chapter for an academic hernia program follows patients throughout their entire cycle of care. The team will provide local management for the care processes, measuring and being accountable for costs, quality, satisfaction, and other outcome measures throughout this entire care cycle. The data collected will allow for better decision making within this full cycle of care. An example of the use of CCQI and patient process documentation would be the selection of hernia mesh for hernia repair. Currently, there are no clear documented guidelines for the selection of hernia mesh. By being able to look at full patient cycles of care for multiple patients, better decisions in the selection of hernia mesh can be made. This can potentially reduce complications such as recurrence, chronic pain, and mesh infections which could require reoperation and removal of the mesh. Through the continuous learning and improvement of a CCQI model, the quality and satisfaction of care can be improved at the same time that the overall cost of care can be lowered. Because of the increasing complexity and pace of change in health care, and our world, this is a never-ending iterative process.

Adapting These Concepts to the Community Setting

It is clear that in a small private- or hospital-based practice, a general surgeon will not have the resources to implement a hernia program using the academic model described in this chapter. However, many of the principles of care coordination and continuous clinical quality improvement can be implemented over time. One goal of our hernia program is to develop software for hernia care processes that can be freely available to surgeons and hospitals. This software, which will be adaptable to the local environment, will help facilitate its implementation for hernia care. Until the software is available, surgeons who desire to be leaders of a hernia team can identify potential team members. These individuals might be current office staff, hospital employees, former patients, family members, or others within the community (several of our team members are former patients who volunteer their time). With a team identified, the dynamic care processes can be defined. These evidence-based care processes and outcome measures that determine value (quality, satisfaction, financial, etc.) will be the starting point for offering care to hernia patients in this model. When patients are cared for guided by these processes, the data that is generated can then be used to learn and to improve these processes.

There are a number of principles for implementing this locally. One of the most critical principles is to develop a true team environment. As a surgeon and leader of a hernia team, it will be necessary to cultivate a safe environment for the team in order to allow all team members to speak freely, without risk of being treated inferiorly. Clearly, each member of the team will have different levels of medical knowledge; however, each member's perspective should be treated as valuable. The ability for all members of the team to speak up can have significant benefits for patient safety and opportunities for innovation. The patient and family perspectives are especially important because of the unique experience of actually going through the cycle of care. It is important to have an open mind and be driven by the outcomes rather than preconceived beliefs. This will not necessarily be easy and will take time.

Another important principle is to not make reactionary decisions. If the first time a new mesh is used and the patient has a recurrence, it is not necessarily a bad mesh. There might be technical issues (learning curve with a new product), patient selection issues, or other factors that generated a poor outcome. Looking at the outcomes with the team will help to prevent reactionary decisions. Most importantly, whatever decisions are made to change processes, they should be measured by looking at the outcomes after the process change has been made.

The following steps can be used to implement a hernia program:

1. Identify a core team.
2. Define dynamic care processes and outcome measures – the types of hernia patients your program will care for, procedure to offer, and types of patients and hernia complications (such as

chronic pain after hernia repair) your program will refer (it will be helpful to identify appropriate surgeons and other hernia programs to which the team can refer patients that your hernia program decides not to care for).

3. Begin to see patients in this hernia program model—allow patients to view the processes and outcomes as they are generated to help them make decisions throughout their cycle of care (shared decision process).
4. Generate outcomes data and identify errors, complications, and anomalies (good and bad) during the patients' cycle of care.
5. Have regular team meetings to review these outcomes and look for opportunities to improve the care processes. These CQI meetings have replaced traditional M&M conference at our new academic medical center.
6. Develop and support extended team members (in the OR, on the floor, etc.) and care communities (former patients and others interested in your hernia program) that can help support the care coordination and continuous learning and improving which are the foundations of this model for hernia care.
7. Have fun! Building a team and a community that cares for each other can be an incredibly rewarding experience. When implemented, this model has the potential to not only improve the value of patient care but also improve the working environment and behavior of the entire care team.

Summary

The decision to implement a hernia program should be made as a commitment to care for patients with hernia problems. No hernia program, ours included, can serve all hernia patients and provide every option for care. It will be important to identify a core hernia team and define the care processes that your team will offer to patients. These care processes should be evidence-based. Outcome measures should be identified and collected that will determine the value of care provided. These will need to be measured not only for a portion of care but also for the entire cycle of care. Applying continuous learning and clinical quality improvement principles will ensure that the care provided by your program will generate better outcomes and better value over time.

References

1. Elhauge E, editor. The fragmentation of the US health care system: causes and solutions. New York: Oxford University Press, Inc.; 2010.
2. Stange K (ed) The problem of fragmentation and the need for integrative solutions. Ann Fam Med. 2009;7(2):100–3.
3. Breen AM, Burton-Houle T, Aron DC. Applying the theory of constraints in health care: Part 1 - The philosophy. Qual Manag Health Care. 2002;10(3):40–6.
4. Plsek P, Greenhalgh T. The challenge of complexity in health care. BMJ. 2001;323:625–8.
5. Weinberg DB, etal. Beyond our walls: impact of patient and provider coordination across the continuum on outcomes for surgical patients. Health Serv Res. 2007;42(1):7–24.
6. Welker J, Huston M, McCue J. Antibiotic timing and errors in diagnosing pneumonia. Arch Intern Med. 2008;168(4):351–6.
7. Hawk MT, et al. Surgical site infection prevention time to move beyond the surgical care improvement program. Ann Surg. 2011;254:494–501.
8. Stahel PF, et al. Wrong-site and wrong-patient procedures in the universal protocol era. Arch Surg. 2010;145(10):978–84.
9. The NICE-SUGAR Study Investigators. Intensive versus conventional glucose control in critically ill patients. N Engl J Med. 2009;360:1283–97.
10. Pines J, Isserman J, Hinfey P. The measurement of time to first antibiotic dose for pneumonia in the emergency department: a white paper and position statement prepared for the American Academy of Emergency Medicine. J Emerg Med. 2009;37(3):335–40.
11. Nicholas L, et al. Hospital process compliance and surgical outcomes in medicare beneficiaries. Arch Surg. 2010;145(10):999–1004.
12. Drake D, Cohen A, Cohn J. National hospital antibiotic timing measures for pneumonia and antibiotic overuse. Qual Manag Health Care. 2007;18(2):113–22.
13. Bogner H, et al. Integrated management of type 2 diabetes mellitus and depression treatment to improve medication adherence: a randomized controlled trial. Ann Fam Med. 2012;10(1):15–22.
14. Edgren L. The meaning of integrated care: a systems approach. Int J Integr Care. 2008;8:e68.
15. Kaplan RS, Porter ME. How to Solve the Cost Crisis in Healthcare. Harv Bus Rev. 2011;89(9):46–52.
16. Black AD, et al. The impact of eHealth on the quality and safety of health care: a systematic overview. PLoS Med. 2011;8(1):e100387. doi:10.1371/journal pmed.100387.

2. Prosthetic Choice in Open Inguinal Hernia Repair

Lisa C. Pickett

While non-mesh repairs can be performed safely in experienced hands with standardized technique, such as the Shouldice (1), tension-free repairs with mesh placement have become the gold standard for the open repair of inguinal hernias (2). Traditionally, there has been concern about the placement of mesh in an acute/incarcerated hernia, but this appears to be safe (3), even in the context of bowel necrosis (4). Internet search of hernia mesh reveals countless brands and types of mesh for the repair of inguinal hernias. Mesh materials vary by source. There are absorbable and permanent synthetic meshes, allograft material, and xenograft material. In addition, mesh is sold in flat sheets, precut segments, and three-dimensional forms. Some mesh products include additional components to resist adhesions, to allow for fixation, or to prevent infection.

Webster's dictionary defines mesh as "that which entangles us" (5). This is not truer than in inguinal hernia repair. Millions of inguinal hernia repairs are performed in the world annually, predominantly open, with every variety of prosthetic, from polyester and polypropropylene to mosquito netting in some parts of the world (6). In fact, a recent study demonstrates no significant difference in outcomes between sterile mosquito nets and standard commercial mesh, which cost 1,000 times more! (7)

History

Initial management of inguinal hernias required external management with bandages, then trusses, first created by French surgeon Guy de Chauliac and then by Ambroise Pare, and subsequently a variety of plugs

B.P. Jacob and B. Ramshaw (eds.), *The SAGES Manual of Hernia Repair*,
DOI 10.1007/978-1-4614-4824-2_2,

to occlude the internal ring (8). Surgical intervention was first performed by Bassini, without any prosthetic, in 1884. The "Bassini repair" was documented with 2.6% mortality and 3.1% recurrence in 227 patients with 98% follow-up at 4.5 years (9). As experience with this procedure widened, a variety of types of wire and suture were utilized to reinforce the abdominal wall (10). Subsequently, early forms of mesh were created and implanted. These consisted of stainless steel, which was too stiff; nylon, which disintegrated too rapidly; and then polypropylene (11–13). At this point, mesh was simply used to buttress or reinforce suture repairs.

Mesh Utilized in Tension-Free Repairs

Usher was the first to introduce significant changes in the conceptual repair of hernias, utilizing mesh to bridge the hernia gap, instead of just buttress a repair performed under tension. Thus, the first description of a tension-free hernia repair was presented: "If mesh is used to bridge the defect instead of reinforcement for tissues approximated under stress, this factor of tension is eliminated, and recurrence becomes less likely" (14). The next mission was to identify the ideal location to place the mesh. Irving Lichtenstein performed and presented an updated tension-free hernia repair with mesh placed anterior to the transversalis fascia in 1980, and this "Lichtenstein repair" has become accepted as a standard hernia repair which is simple to perform, can be safely conducted under local anesthesia, and has acceptable rates of complication and time for recovery (15–17).

Preperitoneal Mesh

The main concern of these repairs remained the forces of abdominal pressure on that location of mesh placement. There was a concern that these forces increase the risk of recurrence for mesh placed anterior to the fascia, instead of the preperitoneal location. Thus, a line of repairs was proposed for mesh placed in the preperitoneal location, either via laparoscopic placement or through open repair (18–20).

A subset of these repairs also includes a prosthetic inserted into the internal ring, either alone or with a hernia patch, to help prevent recurrence (21, 22) (Fig. 2.1). Plugs can be visualized via laparoscopy or CT scan. Radiographically, it appears as a smooth round or oval hypodense mass close to the inferior epigastric artery, confirming the importance of radiologist's knowledge of past surgical history when reviewing scans (23). There are multiple reports of mesh migration from the intended

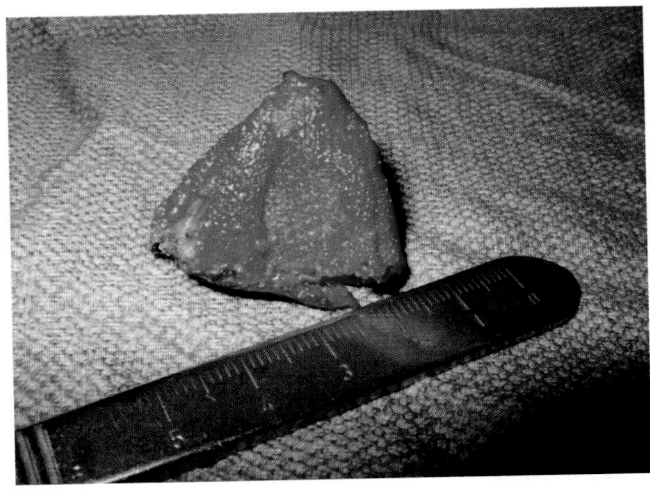

Fig. 2.1. Plug, removed for chronic pain.

location, including a case report of intraperitoneal migration of a mesh plug with a small intestinal perforation (24).

To address this risk, in 1998, Gilbert and Graham introduced a double-layered device, which sits in the inguinal defect, combining a small plug with both a subaponeurotic component and preperitoneal patch, all formed of polypropylene. This mesh is called the Prolene Hernia System (PHS). The PHS incorporates the goal of decreased suture placement with mesh placed in the preperitoneal location. The material is polypropylene and placed via open technique (25). Results have been evaluated and demonstrate 1% recurrence and 2% chronic pain with a mean follow-up of 49 months (26). Longitudinal follow-up has demonstrated 2.3% recurrence and 1.8% chronic pain at 5.5 year follow-up. (27) Comparison of flat polypropylene mesh and PHS at 1 year demonstrates that the PHS surgery takes 15 min longer, on average, and there was no difference in pain, return to activity, complication, or recurrence. (28)

Nonabsorbing synthetic mesh is available in ePTFE (Gortex®), which is seldom used in the groin, and porous sheets such as polypropylene, polyester, and Ultrapro. Porous mesh is further divided into light-, medium-, and heavyweight mesh, based upon the density of the mesh fibers.

Lightweight mesh has been compared with heavyweight, and the recent data has demonstrated some benefit in lightweight mesh. Lightweight mesh has been shown to result in reduced chronic groin pain at the operation site, although there was no associated increase in quality of life in one study (29). In a separate study, reduced postoperative pain and recurrence in the short term was found but there was no statistical difference in recurrence rate at longer-term follow-up (30). Mesh can also be combined with absorbable elements to create ultralightweight mesh, such as Ultrapro®. A literature search was performed using Medline, Embase, and Cochrane databases to identify relevant randomized controlled trials, and comparative studies looked at long-term complications of prosthetic meshes, specifically comparing partially or completely absorbable meshes with conventional nonabsorbable mesh. The primary outcomes reviewed included hospital stay, time taken to return to work, seroma, hematoma, wound infection, groin pain, chronic pain, foreign body sensation, recurrence, and testicular atrophy. It was concluded that absorbable and nonabsorbable mesh repairs of inguinal hernias do not afford significant benefit, but lightweight mesh was associated with a significant reduction in prolonged pain and foreign body sensation. (31) An additional meta-analysis reviewed Vypro II (large pore) and standard polypropylene mesh for inguinal hernia repair, looking at recurrence, pain, urinary tract infection, seroma, foreign body sensation, and testicular atrophy. This analysis found a difference only in the sensation of a foreign body, which was reduced in the large-pore mesh (32).

Self-Fixation Mesh

A more recent addition has been mechanisms of self-fixation to avoid the placement of sutures, which have been implicated in increased pain (Fig. 2.2). A randomized study of self-fixing mesh demonstrates decreased operative time, decreased pain postoperative day 1 by visual analog pain score, and decreased cumulative dose of postoperative pain medicine over standard mesh secured with sutures. (33) Another similar study that assessed pain after the use of a self-adhesive, light mesh with reduced sutures demonstrates reduced early postoperative pain compared with conventional prosthesis (34) and a rat model with similar mesh demonstrates no harmful influence on the ductus deferens in the rat model (35).

Absorbable Mesh

Synthetic mesh is available as an absorbable prosthetic for use in highly contaminated situations. Vicryl® and Dexon are examples of this type of mesh. These products remain intact for just a few weeks and, therefore, are associated with high recurrence rates and are, therefore, generally reserved for grossly contaminated cases.

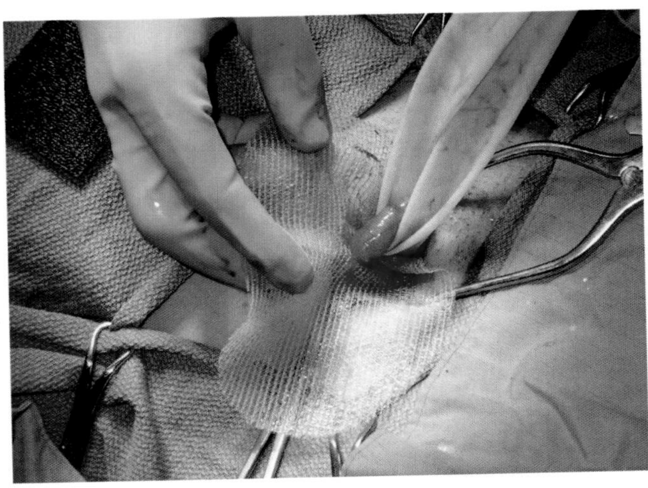

Fig. 2.2. Self fixation mesh.

Biologic Mesh

Biologic mesh is available for patients who are at high risk of infection. Allografts, including Alloderm®, have limited experience and use in the groin. Xenografts are biologics derived from nonhuman dermis, often bovine or porcine. They are harvested cells, essentially an acellular collagen, supported by chemical processes for stabilization. Permacol mesh and Surgisis mesh are examples of xenografts. Additional biologics have been studied (36), but there is little human data and no long-term human outcomes available. As in all prosthetics, allergies and religious and cultural beliefs need to be taken into consideration in the surgical placement of biologic products.

Data on outcomes of hernia repair relative to type of mesh are available in terms of ease of use, durability/recurrence, and long-term chronic pain. See Table 2.1 for a summary of advantages/disadvantages of each mesh type.

In final summary, there are innumerable types, shapes, and components of mesh. Each carries a unique profile of benefits and risks. There is short-term data suggesting better surgeon ease of placement and reduced pain with both lightweight and self-fixation meshes. Long-term results remain unchanged, and biologic grafts remain relatively unstudied. It would seem that surgeons should select a mesh which they feel comfortable

Table 2.1. Advantages/disadvantages of each mesh type.

Mesh		Advantages	Disadvantages
Lichtenstein-type	Heavyweight porous	Safe, well studied	More acute pain Likely more chronic pain
	Lightweight porous	Less acute pain Likely less chronic pain	None
	Porous plus absorbable component	No difference with addition of absorbable material	Increased cost
	Porous with self-fixation component	Less acute pain Possible less chronic pain	Increased cost Less long-term data
	Plug and patch	Helps overcome the force of abdominal pressure	Learning curve Potential increase in chronic pain
	Collagen scaffold	Ability to place in patients high risk for infection Cross-linked have better durability	Increased cost Little long-term data
Preperitoneal	Mesh with a memory ring	Ease of placement Location helps overcome the force of abdominal pressure Less acute pain	Possible migration Increased cost
	Plug	Easy to place with experience Some data suggest it decreases recurrence	Learning curve Plug migration Potential increase in chronic pain
	Prolene Hernia System	Low recurrence Well studied	Learning curve Cost

placing, place these meshes consistently to improve their comfort with the devices, and follow these patients prospectively for outcomes. It is likely that in this complex field, there is not one right mesh for each patient.

References

1. Shouldice EE. The treatment of hernia. Ontario Med Rev. 1953;20:670.
2. Scott NW, McCormack K, Graham, P et al. Open mesh versus non-mesh for repair of femoral and inguinal hernia. Cochrane Database Syst Rev. 2002;CD002197
3. Nieuwenhuizen J, van Ramshort GH, Ten Brinke JG, de Wit T, van der Harst E, Hop WC, Jeekel J, Lange JF. The use of mesh in acute hernia: frequency and outcome in 99 cases. Hernia. 2011;15(3):297–300.
4. Atila K, Guler S, Inal A, Sokmen S, Karademir S, Bora S. Prosthetic repair of acutely incarcerated groin hernias: a prospective clinical observational cohort study. Langenbecks Arch Surg. 2010;395:563–8.
5. Merriam-Webster. Webster's Dictionary. Springfield, MA; 2000
6. Shillcutt SD, Clarke MG, Kingsnorth AN. Cost-effectiveness of groin hernia surgery in the Western Region of Ghana. Arch Surg. 2010;145:954–61.
7. Yang J, Papandria D, Rhee D, Perry H, Abdullah F. Low-cost mesh for inguinal hernia repair in resource-limited settings. Hernia. 2011;15(5):485–9.
8. Stoppa R, Wantz GE, Munegato G, Pluchinotta A. Hernia Healers in illustrated history. Villacoublay: Arnette; 1998.
9. Bassini E. Ueber de behandlung des listenbrunches. Arch F Klin Chir. 1890;40:429–76.
10. Halstead WS. Reporting of twelve cases of complete radical cure of hernia by Halstead's method of over two years standing. Silver wire sutures. Johns Hopkins Hosp Bull V:98–99.
11. Babcock WW. The range of usefulness of commercial stainless steel cloths in general and special forms of surgical practice. Ann West Med Surg. 1952;6:15–23.
12. Moloney GE, Grill WG, Barclay RC. Operations for hernia: technique of nylon darn. Lancet. 1948;2:45–8.
13. Handley WS. A method for the radical cure of inguinal hernia (darn and stay-lace method). Practitioner. 1918;100:466–71.
14. Read RC. Francis C. Usher, herniologist of the twentieth century. Hernia. 1999;3:167–71.
15. Lichtenstein IL, Shulman AG. Ambulatory outpatient hernia surgery. Including a new concept, introducing tension-free repair. Int Surg. 1986;71:1–4.
16. Muldoon RL, Marchant K, Johnson DD, Yoder GG, Read RC, Hauer-Jensen M. Lichtenstein vs anterior preperitoneal prosthetic mesh placement in open inguinal hernia repair: a prospective randomized trial. Hernia. 2004;8(2):98–103.
17. Kurzer M, Belsham PA, Kark AE. The Lichtenstein repair. Surg Clin North Am. 1998;78:1025–46.
18. Estrin J, Lipton S, Block IR. The posterior approach to inguinal and femoral hernias. Surg Gynecol Obstet. 1963;116:547–50.
19. Tinkler LF. Preperitoneal prosthetic herniorrhaphy. Postgrad Med J. 1969;45:665–7.

20. Yoder G, Read RC, Barone GW, Hauer-Jensen M. Preperitoneal prosthetic placement through the groin. Surg Clin North Am. 1993;73:545–55.
21. Shore IL, Lichtenstein JM. Simplified repair of femoral and recurrent inguinal hernias by 'plug' technique. Am J Surg. 1974;28:439–44.
22. Rutkow AW, Robbins IM. The mesh plug hernioplasty. Surg Clin North Am. 1993;75:501–12.
23. Aganovic L, Ishioka KM, Hughes CF, Chu PK, Cosman BC. Plugoma: CT findings after prosthetic plug inguinal hernia repairs. J Am Coll Surg. 2010;211(4):481–4.
24. Tian MJ, Chen YF. Intraperitoneal migration of a mesh plug with a small intestinal perforation: report of a case. Surg Today. 2010;40(6):566–8.
25. Gilbert A. Combined anterior and posterior inguinal hernia repair: intermediate recurrence rates with three groups of surgeons. Hernia. 2004;8:203–7.
26. Mottin CC, Ramos RJ, Ramos MJ. Using the Prolene Hernia System (PHS) for inguinal hernia repair. Rev Col Bras Cir. 2011;38(1):24–7.
27. Faraj D, Ruurda JP, Olsman JG, van Geffen HJ. Five-year results of inguinal hernia treatment with the Prolene Hernia System in a regional training hospital. Hernia. 2010;14(2):155–8.
28. Sutalo N, Maricic A, Kozomara D, Kvesic A, Stalekar H, Trninic Z, Kuzman Z. Comparison of results of surgical treatments of primary inguinal hernia with flat polypropylene mesh and three-dimensional prolene (PHS) mesh-one year follow up. Coll Antropol. 2010;34 Suppl 1:29–33.
29. Nikkolo C, Lepner U, Murrus M, Vaasna T, Seepter H, Tikk T. Randomised clinical trial comparing lightweight mesh with heavyweight mesh for inguinal hernioplasty. Hernia. 2010;14(3):253–8.
30. Smietanski M, Bury K, Smietanska IA, Owczuk R, Paradowski T. Five year results of a randomized controlled multi-centre study comparing heavy-weight knitted versus low-weight, non-woven polypropylene implants in Lichtenstein hernioplasty. Hernia. 2011;15(5):495–501.
31. Markar SR, Karthikesalingam A, Alam F, Tang TY, Walsh SR, Sadat U. Partially or completely absorbable versus nonabsorbable mesh repair for inguinal hernia: a systematic review and meta-analysis. Surg Laparosc Endosc Percutan Tech. 2010;20(4):213–9.
32. Gao M, Han J, Tian J, Yang K. Vypro II mesh for inguinal hernia repair: a meta-analysis of randomized controlled trials. Ann Surg. 2010;251(5):838–42.
33. Kapische M, Schultze H, Caliebe A. Self-fixating mesh for the Lichtenstein procedure-a prestudy. Arch Surg. 2010;395(4):317–22.
34. Torcivia A, Vons C, Barrat C, Dufour F, Champault G. Influence of mesh type on the quality of early outcomes after inguinal hernia repair in ambulatory setting controlled study: Glucamesh vs Polypropylene. Langenbecks Arch Surg. 2011;396(2):173–8.
35. Kilbe T, Hollinsky C, Walter I, Joachim A, Rulicke T. Influence of a new self-gripping hernia mesh on male fertility in a rat model. Surg Endosc. 2010;24(2):455–61.
36. Arslani N, Patrlj L, Kopljar M, Rajkovic Z, Altarac S, Papes D, Stritof D. Advantages of new materials in fascia transversalis reinforcement for inguinal hernia repair. Hernia. 2010;14(6):617–21.

3. Prosthetic Choice in Laparoscopic Inguinal Hernia Repair

Emily L. Albright and J. Scott Roth

Inguinal hernia repair is one of the most common procedures performed by a general surgeon. The management of inguinal hernias has undergone many changes in the last five decades. The advent of prosthetic materials has decreased the recurrence rate compared to primary repair [1]. The age of laparoscopy has brought new techniques with well-defined benefits including a reduction in pain, lower wound infection rates, and a shortened return to normal activities [2–4]. With all these advances have come many choices for the practitioner today regarding prosthetic materials that differ in terms of weight, burst strength, material composition, and inflammatory response. This chapter aims to examine the different prosthetics available and delineate their benefits and shortcomings, specifically relating to laparoscopic inguinal hernia repair.

Synthetic Overview

Prosthetic materials were developed to reinforce hernia repairs and prevent recurrence. The three most common synthetic prosthetics used today are polypropylene, polyester, and PTFE, and they were all developed at roughly the same time. Polyester polymers were first introduced in the United States in 1946; in 1956, Wolstenholme described the use of polyester to repair inguinal hernias [5]. Polypropylene is the most commonly used prosthetic in the United States following its introduction in 1958 by Usher [6]. At the time of its introduction, there were many advantages over the metal meshes that were currently in use.

B.P. Jacob and B. Ramshaw (eds.), *The SAGES Manual of Hernia Repair*,
DOI 10.1007/978-1-4614-4824-2_3,

It had a high tensile strength, was less affected by infection, and was infiltrated by connective tissue when implanted into an animal model. Just 4 years after its introduction, polypropylene was being used by 20% of surgeons for complicated hernia repair [6]. Polytetrafluoroethylene (PTFE) was initially developed by DuPont in 1938 and began to be used in hernia repair in the 1950s. In the 1960s, a process was developed to expand PTFE to produce a uniform structure with improved mechanical strength (ePTFE) [6]. This ePTFE was used not only for abdominal wall reconstruction but also for vascular grafts. When laparoscopic inguinal hernia repair was developed, technology had already made multiple alterations to the three basic polymers—polypropylene, polyester, and PTFE. They each have separate chemical structures and handling properties. It is these differences in texture and porosity that lead to differences in tissue reaction.

Polypropylene

Polypropylene is a thermoplastic polymer consisting of an ethylene with an attached methyl group (Fig. 3.1). It is hydrophobic, electrostatically neutral, and resistant to significant biologic degradation. The biologic reactivity of polypropylene depends on the weight, filament size, pore size, and architecture, in addition to the individual host response. Not all polypropylene prosthetics are equal as structure can alter outcome. In one study comparing various polypropylene, they found that patients with a monofilament polypropylene took significantly longer to return to work, had higher pain scores, and more impairment in everyday activities compared to patients that had a multifilament polypropylene [7]. By utilizing knitted versus woven materials, the flexibility can also be altered [8]. Pore size is also variable between different manufacturers. Pores should be at least 75–100 μm to prevent against infection [9].

Current debate exists regarding the optimal density of polypropylene. Normal intra-abdominal pressure ranges from 1.8 mmHg when supine up to 171 mmHg when jumping [10]. Laboratory data indicates that a prosthetic should withstand at least 16 N/cm strain to prevent disruption based on normal physiologic forces [11]. Many of the original polypropylene prosthetics provide much greater strength than this. Heavyweight meshes were designed to provide maximal strength with thick fibers, small pores, and a high tensile strength. Prosthetic materials have also been found to be inappropriately stiff when compared to the

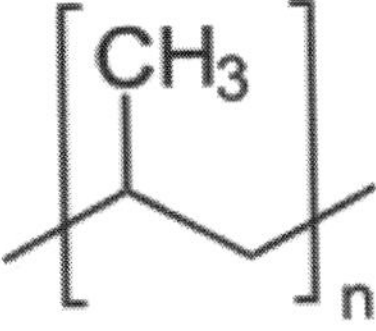

Fig. 3.1. Polypropylene.

normal elasticity of the abdominal wall [11]. Based on this, there has been a move to decrease the density of polypropylene implanted to provide adequate strength while reducing the amount of foreign material.

One outcome that is of particular interest is the effect of the use of lightweight mesh has on postoperative pain. Proponents of lightweight mesh cite less pain and less mesh sensation as benefits. However, this has not been universally seen in all studies. One study in particular compared lightweight polypropylene mesh with a heavyweight polypropylene mesh in patients undergoing laparoscopic bilateral inguinal hernia repair [12]. Lightweight polypropylene was placed in one groin and heavyweight in the contralateral groin. They found that patients could detect a difference and reported less pain on the side with the lightweight polypropylene. In contrast, a comparison of patients undergoing laparoscopic inguinal hernia repair with either a lightweight or heavyweight mesh was published just 1 year later. This study did not find a difference in pain or discomfort at 4- or 15-month follow-up between lightweight and heavyweight prosthetics. They also did not show a difference in awareness of the mesh or stiffness of the groin [13]. There are many more studies comparing lightweight mesh to heavyweight mesh. Some demonstrate an improvement in postoperative pain [14–17]. However, not all series show this difference [18].

While long-term pain and pain in the early postoperative period are important to consider when considering a prosthetics, long-term durability and hernia recurrence are equally important. Many of the opponents to lightweight prosthetics express concern for increasing recurrence. In one study, at 12-month follow-up of open inguinal hernia repair, there was a significant increase in recurrence in patients with a lightweight polypropylene mesh compared to traditional polypropylene [16]. Multiple other studies fail to demonstrate an increased recurrence rate [14, 15, 17]. When lightweight mesh is used specifically for laparoscopic inguinal hernia repair, no difference in hernia recurrence was identified [12, 13, 18]. Whether the concern for an increase in hernia recurrence is justified remains to be seen as long-term follow-up continues.

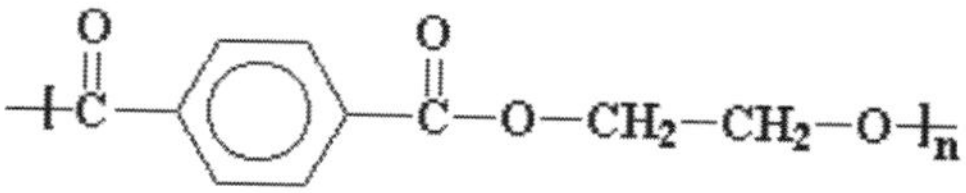

Fig. 3.2. Polyester.

$$\left[\overset{O}{\overset{\|}{C}} - C_6H_4 - \overset{O}{\overset{\|}{C}} - O - CH_2 - CH_2 - O \right]_n$$

Polyester

Polyester is a category of polymers that contain an ester in the main chain (Fig. 3.2) and has many applications in daily life, from clothing to jet engines. While polypropylene is used extensively for hernia repair, polyester is also commonly used. Multiple studies exist comparing these two materials. One study compared patients that had previously undergone laparoscopic inguinal hernia repair either with polypropylene or polyester prosthetic [19]. A phone survey was conducted on patients with a minimum of a 1-year follow-up with questions focused on pain, perception of the mesh, return to work, and satisfaction. In this study, there was an increase in chronic inguinal pain, feeling of a lump, and feeling the mesh in the polypropylene group compared to the polyester group. There was no difference in recurrence rate. Another study citing the benefits of polyester prosthetics was in a series of 337 patients undergoing laparoscopic inguinal hernia repair with polyester mesh [20]. After a mean follow-up of 11 months, there were no recurrences, no mesh infections, and chronic pain in three patients. Despite multiple studies, there exists no clear benefit of polypropylene versus polyester, and choice remains based on surgeon preference.

One concern regarding the use of polyester prosthetics is the degradation that occurs over time. In one study examining explanted polyester vascular grafts, there was hydrolytic degradation of the grafts with increasing time implanted [21]. Further analysis showed that polyester grafts lost 31.4% of their burst strength at 10 years and 100% in 25–39 years. The earliest graft failure in this study was after 19 years. If the same is true of polyester grafts for inguinal hernia repair, this clearly would not be a problem for an inguinal hernia repair in a 90-year-old patient but would affect an 18-year-old patient.

Polytetrafluoroethylene

Polytetrafluoroethylene is a synthetic polymer of tetrafluoroethylene consisting of carbons and fluorines with multiple applications (Fig. 3.3). It is most well-known by the brand name Teflon and can be found as a

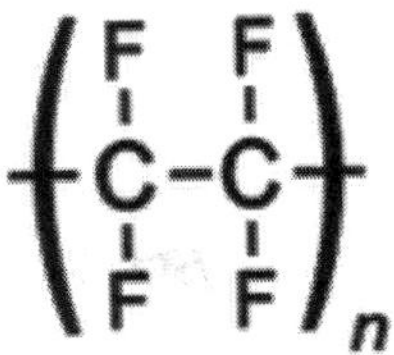

Fig. 3.3. Polytetrafluoroethylene.

nonstick coating for pans, a lubricant in gears, and a roofing material. In the medical profession, PTFE is used for hernia repair as well as in vascular grafts.

With the increasing usage of polypropylene and polyester prosthetics, PTFE is not used as frequently for inguinal hernia repair. However, when laparoscopic techniques were first introduced for inguinal hernia repair, PTFE prosthetics played a key role in intraperitoneal onlay mesh repair (IPOM). Results of a prospective study looking at the ePTFE peritoneal onlay laparoscopic inguinal hernioplasty were published in 1996 [22]. Over a period of 2.8 years, 351 patients underwent repair. They found that on average patients only required 24 h of analgesics, returned to work in 7.7 days for unilateral repairs, and returned to work in 10.1 days for bilateral repairs. There were 13 patients in the series with persistent neuralgia and 17 patients with recurrences (3.8%). Another prospective trial comparing IPOM with ePTFE to an open repair reported an even higher recurrence rate of 43% [23]. It is likely that these recurrence rates contributed to the decline in the use of PTFE for laparoscopic inguinal hernia repair.

In addition to the concern for hernia recurrence is the risk of infection associated with the use of PTFE. When the pore size of a prosthetic is less than 10 μm, macrophages and neutrophils are too large to enter and cannot eliminate bacteria [24]. When PTFE does become colonized, removal is mandatory in order to manage the infection. The small pore size of PTFE also impacts the formation of postoperative seromas. There is insufficient molecular permeability for fibrinous and proteinaceous materials to be cleared [24].

Barrier Prosthetics and Composite Prosthetics

In addition to prosthetics that are pure synthetic material or pure biologic material, there are a variety of prosthetics that combine various materials. One example is beta-glucan-coated polypropylene prosthetics.

Beta-glucan is a plant product that is used to promote healing and also has an immunomodulatory effect. In published series, using beta-glucan-coated polypropylene resulted in a decrease in the incidence of chronic pain compared to polypropylene alone and a low incidence of recurrence at 2 years (1.9%) [25, 26].

Other prosthetics combine permanent material with a barrier layer to prevent adhesions to one side. This type of prosthetic is particularly useful if the peritoneum has been violated and is not available to separate the prosthetic from intra-abdominal contents. Barriers can be placed on one side or both sides of the mesh. Typically, the barrier layer is designed to allow adequate time for a neo-peritoneum to develop prior to their degradation. The previously mentioned prosthetics, including polypropylene, polyester, lightweight and heavyweight, all have an alternative with a barrier layer. The majority of the data regarding prosthetics with a barrier layer focuses on their use in ventral hernia repair where they are more likely to be intact with intra-abdominal contents.

In an effort to decrease the amount of permanent foreign material, composite materials have been developed that combine polypropylene with absorbable materials. One example is a composite mesh of polypropylene with polyglactine. While the polypropylene is permanent, the polyglactine fibers are resorbed in approximately 60 days. In studies comparing polyglactine-polypropylene composite with polypropylene alone in open inguinal hernia repair, there was no difference in perioperative complications, postoperative pain, or recurrence [27–29]. These results were similar when polyglactine-polypropylene was compared to polypropylene alone in laparoscopic inguinal hernia repair with no difference in pain, return to normal daily activities, and recurrence [7, 30–32]. Polyglactine-polypropylene is smoother than polypropylene and thus has different handling characteristics. However, this does not translate into a difference in operating times or subjective assessment of difficulty of mesh placement [31].

In addition to polyglactine, there are other alternatives to an absorbable component combined with polypropylene. One such example is polyglecaprone 25. When polypropylene was compared to a polyglecaprone 25-polypropylene composite in an animal model, there was a decrease in the inflammatory and fibrotic reaction; however, it was not statistically significant [33]. As we search for the optimal mesh, there are likely to be more combined prosthetics developed in addition to those mentioned here.

Prosthetics have also been altered to decrease the need for fixation. One example is a polypropylene mesh with a nitinol frame [34]. Another example is a titanium-coated monofilament polypropylene mesh that has been shown to have a recurrence rate of 0.4%, persistent inguinal pain in 3.8%, and groin stiffness in 1.7% after a 7-week follow-up [35].

As humans are two-dimensional structures, there has been an effort to manufacture prosthetics that conform to the contours of the human body and avoid the need for fixation. One study looking at mesh fixation showed it to be associated with a longer hospital stay and more narcotic analgesia requirements [36]. In a retrospective review of 212 transabdominal pre-peritoneal herniaplasties using a three-dimensional mesh, 94% of patients had returned to normal activities by 3 weeks. Mesh fixation was used in 19% of the cases in this series. They did not find that bilateral repair or fixation altered recovery. Only four patients in the series had minor pain or numbness. With a mean follow-up of 23 months, there was only one recurrence. They concluded that an anatomically contoured prosthetic had minimal risk of neuropathy, had a low recurrence rate, and often does not require fixation [37]. A second series looking at an anatomically contoured prosthetic in 390 patients had similar results [38]. At 2 years, there were three recurrences, and 43 patients reported minor parietal pain.

Biologic Prosthetics

Biologic prosthetics are designed as either allografts (from human tissue) or as xenografts (from animal tissue). Available animal products are porcine and bovine. In addition to what species a biologic material is from, they also differ on what part is harvested, including dermis, small intestinal submucosa, and pericardium. The role of biologic materials in any hernia repair has mainly been limited to infected surgical fields. For laparoscopic inguinal hernia repair, there exists limited data examining the role of biologic prosthetics, and research examining their role is ongoing. Recently, the design of a study comparing the use of lightweight polypropylene to cross-linked porcine dermis was published [39]. Currently, 172 men are enrolled in the study, and data are being collected. Other studies have focused on the feasibility of using biologic prosthetics for inguinal hernia repair [40–42].

There are concerns regarding the use of biologic prosthetics for laparoscopic inguinal hernia repair, namely, the risk of recurrence. For laparoscopic inguinal hernia repair, all prosthetics are placed in a bridging manner. In incisional hernia repair, when biologic prosthetics are used in a bridging manner, there is an 80% recurrence rate [43]. In this study, there is no comment on size of hernia defect, but generally incisional hernias have a larger defect size than inguinal hernias. The risk of recurrence with a bridging biologic prosthetic in laparoscopic inguinal hernia repair would not be expected to be as high as in incisional hernia repair but still expected higher than a synthetic material. In a prospective series of 11 patients undergoing laparoscopic inguinal hernia repair using a biologic prosthetic, there was one recurrence (9%) with a mean follow-up of 14.5 months [40].

Advantages of biologic materials for inguinal hernia repair are mainly focused on postoperative pain. In a randomized trial comparing polypropylene to a biologic prosthetic derived from small intestine submucosa, while there was no difference to the incidence in postsurgical pain, there was a significant decrease in the degree of pain and a lower proportion of patients that took pain medications [44].

Summary

There exists a multitude of options available to surgeons today. While there are multiple prosthetics that have proven their longevity over the years, multiple new prosthetics enter the market each year. The choice of prosthetic used for laparoscopic hernia repair must be tailored to the individual patient. Clearly there is not one prosthetic that fits all patients or situations.

References

1. Vrijland WW, van den Tol MP, Luijendijk RW, Hop WCJ, et al. Randomized clinical trial of non-mesh versus mesh repair of primary inguinal hernia. Br J Surg. 2002;89:293–7.
2. Johansson B, Hallerback B, Glise H, Anesten B, et al. Laparoscopic mesh versus open preperitoneal mesh versus conventional technique for inguinal hernia repair: a randomized multicenter trial (SCUR hernia repair study). Ann Surg. 1999;230:225–31.
3. Karthikesalingam A, Markar SR, Holt PJE, Praseedom RK. Meta-analysis of randomized controlled trials comparing laparoscopic with open mesh repair of recurrent inguinal hernia. Br J Surg. 2010;97:4–11.
4. Langeveld HR, van't Reit M, Weidema WF, Stassen LP, et al. Total extraperitoneal inguinal hernia repair compared with Lichtenstein (the LEVEL-Trial). Ann Surg. 2010;251:819–24.

5. Wolstenholme JT. Use of commercial Dacron fabric in the repair of inguinal hernias and abdominal wall defects. Arch Surg. 1956;73:1004–8.
6. DeBord JR. The historical development of prosthetics in hernia surgery. Surg Clin North Am. 1998;78:973–1006.
7. Langenbach MR, Schmidt J, Zirngibl H. Comparison of biomaterials: three meshes and TAPP for inguinal hernia. Surg Endosc. 2006;20:1511–7.
8. Cobb WS, Peindl RM, Zerey M, Carbonell AM, Heniford BT. Mesh terminology 101. Hernia. 2009;13:1–6.
9. Weyhe D, Belyaev O, Muller C, Meurer K, Bauer KH, et al. Improving outcomes in hernia repair by the use of light meshes – a comparison of different implant constructions based on a critical appraisal of the literature. World J Surg. 2007;31:234–44.
10. Cobb WS, Burns JM, Kercher KW, Matthews BD, et al. Normal intraabdominal pressure in healthy adults. J Surg Res. 2005;129:231–5.
11. Junge K, Klinge U, Prescher A, Giboni P, et al. Elasticity of the anterior abdominal wall and impact for reparation of incisional hernias using mesh implants. Hernia. 2001;5:113–8.
12. Agarwal BB, Agarwal KA, Mahajan KC. Prospective double-blind randomized controlled study comparing heavy- and lightweight polypropylene mesh in totally extraperitoneal repair of inguinal hernia: early results. Surg Endosc. 2009;23:242–7.
13. Khan LR, Liong S, de Beaux AC, Kumar S, Nixon SJ. Lightweight mesh improves functional outcome in laparoscopic totally extra-peritoneal inguinal hernia repair. Hernia. 2010;14:39–45.
14. Bringman S, Wollert S, Osterberg J, Smedberg S, et al. Three-year results of a randomized clinical trial of lightweight or standard polypropylene mesh in Lichtenstein repair of primary inguinal hernia. Br J Surg. 2006;93:1056–9.
15. Nikkolo C, Lepner U, Murruste M, Vaasna T, Seepter H, Tikk T. Randomized clinical trial comparing lightweight mesh with heavyweight mesh for inguinal hernioplasty. Hernia. 2010;14:253–8.
16. O'Dwyer PJ, Kingsnorth AN, Molloy RG, Small PK, et al. Randomized clinical trial assessing impact of a lightweight or heavyweight mesh on chronic pain after inguinal hernia repair. Br J Surg. 2005;92:166–70.
17. Post S, Weiss B, Willer M, Neufang T, Lorenz D. Randomized clinical trial of lightweight composite mesh for Lichtenstein inguinal hernia repair. Br J Surg. 2004;91:44–8.
18. Khan LR, Kumar S, Nixon SJ. Early results for new lightweight mesh in laparoscopic totally extra-peritoneal inguinal hernia repair. Hernia. 2006;10:303–8.
19. Shah BC, Goede MR, Bayer R, Buettner SL, et al. Does type of mesh used have an impact on outcomes in laparoscopic inguinal hernia? Am J Surg. 2009;198:759–64.
20. Ramshaw B, Abiad F, Voeller G, Wilson R, Mason E. Polyester (Parietex) mesh for total extraperitoneal laparoscopic inguinal hernia repair. Surg Endosc. 2003;17:498–501.
21. Riepe G, Loos J, Imig H, Schroder A, et al. Long-term in vivo alterations of polyester vascular grafts in humans. Eur J Vasc Endovasc Surg. 1997;13:540–8.

22. Toy FK, Moskowitz M, Smott RT, Pleatman M, et al. Results of a prospective multicenter trial evaluating the ePTFE peritoneal onlay laparoscopic inguinal hernioplasty. J Laparoendosc Surg. 1996;6:375–86.
23. Kingsley D, Vogt DM, Nelson T, Curet MJ, Pitcher DE. Laparoscopic intraperitoneal onlay inguinal herniorrhaphy. Am J Surg. 1998;176:548–53.
24. Amid PK. Classification of biomaterials and their related complications in abdominal wall hernia surgery. Hernia. 1997;1:15–21.
25. Champault G, Barrat C. Inguinal hernia repair with beta glucan coated mesh: results at two-year follow up. Hernia. 2005;9:125–30.
26. Champault G, Bernard C, Rizk N, Polliand C. Inguinal hernia repair: the choice of prosthesis outweighs that of technique. Hernia. 2007;11:125–8.
27. Bringman S, Heikkinen TJ, Wollert S, Osterberg J, et al. Early results of a single-blinded, randomized, controlled Internet-based multicenter trial comparing Prolene and Vypro II mesh in Lichtenstein hernioplasty. Hernia. 2004;8:127–34.
28. Bringman S, Wollert S, Osterberg J, Smedberg S, et al. One year results of randomized controlled multi-centre study comparing Prolene and Vypro II-mesh in Lichtenstein hernioplasty. Hernia. 2005;9:223–7.
29. Khan N, Bangash A, Sadiq M, Hadi AU, Hamid H. Polyglactine/polypropylene mesh vs. propylene mesh: Is there a need fo newer prosthesis in inguinal hernia? Saudi J. Gastroenterology. 2010;16:8–13.
30. Bringman S, Wollert S, Osterberg J, Heikkinen T. Early results of a randomized multicenter trial comparing Prolene and VyproII mesh in bilateral endoscopic extraperitoneal hernioplasty (TEP). Surg Endosc. 2005;19:536–40.
31. Heikkinen T, Wollert S, Osterberg J, Smedberg S, Bringman S. Early results of a randomized trial comparing Prolene and VyproII-mesh in endoscopic extraperitoneal inguinal hernia repair (TEP) of recurrent unilateral hernias. Hernia. 2006;10:34–40.
32. Junge K, Rosch R, Krones CJ, Klinge U, Mertens PR, et al. Influence of polyglecaprone 25 (Monocryl) supplementation on the biocompatibility of a polypropylene mesh for hernia repair. Hernia. 2005;9:212–7.
33. Torres-Villalobos G, Sorcic L, Ruth GR, Andrade R, et al. Evaluation of the rebound hernia repair device for laparoscopic hernia repair. JSLS. 2010;14:95–102.
34. Tamme C, Garde N, Klingler A, Hampe C, Wunder R, Kockerling F. Totally extraperitoneal inguinal hernioplasty with titanium-coated lightweight polypropylene mesh. Surg Endosc. 2005;19:1125–9.
35. Koch CA, Greenlee SM, Larsan DR, Harrington JR, Farley DR. Randomized prospective study of totally extraperitoneal inguinal hernia repair: Fixation versus no fixation of mesh. JSLS. 2006;10:457–60.
36. Bell RCW, Price JG. Laparoscopic inguinal hernia repair using an anatomically contoured three-dimensional mesh. Surg Endosc. 2003;17:1784–8.
37. Pajotin P. Laparoscopic groin hernia repair using a curved prosthesis without fixation. Le Journal de Celio-Chirurgie. 1998;28:64–8.
38. Bellows CF, Shadduck PP, Helton WS, Fitzgibbons RJ. The design of an Industry-sponsored randomized controlled trial to compare synthetic mesh versus biologic mesh for inguinal hernia repair. Hernia. 2011;15:325–32.

39. Agresta F, Bedin N. Transabdominal laparoscopic inguinal hernia repair: is there a place for biologic mesh? Hernia. 2008;12:609–12.
40. Ansaloni L, Catena F, Gagliardi S, Gazzotti F, et al. Hernia repair with porcine small-intestinal submucosa. Hernia. 2007;11:321–6.
41. Fine A. Laparoscopic repair of inguinal hernia using Surgisis mesh and fibrin sealant. JSLS. 2006;10:461–5.
42. Jin J, Rosen MJ, Blatnik J, McGee MF, et al. Use of acellular dermal matrix for complicated ventral hernia repair: does technique affect outcome. J Am Coll Surg. 2007;205:654–60.
43. Ansaloni L, Catena F, Coccolini F, Gazzotti F, et al. Inguinal hernia repair with porcine small intestine submucosa: 3-year follow-up results of a randomized controlled trial of Lichtenstein's repair with polypropylene mesh versus Surgisis Inguinal Hernia Matrix. Am J Surg. 2009;198:303–12.

Part II
Techniques for Inguinal Hernia Repair

4. Technique: Lichtenstein

David C. Chen and Parviz K. Amid

Lichtenstein Tension-Free Operation for the Repair of Unilateral and Bilateral Inguinal Hernias

Lichtenstein "tension-free" hernia repair, a term coined by our group, began as a protocol-driven project in 1985 and evolved to its current standard procedure in the late 1980s [1, 2]. Standard tissue repair to close the abdominal wall defect had changed little in the hundred years since Bassini introduced the modern era of herniorrhaphy in 1887. Several modifications of tissue repair introduced by Shouldice, McVay, and others helped to refine this method, but overall recurrence rates remained in the range of 10–15%. In the "tension-free" method, synthetic mesh is placed between the external and internal oblique layers eliminating the need to pull the tissues together under tension. The advantages of this method have been extensively defined and resulted in a paradigm shift in hernia repair with "tension-free" repair accepted as the standard of care.

In the 1990s, variations on this concept of "tension-free" repair led to several different preperitoneal open and laparoscopic approaches. Some have demonstrated relative equivalency, but none have proven to be superior. While "tension-free" repair using mesh has markedly reduced the recurrence rate, chronic pain after all varieties of both open and laparoscopic hernia repair is a continuing concern. This chapter describes the sequential steps of the Lichtenstein "tension-free" operation for the repair of unilateral and bilateral [3] inguinal hernias. Special attention is given to groin neuroanatomy and correct nerve handling to minimizing the risk of chronic postoperative pain.

B.P. Jacob and B. Ramshaw (eds.), *The SAGES Manual of Hernia Repair*,
DOI 10.1007/978-1-4614-4824-2_4,

Post-Herniorrhaphy Inguinodynia

While the rates of recurrence associated with inguinal hernia repair dramatically decreased after "tension-free" methods became standard practice, the incidence of postoperative inguinodynia remains a major concern. According to a Danish nationwide study, the rate of post-herniorrhaphy chronic pain is independent of the method of the hernia repair (tissue repair, open mesh repair, or laparoscopic mesh repair) [4]. Based on the classification of pain by the International Association for the Study of Pain (IASP), post-herniorrhaphy inguinodynia can be broadly divided into nociceptive and neuropathic pain.

Nociceptive pain is caused by activation of nociceptors by nociceptive molecules due to tissue injury or inflammatory reaction. These signals are then transmitted to the brain via A-delta and C-fibers. Nociceptive pain can be reduced by gentle tissue handling and using local anesthesia to reduce production of nociceptive molecules.

Neuropathic pain is caused by direct nerve injury such as myelin undulation, myelin separation, axon crystallization, and other structural changes of nerve fibers due to direct contact of nerves with mesh and/or nerve entrapment by sutures, staples, tacks, folded mesh, or meshoma [5]. Neuropathic pain can be reduced from the reported range of 6–8% to less than 1% by careful nerve handling to avoid destruction of the protective layers of the nerves during open repair [6, 7], by avoiding placement of mesh in the parietal compartment of the preperitoneal space, by adequate mesh fixation, and by preventing mesh wrinkling and meshoma formation during laparoscopic and open preperitoneal inguinal hernia repair [8, 9].

Groin Neuroanatomy

There are three nerves within the inguinal canal (Fig. 4.1). The *ilioinguinal nerve* is located over the spermatic cord, covered and protected from the mesh by the investing fascia of the internal oblique muscle (Fig. 4.2). This protective fascia should not be damaged by removing the nerve from its natural bed. Removing the ilioinguinal nerve from its native position over the cord and placing it below the inguinal ligament, which was the teaching of a prior era, destroys the protective fascia of the nerve and risks perineural scaring and direct contact of the nerve with mesh.

The genital branch of the genitofemoral nerve is located under the cord (Fig. 4.1), covered and protected from direct contact with mesh by

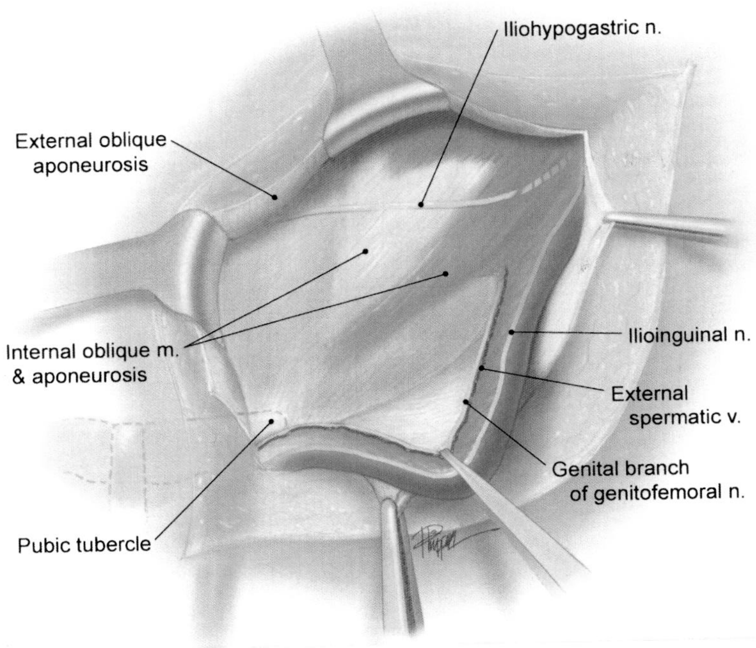

Fig. 4.1. Neuroanatomy of the left inguinal canal. Pubic tubercle on the left.

the deep cremasteric fascia. Although small and difficult to see, its location can be determined by the easily visible "blue line" of the external spermatic vein that is always adjacent to the nerve (Fig. 4.3). To assure safety of the nerve, it must be kept with the spermatic cord while the cord is separated from the inguinal floor using a blunt dissector such as peanut under direct visualization. Grasping the cord with thumb and index finger and bluntly finger dissecting this off the floor is excessively traumatic and should be avoided. This may damage the deep cremasteric fascia which can lead to perineural scaring and direct contact of the genital nerve with the implanted mesh. In addition it results in direct contact of the vas and sensory nerve fibers of the testicle (paravasal nerve fibers) within the covering sheath of the vas (lamina propria of the vas) that can lead to orchialgia [10], azoospermia [11], and dysejaculation.

The iliohypogastric nerve is located between the external and internal oblique layers, covered and protected from mesh by the investing fascia of the internal oblique muscle (Fig. 4.1). The key step to exposing the

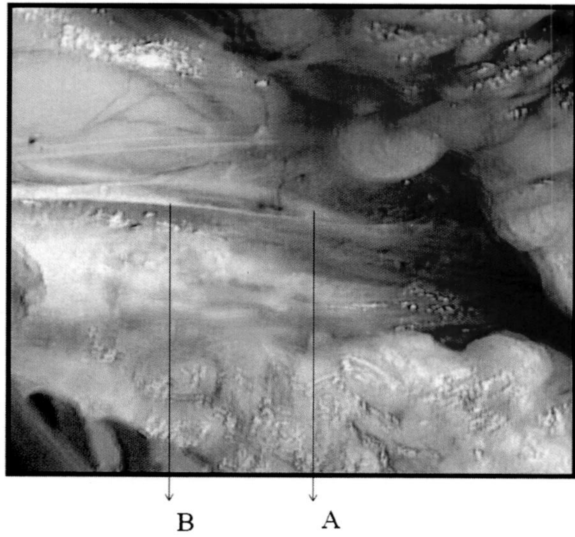

Fig. 4.2. Left ilioinguinal nerve (A). Pubic tubercle on the left. Investing fascia of the internal oblique muscle covering and protecting the nerve (B).

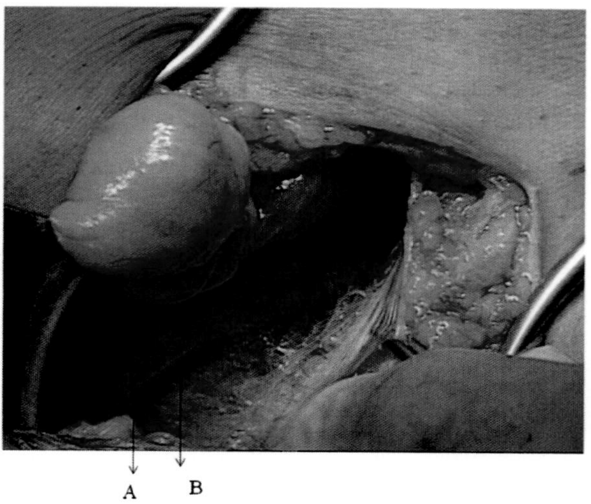

Fig. 4.3. Left genitofemoral nerve (A). Pubic tubercle on the left. The "blue" line of the external spermatic vein (B).

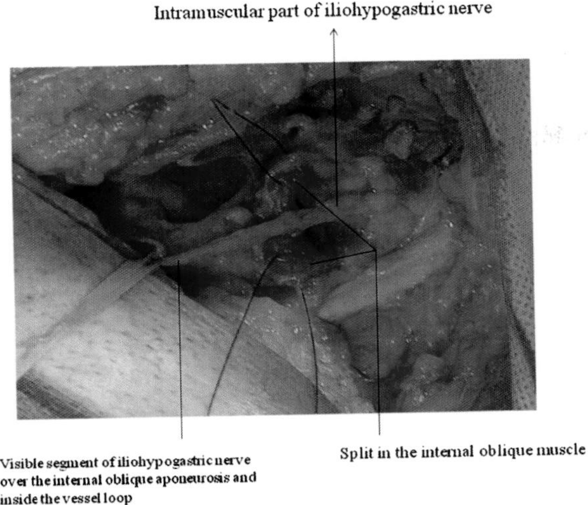

Fig. 4.4. Left iliohypogastric nerve. Pubic tubercle on the lower part of the left side.

iliohypogastric nerve is opening the anatomic cleavage between the internal and external oblique layers high enough to expose the internal oblique aponeurosis. This simple step readily exposes the iliohypogastric nerve. The iliohypogastric nerve has an easily visible part over the internal oblique aponeurosis and muscle (Fig. 4.4). There is also a hidden segment that runs inferiorly and laterally within the internal oblique muscle (Fig. 4.4 and dotted line in Fig. 4.1). This segment of the iliohypogastric nerve is the most vulnerable neural structure of the inguinal area because it is not visible within the operative field [10]. Suturing through the internal oblique muscle, or the so-called conjoined tendon, for its fixation to the inguinal ligament, flat mesh, or plug has the potential risk of injuring the intramuscular segment of the nerve with the needle or entrapping it by the suture.

Operative Technique

The procedure is performed under local anesthesia [12], which is our preferred choice for all reducible adult unilateral and bilateral [2] inguinal hernias. It is safe, simple, effective, economical, and without the normal side effects of general anesthesia such as nausea, vomiting, and urinary retention. Furthermore, local anesthesia administered prior to making the incision produces a preemptive and prolonged analgesic effect via inhibition of the buildup of local nociceptive molecules [12].

A 5–6 cm skin incision, which starts from the pubic tubercle and extends laterally following a Langer's line, provides excellent exposure to both the pubic tubercle and the internal ring. The incision is carried down through Scarpa's fascia to the external oblique aponeurosis. The external oblique aponeurosis is opened in the direction of its fibers down through the external ring. The lower leaf of the external oblique (the inguinal ligament) is freed from the spermatic cord. The ilioinguinal nerve can usually be identified coursing with the spermatic cord immediately upon lifting the external oblique aponeurosis, and care is taken to preserve this structure during exposure. The upper leaf of the external oblique is then freed from the underlying internal oblique muscle until the internal oblique aponeurosis is exposed (Fig. 4.1). The anatomic cleavage between these two layers is avascular, and the dissection can be performed rapidly and atraumatically. High separation of these layers allows for visualization of the iliohypogastric nerve and internal oblique aponeurosis. This dissection also creates ample space for insertion of a sufficiently wide sheet of mesh that can overlap the internal oblique well above the upper margin of the inguinal floor.

The cord with its cremaster covering is separated from the floor of the inguinal canal and the pubic bone for a distance of approximately 2 cm beyond the pubic tubercle (Fig. 4.1). The anatomic plane between the cremasteric muscle and attachment of rectus sheath to the pubic bone is avascular. Strictly dissecting within this plane avoids the risk of damaging testicular blood flow. When lifting the cord, care should be taken to include the ilioinguinal nerve, the easily visible blue external spermatic vein, and the genital nerve with the cord. This assures that the genital nerve, which is always in juxtaposition to the external spermatic vessels, is securely preserved.

The internal ring is always explored to identify the presence of an indirect hernia sac. The cremasteric muscle layer is opened anteriorly and incised longitudinally approximately 3–4 cm at the level of the deep ring to access the cremasteric compartment. Complete stripping and resection of the cremasteric fibers are unnecessary and can result in direct exposure of the genital nerve, vas deferens, and paravasal nerves to the mesh, resulting in chronic groin and testicular pain.

Indirect hernia sacs are identified and freed from the cord using the electrocautery tip as a dissector with or without energy and gentle traction. The sac is freed to a point beyond its neck and is inverted into the properitoneal space without ligation. Because of mechanical pressure and ischemic changes, ligation of the highly innervated peritoneal sac is a major cause of acute postoperative pain. *It has been demonstrated that nonligation of the indirect hernia sac does not increase the chance of recurrence.* To minimize the risk of postoperative ischemic orchitis, complete nonsliding scrotal hernia sacs are transected at the midpoint of the canal, leaving the distal portion of the sac in place. However, the anterior wall of the distal sac is incised to prevent postoperative hydrocele formation. If the internal ring is too large, it can be tightened using one or two Marcy Sutures placed on the transversalis fascia at the deep ring.

The floor of the inguinal canal inferomedial to the inferior epigastric vessel is evaluated for evidence of a direct hernia. If large with a narrow neck, the direct sac is inverted using a purse string suture. If large with a wide base, the sac is inverted with an absorbable suture placed along the transversalis fascia. For this purpose, the lower edge of the internal oblique muscle should not be included in the suture under tension as in the classic Bassini operation preserving the "tension-free" principle of this repair. A thorough exploration of the groin is necessary to rule out coexisting intraparietal (interstitial), low-lying spigelian, or femoral hernias. The femoral ring is routinely evaluated via the space of Bogros through a small opening in the canal floor.

A 7×15 cm sheet of mesh is used to repair the floor of the inguinal canal. We prefer monofilament, macroporous, polypropylene meshes because the monofilament structure does not perpetuate or harbor infection. The medial corner of the mesh is tailored to its standard shape, (Fig. 4.5) which resembles the tracing of a footprint, with a lower sharper angle to fit into the angle between the inguinal ligament and the rectus sheath and an upper wider angle to spread over the rectus sheath. With the cord retracted upward, the sharper corner is sutured with a nonabsorbable monofilament suture material or stapled to the rectus sheath above its insertion to the pubic bone and overlapping the bone by 1–2 cm (Fig. 4.6). This is a crucial step in the repair because failure to cover this bone with the mesh can result in recurrence of the hernia. The periosteum of the bone is avoided. This is continued as a continuous running suture or intermittent staples attaching the lower edge of the mesh patch to the inguinal ligament up to a point just lateral to the internal ring (Fig. 4.6). Suturing or stapling the mesh beyond this point is unnecessary and could injure the femoral nerve. If there is a concurrent femoral hernia, it can be fixed using a modification in which the mesh is also sutured to the Cooper ligament 1–2 cm below the suture line with the inguinal ligament in order to close

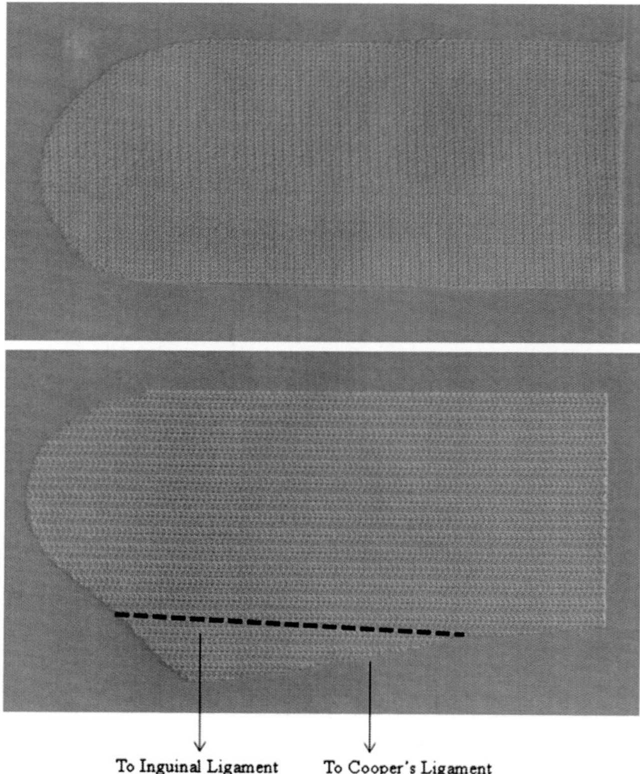

Fig. 4.5. Standard mesh: 7 cm × 15 cm (*top*). Modified mesh with a triangular extension for the repair of a coexisting femoral hernia (*bottom*).

the femoral ring. Alternatively, the mesh can be tailored to have a triangular extension from its lower edge. The lateral aspect of the triangular extension is sutured to the Cooper ligament, and the body of the mesh is sutured to the inguinal ligament along the dotted line (Fig. 4.5) obliterating the defect in the femoral canal.

A slit is made at the lateral end of the mesh, creating two tails, a wider one (two-thirds of the width) above and a narrower one (one-third of the width) below. The wider upper tail is grasped with forceps and passed toward the head of the patient from underneath the spermatic cord; this positions the cord between the two tails of the mesh (Fig. 4.7). The upper tail is crossed and placed over the lower tail and held with a hemostat (Fig. 4.8). With the cord retracted downward and the upper leaf of the external oblique aponeurosis retracted upward, the upper edge of

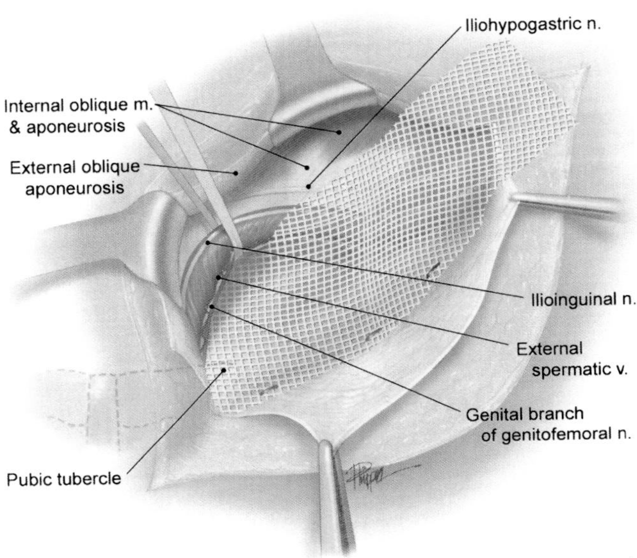

Fig. 4.6. With the cord retracted upward, the lower edge of the mesh with a 2 cm extension medial to the pubic tubercle is fixed to the inguinal ligament. The medial corner of mesh is fixed to the insertion of rectus sheath on the pubic bone away from the pubic tubercle.

the mesh patch is sutured in place with two interrupted absorbable sutures or stapled, one to the rectus sheath and the other to the internal oblique aponeurosis just medial to the internal ring (Fig. 4.8). Occasionally, the course of the iliohypogastric nerve passes against the upper edge of the mesh. In this case, a slit in the mesh will accommodate the nerve. If in doubt, the nerve can be resected with proximal-end ligation to prevent traumatic neuroma formation and implantation within the fibers of the internal oblique muscle to keep the stump of the nerve away from the future scarring within the operative field. Suturing or stapling the upper edge of the mesh to the internal oblique muscle should be avoided to prevent injuring the intramuscular segment of the iliohypogastric nerve.

Using a single nonabsorbable monofilament suture or staple, the lower edges of each of the two tails are fixed to the inguinal ligament just lateral to the completion knot of the lower running suture, leaving adequate space for the passage of the spermatic cord (Fig. 4.9). The excess patch on the lateral side is trimmed, leaving at least 5 cm of mesh beyond the internal ring. This is tucked underneath the external oblique aponeurosis (Fig. 4.9). Fixation of the tails of the mesh to the internal

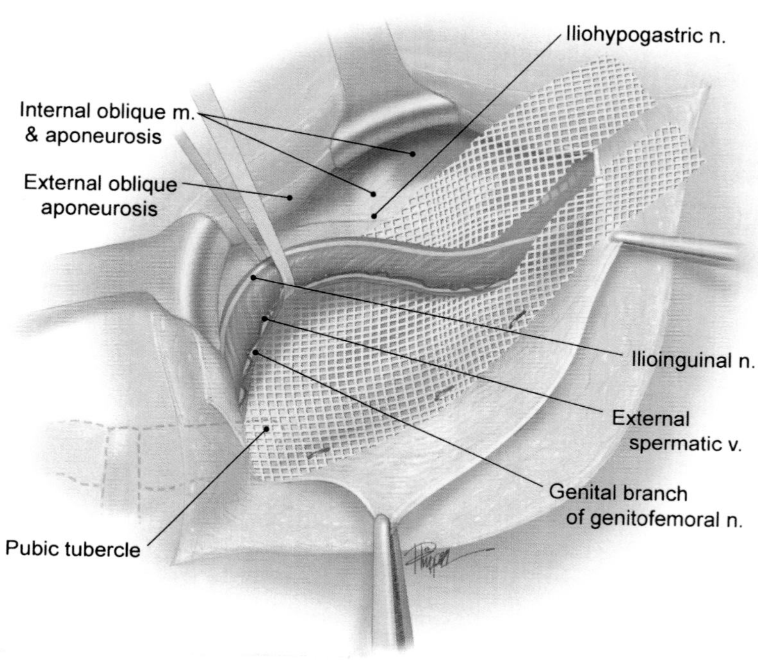

Fig. 4.7. A slit is made at the lateral end of the mesh forming two tails. The spermatic cord is placed in between the two tails.

oblique muscle, lateral to the internal ring, is unnecessary and could result in entrapment of the ilioinguinal nerve with the fixation suture or staple. The aponeurosis of the external oblique is then closed over the cord with an absorbable suture. The skin may be closed with an absorbable subcuticular suture or staples completing the repair.

Evidence-Based Medicine: The Role of the Lichtenstein "Tension-Free" Hernia Repair

Since the introduction of the open "tension-free" hernioplasty in 1984, the operation has been evaluated and compared with other types of hernia repairs in numerous studies with regard to postoperative pain,

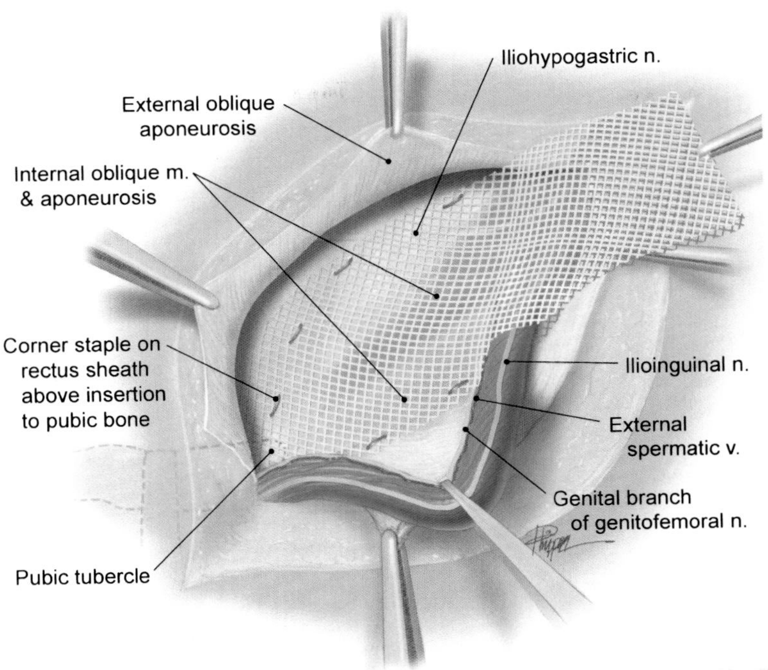

Fig. 4.8. With the cord retracted downward, the tails of the mesh are crossed and held in place with a clamp. The upper edge of the mesh is sutured or stapled to the internal oblique aponeurosis.

postoperative time off work, complications, costs, and, most significantly, recurrence rate. According to the 2009 European Hernia Guidelines prepared by 14 renowned European hernia experts based on the review of 324 published clinical trials, the Lichtenstein technique introduced in 1984 is currently the best evaluated and most popular of different open mesh techniques. It is reproducible with minimal morbidity; it can be performed in the outpatient setting under local anesthesia and has low recurrence rates in long-term follow-up [13]. Results of nonexpert surgeons and supervised residents using the Lichtenstein repair for primary inguinal hernias showed comparable excellent results underscoring the ease, safety, and reproducibility of this technique [14].

A Cochrane review of 20 randomized trials comparing Lichtenstein repair to tissue repair demonstrated a shorter length of hospital stay, quicker return to usual activities, less chronic pain, and significantly

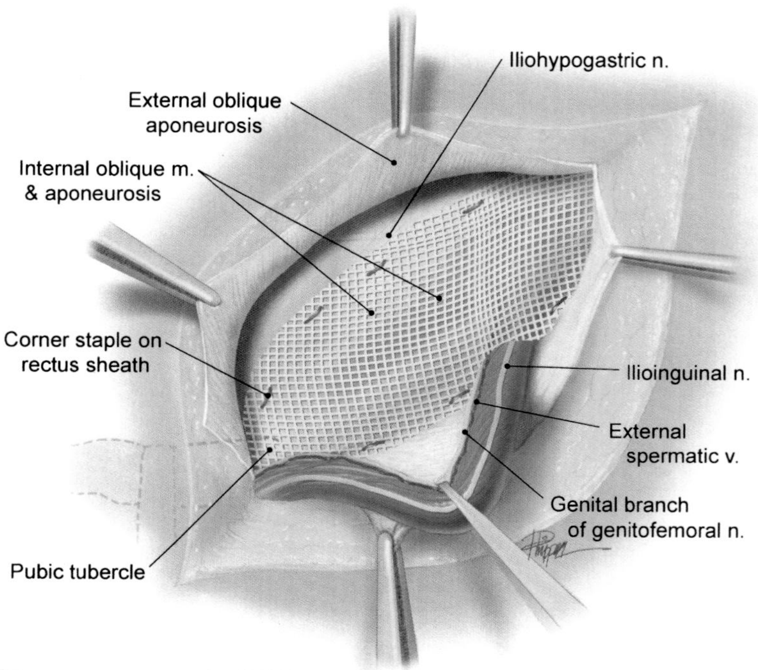

Fig. 4.9. The lower edges of the two tails are sutured to the inguinal ligament, providing adequate space for the passage of the cord. The end of the mesh is tucked under the external oblique aponeurosis.

fewer hernia recurrences. The use of the Lichtenstein "tension-free" mesh repair is associated with a reduction in the risk of recurrence of between 50% and 75% [15]. Comparison between Lichtenstein and laparoscopic total extraperitoneal (TEP) mesh repair demonstrates more equivalency with recommendations for both operations under certain conditions.

The randomized controlled "LEVEL" trial concluded that the *TEP* procedure compared to Lichtenstein repair was associated with less subjectively reported acute postoperative pain and faster recovery of daily activities and return to work by approximately half a day. Both of these results did not affect quality of life indicators, and pain levels were low in both groups after 1 week. Recurrence rates and chronic pain were comparable [16]. These benefits should be weighed in relation to the added operative costs, increased intraoperative adverse events, need for general anesthesia, elevated learning curve, and significant difficulty with addressing inguinodynia in patients in which mesh is placed in the preperitoneal compartment. Grade *A* recommendations of the European Hernia Guidelines state that "For adults with primary unilateral and bilateral inguinal hernias, Lichtenstein or endoscopic repairs are both recommended, endoscopic repair only if expertise is available" [13].

References

1. Amid PK, Shulman AG, Lichtenstein IL. Critical scrutiny of the open tension-free hernioplasty. Am J Surg. 1993;165:369–71.
2. Amid PK. Lichtenstein tension-free hernioplasty: Its inception, evolution, and principles. Hernia. 2004;8:1–7.
3. Amid PK, Shulman AG, Lichtenstein IL. Simultaneous repair of bilateral inguinal hernias under local anesthesia. Ann Surg. 1996;223(3):249–52.
4. Bay-nielsen M, Perkins FM, et al. Pain and functional impairment 1 year after inguinal herniorrhaphy: a nationwide questionnaire study. Ann Surg. 2001;233(1):1–7.
5. Amid PK. Radiological images of meshoma: a new phenomenon after prosthetic repair of abdominal wall hernia. Arch Surg. 2004;139:1297–8.
6. Wijsmuller AR, Lang JFM, et al. Surgical technique preventing chronic pain after Lichtenstein hernia repair; state of the art vs. daily practice in the Netherlands. Hernia. 2007;11:147–51.
7. Alfieri S, Rotandi F, et al. Influence of preservation versus division of ilioinguinal, iliohypogastric, and genital nerves during open mesh herniorrhaphy. Prospective multicenter study of chronic pain. Ann Surg. 2006;243(4):553–8.
8. Mirilas P, Anastasia M, Skandalakis JE. Secondary internal inguinal ring and associated surgical planes: surgical anatomy, embryology, application. J Am Coll Surg. 2008;206(3):561–70.
9. Amid PK, Hiatt JR. Surgical anatomy of the preperitoneal space. J Am Coll Surg. 2008;707(2):295.
10. Amid PK. New understanding of the causes and surgical treatment of postherniorrhaphy inguinodynia and orchialgia. J Am Coll Surg. 2007;205:381–5.
11. Peiper C, Junge K, Klinge U, Strehlau E, Ottinger A, Schumpelick V. Is there a risk of infertility after inguinal mesh repair? Experimental studies in pig and rabbit. Hernia. 2006;10(1):7–12.
12. Amid PK, Shulman AG, Lichtenstein IL. Local anesthesia for inguinal hernia repair step-by-step procedure. Ann Surg. 1994;220(6):735–7.
13. Simons MP, Aufenacker T, Bay Nielsoen M, et al. European Hernia Society guidelines on the treatment of inguinal hernia in adult patients. Hernia. 2009;13:343–403.
14. Shulman AG, Amid PK, Lichtenstein IL. A survey of non-expert surgeons using the open tension-free mesh patch repair for primary inguinal hernias. Int Surg. 1995;80(1):35–6.

15. Scott NW, McCormack K, Graham P, Go PM, Ross SJ, Grant AM. Open mesh versus non-mesh for repair of femoral and inguinal hernia. Cochrane Database Syst Rev. 2002;4:CD002197
16. Langeveld HR, van't Riet M, Weidema WF, Stassen LP, Steyerberg EW, Lange J, Bonjer HJ, Jeekel J. Total extraperitoneal inguinal hernia repair compared with Lichtenstein (the LEVEL-Trial): a randomized controlled trial. Ann Surg. 2010;251(5):819–24.

5. Technique: Plug and Patch

Carl Doerhoff

Children intuitively love to put pegs in holes. Perhaps the most famous example of this is the story of the little Dutch boy who plugged a dike with his finger. Was he aware that the act prevented a disaster, or was he just interested in plugging a hole? The documented history of hernia hole plugging begins in 1836 with Pierre Nicolas Gerdy [1], a Parisian surgeon, who believed that an inguinal canal could be "plugged" by inverting a fold of scrotal skin. As a result of inflammation, the inguinal canal would close. The first documented device was an external wooden plug used by C.W. Wutzer, professor of surgery in Bonn, in 1841 [2]. The plug was used to advance the testicle and scrotal skin through the hernia defect. Again, inflammation and scar was the rationale for the repair.

In 1886, William Macewen of Glasgow conceptualized the first use of an autologous internal plug. Macewen reported 33 patients on whom he imbricated the hernia sac and advanced it through the internal ring as a "plug" [3]. He started at the distal end of the sac and passed a suture toward the internal ring, imbricating the sac much like threading a worm onto a hook. When he pulled on the suture, the sac would become pleated "like a curtain." He placed the "plug" through the internal ring and tightened the ring medially with suture. In 1956, Sir Francis Usher used a flat sheet of prosthetic polypropylene mesh (Marlex) to bridge a hernia defect. His creativity catapulted hernia repair to a new dimension, creating the opportunity for someone to forge a prosthetic device.

Lichtenstein Cylindrical Plug

In 1968, Lichtenstein began plugging femoral and recurrent hernias with a rolled plug of Marlex mesh. He fashioned a 2 cm×5 cm strip of Marlex and rolled it into a cylinder [4] (Fig. 5.1). He placed the "cigarette" plug into

B.P. Jacob and B. Ramshaw (eds.), *The SAGES Manual of Hernia Repair*,
DOI 10.1007/978-1-4614-4824-2_5,

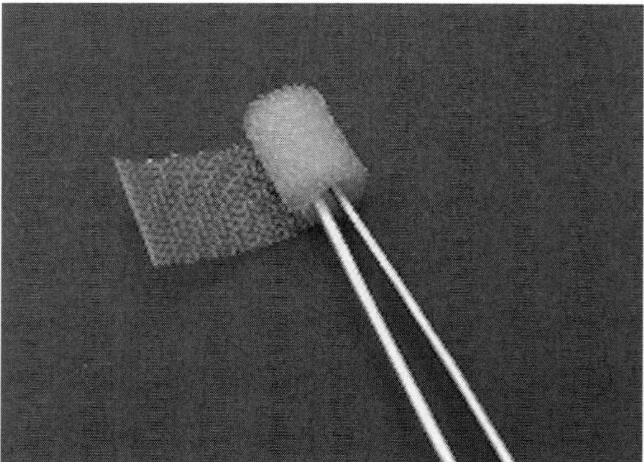

Fig. 5.1. Lichtenstein plugged femoral and recurrent hernias with a rolled plug of Marlex mesh.

the femoral defect and used two nonabsorbable sutures to hold the plug in place. In 1974, Lichtenstein reported his experience with femoral and recurrent hernias using the plug for repair. He pointed out that a recurrence from a sutured repair occurred either medial at the pubis or lateral at the internal ring. He realized that these are the two weakest areas of a sutured repair, since there is no other stitch medial nor lateral to either area to reduce tension or bolster the end stitch. Because the rest of the floor repair remained strong and intact, he used only the cylindrical plug as the repair.

In 1990, Lichtenstein reported 20 years of experience with the cigarette plug repair. Using a 2 cm×20 cm cylinder of mesh [5]. He stated, "Where larger defects are encountered, a second or third strip is employed around the first to fatten the plug as needed." He inserted the tightly rolled plug flush or just beneath the defect. The plug would uncoil until it filled the defect. Lichtenstein used several interrupted nonabsorbable sutures to hold the plug in place. He reported 1,402 patients repaired by this technique with a failure rate of only 1.6%.

Gilbert Plug and Swatch

In 1989, Gilbert published his classification of five types of inguinal hernias. He studied the anatomic differences of the five defects. Types 1, 2, and 3 were classified as indirect. Types 4 and 5 were direct. The type

1 indirect hernia had a snug internal ring with the canal floor intact. The type 2 indirect had a moderately enlarged internal ring and admitted one to two fingers, but the floor was intact. The type 3 indirect hernia had a large indirect defect admitting two or more fingers. Because of the large type 3 indirect defect, the inguinal floor was also incompetent. Its repair required reconstruction of both the floor and the internal ring. The type 4 direct hernia was a "large or full blowout defect of the inguinal floor [6]." The internal ring was intact. The type 5 direct hernia was a diverticular defect usually no larger than one finger, and the internal ring was intact. As Gilbert meticulously created his classification system, he also created an intricate system of repairing each hernia according to type. From 1984 to 1987, he used Marlex mesh to repair each of the five types of hernias. For the type 1 hernia, the indirect sac was invaginated. A Marlex flat mesh or "swatch" was placed over the inguinal floor to reinforce it against future herniation. The overlay swatch was not sutured but, instead, held in place by approximating the transverse aponeurotic arch to Poupart's ligament over the swatch, using a two-layer continuous 3-0 Prolene. For the type 2 indirect hernia, Gilbert borrowed Lichtenstein's idea of using a rolled Marlex cylindrical plug [7]. The hernia sac was invaginated, and the plug was placed through the internal ring and held there with two stitches. Again, an overlay mesh was placed, prophylactically, reinforcing the floor. For type 3 hernias (large enough to be scrotal and sliding), both the internal ring and the floor required reconstruction. A cylindrical plug was placed through the internal ring. The floor was opened, and an underlay graft was placed in the preperitoneal space. Tissue was sutured over the graft. For type 4 hernias, the entire floor was opened and reconstructed—identical to type 3 hernias. Later, an overlay graft was also added. The type 5 diverticular direct defect was repaired using a Marlex plug-graft and an adjunctive Marlex overlay graft. For small recurrent hernias, only a rolled Marlex plug-graft was used for the repair.

The configuration of the plug also changed over time. In some patients, "the plug was annoyingly palpable [8]." Subsequently, the hand-rolled plug was then placed deeper, completely through the internal ring into the preperitoneal space, and allowed to unravel against the anterior abdominal wall; however, the plug did not consistently unroll, and still some patients reported feeling the wad of mesh. Gilbert was dissatisfied that the mesh did not always unroll but remained coiled, causing scarring and discomfort. To correct this, he began with a 2.5 in. × 2.5 in. square piece of flat mesh, next, cut the radius, and then folded the mesh into a closed umbrella configuration (Fig. 5.2). He placed the closed umbrella,

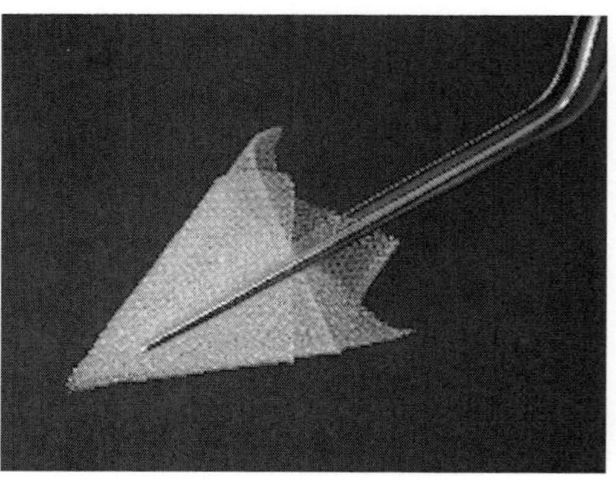

Fig. 5.2. Gilbert used Marlex mesh to repair each of the five types of hernias.

point first, completely through the internal ring. The umbrella was allowed to unfold, anticipating it would lay flat in the preperitoneal space. The flattened umbrella did not require suture fixation. This very intricate system was successful in terms of low recurrence rates and became known as Gilbert's sutureless umbrella plug repair.

Rutkow-Robbins Hand-Rolled Umbrella/Cone Plug

Rutkow and Robbins modified the Gilbert classification [9, 10], enlarging the dimensions of the type III hernia and adding pantaloon (type VI) and femoral hernias (type VII). Type I indirect has a tight internal ring. Type II indirect hernia has a moderately enlarged internal ring. Type III indirect hernia has a patulous internal ring greater than 4 cm and occupies most of the inguinal floor. Type IV direct hernia is a fusiform defect of the entire inguinal floor. A type IV hernia is essentially the same as a type III defect, except the defect begins medial to the epigastric vessels. Type V is a diverticular defect within the inguinal floor, type VI is a pantaloon indirect and direct hernia, and type VII is a femoral hernia.

In 1989, Rutkow and Robbins used a hand-fashioned umbrella plug for their first sutureless repair of a type I indirect hernia. At 1 week post-op, the patient had markedly less discomfort than Rutkow and Robbins observed in their previous 3,000 sutured hernioplasties. They proceeded to repair small indirect hernias (type I and II) with a plug.

Because there was no shutter mechanism for a type III indirect hernia, they made larger umbrellas and partially opened the umbrella plug. The cone was placed point first and advanced until the widest portion of the cone was at the level of the defect. At this level, the plug was fixated with three to six interrupted absorbable stitches. The stitches were not deep into the tissue, simply sustaining the plug in the appropriate position. A larger plug was used for type IV defects. Type IV defects sometimes required a second plug. Pantaloon defects often required two or even three cone-shaped plugs sutured together, shoulder to shoulder. Rutkow and Robbins believed that the plug was the repair and an overlay flat mesh was optional. Later, an overlay mesh was routinely used to prevent a new hernia. The flat mesh was laid over the internal oblique and directed toward the pubis. The overlay mesh was not sutured to tissue. A slit was cut laterally for the cord, and the tails were sutured to themselves around the cord. For type III indirect and type IV direct hernias, multiple sutures were used to secure the plug.

By the end of 1991, the umbrella plug was used to repair all types of hernias. In 1993, Rutkow and Robbins reported their experience of 1,563 mesh-plug hernioplasties from January 1989 through December 1992. Their recurrence rate was 0.1%. They had standardized the mesh-plug inguinal hernia technique for all indirect, direct, and femoral hernias.

Bard PerFix Plug

In 1993, Rutkow and Robbins participated with C.R. Bard Company to develop a preformed plug out of Marlex mesh (PerFix) [11–14] (Fig. 5.3). The tip of the PerFix plug was more rounded in contrast to the sharply pointed cone plug. The outer portion of the PerFix plug was fluted. To reduce the likelihood of contracture and to provide bulk, eight mesh petals were placed inside the shuttlecock-looking device. Eventually, four plug sizes were offered. A 3 cm×6 cm overlay mesh was provided with the plug. This standardized the plug/patch device so that it could be used by any surgeon.

Rutkow and Robbins stated: "The less we dissect, the better the result." They made a 4- to 6-cm oblique incision with a knife. All other dissection, including mobilization of the sac, was with electrocautery. If the ilioinguinal or genitofemoral nerves were identified, they were preserved, but they were not intentionally looked for. The cord was mobilized, and the sac was dissected "high" through the internal ring.

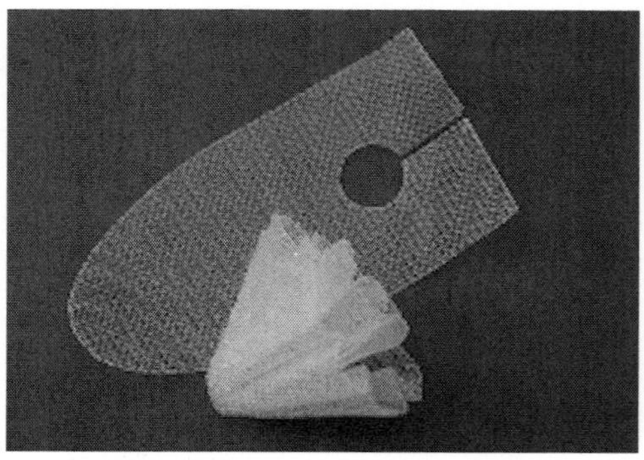

Fig. 5.3. Rutkow and Robbins participated with C.R. Bard Company to develop a preformed plug out of Marlex mesh (PerFix).

The sac was not opened and not ligated. The appropriate size of mesh plug was inserted. For small indirect hernias, one to two interrupted 3-0 polyglactin (Vicryl) sutures were used. In larger indirect and large direct hernias, the plug was secured with 8–10 stitches. If necessary, petals could be removed to reduce the bulk—especially for thin, athletic patients. For large direct hernias and for pantaloon hernias, two or more plugs were used, and the plugs were sutured to each other. A 3×6 cm precut flat Marlex mesh was placed over the floor for reinforcement. A single absorbable stitch brought the tails together around the cord. The patch was laid over the internal oblique, and the cord passed anterior to the mesh. The mesh itself was not sutured to underlying tissue. For femoral hernias, an infrainguinal approach was made. Petals were removed from a small plug. If the hernia sac could not be reduced, it was transected and ligated. A small plug was held in place by suturing it to surrounding tissue.

For recurrent hernias, the rule was to dissect even less. First, they exposed the defect, making no attempt to dissect through fused layers. The spermatic cord was not mobilized unless it was necessary to expose the defect. The appropriate size plug was held in place with multiple interrupted stitches. The onlay patch could be used only if there was sufficient room for placement.

Between 1989 and 1997, Rutkow and Robbins performed 3,268 mesh-plug hernioplasties. 88% were primary repairs. 12% were recurrent repairs. This included 1,708 hand-rolled Marlex umbrella/cone plugs and 1,560 PerFix preformed plugs. The use of the PerFix plug further decreased their operating time by 4 min. The skin-to-skin operating time was 17 min for primary hernioplasty and 20 min for recurrent hernioplasty. 95% of all patients returned to daily activities within 3 days of their operation. Of the 2,861 initial indirect and direct repairs, there was less than a 1% recurrence rate. Of the 32 patients with primary femoral hernioplasty, there were no recurrences. To repair a recurrent hernia, there was a 3% chance of recurrence. For a multiply recurrent hernias, there was a 9% risk of recurrence, and an alternative repair (preperitoneal, Stoppa, or laparoscopic) was recommended.

Prospective and randomized studies support the simplicity, effectiveness, and economical advantage of the Rutkow and Robbins technique of PerFix plug/patch, demonstrating no statistical increase of recurrence rate or long-term groin pain [15–20].

Complications of the Plug-Patch

Any operation can have complications, and plug and patch is no exception. Complications are lessons to be learned. Unfortunately, the standardized operation by Rutkow and Robbins has been liberally modified by surgeons performing plug-patch hernioplasty. Certainly, some of the complications are related to technical errors—improper placement, fixation, or patient selection. There are multiple anecdotal reports of plug erosion and migration [21–27]. Because the point of the plug stretches the peritoneum, it is possible that the tip of the plug either creates a break in the peritoneum at the time of insertion or the peritoneum thins over time, exposing the plug to the abdominal cavity. Plugs have caused deep vein thrombosis, migrated into the scrotum, eroded in the bladder, iliac vessels, and intestine.

Some complications are related to mesh shrinkage. Amid [28] reports flat mesh will lose 20% of its size secondary to scar. According to LeBlanc [29], "a cone will lose 70% of its volume if it loses 20% of its surface area, thereby adversely affecting its ability to fill a defect." Mesh will shrink regardless of whether absorbable or nonabsorbable sutures are used. As the plug separates from the defect, it increases the likelihood of recurrence or frees the plug for potential migration.

While it has been alleged that the plug may cause long-term neuralgia, the direct correlation is difficult to prove. Numbness may follow any incision, and post-herniorrhaphy pain may be due to nerve injury or entrapment. Despite the reported low incidence of chronic pain by Rutkow and Robbins, other surgeons have not been able to duplicate their results [30]. LeBlanc polled 26 members of the American Hernia Society who reported 9% of their patients had pain that interfered with their lifestyle. Palot et al. [31] found a 6.3% incidence of inguinodynia with plug-patch.

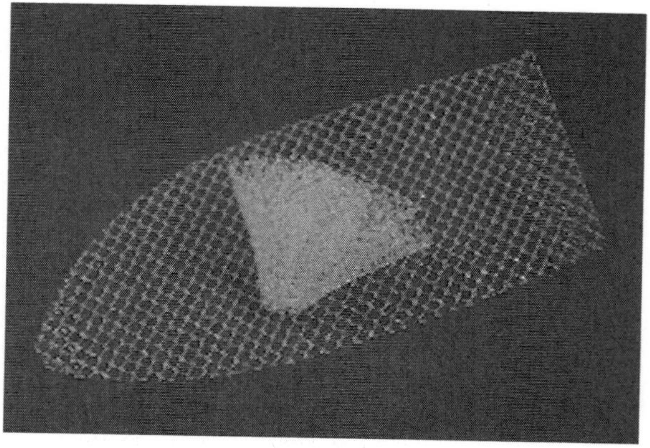

Fig. 5.4. For surgeons who believed that heavyweight mesh was linked to inguinodynia, Bard introduced the PerFix Light Plug in 2010.

For surgeons who believed that heavyweight mesh was linked to inguinodynia, Bard introduced the PerFix Light Plug in 2010 (Fig. 5.4). Bard fashioned the macroporous PerFix Light Plug from polypropylene mesh weighing 59 g/m^2 with a pore size of 0.48 mm^2. The overlay measures 5.8 cm × 14 cm. The original PerFix plug is made from polypropylene, weighing 115 g/m^2 with a pore size of 0.4 mm^2. Its overlay is 4.6 cm by 8.9 cm.

Millikan Modified Mesh-Plug Hernioplasty

In 1997, Dr. Keith Millikan modified the PerFix plug hernioplasty [32]. Millikan noted that Rutkow and Robbins positioned the fluted portion of the plug to the edge of the defect, causing the plug to protrude further than necessary toward the abdominal cavity. Millikan inserted the entire plug through the defect, but instead of suturing the fluted edge to the defect allowed the fluted portion to lay much flatter in the preperitoneal space extending away from the defect. The plug was secured by its petals. This method of flattening the plug appeared to have several benefits: wider overlap of the defect and less protrusion of the tip toward the abdominal cavity.

In 2003, Millikan reported results of 1,056 patients who underwent primary unilateral herniorrhaphy. For type I and type II indirect hernias, the inside petals of a large plug were sutured to the internal oblique portion of the internal ring. For type III indirect and type IV and V direct hernias, an extra-large plug was used. Petals were sutured to the conjoined tendon, Cooper's ligament, and the shelving edge of the inguinal ligament. Monofilament permanent sutures were used for plug fixation for types III, IV, and V. The onlay mesh was placed around the cord and the tails secured with a stitch. The mesh itself is not suture fixated. At 1 year, recurrence rate was 0.1%. 95.9% of patients had returned to normal activities by the third postoperative day. The incidence of postoperative groin pain was only 0.5%. There were no reports of erosion or migration.

Atrium ProLite Mesh and ProLoop

In 1997, Atrium provided the plug-patch surgeon another alternative. The ProLite self-forming plug consists of three circular layers of ProLite mesh made from polypropylene mesh weighing 85 g/m^2 (Fig. 5.5). The three layers are welded at 3, 6, 9, and 12 o'clock. A central tab has been added that can be grasped, facilitating insertion. The circular mesh forms a conical plug as it is introduced through a hernia defect. Dr. Goldstein recommended suturing the plug in place with interrupted monofilament sutures [33, 34].

In 2001, Atrium introduced the ProLoop plug (Fig. 5.6). ProLoop is a preformed polypropylene plug that has 30% less polypropylene than the PerFix plug. The ProLoop plug has multiple protruding monofilament loops that reportedly keep the plug from deforming as it is inserted through the defect. The loops reduce contact of the plug with surrounding tissue—in hopes of reducing mesh/plug shrinkage, hardening, and contracture. The intent is to decrease the incidence of long-term groin pain. Two overlay patches are available: One is an oval pointed patch measuring 4.6 cm × 8.9 cm with a lateral slit, and the other is a blunted 5.0 cm × 8.9 cm overlay with a caudal slit.

A study by Sanders [35] randomized 239 patients between Lichtenstein repair, PerFix plug and patch, and ProLoop plug-and-patch repair of primary inguinal hernias. No significant statistical differences in recurrence rates, complications, or inguinodynia were noted. Recurrence rate for the ProLoop plug was 2.1%, for the PerFix plug 1%, and 2% for Lichtenstein repair. All procedures were performed under local anesthesia with 100 mg diclofenac suppository given 1 h preoperatively. Operative times were comparable: 32.9 min for the ProLoop plug, 31.1 min for the

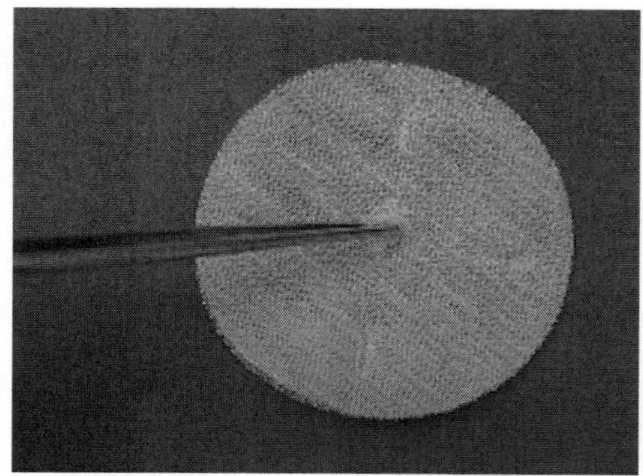

Fig. 5.5. The Atrium ProLite self-forming plug consists of three circular layers of ProLite mesh made from polypropylene mesh weighing 85 g/m^2.

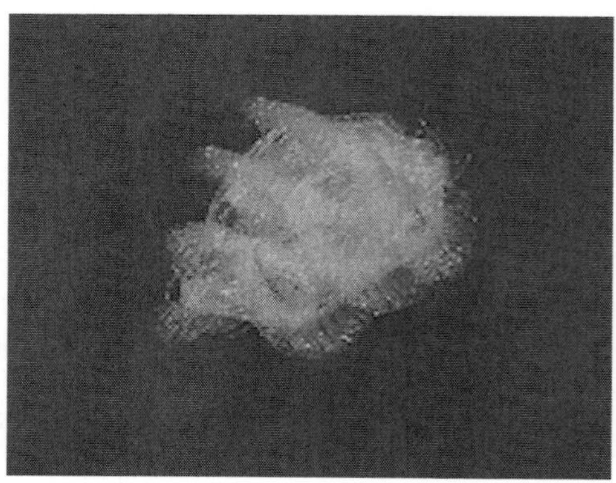

Fig. 5.6. In 2001, Atrium introduced the ProLoop plug.

PerFix plug, and 32.8 min for the Lichtenstein tension-free mesh repair. By comparison to the Rutkow study of 2,060 patients that had a 1% recurrence for primary hernia repair and 2% for recurrent hernia repair at 6 years, Sanders suggested that surgery in a highly specialized center for inguinal hernia repair by higher volume surgeons would have a lower recurrence rate.

Ethicon Ultrapro Plug and Patch

In 2007, Ethicon introduced a double-sided low-profile plug that works well for hernia defects that are 3 cm and smaller. The plug looks like a circular plate (anchor) connected to a shallow bowl (rim) (Fig. 5.7). For a large plug, the preperitoneal portion or "anchor," measures 5 cm in

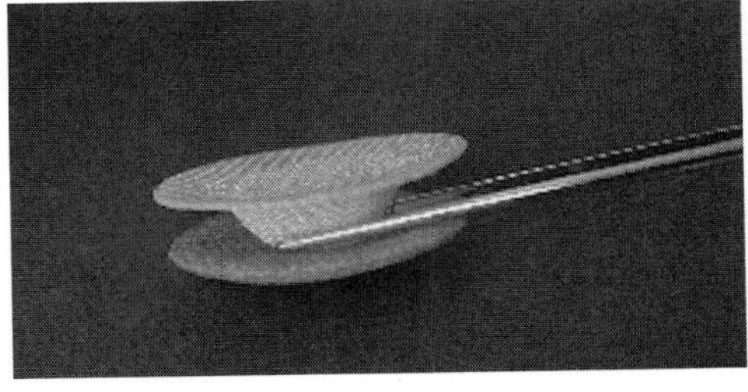

Fig. 5.7. In 2007, Ethicon introduced a double-sided low-profile plug, the Ethicon Ultrapro Plug, that works well for hernia defects that are 3 cm and smaller.

diameter. Once inserted, the anchor lies flat in the preperitoneal space. The flat and flexible anchor is unlikely to erode through peritoneum. The inguinal floor portion or "rim" measures 5 cm in diameter. The rim lies on top of the inguinal floor. For indirect hernias, if a wedge of the rim is removed, it keeps the rim from lying on top of the cord and tilting the position of the rim.

The plug is 25% PROLENE* (polypropylene) and 75% MONOCRYL* (poliglecaprone 25). The prolene portion of the plug is lightweight mesh 28 g/m^2. The weight of the large plug before absorption is 2.82 g. The absorbable component improves handling characteristics and absorbs in 120 days. The weight of the large plug postabsorption is only 0.26 g.

The overlay patch is 25% ULTRAPRO* (31 g/m^2 and intertwined with MONOCRYL*) and measures 7.5 cm × 12 cm. Usually, the patch can be placed without trimming. A slit for the cord can be fashioned lateral or caudal.

Three or four absorbable sutures are used to "position" the overlay patch. The first stitch attaches the patch to the rectus fascia, assuring a 1.5–2 cm overlap medially. Lateral to that, two of the stitches will incorporate the overlay patch, the rim of the plug, and together are affixed to the iliopubic tract (Fig. 5.8).

Holzheimer, RG reported about early outcomes for outpatient inguinal hernia repair among 16 specialized hernia centers in Germany. A register was introduced on October 1, 2009, with an online hernia database (www.qs-leistenhernie.de) [36]. By poster at the International Ambulatory Surgery conference, Koch reported early results of 1,322 cases. 57% had UHS (UltraPro Hernia System) and 43% UPP. At 12 weeks, the recurrence rate was 0.7%, inguinal pain 2.3%, and testicular pain 0.7%. Their early conclusion was that the "incidence of pain" was comparable or less than other repairs. The ongoing database will provide continuous documentation and quality control in hernia surgery. Since introduction of UPP, more than 200,000 procedures have been performed worldwide.

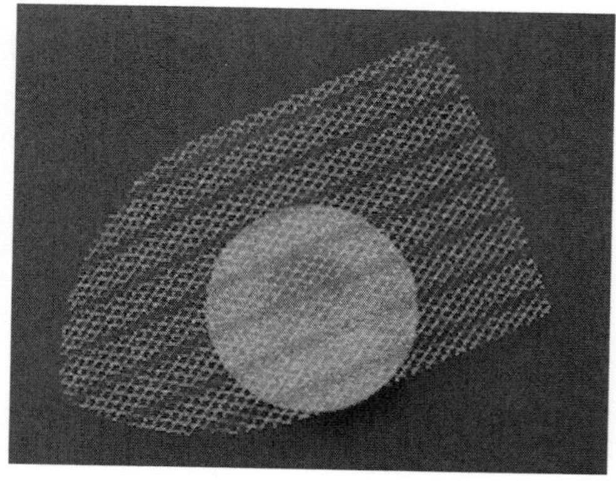

Fig. 5.8. Three or four absorbable sutures are used to "position" the overlay patch of the Ultrapro Plug. The first stitch attaches the patch to the rectus fascia assuring a 1.5–2 cm overlap medially. Lateral to that, two of the stitches will incorporate the overlay patch, the rim of the plug, and together are affixed to the iliopubic tract.

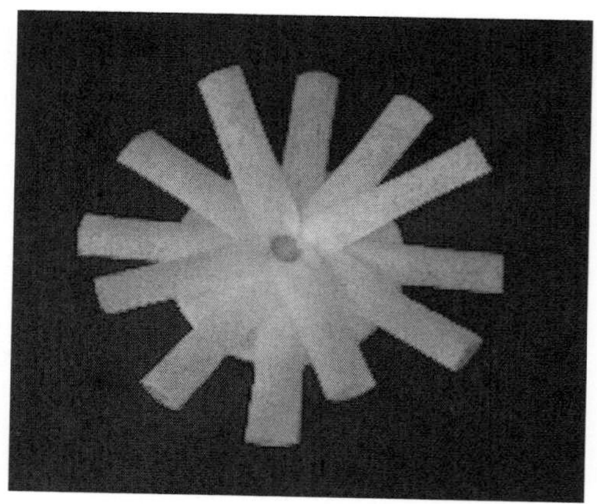

Fig. 5.9. In 2004, Gore introduced the Gore Bioabsorbable Hernia Plug.

Gore Bioabsorbable Hernia Plug

In 2004, W. L. Gore introduced a synthetic, completely absorbable hernia plug (Fig. 5.9). It is made of 67% polyglycolic acid (PGA) and 33% trimethylene carbonate (TMC)—the same material composition as Maxon suture. After implantation, the plug retains 70% tensile strength at 3 weeks, 0% tensile strength at 6 weeks, and is completely absorbed by 6 months. Following repair with the Gore plug and overlay patch, four studies show an impressively low incidence of long-term groin pain [37–40]. For implantation, the plug is placed entirely within the preperitoneal space and allowed to lay as flat as possible. The porous surface of the material "sticks" to surrounding tissue. The plug requires no fixation. Since the plug completely absorbs, there is absolutely no risk of migration or erosion. The plug keeps the hernia reduced as the overlay mesh incorporates. In doing so, less fixation is needed for the overlay patch. For the overlay patch, good selections are macroporous polypropylene, hydrophilic polyester, or self-adhesing polyester.

Lessons Learned and Opinions

The 3D plug and patches available to the surgeon allow the surgeon to tailor the plug and patch to best fit the needs for initial inguinal hernia repair. Patients with a defect of 3 cm or smaller are excellent candidates for plug-and-patch repair. Poor candidates for plug and patch are patients with giant hernias, large recurrent hernias, multiply recurrent hernias, and obese patients where subcutaneous fat is greater than 5–6 cm.

LeBlanc stated, "Simplicity should not be confused with complacency." Some are quick to correlate the plug with pain. A surgeon should understand the plug-and-patch repair in its entirety. Components of the procedure are a combination of mesh and technique. Inguinodynia seemingly must come from one of four sources: Dissection, the plug, overlay patch, or fixation. It is a surgeon's responsibility/obligation to properly identify and not injure nerves. However, if a nerve interferes with flat placement of the overlay, the nerve should be transected and ligated. Whatever plug material is used, its preperitoneal deployment should be larger than the defect it traverses. Cone-shaped mesh plugs require suture fixation. For cone mesh plugs, migration might be a concern. A single nonabsorbable loose stitch between the overlay patch and plug should prevent any risk of plug migration. When covering the myopectineal orifice, the bigger the patch, the better. The overlay patch should extend 1.5–2 cm medial to the pubis and 3–4 cm lateral to the internal ring. Since the plug reduces the hernia immediately with implantation, the overlay need only be positioned correctly—not fixated. Surgeons have the option of using loose stitches, fibrin sealant, or nothing at all.

Plug and patch has a short learning curve and a proven track record for low recurrence. As a result of modifications of plug-and-patch materials and techniques, this durable procedure has culminated in fewer and fewer complications with a decreasing incidence of inguinodynia. The plug-patch will remain a popular choice for inguinal hernia repair for years to come.

References

1. Gerdy PN. Nouvelles operations pour guerir radicalement les hernies due ventre. Gaz Hop. 1836;1:10.
2. Wutzer CW. Ueber radicale Heilung beweglicher Leisten-Bruche. In: Naumann MEA, Wutzer CW, Kilian HF, editors. Organ fur die gasmmte Heilkunde. Henry and Cohen: Bonn; 1841. p. 1.
3. Macewen W. On the radical cure of oblique inguinal hernia by internal abdominal peritoneal pad, and the restoration of the valved form of the inguinal canal. Ann Surg. 1886;4:89.
4. Lichntenstein IL, Shore JM. Simplified repair of femoral and recurrent inguinal hernias by a "Plug" technique. Am J Surg. 1974;128:439–44.
5. Shulman AG, Amid PK, Lichtenstein IL. The plug repair of 1402 recurrent inguinal hernias. Arch Surg. 1990;125:265–7.
6. Gilbert AI. An anatomic and functional classification for the diagnosis and treatment of inguinal hernia. Am J Surg. 1989;157:331–3.
7. Gilbert AI. Overnight hernia repair: updated considerations. South Med J. 1987;80(2):191–5.
8. Gilbert AI. Generations of the plug and patch repair: its development and lessons from history, mastery of surgery. 5th ed. Philadelphia, PA: Lippincott Williams & Wilkins; 2007. p. 1940–3. Chapter 177.
9. Rutkow IM, Robbins AW. "Tension-free" inguinal herniorrhaphy: a preliminary report on the "mesh plug" technique. Surgery. 1993;114(3):3–8.
10. Robbins AW, Rutkow IM. The mesh-plug hernioplasty. Surg Clin North Am. 1993;73(3):501–11.
11. Rutkow IM, Robbins AW. The marlex mesh perfix plug groin hernioplasty. Eur J Surg. 1998;164:549.
12. Robbins AW, Rutkow IM. Mesh plug repair and groin hernia surgery. Surg Clin North Am. 1998;78(6):1007–23.
13. Robbins AW, Rutkow IM. Open mesh plug hernioplasty: the less invasive procedure. In: Szabi Z, Lewis JE, Fantini GA, et al., editors. Surgical technology international. 5th ed. San Francisco: Universal Medical Press; 1996. p. 87–90.
14. Rutkow IM, Robbins AW. The mesh plug technique for recurrent groin herniorrhaphy: a nine year experience of 407 repairs. Surgery. 1998;124(5):844–7.
15. Goyal S, Abbasakoor F, Stephenson BM. Experience with the preperitoneal 'plug and patch' inguinal hernia repair. Br J Surg. 1999;86:1284–5.
16. Bringman S, Ramel S, Nyberg B, Anderberg B. Introduction of herniorrhaphy with mesh plug and patch. Eur J Surg. 2000;166:310–2.
17. Isemer FE, Dathe V, Peschka B, Heinze R, Radke A. Rutkow perfix-plug repair for primary and recurrent inguinal hernias-a prospective study. Surg Technol Int. 2004;12:129–36.
18. Huang CS, Huang CC, Lien HH. Prolene hernia system compared with mesh plug technique: a prospective study of short- to mid-term outcomes in primary groin hernia repair. Hernia. 2005;9:167–71.

19. van Nienhuijis SW, Oort I, Keemers-Gels ME, Strobbe JA, Rosman C. Randomized clinical trial comparing the prolene hernia system, mesh plug repair and Lichtenstein method for open inguinal hernia repair. Br J Surg. 2005;92:33–8.
20. Dalenback J, Anderson C, Anesten B, Bjorck S, Eklund S, Magnusson O, Rimback G, Stenquist B, Wedel N. Prolene hernia system, Lichtenstein mesh and plug-and-patch for primary inguinal hernia repair: 3 year outcome of a prospective randomized controlled trial. Hernia. 2009;13:121–9.
21. Cristaldi M, Pisacreta M, Elli M, Valgo GL, Danelli PG, Sampietro GM, Taschieri AM. Femoro-popliteal by-pass occlusion following mesh-plug for prevascular femoral hernia repair. Hernia. 1997;1:197–9.
22. Dieter RA. Mesh plug migration into scrotum: a new complication of hernia repair. Int Surg. 1999;84:57–9.
23. Chuback JA, Singh RS, Sills C, Dick LS. Small bowel obstruction resulting from mesh plug migration after open inguinal hernia repair. Surgery. 2000;127:475–6.
24. Tokunaga Y, Tokuka A, Ohsumi K. Sigmoid colon diverticulosis adherent to mesh plug migration after open inguinal hernia repair. Curr Surg. 2001;58(5):493–4.
25. Moorman ML, Price PD. Migrating mesh plug: complication of a well established hernia repair technique. Am J Surg. 2004;70:298–9.
26. Jeans S, Williams G, Stephenson B. Migration after open mesh plug inguinal hernioplasty: a review of the literature. Am Surg. 2007;73:207–9.
27. Murphy JW, Misra DC, Silverglide B. Sigmoid colonic fistula secondary to Perfix-plug, left inguinal hernia repair. Hernia. 2006;10:436–8.
28. Amid PK, Lichtenstein IL. Long-term result and current status of the Lichtenstein open tension-free hernioplasty. Hernia. 1998;2:89–94.
29. LeBlanc KA. Complications associated with the plug and patch method of inguinal herniorrhaphy. Hernia. 2001;5:135–8.
30. Kingsnorth AN, Hyland ME, Porter CA, Sudergren S. Prospective double-blind randomized study comparing Perfix plug-and-patch with Lichtenstein patch in inguinal hernia repair: one year quality of life results. Hernia. 2000;4:255–8.
31. Palot JP, Avisse C, Cailliez-Tomasi JP, Greffler D, Flament JB. The mesh plug repair of groin hernias: a three-year experience. Hernia. 1998;2:31–4.
32. Millikan K, Cummings B, Doolas A. The millikan modified mesh-plug hernioplasty. Arch Surg. 2003;138:525–30.
33. Goldstein HS. A university experience using mesh in inguinal hernia repair. Hernia. 2002;5:182–5.
34. Goldstein HS, Rabaza JR, Gonzalez AM, Verdeja JC. Evaluation of pain and disability in plug repair with the aid of a personal digital assistant. Hernia. 2003;7:25–8.
35. Sanders DL, Samarakoon DH, Ganshirt SW, Porter CS, Kingsnorth AN. A two-centre blinded randomized control study comparing the Lichtenstein patch. Perfix plug and ProLoop plug in the repair of primary inguinal hernia. Hernia. 2009;13: 499–503.
36. Holzheimer RG. First results of Lichtenstein hernia repair with Ultrapro-mesh as cost saving procedure–quality control combined with a modified quality of life questionnaire (SF-36) in a series of ambulatory operated patients. Eur J Med Res. 2004;9(6):323–7.

37. DeBord JR, et al. Two year results: reducing chronic pain utilizing GORE Bioabsorbable Hernia Plug in inguinal herniorrhaphy. Poster presented at the 94th annual clinical congress of the American College of Surgeons; 2008 Oct; San Francisco, CA.
38. Arnaud JP, et al. 1-year preliminary results: RESOLUT study. Poster presented at the 4th join society congress of the European Hernia Society/American Hernia Society; 2009 Sept; Berlin, Germany.
39. Manno AM, et al. Prospective randomized trial comparing polypropylene and new biomaterials in plug and patch surgery for inguinal hernia. Hernia. 2011;15:S6. Abstract retrieved from http://www.springer.com/medicine/surgery/journal/10029.
40. Misra DC. Open pre-peritoneal prosthetic mesh repair for inguinal hernia repair: preliminary experience at 1 year. Poster presented at the 14th annual hernia repair meeting; 2011 Mar; San Francisco, CA.

6. Technique: Laparoscopic TEP

Guy Voeller and Benjamin S. Powell

Indications

Open inguinal hernia repair is one of the most common surgical procedures performed. Laparoscopic repair of inguinal hernia gives excellent results when performed by surgeons expert in the technique and is estimated to make up between 15 and 30% of inguinal hernia repairs in the USA. We believe, however, a good herniologist should have multiple options to offer his/her patients. Most hernia repair methods, both open and laparoscopic, have literature supporting a very low recurrence rate when using mesh. The majority of data does show that the laparoscopic repair leads to less acute pain and quicker recovery, but most importantly, when done correctly, the risk of chronic pain is lower for the laparoscopic repair. Most patients referred for repair are symptomatic, and we advocate fixing all symptomatic inguinal hernias if the patient can tolerate surgery. If the patient is asymptomatic, then we will discuss watchful waiting realizing that many will eventually become symptomatic. We perform both laparoscopic and open repairs for inguinal hernia in the range of 250 per year. For a surgeon to become comfortable with the laparoscopic repair, it requires a significant amount of repetition to become proficient enough to have almost no morbidity and to have low long-term recurrence rates. We believe TEP inguinal hernia repair can be used in the following instances:

1. Unilateral hernias: Some believe only recurrent or bilateral hernias should be done with the laparoscope. We disagree. We believe that the *only* way to become proficient at lap repair is to learn the technique on the unilateral, virgin inguinal hernia. The recurrent hernia can have scar tissue that distorts anatomy and makes the case more difficult. Bilateral repairs will take a long time until the learning curve is shortened, and thus, it can be very frustrating for

B.P. Jacob and B. Ramshaw (eds.), *The SAGES Manual of Hernia Repair*,
DOI 10.1007/978-1-4614-4824-2_6,

the novice surgeon. Lastly, when done properly, the unilateral repair makes for a very satisfied patient.

2. Recurrent hernia: This is the ideal hernia to repair if the prior repair was done open since the surgeon is avoiding all the scar tissues left from the previous repair.
3. Bilateral hernias: These hernias probably have the most benefit for repair of all indications for obvious reasons.

Contraindications

The only absolute contraindication for TEP inguinal hernia repair is inability to tolerate general anesthesia. For these patients, we recommend open repair under local anesthesia with mesh. We also believe that in patients that have had previous preperitoneal surgery such as prostate removal, the TEP approach is too difficult, and even though studies show it is possible, it has higher risks than an open operation in virgin tissues. In addition, if the hernia cannot be completely reduced such as large scrotal hernias, we will opt for the easier to do open approach. We will perform the TEP repair in large, older teenagers if the hernia is significant in size and requires mesh.

Lastly, in men in whom there is concern about elevated PSA levels and prostate cancer, they should be told that the TEP may make preperitoneal prostate removal more difficult in some cases, depending on the mesh used and the experience of the urologist. Even though studies show that in expert hands preperitoneal prostate removal is readily done after a previous TEP repair, this should be discussed at length with this patient population.

Patient Positioning and Room Setup

Patient positioning for laparoscopic inguinal hernia repair is the same for TAPP and TEP inguinal hernia repair.

1. The patient is positioned supine on the operating table, with both arms tucked at his or her sides. Having the arms tucked allows for adequate room for the surgeon and other assistants to stand.
2. The video monitor is placed at the foot of the table.

3. A Foley catheter can be placed if so desired to decompress the bladder; we only place 5 cm^3 of fluid in the Foley balloon. There have been reports of bladder injury, and one mechanism may be sheer force between the Foley balloon with 10 cm^3 and the preperitoneal distention balloon. The bladder must be totally decompressed to place the mesh far down over Cooper's ligament, especially in direct hernias. Voiding prior to surgery is not adequate since anesthesia begins giving fluids that quickly fill the bladder and thus limit proper placement of the mesh down over the pubic bone.
4. The assistant stands on the side of the hernia to hold the camera, while the operative surgeon stands on the opposite side.

Pertinent Anatomy

A thorough knowledge of preperitoneal anatomy is required to perform an excellent TEP. Complete visualization of the myopectineal orifice is accomplished with the laparoscope, and any type of groin hernia is adequately visualized (Fig. 6.1). Initial dissection of a TEP

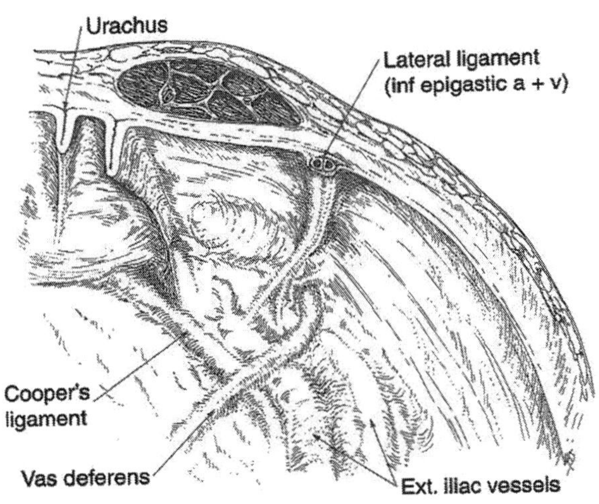

Fig. 6.1. Male groin anatomy. In the female, the round ligament of the uterus leaves the internal ring (From Scott-Conner CE, ed. The SAGES Manual: Fundamentals of Laparoscopy, Thoracoscopy, and GI Endoscopy, 2nd Ed., New York, Springer, 2006, with permission of Springer Science+Business Media).

hernia begins in the posterior rectus space. This space becomes the preperitoneal space below the arcuate line and is continuous with the space of Retzius of the pelvis. Some authors have used phrases such as "triangle of pain" and "triangle of doom"; however, we believe these terms should be used sparingly. There is a large amount of variability of the iliac artery and nerves in this region; hence, a thorough understanding of this region and its variabilities is paramount to avoid complications. In some 3,000 TEP repairs, we have not had an injury to bladder, colon, or iliac artery or vein, showing that this operation can be done safely if the surgeon learns the anatomy. Understanding the anatomy depicted in Fig. 6.1 is the key to a successful TEP repair. Key landmarks are necessary to keep orientation in this small space. A surgeon needs to recognize the pubic bone, Cooper's ligament, inferior epigastric vessels, and cord structures if they are to adequate and safely perform TEP procedures.

Operative Approach

1. After patient positioning, an infraumbilical incision is made in the midline. Dissection is carried down to the fascia with S-shaped retractors. We prefer to incise the rectus sheath on the same side as the hernia.
2. A longitudinal incision in the rectus sheath is made just off midline on the side of the hernia. A hemostat is used to widen incision to accommodate an S-shaped retractor behind the rectus sheath. The rectus muscle is then retracted laterally.
3. A balloon dissector is used next to facilitate dissection in the preperitoneal space. We prefer the original round unilateral balloon since it will not tear the epigastric vessels or damage tissue layers as can the bilateral balloon. While the dissection can be done without the balloon, we have found it is quicker, more uniform, and less bloody when the balloon is used.
4. The balloon dissector is passed along the posterior sheath until it contacts the pubic bone. Once the pubis is felt with the balloon dissector, the balloon is insufflated under direct vision with the laparoscope. Careful placement of the dissector is key so as not to tear the peritoneum or cause bleeding along the pubic bone.

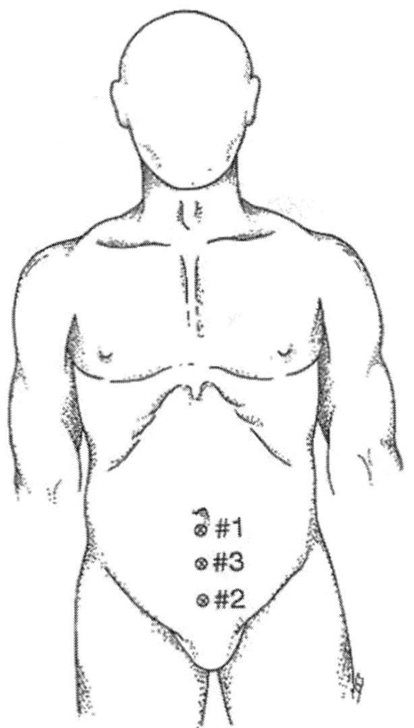

Fig. 6.2. Trocar placement for TEP (From Scott-Conner CE, ed. The SAGES Manual: Fundamentals of Laparoscopy, Thoracoscopy, and GI Endoscopy, 2nd Ed., New York, Springer, 2006, with permission of Springer Science+Business Media).

5. The balloon dissector is removed, and a balloon-tipped trocar is placed into the retrorectus space. Carbon dioxide is then used to insufflate the preperitoneal space. Lower pressures of 12 mmHg are used to prevent subcutaneous emphysema which will compromise the operative space.
6. A 45° 10-mm laparoscope is used, and two more 5-mm trocars are placed. The first 5-mm trocar is placed suprapubic, and the second is placed halfway between the other two trocars (Fig. 6.2). The 45° laparoscope allows the surgeon to mimic the open repair as described by Rives, i.e., sweeping the peritoneum back to the level of the umbilicus. The patient is then placed in Trendelenburg position.
7. Initial dissection is done to clear off tissue along the pubic bone to clearly visualize Cooper's ligament. In direct hernias, this means reducing the fat from the defect and pushing the transversalis sac back down into the defect. If the patient has a low insertion of the arcuate line, this is cut at this time and retracted to the level of the umbilicus.

8. The lateral space is then dissected to allow for adequate placement of the mesh. The peritoneum must be dissected off of the cord, anterior abdominal wall, and the retroperitoneum. The peritoneum overlying the psoas is swept cephalad so that the mesh will lie on the muscle.
9. During this dissection, the nerves are often seen. Care should be taken at this point to leave a fat layer on the abdominal wall to minimize bleeding and possible damage to these nerves. Once the lateral space has been dissected free, attention is then turned to dissection of the cord structures. The peritoneum is usually pulled medially and cord structures swept laterally. This allows the surgeon to see the proper plane which is between the peritoneum and the vessels on the vas deferens.
10. Any hole in the peritoneum can be dealt with by decreasing the insufflation pressure to 10 mmHg, and if necessary, a Veress needle can be placed into the peritoneal cavity above the umbilicus for decompression. Holes in the peritoneum do not need to be closed as long as the CO_2 is evacuated completely from the peritoneal cavity. Once this is done, the edges of the defect come together and heal quickly.
11. We use a polyester mesh (Parietex™) for the repair since Rives and Stoppa believed it was soft and readily would contour to all the curves of the preperitoneal space (unlike polypropylene). Our mesh is anatomically shaped (there are right and left meshes) and specifically designed for laparoscopic placement in the preperitoneal space. The key is to do a large dissection of the space so the mesh simply falls over the myopectineal area with coverage of all potential hernia defects.
12. The mesh is positioned so that there is adequate coverage of both the direct and indirect spaces. Direct hernias must have the mesh extending at least 2 cm beyond the defect in all directions. More important than an overlap of 2 cm, the medial extent of the mesh should be aligned or even pass the midline of the abdomen, and if bilateral, both medial aspects of each mesh should overlap in the midline. It is imperative to understand that the medial extent of large direct defects can extend to within 2 cm of the midline. We use an onlay technique over the cord structures and do not keyhole our mesh, mimicking the original open repair of Rives (Fig. 6.3).
13. While some believe the mesh does not need to be fixated, we believe in most situations, at least some fixation is key for

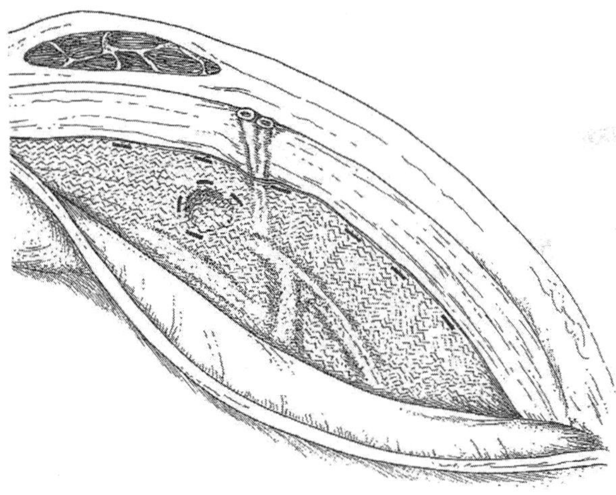

Fig. 6.3. Mesh placement for TEP inguinal hernia repair (From Scott-Conner CE, ed. The SAGES Manual: Fundamentals of Laparoscopy, Thoracoscopy, and GI Endoscopy, 2nd Ed., New York, Springer, 2006, with permission of Springer Science+Business Media).

long-term success. Rives and Stoppa both sutured the mesh when they described the open preperitoneal technique, and we try to mimic what they described. Kes, Schwab, and Katkhouda all have shown the mesh does move and migrate and is displaced without fixation. The Tisseel™ brand of fibrin glue works the best as a true adhesive and is our choice for use in our TEP repair, and so the remainder of this section will focus on our technique with the use of glue. That being said, the editors of this manual point out that there are a variety of ways of fixing the mesh other than the use of glue (permanent tacks, absorbable tacks, self-gripping mesh, no fixation), and all methods can produce optimal outcomes in the hands of someone experienced in that technique.

The fibrin glue works very well with the pore size and flexibility of the mesh. The use of the fibrin glue is an off label use of the product, but it has been used for years in Europe for hernia repair, and we have used it since 2003 for our TEP repairs. Not all fibrin glue is the same, and not all meshes work well with fibrin glue. The fibrin glue dries immediately and disappears in a few weeks postoperatively. The advantage of the glue is we can mimic the open repair as described by Rives and fix the mesh over the psoas, the cord, and other areas where mechanical fixation is not safe. We do NOT use the spray applicator but prefer to use the white applicator made by Baxter.

14. Once the glue has dried, the pneumoperitoneum is evacuated, and we watch the peritoneum and abdominal contents fall onto the mesh. The fascial defect in the anterior rectus is closed with a 0 vicryl suture. The skin is then closed with sutures, and sterile dressing is applied. Early unrestricted activity is important, and following this technique, most patients have rather rapid recoveries and return to usual daily activities.

Complications

Complications from TEP repair should be extremely rare and will be thoroughly covered in a separate chapter in this manual. Catastrophic complications such as major vascular, visceral, or cord injuries should be virtually nonexistent in experienced hands, and we have yet to experience these complications. Mesh infections should be few, if at all with TEP repair. This section will discuss some of the complications that are seen and their management.

Vascular Injuries

External iliac vessel injury is by far the most dreaded vascular complication and requires immediate repair. More common vessel injuries include inferior epigastric or spermatic vessel injury. These can often be controlled with either clips or cautery. Vessels along the pubic bone making up the "corona mortis" can also bleed, leading to massive preperitoneal hematoma postoperatively. Care must be used when dissecting along the pubic bone to prevent this complication. Obturator vessels need to be avoided as well.

Nerve Injury

A thorough knowledge of the nerves of the inguinal region is required to perform this procedure well and to minimize inguinodynia. The femoral branch of the genitofemoral nerve and branches of the femoral nerve, as well as the lateral cutaneous nerve of the thigh, are at risk for damage. We no longer tack with our repairs and feel that these complications should be infrequent. If tacks are used, these nerves should be carefully avoided.

Other

Urinary retention or hematuria tends to be one of the more common immediate sequelae after TEP repair. It is usually self-limited but might require replacement of a urinary catheter. Bladder injury should be rare and immediately repaired if seen.

Hernia recurrence is very rare with this approach. This can be due to a number of factors. Incomplete dissection, missed hernias, inadequate mesh coverage, and mesh displacement are all thought to lead to hernia recurrence.

Mesh-related complications are very infrequent in our experience. Prophylactic antibiotics are not required with TEP, and we have not experienced any known mesh infections in our patients. The TEP procedure also keeps the mesh away from intraabdominal structures; hence, erosion and adhesion formation that is possible with a TAPP approach should be minimal with a TEP.

Conclusions

TEP inguinal hernia repair gives excellent results for all types of inguinal hernias. Knowledge of anatomy, gentle dissection, and hundreds of repairs are required for minimal morbidity and low recurrence rates.

Suggested Reading

1. Ceccarelli G, Casciola L, Pisanelli MC, Bartoli A, Di Zitti L, Spaziani A, Biancafarina A, Stefanoni M, Patriti A. Comparing fibrin sealant with staples for mesh fixation in laparoscopic transabdominal hernia repair: a case control-study. Surg Endosc. 2008;22(3):668–73.
2. Clarke T, Katkhouda N, Mason RJ, Cheng BC, Algra J, Olasky J, Sohn HJ, Moazzez

A, Balouch M. Fibrin glue for intraperitoneal laparoscopic mesh fixation: a comparative study in a swine model. Surg Endosc. 2011;25(3):737–48.

3. Descottes B, Bagot d'Arc M. Fibrin sealant in inguinal hernioplasty: an observational multicentre study in 1,201 patients. Hernia. 2009;13(5):505–10.
4. Katkhouda N, Mavor E, Friedlander MH, Mason RJ, Kiyabu M, Grant SW, Achanta K, Kirkman EL, Narayanan K, Essani R. Use of fibrin sealant for prosthetic mesh fixation in laparoscopic extraperitoneal inguinal hernia repair. Ann Surg. 2001;233(1):18–25.
5. Novik B. Randomized trial of fixation vs nonfixation of mesh in total extraperitoneal inguinal hernioplasty. Arch Surg. 2005;140(8):811–2. author reply 812.
6. Novik B, Hagedorn S, Mörk UB, Dahlin K, Skullman S, Dalenbäck J. Fibrin glue for securing the mesh in laparoscopic totally extraperitoneal inguinal hernia repair: a study with a 40-month prospective follow-up period. Surg Endosc. 2006;20(3):462–7.
7. Olmi S, Scaini A, Erba L, Bertolini A, Croce E. Laparoscopic repair of inguinal hernias using an intraperitoneal onlay mesh technique and a Parietex composite mesh fixed with fibrin glue (Tissucol). Personal technique and preliminary results. Surg Endosc. 2007;21(11):1961–4.
8. Ramshaw BJ, Tucker JG, Mason EM, Duncan TD, Wilson JP, Angood PB, Lucas GW. A comparison of transabdominal preperitoneal (TAPP) and total extraperitoneal approach (TEP) laparoscopic herniorrhaphies. Am Surg. 1995;61:279–83.
9. Ramshaw BJ, Tucker JG, Conner T, Mason EM, Duncan TD, Lucas GW. A comparison of the approaches to laparoscopic herniorrhaphy. Surg Endosc. 1996;10:29–32.
10. Ramshaw B, Abiad F, Voeller G, Wilson R, Mason E. Polyester (Parietex) mesh for total extraperitoneal laparoscopic inguinal hernia repair: initial experience in the United States. Surg Endosc. 2003;17(3):498–501.
11. Taylor C, Layani L, Liew V, Ghusn M, Crampton N, White S. Laparoscopic inguinal hernia repair without mesh fixation, early results of a large randomised clinical trial. Surg Endosc. 2008;22(3):757–62.
12. Topart P, Vandenbroucke F, Lozac'h P. Tisseel versus tack staples as mesh fixation in totally extraperitoneal laparoscopic repair of groin hernias: a retrospective analysis. Surg Endosc. 2005;19(5):724–7.
13. Voeller GR. Management of peritoneal tear during endoscopic extraperitoneal inguinal hernioplasty. Surg Endosc. 2003;17(8):1335. author reply 1336.
14. Voeller GR, Mangiante EC, Britt LG. Preliminary evaluation of laparoscopic herniorrhaphy. Surg Laparosc Endosc. 1993;3(2):100–5.

7. Technique: Laparoscopic TAPP and IPOM

William S. Cobb IV

The ideal inguinal hernia repair should provide adequate coverage of the myopectineal orifice of Fruchaud with durable results that are reproducible when taught to other surgeons. While a low recurrence rate is desirable, the incidence of long-term groin pain must be considered as well. Placing mesh posterior to the defect utilizes the intra-abdominal pressures to support the repair. Additionally, the transabdominal laparoscopic approach provides excellent visualization of the inguinal region from a vantage point that all surgeons are comfortable with.

Anatomy

A successful laparoscopic inguinal hernia repair relies on the surgeon's grasp of the inguinal anatomy, particularly from a posterior vantage point. The laparoscopic repair of groin hernias provides minimal access but not minimal invasion. It is imperative to understand the location of the iliac vessels, genitofemoral and lateral femoral cutaneous nerves, and bladder to avoid catastrophic complications. Other landmarks of the posterior abdominal wall and inguinal region assist in describing the repair correctly (Fig. 7.1).

The umbilical ligaments are important landmarks for the TAPP inguinal hernia repair. The median umbilical ligament consists of the atretic urachus and courses from the dome of the bladder to the umbilicus. The paired medial and lateral umbilical ligaments are folds of the peritoneal that contain the obliterated umbilical arteries and the inferior epigastric vessels, respectively.

B.P. Jacob and B. Ramshaw (eds.), *The SAGES Manual of Hernia Repair*,
DOI 10.1007/978-1-4614-4824-2_7,

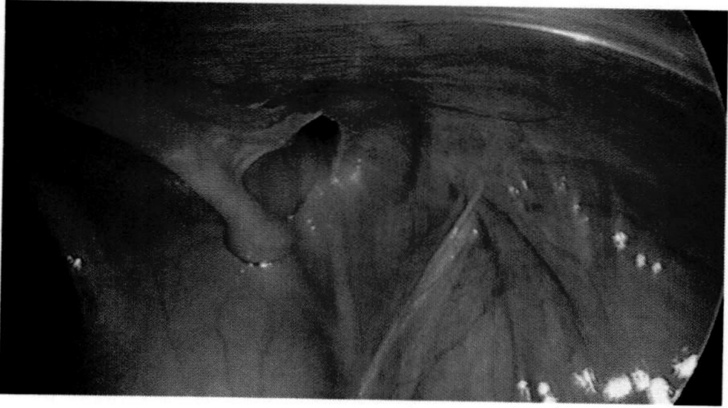

Fig. 7.1. The anterior abdominal wall and inguinal region from the intra-abdominal perspective.

Once the peritoneum is peeled away, the inferior epigastric vessels are uncovered. These vessels are important landmarks, which lead inferiorly to the iliac vessels. Medially, the prevesical space of Retzius is entered anterior to the bladder. The pectineal ligament (Cooper's) is identified medially. Just superior to pectineal ligament courses the "corona mortis" which is a direct branch of the iliacs. Frequently, an accessory obturator vessel traverses the pectineal ligament. These vessels must be appreciated and respected to avoid potential complications.

The iliopubic tract is a thickening of the inferior margin of the transversalis fascia. It parallels the course of the more superficial inguinal ligament, running from the pubic tubercle to the anterior superior iliac spine. Fixation devices should not be placed below the iliopubic tract to avoid damage to nerves and major vessels.

Preoperative Considerations

All patients with a groin hernia can be considered for a laparoscopic repair. The laparoscopic approach is preferred in bilateral inguinal defects, recurrent defects following an anterior repair, and inguinal defects with concomitant pathology requiring laparoscopy. Larger inguinoscrotal defects are certainly more challenging for a laparoscopic approach and should be avoided early in one's experience.

Candidates for a laparoscopic inguinal hernia repair should be able to tolerate general anesthesia. Absolute contraindications include active intra-abdominal infection or peritonitis. Relative contraindications include coagulopathy, ascites, and previous retropubic dissection.

The preoperative consultation should include discussion of potential complications. Patients should be provided with the risks vs. benefits of both laparoscopic and open repairs and then allowed to choose. The purported benefits of the laparoscopic repair include earlier return to activity, the ability to diagnose occult hernias, and potentially less chronic groin pain.

Intraoperative Setup

Equipment needs for a laparoscopic inguinal herniorrhaphy include a standard laparoscopic instrument set. The Maryland dissector and blunt-tipped fine-toothed graspers are all that are typically needed for dissection. The endoshears are necessary and are attached to the electrocautery cord.

The patient is asked to void his bladder prior to being brought back to the operating suite. A urinary catheter is usually not necessary. The intraoperative fluids are held to less than one liter if possible to prevent potential urinary retention.

Patients receive prophylaxis for deep venous thrombosis in the form of sequential compression devices and subcutaneous heparin. A first-generation cephalosporin is given preoperatively.

The patient is prepped and draped for possible conversion to an open repair. The patients' arms are carefully padded and tucked at the sides bilaterally. The surgeon stands on the side opposite the inguinal hernia. The dissecting instrument is held in the hand of the same side as the hernia (i.e., a right-sided defect is a right-handed repair and vice versa). The video monitors are placed at the patients' feet (Fig. 7.2).

Operative Technique: TAPP

Initial entry should be achieved per the surgeon's comfort level. Trocars are placed at the infraumbilical fold (12 mm) and just lateral to the edge of the rectus muscle at the level of the umbilicus bilaterally (5 mm). A long-acting local anesthetic is injected at the trocar sites prior to making the incision. We prefer a cutdown, umbilical stalk technique for initial entry at the umbilicus. A 5-mm 30° laparoscope is placed on

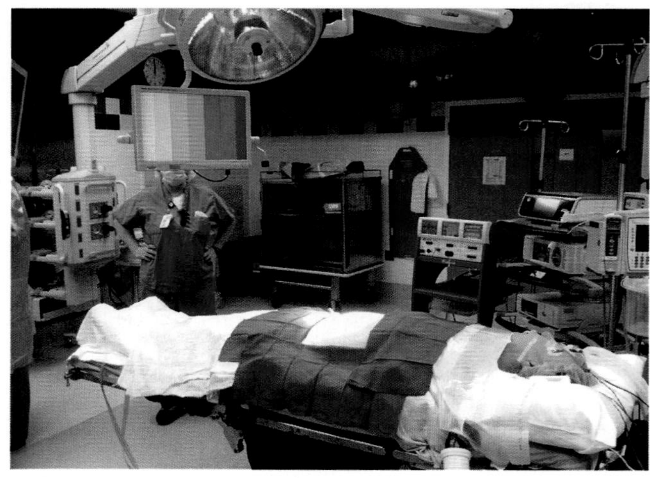

Fig. 7.2. Operating room setup for a laparoscopic TAPP inguinal herniorrhaphy.

the side of the hernia and held by the assistant. Inspection of the bilateral inguinal regions is performed to assess for occult defects. The patient is placed in Trendelenburg position to allow for the intra-abdominal contents to “fall away.”

Dissection begins at the level of the medial umbilical ligament. Beginning the dissection high on the abdominal wall just inferior to the umbilicus allows for the creation of a sizable, preperitoneal pocket which makes placement of mesh easier. The Maryland dissector is used to retract posteriorly, and the shears are used to open up the peritoneum. Ideally, the plane between the parietal peritoneum and the transversalis fascia is developed. With continued gentle retraction posteriorly, the endoshears can be used to bluntly open up the preperitoneal space with countertraction. Medially, the space of Retzius is developed, and the bladder flap is lowered. Laterally, the fat is carefully stripped off of the peritoneum.

Attention is then directed to the hernia sac. Reduction of the hernia sac depends on the type of defect. In direct defects, the peritoneal sac is teased away from the attenuated transversalis fascia or “pseudosac.” The pectineal ligament is uncovered medially until the femoral canal is identified. The “corona mortis” and any accessory obturator vessels should be visualized prior to placing tacks into Cooper’s ligament.

For indirect hernias, the sac dissection is more involved as it requires identification and preservation of the vas deferens and gonadal vessels

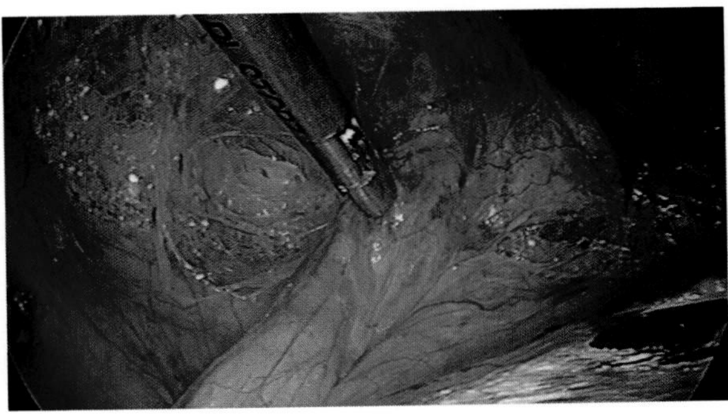

Fig. 7.3. In direct defects, the sac is reduced while preserving the vas deferens and gonadal vessels.

(Fig. 7.3). In the female patient, this dissection is simplified by dividing the round ligament. Smaller indirect sacs can be dissected free of the cord structures and completely reduced. With large indirect sacs and especially inguinoscrotal hernias, the sac can be dissected free of the vas deferens and gonadal vessels and then divided. This maneuver may result in postoperative seroma but does reduce the risk of ischemic orchitis.

Once the sac is reduced, the cord structures are skeletonized off the peritoneum to the level of the psoas muscle. This dissection provides for a large peritoneal pocket for mesh placement and importantly reduces the risk of an inferior recurrence. Development of the pocket inferiorly is best achieved by grasping the peritoneum and retracting in inward while teasing away the retroperitoneal attachments.

After an adequate-sized preperitoneal pocket has been developed, a mesh is brought onto the field for reinforcement of the myopectineal orifice. A tissue-separating or barrier-type mesh is not necessary because of the protection provided by the peritoneum. A flat, uncoated polyester or polypropylene-based material works well in the groin. Macroporous, lightweight materials are preferred for enhanced ingrowth and potential reduction in pain. Typically, a mesh measuring 12×15 cm is utilized. There is no need to slit the mesh. The blunt-tipped graspers are well-suited to manipulate the mesh and avoid having the tips of the finer-tipped Maryland grasper get caught in the interstices of the macroporous meshes. The mesh should provide adequate coverage of the indirect and direct inguinal spaces as well as the femoral space. The inferior edge of the mesh should lie flush against the retroperitoneum and not curl under when the peritoneum is elevated (Fig. 7.4).

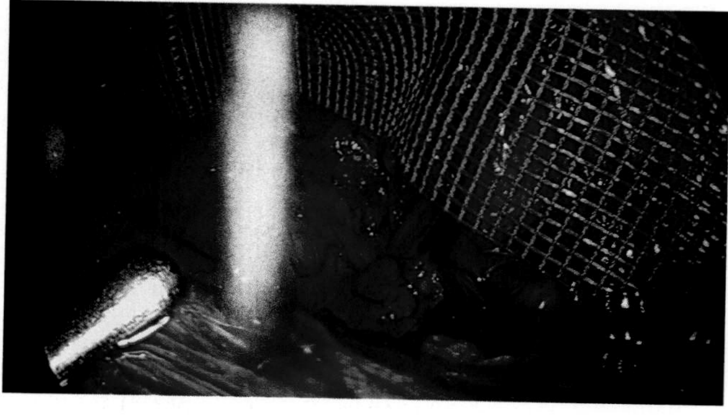

Fig. 7.4. The inferior edge of the mesh should not move when the peritoneal flap is elevated.

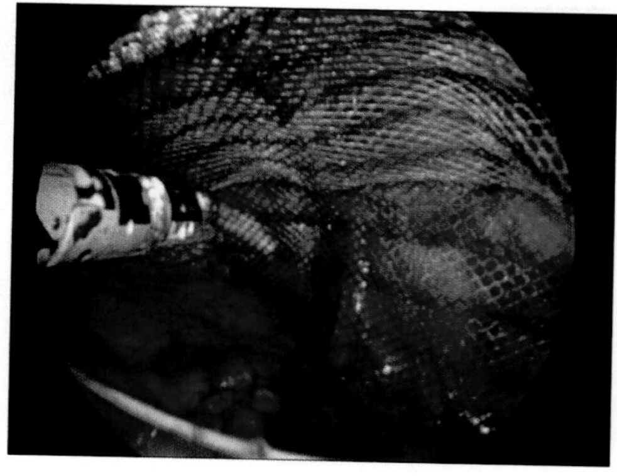

Fig. 7.5. Mesh covers the myopectineal orifice and is secured with staples placed above the iliopubic tract.

Mesh fixation can be achieved with mechanical devices (staples or tacks) or fibrin sealants. Staples are placed on Cooper's ligament at 2–3 points and to the anterior abdominal wall where the tip of the tacker can be palpated in 2–3 additional spots. By palpating the tip of the fixation device, one avoids firing fixation constructs below the iliopubic tract, which can damage nerves or vessels (Fig. 7.5).

The repair is completed by re-approximating the peritoneal flap. Closure is achieved with suture, staples, or tacks. Staples are preferred. They are not driven into the abdominal wall, thereby minimizing trauma, and they save time as compared to suturing. Hemostasis is confirmed and the integrity of the peritoneal closure is assessed. Any additional tears in the peritoneum that occurred during the dissection can be closed with the stapler or suture. The trocars are removed under laparoscopic visualization to ensure no injury or bleeding from the inferior epigastric vessels. The fascial defect at the umbilicus is closed with an absorbable suture using a suture-passer device.

Operative Technique: IPOM

The intraperitoneal onlay mesh (IPOM) procedure for inguinal hernias is a transabdominal approach as well. The technique is similar to the laparoscopic repair of ventral hernias and involves the placement of a tissue-separating mesh against an intact peritoneum. The IPOM technique of inguinal herniorrhaphy avoids the preperitoneal dissection required with the TAPP repair and simplifies the transabdominal placement of mesh in the groin. The IPOM repair of inguinal hernias was initially described utilizing uncoated polypropylene mesh; however, with the advances in mesh technology, a coated, barrier mesh is preferred. Patient preparation, operating room setup, and trocar positioning are similar to the TAPP repair. A urinary catheter is routinely placed for bladder decompression.

The bilateral myopectineal orifices are examined for the presence of inguinal and femoral defects. The sac in direct or indirect defects is inverted with gentle external pressure. The peritoneum is then excised approximately 1–2 cm from the base of the defect. The peritoneum is excised circumferentially to reduce the sac. The gonadal vessels and vas deferens are identified to avoid injury during this portion of the dissection. Dissection of the sac allows for removal of cord lipomas as well. Just as with the TAPP technique, large inguinoscrotal sacs are left intact after removing the peritoneum from the base of the defect (i.e., "ringing the neck" of the hernia sac).

A coated, barrier mesh measuring 12 × 15 cm is selected. The mesh is introduced through the 12-mm umbilical trocar. The mesh is oriented in the groin to provide coverage of both inguinal and femoral spaces with at least 3 cm of overlap of the hernia defect. The suture passer is then utilized to pass transabdominal sutures through the midpoint of the upper edge of the mesh and in each of the superior corners of the mesh. These three sutures are secured to fixate the mesh. The hernia stapler is then used to fixate the lateral and inferior aspects of the prosthesis. Medially, the mesh is fixated to the pectineal (Cooper's) ligament. The lateral side of the mesh is fixated by palpating the tip of the stapler externally during deployment. Fixation constructs are placed approximately 1 cm apart. Inferiorly, the staples are placed lightly and approximately 2 cm apart to minimize potential damage to nerves and vessels. Here, the staples should be fired in a vertical orientation to avoid nerve entrapment. Fixation constructs should not be placed just inferior to the internal ring to avoid damage to the cord structures.

Complications

Similar to open inguinal herniorrhaphy, complications following transabdominal, laparoscopic inguinal repair are typically rare and minor when they do occur. Nevertheless, a transabdominal approach does create the possibility of more serious complications that are typically not of concern with an anterior groin approach.

Urinary retention can occur following any inguinal repair. Patients with benign prostatic hypertrophy and bilateral repairs result in a higher incidence of urinary retention. Bladder decompression with a urinary catheter is usually all that is required.

Seromas can occur particularly with larger defects and when the sac is not completely reduced. They are almost always painless and self-limiting. Rarely aspiration is required for excessively large fluid collections.

Wound and mesh infections are almost unheard of following laparoscopic inguinal hernia repair and typically imply a break in surgical technique. Ecchymosis of the groin and testicle can occur following the repair; however, erythema raises the concern for potential staphylococcal contamination. If concern for a mesh infection is present, computed tomography of the pelvis is indicated.

Early postoperative small bowel obstruction can occur if the peritoneal closure breaks down and bowel herniation occurs. Any patient with persistent postoperative nausea and vomiting should raise concern, and appropriate radiographic studies should be obtained.

Serious complications can arise during and after laparoscopic inguinal herniorrhaphy. Major vascular and visceral injuries can occur with trocar placement or during dissection. The best management of such injuries depends on the comfort level of the surgeon. The patient's lower abdomen and thighs should be prepped and draped as if performing an open inguinal hernia repair to allow for rapid conversion to a groin incision or lower midline incision if such complications occur. For bowel or bladder injuries, the repair can be performed either laparoscopically or open. Bladder injuries are repaired with an absorbable suture in two layers. A urinary catheter is placed and left in place for 7 days. A contrast study of the bladder is obtained prior to removal of the catheter. The decision to place a synthetic mesh in the face of bowel or bladder injury depends on the degree of contamination. The literature supports the use of a lightweight, macroporous synthetic mesh with minimal contamination of urine or enteric contents. Biologic and bioresorbable materials can be utilized if a synthetic mesh is not desired.

Long-term complications following laparoscopic inguinal hernia repair consist of recurrence and trocar site hernias. The recurrence rates following the laparoscopic approach as compared to the open technique have been long debated in the literature and are difficult to interpret. What is clear is that the laparoscopic TAPP repair can provide recurrence rates comparable to open mesh-based repairs in the hands of experts. Additionally, the learning curve for the laparoscopic approach to inguinal hernias is much greater than for open repairs. Some authors suggest that the learning experience may be as high as 250 cases. The growing number of advanced laparoscopic training programs and proper instruction of the technique have probably reduced this number, but it is still a more difficult repair to grasp than the open repair.

Further Reading

1. Colburn GL, Brick WG, Gadacz TR, et al. Inguinal anatomy for laparoscopic herniorrhaphy, part I: the normal anatomy. Surg Rounds. 1995;18:189–98.
2. Franklin ME, Diaz-Elizondo JA. The intraperitoneal onlay mesh procedure for groin hernias. In: Fitzgibbon's Jr RJ, Greenburg AG, editors. Nyhus & condon's hernia. 5th ed. Philadelphia, PA: Lippincott Williams & Wilkins; 2002. p. 269–76.
3. Neumeyer LA, Gawande AA, Wang J, et al. Proficiency of surgeons in inguinal hernia repair: effect of experience and age. Ann Surg. 2005;242:344–52.
4. Wauschkuhn CA, Schwarz J, Boekeler U, Bittner R. Laparoscopic inguinal hernia repair: gold standard in bilateral hernia repair? Results of more than 2800 patients in comparison to literature. Surg Endosc. 2010;24:3026–30.

8. Strangulated Inguinal Hernia

Jonathan P. Pearl and E. Matthew Ritter

Strangulated inguinal hernias occur when the contents of a hernia are deprived of adequate blood supply. This may occur in both acutely and chronically incarcerated hernias. Strangulation is quite rare, but when it occurs, it is a true hernia emergency necessitating immediate operation. The mortality rate in strangulated inguinal hernias may be as high as 30%.

Pathophysiology

Strangulation represents a continuum from incarceration of hernia contents to vascular compromise to tissue necrosis if the condition goes untreated. Hernia contents become incarcerated within the hernia ring with resulting tissue edema. Increasing edema and interstitial pressure cause venous stasis with concomitant impairment of perfusion across the capillaries. This can lead to necrosis and eventual perforation. One study showed that risk of strangulation increased significantly if symptoms had persisted for more than 6 h prior to presentation for medical care.

All groin hernias are susceptible to strangulation, with most series reporting a preponderance of right-sided indirect hernias. Strangulation might occur in femoral hernias in greater proportion to their incidence because of the lack of elasticity of the femoral canal. Similarly, obturator hernias also carry an increased risk of incarceration and strangulation as evidence by the fact that as many as 90% of patients with obturator hernias present with a small bowel obstruction due to incarceration. Small bowel and greater omentum are the most commonly strangulated organs, but there are reports of strangulated vermiform appendixes (Amyand's hernia), colon, bladder, ovary, and uterus (Fig. 8.1).

B.P. Jacob and B. Ramshaw (eds.), *The SAGES Manual of Hernia Repair*,
DOI 10.1007/978-1-4614-4824-2_8,

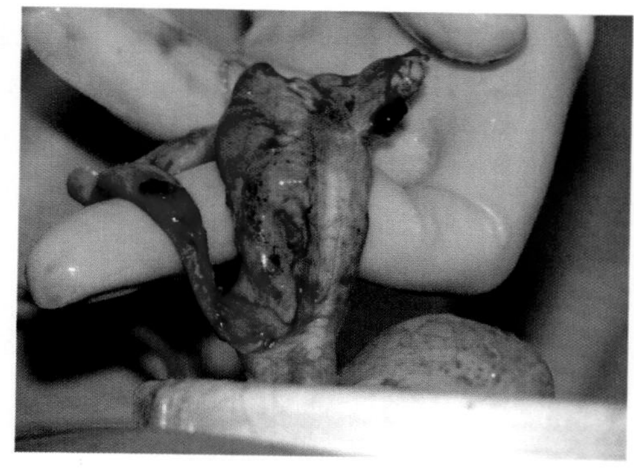

Fig. 8.1. Necrotic appendix secondary to a strangulated right-sided obturator hernia.

Presentation and Diagnosis

Men vastly outnumber women with strangulated hernias, likely because of the higher incidence of hernias in men. Strangulated femoral hernias are more common in women. The median age of patients with strangulated hernias is approximately 60 years, although strangulation has been reported in all ages from pediatric patients to nonagenarians.

The most common presenting symptom is acute groin pain with an accompanying bulge. Patients with strangulated bowel may also present with nausea or vomiting, fevers, chills, or malaise. Neglected strangulated hernias may lead to bowel perforation with attendant hemodynamic instability. In rare cases, bowel perforation may result in scrotal fecal fistula.

On examination, the hernia bulge is usually evident on inspection. The overlying skin may be erythematous. A tender mass will be palpable either cephalad or caudad to the inguinal ligament, depending on the type of hernia.

A thorough history and physical examination are usually sufficient to establish the diagnosis of incarcerated inguinal hernia, and strangulation may be suspected based on tenderness, skin erythema, fever, or leukocytosis. Extrapolating from data from strangulated bowel obstructions, it may be difficult to discern incarceration from strangulation based on clinical findings alone.

When the diagnosis is uncertain from the history and physical examination, radiologic imaging may be useful. Plain abdominal radiographs may show evidence of a bowel obstruction. Computed tomography will clearly delineate the incarcerated organ and establish the diagnosis (Fig. 8.2). Vascular compromise of the hernia contents

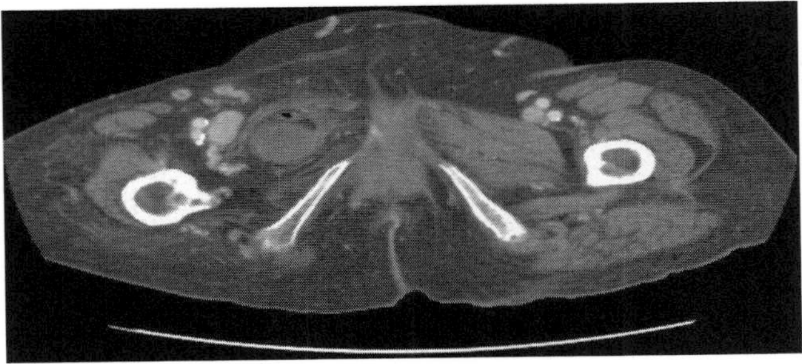

Fig. 8.2. CT scan showing evidence of obturator hernia with surrounding fluid, fat stranding, and tissue edema.

might be suggested by pneumatosis intestinalis, fat stranding, or even free air within the hernia sac.

Reduction of a tender inguinal hernia can be judiciously attempted, especially if the incarceration occurred within a few hours of presentation. However, even reduced hernia contents remain at risk for strangulation if the hernia is reduced en masse. Reduction of strangulated contents can be dangerous since the liberated organ may elaborate inflammatory mediators or even succus entericus due to perforation; therefore, forced reduction of potentially strangulated contents should be avoided. In the case of either an acutely tender incarcerated hernia or a strangulated hernia, immediate operation is indicated.

Operative Approaches

The principles for management of strangulated inguinal hernias are the same regardless of approach: reduction of the hernia contents, inspection of the contents to assess viability, resection of necrotic organs, and repair of the defect. This can be accomplished via an anterior approach, an open preperitoneal approach, or laparoscopically via either a transabdominal or totally extraperitoneal approach.

Strangulated inguinal hernias may be managed using a standard anterior groin incision and repair. After dividing the fascia of the external oblique muscle, the hernia sac will be encountered. The sac should be carefully opened and the hernia contents inspected for viability. If necrotic bowel is discovered, a resection may be performed through the same incision, rather than performing a laparotomy. A tension-free repair will yield the lowest recurrence rate, but there is a concern for mesh infection in the contaminated field. However, there are several studies describing the safe use of polypropylene mesh for the Lichtenstein repair of strangulated hernias. A biologic mesh may also be an option which may minimize the risk of mesh infection.

On occasion, hernia contents may be difficult to reduce via the anterior approach. In this case, after the hernia sac has been opened and the contents inspected, the defect may need to be expanded to allow reduction of the incarcerated contents. For indirect hernias, the deep inguinal ring should be incised medially to avoid injury to the external spermatic artery or vas deferens. Care must be taken to ensure the inferior epigastric vessels are properly ligated to avoid hemorrhagic complication. For direct hernias, a division of the transversalis fascia either medially or laterally may be required. Extensive lateral division also requires awareness of the inferior epigastrics. For femoral hernias, the lacunar ligament may be divided medially or the iliopubic tract superiorly. Laterally, the external iliac vessels prevent extensive dissection.

Induction of general anesthesia may result in spontaneous reduction of incarcerated or strangulated hernia contents. The risk of reduction en masse or reduction of compromised bowel exists; thus, the intra-abdominal contents must be explored. This can be accomplished via low-midline laparotomy or, less invasively, using the laparoscope. A trocar can be inserted through the hernia sac into the abdominal cavity. With the sac secured tightly around the trocar, a pneumoperitoneum can be established. A laparoscopic peritoneal access site remote from the groin may also be chosen with the added benefit of being able to plan further incisions based on the findings. The laparoscope will allow visualization of the abdominal contents. If ischemic bowel is encountered, it can be resected via either laparotomy or via laparoscopic techniques.

Malangoni and Condon first described the preperitoneal repair of strangulated inguinal hernias in 1986. A transverse skin incision is made 2 cm cephalad to the anticipated location of the external inguinal ring. The external oblique, internal oblique, and transversus abdominis muscles are incised, and the preperitoneal space is entered. From this approach, the hernia contents can be easily inspected, resection can be performed, if necessary, and the hernia defect can be repaired. Either a Cooper's ligament or iliopubic tract repair was originally used, but today, a prosthetic might be chosen.

The Henry operation uses a midline infraumbilical incision to access the preperitoneal space. The linea alba is divided below the umbilicus, and the retrorectus space is entered. Below the semilunar line, the

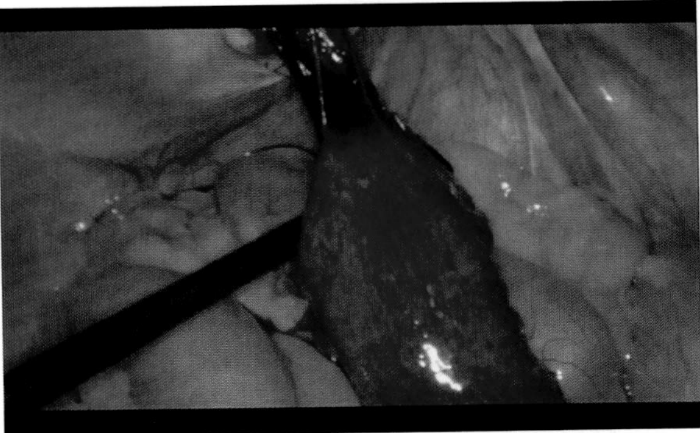

Fig. 8.3. Characteristics of ischemic but ultimately viable bowel from a strangulated inguinal hernia. Note the uniform *red* discoloration. This bowel also demonstrated peristalsis on inspection.

retrorectus space and the preperitoneal space are confluent. Strangulated hernia contents are resected after opening the peritoneum and controlling the necrotic bowel. Repair of the defect was originally described using a tissue repair, but a prosthetic may be a better choice.

Both the transabdominal preperitoneal (TAPP) and the totally extraperitoneal (TEP) laparoscopic repairs have been described for managing incarcerated and strangulated inguinal hernias. Incarcerated inguinal, femoral, and obturator hernias can be approached with the laparoscope. For the TAPP, the abdomen is entered at the umbilicus. Reduction of the hernia contents often requires incision of the hernia ring. For indirect hernias, the ring is incised in a ventrolateral direction to avoid the vas deferens and testicular vessels. For direct and femoral hernias, the ring is enlarged using a ventromedial incision to avoid the femoral vessels.

The transabdominal laparoscopic repair affords an optimal view of intra-abdominal contents to assess viability of the incarcerated organs. If ischemic bowel is encountered, it should not be immediately resected. Assessing bowel viability is usually based on the subjective appearance of the bowel (Figs. 8.3 and 8.4). The bowel can be observed for several minutes to assess for improvement in ischemia following hernia reduction. Signs of resolving ischemia can include improvements in color, regaining normal caliber, and return of visible peristalsis. If the viability is still in question after a period of observation, the bowel may be left in situ and a second-look laparoscopy could be planned for the next 24–72 h. In cases of strangulated small bowel obstructions, second-look laparoscopy has been shown to be safe and can prevent a bowel resection in some patients.

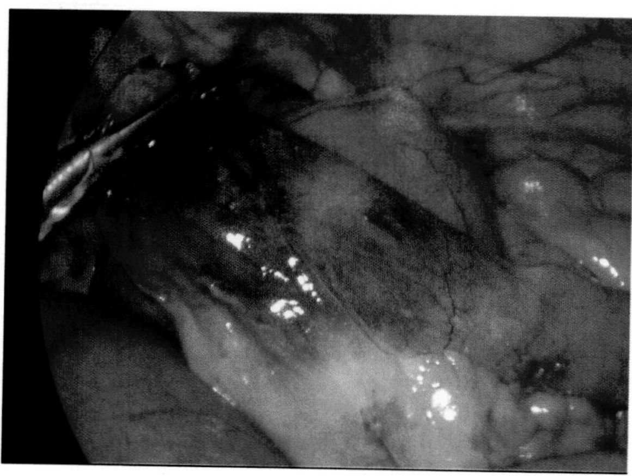

Fig. 8.4. Example of necrotic small bowel from a strangulated inguinal hernia. Note the areas of *deep purple* discoloration and the areas of blanching serosa. The grasper on the *left* is controlling spillage from an area of perforation.

Second-look laparoscopy may be useful in the case of strangulated groin hernias. If the reduced hernia contents are viable or become clearly viable after reduction, repair can proceed via either a TAPP or TEP approach. If the bowel remains ischemic after reduction and hernia repair, it should be resected. This can be accomplished totally laparoscopically or a small directed laparotomy may be performed (Fig. 8.5).

Many surgeons prefer the totally extraperitoneal approach for inguinal hernia repair. The TEP repair affords access to all of the hernia orifices but does not allow the same inspection of the hernia contents as the TAPP. An advantage of the TEP over the TAPP repair is the maintenance of an intact peritoneum to protect the prosthetic from potential contamination. A meta-analysis of TAP and TEPP in incarcerated and strangulated hernias has shown no difference in rates of mesh infection or contamination.

A combined transabdominal and extraperitoneal laparoscopic approach may be ideal. The peritoneal space can be entered either at the umbilicus or the subcostal region. One or two additional trocars may be needed to reduce the hernia contents and inspect their viability. Immediate resection is not recommended unless full thickness necrosis and perforation is present. The trocars can be left in place after evacuation of the pneumoperitoneum and a TEP repair performed using standard techniques. Access to the preperitoneal space can be gained at the umbilicus even if this site was used for initial access to the peritoneal space. Lateral dissection through the same infraumbilical skin incision will expose the anterior rectus sheath. Incision of the anterior sheath with lateral retraction

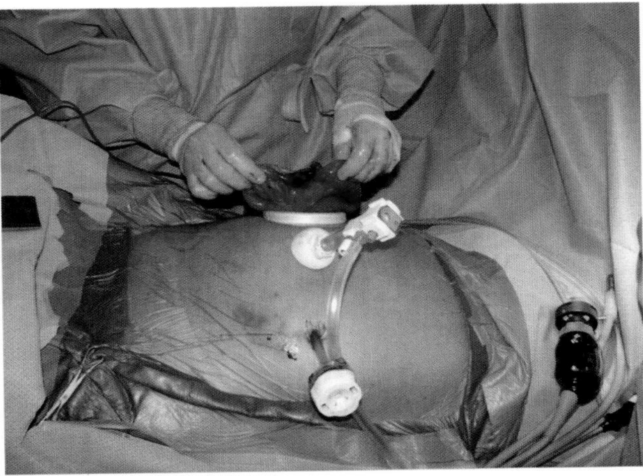

Fig. 8.5 Transperitoneal laparoscopic exploration allows for a minimized and planned laparotomy well away from the groin. This should minimize the chance for local contamination in the area of the prosthetic mesh repair.

of the underlying rectus muscle will allow access to the preperitoneal space well below the level of the initial intraperitoneal trocar. Care should be used to avoid puncture of the peritoneum during groin dissections as this eliminates the potential protection of the mesh provided by an intact peritoneum. At the completion of the TEP, the pneumoperitoneum can be reestablished and the abdominal contents reinspected.

An alternative is to perform the extraperitoneal portion of the hernia repair initially. A standard TEP can be performed with reduction of the incarcerated contents. To adequately inspect the bowel, the abdomen can be entered through the infraumbilical incision after the conclusion of the TEP. Additional transabdominal trocars might be necessary to manipulate the intra-abdominal structures. This approach is best employed when the suspicion of the presence of necrotic contents is low.

Choice of Prosthetic

The controversy around the choice of prosthetic for repair of strangulated hernias begins with the decision as to whether or not to use a prosthetic material at all. Additionally, if a prosthetic repair is chosen,

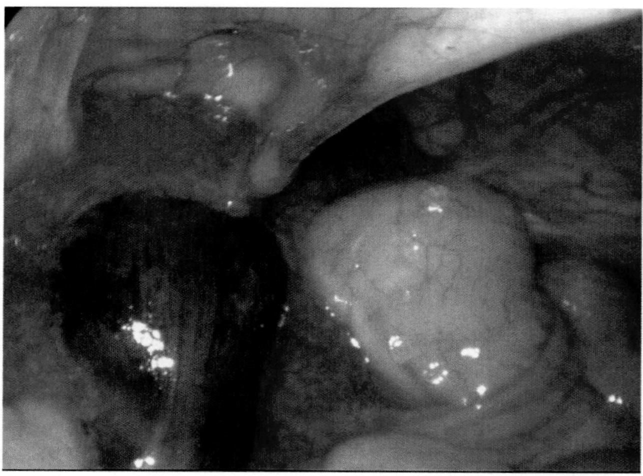

Fig. 8.6. Gross contamination from small bowel perforation secondary to a strangulated obturator hernia. Prosthetic mesh is best avoided in this situation.

which of the overwhelming prosthetic mesh options should be used? A variety of patient and prosthetic factors can help guide this decision-making process. The first and most important factor is the degree of contamination in the operative field. There is general consensus that permanent prosthetic mesh materials should not be placed into heavily contaminated or dirty fields. This scenario would most commonly be encountered if strangulated intestinal contents had progressed to perforation or if perforation had occurred during attempts to reduce the strangulated contents (Fig. 8.6). Less commonly, significant spillage could occur in the operative field during resection and reanastamosis of nonviable viscera. In either scenario, once the field is classified as dirty, a permanent prosthetic should not be used. Another way to think about this scenario is that the hernia itself is no longer the patient's primary problem, and focus should be on treating the bowel and sepsis. The hernia itself can be treated during a later staged repair. Options in this setting include primary repair techniques, use of absorbable prosthetic mesh, or placement of a biologic mesh. In all settings, the source of contamination should be either controlled or well drained to optimize outcomes. While use of prosthetic absorbable mesh essentially ensures hernia recurrence, primary repairs and use of biologic mesh in fields with controlled contamination may result in durable repair. Exact recurrence rates will vary significantly base on individual patient scenarios. There is nothing worse than an infected synthetic in this scenario, and all efforts should be made to prevent this from happening.

In the setting of clean-contaminated cases, or the potential for contamination secondary to the presence of nonviable or marginally viable tissue, there is less agreement on the use of permanent prosthetic mesh for hernia repair. While many surgeons fear the potential for mesh infection in this scenario, the majority of the available evidence supports the safe use of prosthetic mesh material without increased rates of wound or mesh infections. Nearly all types of permanent prosthetic have been successfully used in this setting, including polyester, polypropylene, and expanded polytetrafluoroethylene (ePTFE). Reported strategies to decrease the risks of potential mesh infection include placing the mesh in a tissue plane remote from the area of potential contamination (i.e., preperitoneal) and decontamination of the plane with disinfectant solution such as betadine or chlorhexidine prior to mesh placement. The benefit of these strategies is unclear. Given the long-term benefits of tension-free prosthetic repairs, especially with respect to rates of recurrence, and the available evidence to support its safe use, prosthetic repair should be the option of choice for most surgeons repairing strangulated hernias in the absence of gross contamination of the surgical field.

A final prosthetic-related factor to consider is the timing of prosthetic placement. As discussed above, a "second-look" operative strategy may be employed when the viability of reduced hernia contents is questionable and resection is undesirable, not easily performed, or if the patient's physiologic status dictates the need for an abbreviated operation. If a second-look operation is planned, it is probably best to defer placement of prosthetic until the time of the last operation. The viability of the contents and the presence or absence of contamination in the field at the time of open or laparoscopic reexploration will dictate how or if prosthetic mesh should be used. Additionally, the use of systemic antibiotics to treat infection in the interim between the initial and subsequent operations may decrease the bacterial load in the operative field and potentially reduce mesh-related infectious complications.

Special Considerations: Obturator Hernia

Herniation of intra-abdominal contents through the obturator foramen is an unusual but potentially life-threatening cause of a strangulated groin hernia. These hernias present classically in older women, most

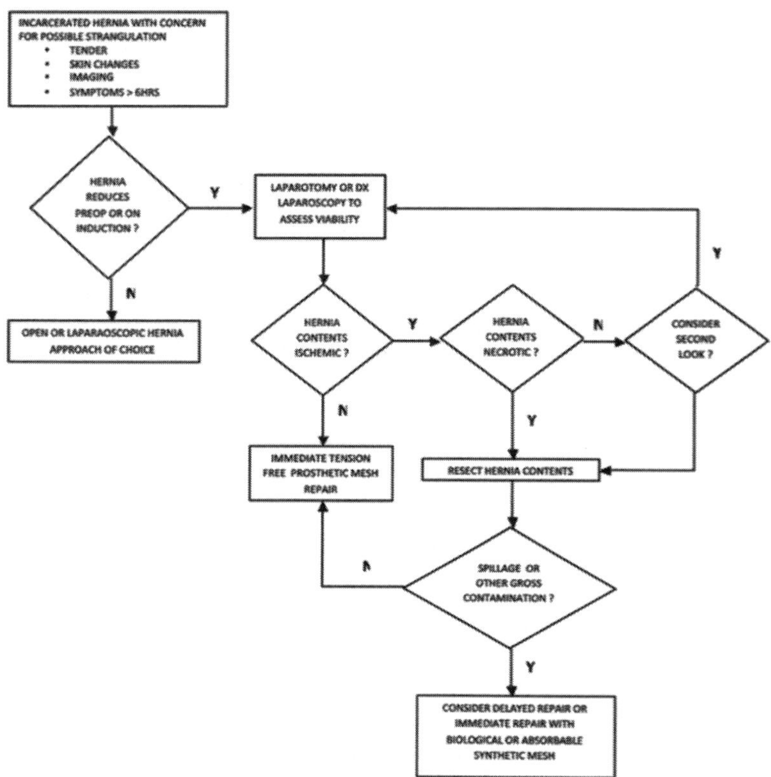

Fig. 8.7 Proposed algorithm for the surgical management of potentially strangulated inguinal hernias.

commonly on the right side, with up to 90% of patients presenting initially with signs and symptoms of a partial or complete small bowel obstruction. Given the subtle signs, the typical lack of a palpable hernia bulge on physical exam and the comorbidities of the elderly affected population, diagnosis of an incarcerated obturator hernia is often delayed or not recognized until strangulation occurs. The mortality rate associated with development of a strangulated obturator hernia has been reported as high as 30%.

When an incarcerated or strangulated obturator hernia is suspected based on history, physical exam, and/or imaging studies, a rapid transperitoneal approach is warranted. This can be done by laparotomy via either a low-midline or Pfannenstiel incision or, in hemodynamically stable patients, via transperitoneal laparoscopic approach. With either approach, visualization of the obturator foramen is facilitated with head-down positioning of the patient on the operating table. Once identified, the contents can typically be gently reduced, taking care to avoid bowel perforation if at all possible. If reduction is difficult, the obturator foramen can be enlarged by incising the obturator membrane inferomedially to avoid injury to the obturator neurovascular bundle.

Once reduced, the decision making follows exactly as outlined above for all potentially strangulated groin hernias. If conditions allow for a permanent prosthetic repair, it is easily done by entering the preperitoneal space and obtaining wide coverage of the obturator defect with prosthetic mesh. In contaminated operative fields, biologic mesh is probably the best option as primary tissue repair at this location is usually not realistic. Temporary exclusion of the obturator defect from the peritoneal cavity with fat plugs, bladder, and bowel has been described but should be considered only if a mesh alternative is not readily available. All potential repairs can be performed via either laparotomy or a laparoscopic approach. An algorithmic overview of the approach to potentially strangulated hernias is presented in Fig. 8.7.

Summary

Strangulated inguinal hernias occur with regularity and pose the risk of serious morbidity and mortality. Prompt recognition and treatment is imperative. The goals of operation for strangulated inguinal hernia are reduction and inspection of hernia contents, resection of necrotic tissue, and repair of the hernia defect. The operative approach can be either conventional using the anterior or preperitoneal approach or laparoscopically using a transabdominal, preperitoneal, or combined technique.

Suggested Reading

1. Bachman S, Ramshaw B. Prosthetic material in ventral hernia repair: how do I choose? Surg Clin North Am. 2008;88:101–12.
2. Berliner SD, Burson LC, Wise L. The Henry operation for incarcerated and strangulated femoral hernias. Arch Surg. 1992;127:314–6.

3. Campanelli G, Nicolosi FM, Pettinari D, Contessini Avesami E. Prosthetic repair, intestinal resection, and potentially contaminated fields: safe and feasible? Hernia. 2004;8:190–2.
4. Malangoni MA, Condon RE. Preperitoneal repair of acute incarcerated and strangulated hernias of the groin. Surg Gynecol Obstet. 1986;162:65–7.
5. Rebuffat C, Galli A, Scalambra MS, Balsamo F. Laparoscopic repair of strangulated hernias. Surg Endosc. 2006;20:131–4.

9. Femoral Hernia

Daniel E. Swartz and Edward L. Felix

Introduction

The femoral hernia, despite accounting for less than 10% of adult groin hernias, is associated with greater risk of incarceration, strangulation, requiring emergency surgery, bowel resection, morbidity and mortality than inguinal hernias. Because the anatomic location is so closely related to the more common inguinal hernia, the diagnosis is often not made until surgery.

Femoral Hernia Facts

Femoral hernias account for 2-8% of inguinal hernias encountered, with an even higher incidence of up to 11% of hernias reported since laparoscopy was first introduced (1).

Femoral hernias occur 2-5 times more often in women than men (62.5% occur in women vs 25% of inguinal hernias) (2). Additionally, they typically occur in older patients with a peak incidence in the sixth decade, and concomitant inguinal hernias are found in up to 51% (3,4). Approximately 27,000 femoral hernia repairs are performed per year in U.S, and 36% of femoral hernias are repaired emergently compared to 5% of inguinal hernias (5). Emergent repair of femoral hernia is associated with up to 30% morbidity, 10% mortality (6,7) and 23% require a bowel resection (5). Once diagnosed, up to 22% of femoral hernias incarcerate by 3 months and up to 45% by 21 months (8).

B.P. Jacob and B. Ramshaw (eds.), *The SAGES Manual of Hernia Repair*,
DOI 10.1007/978-1-4614-4824-2_9,

Anatomic Definitions

The femoral canal is an elliptical cone located medial to the femoral vein extending from the femoral ring superiomedially to the femoral orifice inferolaterally that contains lymphatics, adipose tissue, and commonly the lymph node of Cloquet. The femoral ring (the entrance to the femoral canal) is lined by the iliopubic tract anterosuperiorly, by Cooper's ligament inferoposteriorly and by the femoral sheath laterally. When a femoral hernia is present, an opening known as the femoral orifice is created. The femoral orifice is bounded posteriorly by the pectineal fascia, laterally by the femoral sheath, anteriorly by the superior cornu of the fascia lata, and medially by the fan-shaped fibers of the iliopubic tract. A femoral hernia is the result of a protrusion of preperitoneal fat, bladder or peritoneal sac through the femoral ring. It becomes clinically evident once the exit of the femoral canal, or the femoral orifice, is breached. It is considered an acquired, not a congenital, defect.

Diagnosis

The classic presentation of a femoral hernia is with a main complaint of pain and/or a lump in groin (may be asymptomatic), with physical findings revealing a mass and/or tenderness below inguinal ligament on anteromedial thigh. The differential diagnosis includes inguinal hernia, obturator hernia, lymphadenopathy, lipoma, and pseudohernia which is defined as a nonpathogenic lymph node (Cloquet's node) in extremely

Table 9.1 Distinguishing Inguinal From Femoral Hernia

	Inguinal Hernia	Femoral Hernia
Relation to Pubic Tubercle	Inferolateral	Superomedial (Nyhus)
Have patient cough while examining medial end of inguinal ligament	Hernia Appears Above the Inguinal Ligament	Hernia Appears Below the Inguinal Ligament (Nyhus)
Have patient cough while palpating just lateral to the Adductor Longus Tendon about one fingerbreadth medial to the femoral artery.	Hernia Appears	Hernia Stays Reduced (Hair)

thin patients. An incarcerated groin hernia should raise the physician's suspicion that this might be a femoral hernia as a higher percentage of femoral hernias incarcerate compared to inguinal or any other abdominal wall hernia (9). Other imaging modalities like CT Scan, color Doppler ultrasound, and contast herniography are used, but because the accuracy of these tests are unknown, physicians should generally rely on the physical exam as the primary diagnostic modality. Distinguishing Between Inguinal and Femoral Hernia: see Table 9.1

Three Classic Anatomic Approaches To Treatment

Femoral Approach

The femoral approach was first described by Socin (1879) with a high ligation of the hernia sac but was associated with a high recurrence rate (10). Bassini (1885) added a femoral ring closure with suture after the high sac ligation. Three decades later, Lichtenstein and Shore (1974) recommended a tension-free repair with a polyproplylene plug sutured into the femoral ring followed by placement of an additional mesh to repair inguinal floor (11).

The femoral approach technique begins with an inguinal or subinguinal incision (Fig. 9.1a), where the hernia sac is usually located inferior to external oblique aponeurosis and the lacunar ligament may be divided in cases of incarceration (but counter incision to expose inguinal floor may be required). The hernia sac is dissected, opened for exploration and the contents reduced into the abdominal cavity before the sac is ligated (Fig. 9.1b). The canal is obliterated by suture or mesh plug that is rolled or sutured to inguinal ligament, fascia lata and pectineal fascia (Fig. 9.1c). The femoral approach generally should not be used in strangulated femoral hernias although it requires the least dissection. One advantage of the femoral approach is that it may be performed under local anesthesia, thus making it a preferred approach for high-risk surgical patients.

Inguinal Approach

The inguinal approach was first described by Annandale (1876) and is also associated with a high ligation of the sac (12). Ruggi then described suturing Cooper's Ligament to inguinal ligament (1892) after sac ligation.

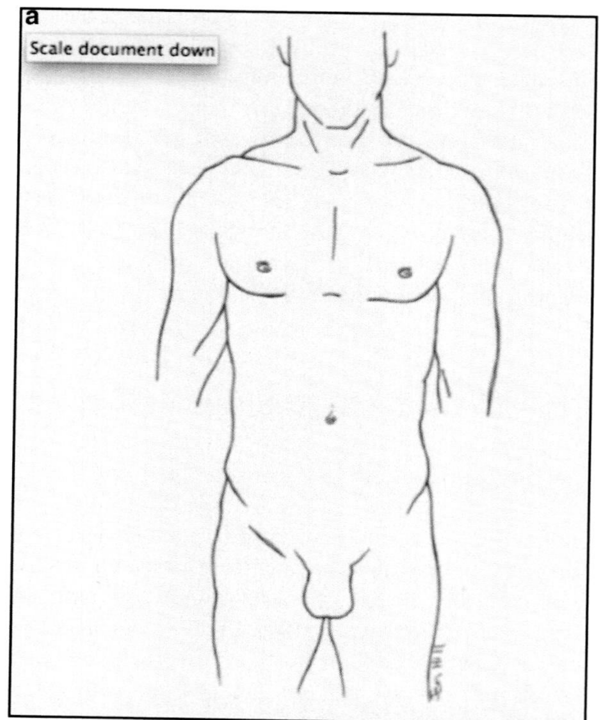

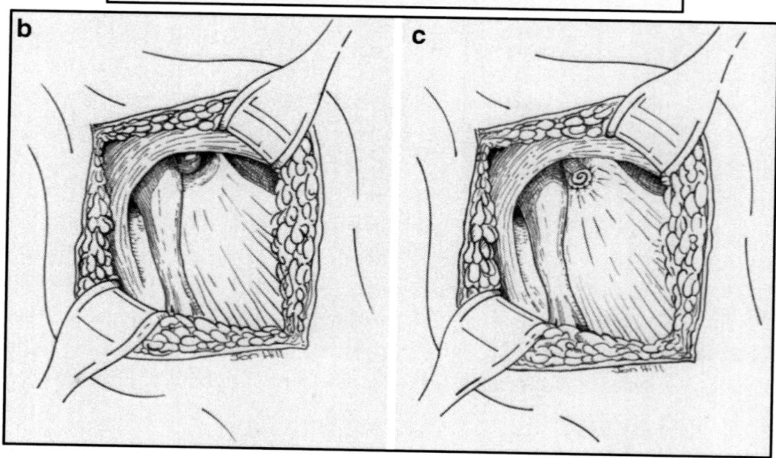

Fig. 9.1 (**a**) Illustration of the skin incision for the femoral approach to repair of a right femoral hernia. (**b**) Illustration of the exposure of a right femoral hernia via the femoral approach. Note the location of the hernia medial to the femoral vein. (**c**) *Cylindrical mesh roll* use to obliterate the femoral canal on a right-sided femoral hernia repair using the femoral approach.

Moschowicz included the use of an inguinal floor repair (included transverse aponeurotic arch) (13). Later, McVay and Anson's (1942) "Cooper's ligament repair" (suturing Cooper's ligament to transverse aponeurotic arch) then became standard repair for femoral and direct inguinal hernias (12). Three decades later, Lichtenstein and Shore (1974) recommended a tension-free repair with a polyproplylene plug sutured into the femoral ring and additional mesh to repair inguinal floor (11). This approach provides excellent exposure of the femoral ring with an opportunity to resect bowel if needed.

Femoral hernia repairs performed via an inguinal incision begin with a traditional inguinal incision that permits routine opening of the inguinal canal via the external oblique aponeurosis, followed by mobilization of the cord with an examination to exclude or repair any concomitant indirect inguinal hernias. Next the inguinal floor can be opened by transecting the transveralis fascia. If incarceration is present, the lacunar ligament and iliopubic tract can be divided at the medial edge of the femoral ring. Incarceration mandates opening of the sac to examine the contents for any evidence of ischemia or gangrene. High ligation of the sac is performed and is then followed by a hernia repair, preferentially with mesh. Suture repair may be selected if prosthetic mesh is contraindicated (gross contamination, strangulation). The main principle is to approximate the iliopubic tract and lacunar ligament to Cooper's ligament with nonabsorbable suture. The inguinal floor will also need to be reconstructed with mesh (preferably) or, rarely, suture approximation (Fig. 9.2).

Preperitoneal Approach

The preperitoneal repair through a low midline incision was also first described by Annandale (1876). Here, the linea alba was opened with blunt dissection of the peritoneum from the pelvis with again, a high ligation of the sac. McEvedy then described a repair where Cooper's ligament is sutured to the conjoined tend on via an oblique incision over the lateral rectus sheath (1950). An additional modification was described by Nyhus who used a transverse incision to approximate Cooper's ligament to the iliopubic tract (1950) and later added polypropylene mesh to buttress the repair. (14) Stoppa (1973) placed large sheet of Dacron mesh over both of the groins (15), while Kugel used a ring-supported mesh placed through a small incision (2003) (16).

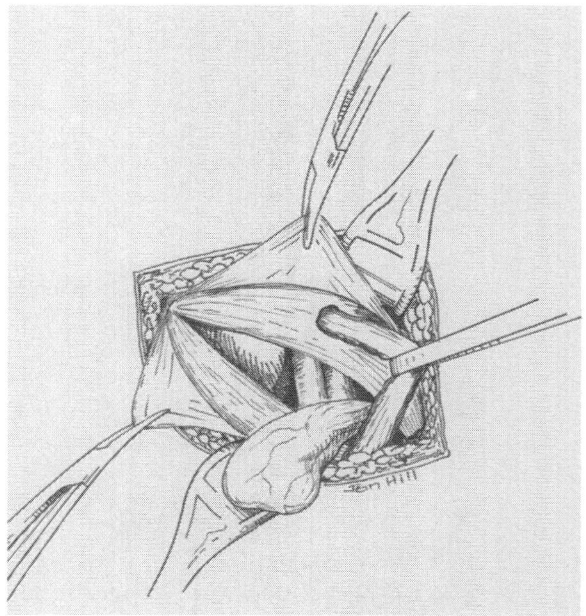

Fig. 9.2 Inguinal approach to the repair of a right femoral hernia. After an exposing the inguinal canal, the inguinal floor is opened to access and repair a femoral hernia.

The preperitoneal approach can also be accomplished by laparoscopy, and the first laparoscopic transabdominal preperitoneal (TAPP) repair was reported by Schultz (1990) (17), while the first laparoscopic totally extraperitoneal (TEP) repair was reported soon afterward (18). The laparoscopic TEP repair should intuitively be avoided in suspected strangulation as the bowel needs a thorough assessment during the repair.

In contrast to laparoscopy, an open preperitoneal approach provides excellent exposure of all potential groin hernia sites and easy access to the intraperitoneal contents. The technique involves making a transverse lower abdominal incision 3 cm cephalad to a routine inguinal incision. The anterior rectus sheath is divided cephalad to the internal ring, and the rectus abdominis is retracted medially. The femoral sac is then reduced (if incarceration is present, the surgeon can incise the iliopubict tract near the medial edge of the femoral ring). Small primary femoral hernias can be suture repaired by approximating Cooper's ligament to the iliopubic tract or repaired with mesh. Primary and recurrent hernias

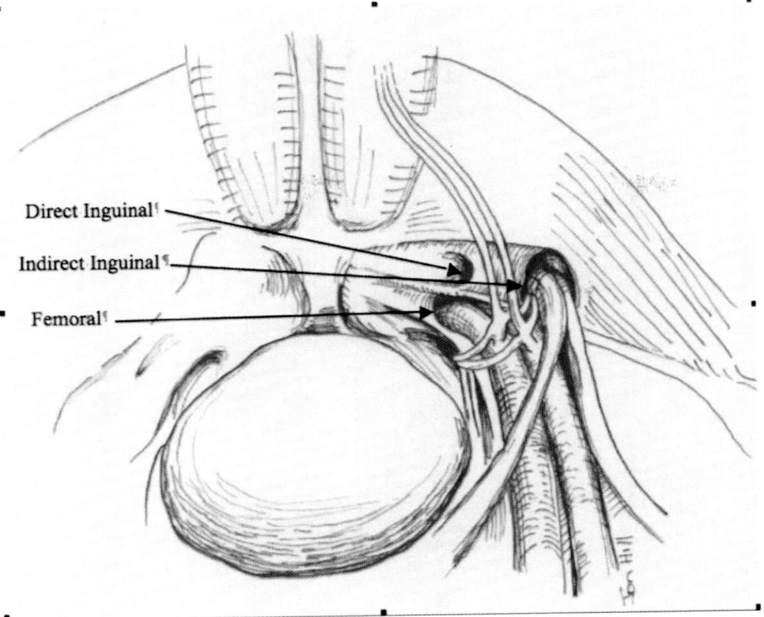

Fig. 9.3 Preperitoneal exposure of the right groin. The femoral hernia is located posterior to the iliopubic tract and medial to the femoral vein. The indirect inguinal hernia is located at the internal ring, while the direct hernia is located in Hesselbach's triangle medial to the epigastric vessels and anterior to the iliopubic tract.

should be repaired with mesh with a 2 -3 cm overlap that also covers the direct and indirect inguinal spaces. Preperitoneal structures and hernia sites are demonstrated in Fig. 9.3.

The laparoscopic TAPP first requires placement of ports (Fig. 9.4a) and establishment of pneumorperitoneum. Next, an intraperitoneal dissection can then be performed by beginning to open the parietal peritoneum 2 cm cephalad to the internal ring. Thorough dissection of retroperitoneal structures is required, including dissection of the iliopubic tract, symphisis pubis, and sometimes a partial bladder dissection into the Space of Retzius, to create enough space for the inferior edge of the mesh. All three potential groin hernia sites must be exposed (Fig. 9.3). Examination for an inguinal canal lipoma must be included. During a TAPP, the incarcerated sac is often reduced, if possible, however sac division with proximal sac ligation is acceptable. If there are incarcerated

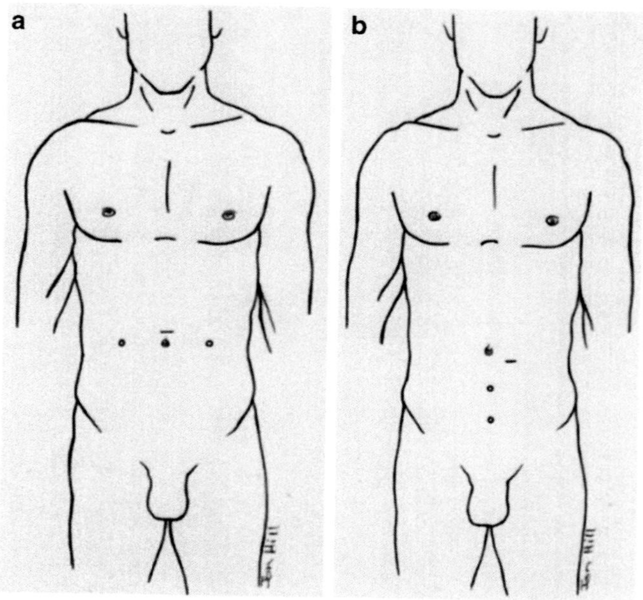

Fig. 9.4 (**a**) Illustration of port placement for a laparoscopic transabdominal preperitoneal (TAPP) groin hernia repair. (**b**) Illustration of port placement for a laparoscopic totally extraperitoneal preperitoneal (TEP) groin hernia repair.

or strangulated contents in a tight femoral ring, to reduce the contents it may be necessary to first divide Lacunar's ligament for 1 – 2 cm heading mediosuperiorly along the transversalis fascia in order to widen the defect and to permit safe reduction of hernia contents. This can be done with a hook cautery or with ultrasonic shears. Careful attention must be made to identify the iliac vein lateral to the hernia and to avoid it's injury. If there are no veins running on the transversalis fascia, a hook cautery can be used to do this maneuver, however ultrasonic shears may also be employed to obtain simultaneous hemostasis if veins are present. We recommend using bipolar cautery on a Maryland grasper to coagulate all small veins in the region first, and then opening the fasica to reduce the contents. The fascia does not have to be closed again at the end of the case when doing this laparoscopically. Once the hernia contents are reduced, the cord structures should be dissected from peritoneum as far posteriorly as possible. Mesh is placed covering all three potential groin hernia sites with overlap. Fixation to Cooper's ligament may be used. Reappoximation of the peritoneum must be performed.

The laparoscopic TEP technique also begins after port placement (Fig. 9.4b) and subrectus preperitoneal dissection with a balloon. The technique is identical to the TAPP repair without the need for peritoneum reapproximation and fixation of mesh is not usually necessary. Technical details are described in other chapters in this manual.

Surgical Caveats

Nonincarcerated, nonstrangulated femoral hernias may be repaired using any of the described approaches. However, incarceration or strangulation of femoral hernias is a relative contraindication to laparoscopic TEP repairs unless the surgeon has tremendous experience with laparoscopic techniques and can explore and assess the bowel intraperitoneally during the case. Strangulation in a femoral or inguinal hernia requiring bowel resection becomes a contraindication to simultaneous permanent synthetic mesh placement. That being said, it has been shown that Franklin et al. reported no recurrences or mesh-related complications over 19 months in 58 patients with strangulated groin hernias with gross contamination repaired with biologic mesh (19).

We feel that despite having a hernia, in the setting of clean-contaminated or contaminated fields, like a bowel strangulation with gangrene during a femoral hernia case, the patient's primary problem becomes that infectious process. A more permanent solution to the hernia defect can be staged at a later time. Attempts that risk a potential synthetic mesh infection should generally be avoided, and absorbable mesh products which are widely available may be more ideal in this situation. Patients should be told to anticipate a hernia recurrence after the mesh is resorbed, at which time an elective repair should be performed.

Most surgeons repair femoral hernias with polypropylene mesh with or without fixation. Laparoscopic hernia repair is increasingly popular since it combines the benefits of laparoscopy (less pain, early return to activities, nonexistent mesh infection rate) and preperitoneal approach (excellent exposure, access to viscera, assessment of all groin hernias). Laparoscopic TEP approach avoids potential intraperitoneal complications (both are equally acceptable). Laparoscopic TAPP preferred for incarceration or previous retroperitoneal pelvic surgery or radiation because of the risk of tearing the peritoneum or incarcerated viscera when performing balloon dissection.

Results

Publications in the literature suggest a post-femoral hernia repair recurrence rate incidence of up to 10%. The femoral approach with plug has been reported to have a higher seroma and foreign body sensation than suture repair. The femoral approach has been shown to miss concomitant inguinal hernias (20). The laparoscopic repair is generally associated with <1% recurrence rates.

Commentary

Femoral hernias occur much less commonly than inguinal hernias (accounting for less than 8% of groin hernias) and are therefore often misdiagnosed as inguinal hernias. This fact has several consequences. First, the anterior approach to groin hernia repair can result in "missing" a femoral hernia unless careful palpation through the inguinal floor is undertaken. One study using a national database of almost 35,000 consecutive groin hernias performed over a three year period found that the incidence of femoral hernias following inguinal hernia repair was 15 times the incidence of primary femoral hernias (21). A preperitoneal approach, either laparoscopic or open, has the advantage of direct visualization of femoral hernias as well as treatment of either femoral or inguinal hernia includes the mesh coverage of the other.

The second consequence of misdiagnosed femoral hernias is that due to their increased likelihood of incarceration with or without strangulation, once diagnosed, a femoral hernia should be repaired. This is because one in three femoral hernias will need to be repaired emergently (compared to 5% of inguinal hernias). The risk of incarceration of a femoral hernia once diagnosed is 22% at three months and 45% at 21 months (8). There is a recent tendency toward watchful waiting in the treatment of small, asymptomatic inguinal hernias but one must be certain that the hernia is inguinal and not femoral because of the high incidence of incarceration in femoral hernias (22, 23).

Which of the three approaches to use for femoral hernia repair largely rests upon surgeon preference and experience. Several caveats, however, exist as listed above which serve as relatively strong contraindications for one or more approaches. Almost all surgeons now embrace a tension-free hernioplasty using prosthetic mesh in all approaches. The only contraindications to prosthetic mesh are gross contamination or bowel resection and, although biologic mesh has been used in these situations, there is not enough data at this time to recommend against primary suture repair. In fact, small primary femoral hernias (without concomitant inguinal hernia) in non-obese patients may be repaired with suture. Polypropylene cylindrical plugs have been associated with a discomforting foreign-body sensation and higher recurrence and seroma rates (20). Incarcerated and strangulated femoral hernias should be approached from either an inguinal or preperitoneal incision if open, or a TAPP repair if laparoscopic. The femoral approach may make reduction difficult and it will prevent adequate assessment of the bowel and resection if needed. Laparoscopic TEP repair in the face of incarceration makes tearing the peritoneum likely which requires conversion to a TAPP if resection of the bowel is needed.

A common conundrum occurs if, upon laparoscopy, no hernia (as evidenced as no peritoneal dimpling) is identified. The peritoneum should be opened and a repair should be performed as planned. Recurrences after failing to identify a retroperitoneal hernia are common. We encourage a meticulous search for an inguinal or femoral lipoma, as well as for other frequent etiologies of the clinical diagnosis of groin hernias is encouraged (24).

At our center, we have repaired over 2000 groin hernias using a laparoscopic approach. Unless a contraindication exists (obliteration of the preperitoneal space from surgery or radiation or a risk of general anesthesia), we routinely employ a laparoscopic approach as this facilitates evaluation and treatment of all potential groin hernia sites including the femoral hernia.

References

1. Babar M, Myers E, Matingal J, Hurley ML. The modified Nyhus-Condon femoral hernia repair. *Hernia* 2010;14:271–285.
2. Crawford DL, Hiatt JR, Phillips EH. Laparoscopy identifies unexpected groin hernias. *Am Surg* 1998;64(10):976–978.
3. Griffin KJ, Harris S, Tang TY, Skelton N, Reed JB, Harris AM. Incidence of contralateral occult inguinal hernia found at the time of laparosocpi trans-abdominal pre-peritoneal (TAPP) repair. *Hernia* 2010;14:345–349.
4. Chan G, Chan CK. Longterm results of a prospective study of 225 femoral hernia repairs: Indications for tissue and mesh repair. *J Am Coll Surg* 2008;207(3):360–367.
5. Dahlstrand U, Wollert S, Nordin P, Sandblom G, Gunnarsson U. Emergency femoral hernia repair. A study based on a national register. *Ann Surg* 2009;249(4):672–676.

6. Garg P, Ismail M. Laparoscopic total extraperitoneal repair in femoral hernia without fixation of the mesh. *JSLS* 2009;13:597–600.
7. Suppiah A, Gatt M, Barandarian J, Heng MS, Perry EP. Outcomes of emergency and elective femoral hernia surgery in four district general hospitals: a 4-year study. *Hernia* 2007;11(6):509–512.
8. Van den Hueval B, Dwars BJ, Klassen DR, Bonjer HJ. Is surgical repair of an asymptomatic groin hernia appropriate? A review. *Hernia* 2011 Epub ahead of print.
9. Bendavid R. Femoral hernia (Part III): An "umbrella" for femoral hernia repair. In: Bendavid, R., ed. *Prostheses and Abdominal Wall Hernias*. Boca Raton, CRC Press, 1994:413.
10. Lau WY. History of treatment of groin hernia. *World J Surg* 2002;26(6):748–759.
11. Lichtenstein IL, Shore JM. Simplified repair of femoral and recurrent inguinal hernias by a "plug" technique. *Am J Surg* 1974;128(3):439–444.
12. Read RC. British contributions to modern herniology of the groin. *Hernia* 2005;9(1): 6–11.
13. Moschowitz AV. Femoral hernia; a new operation for radical cure. *New York J Med* 1907;21:1087.
14. Nyhus LM, Condon RE, Harkins HN. Clinial experiences with preperitoneal hernia repair for all types of hernia of the groin. *Am J Surg* 1960;100:233–244.
15. Stoppa R, Petit J, Abourachid H, et al. Procede original de plastie des hernia de l'aine: L'Interposition sous fixation d'une prothese en tulle de Dacron par voie mediane sous-peritoneale. *Chirurgie* 1973;99(2):119–23.
16. Kugel, RD. The Kugel repair for groin hernias. Surg Clin N Am. 2003;83(5): 1119–1139.
17. Schultz LS, Graber JN, Peritrafitta J, Hickok DF. Early results with laparoscopic inguinal herniorrhaphy are promising. *Clin Laser Mon* 1990;8(7):103–5.
18. McKernan, JB, Laws, HL. Laparoscopic repair of inguinal hernias using a totally extraperitoneal prosthetic approach. *Surg Endosc* 1993;7(1):26–28.
19. Franklin ME Jr, Gonzalez JJ, Glass JL. Use of porcine small intestinal submucosa as a prosthetic device for laparoscopic repair of hernias in contaminated fields: 2-year follow-up. *Hernia* 2004;8(3):186–189.
20. Chen J, Lv Y, Shen Y, Liu S, Wang M. A prospective comparison of preperitoneal tension-free open herniorrhaphy with mesh plug herniorrhaphy for the treatment of femoral hernias. *Surgery* 2010;148:976–981.
21. Mikkelsen T, Bay-Nielsen M, Kehlet H. Risk of femoral hernia after inguinal herniorrhaphy. *Brit. J. Surg*. 2002;89(4):486–488.
22. Fitzgibbons RJ Jr, Giobbie-Hurder A, Gibbs JO et al. Watchful waiting vs repair of inguinal hernia in minimally symptomatic men: a randomized clinical trial. *JAMA* 2006;295(3):285–292.
23. O'Dwyer, P.J., Norrie, J., Alani, A., et al.: Observation or operation for patients with an asymptomatic inguinal hernia: a randomized clinical trial. *Ann Surg* 2006;244(2): 167–173.
24. Hollinsky C, Sandberg S. Clinically diagnosed groin hernias without a peritoneal sac at laparoscopy – what to do? *Am J Surg* 2010;199(6):730–735.

Part III
Outcomes and Complications Following Inguinal Hernia Repair

10. Results of Laparoscopic Repair of Inguinal Hernia

Daniel Marcus

The Evolution of the Laparoscopic Technique

The surgical history of inguinal hernias dates back to ancient Egypt. From Bassini's heralding of the modern era to today's mesh-based open and laparoscopic repairs, this history parallels closely the evolution in anatomical understanding and development of the techniques of general surgery. The evolution of minimally invasive approach to the repair of inguinal hernias began in the early 1990s as the revolution of laparoscopic surgery began. The introduction of laparoscopic cholecystectomy was the first of many procedures in general surgery tried by surgeons via laparoscopic technique. The laparoscopic technique began with the IPOM (intraperitoneal placement of mesh). This technique was first to be published, seemed appealing because the simple procedure could be adapted by surgeons easily (reference by early studies). It soon became clear that this technique was fraught with issues due to high risk of complications and recurrence. Early reports revealed a recurrence rate of 43% at 41 months compared to 15% to conventional anterior repair [1].

The next technique to be promoted for inguinal hernia repair was the transabdominal preperitoneal approach or TAPP. This mirrored the established technique of laparoscopy which was becoming the norm for many procedures.

The totally extraperitoneal or TEP technique followed the TAPP as the evolution in inguinal hernia repair continued. This allows the surgeon to avoid any dissection inside the abdomen and therefore minimize the risk of injury in the short term and adhesion between the mesh and the bowel in the long term.

Accounting for 75% of all abdominal wall hernias, and with a lifetime risk of 27% in men and 3% in women, inguinal hernia repair is one of the

B.P. Jacob and B. Ramshaw (eds.), *The SAGES Manual of Hernia Repair*,
DOI 10.1007/978-1-4614-4824-2_10,

most commonly performed surgeries in the world [2]. In the United States, inguinal herniorrhaphy accounts for approximately 800,000 cases annually.

Most randomized studies comparing laparoscopy to open repair have confirmed the following findings [3, 4]:

Pros:

- Reduced postoperative pain
- Earlier return to work

Cons:

- Increased cost
- Lengthier operation
- Steeper learning curve
- Higher recurrence and complication rates early in a surgeon's experience

Although open, mesh-based, tension-free repair remains the criterion standard, laparoscopic herniorrhaphy, in the hands of adequately trained surgeons, produces excellent results comparable to those of open repair [4]. In a comparison of open repair with laparoscopic (totally extraperitoneal patch) repair, Eklund et al. found that 5 years postoperatively, 1.9% of patients who had undergone laparoscopic repair continued to report moderate or severe pain compared with 3.5% of those in the open repair group [5].

Definitions

Laparoscopic inguinal herniorrhaphy can refer to any of the following three techniques:

Totally extraperitoneal (TEP) repair: See the sections below for a detailed description of this technique.

Transabdominal preperitoneal (TAPP) repair: The abdomen is accessed, and pneumoperitoneum is achieved using standard laparoscopic techniques. The preperitoneal space is then exposed transabdominally by sharply incising and bluntly stripping the peritoneum that overlies the inguinal anatomy. A mesh is then deployed and fixed in place as with the TEP technique and the peritoneum returned to its anatomical position.

Intraperitoneal onlay mesh (IPOM) repair: A dual-layer mesh is placed over the myopectineal orifice transabdominally and fixed in place. The preperitoneal space is not entered, and minimal dissection is carried out.

TEP and TAPP

The most commonly performed laparoscopic techniques are the TEP and TAPP repairs [6, 7]. Laparoscopic hernia repair was first described by Ger in 1990, who placed a simple mesh plug in the defect [8]. The technique has undergone a significant metamorphosis during the last few years. Currently, there are two types of laparoscopic hernia repair: the transabdominal preperitoneal (TAPP) repair (as described in this chapter) and the totally extraperitoneal (TEP) repair. The TEP involves creation of an extraperitoneal space posterior to the inguinal canal either with a Veress needle or more commonly a balloon and placement of a mesh in a similar fashion to the TAPP repair. The TEP may have some advantages over the TAPP in terms of postoperative pain and reduced potential for intraperitoneal complications but does require a high level of technical skill associated with a considerable learning curve. Many surgeons initially learned the TAPP technique as it was considered easier and was the first technique introduced after the IPOM. With the introduction of the TEP method with the preperitoneal balloon dissection, many began to prefer this technique. The theoretical advantages of the TEP were the fact that the peritoneum is totally avoided, thereby reducing greatly the risk of adhesions to the bowel by the mesh. Those who prefer TAPP repairs believe they are technically easier, provide a better view of the anatomy, and do not require further equipment beyond that normally available in most departments performing laparoscopic cholecystectomy. Several studies have demonstrated a clear advantage of laparoscopic hernia repair over open repair in terms of reduced postoperative pain and earlier return to work and normal activities. Despite this, the laparoscopic approach has been slow to gain popularity among many surgeons. This is due to a number of factors. Firstly, more advanced technical skills are required compared with a Lichtenstein repair. Most surgeons who have not had special training, i.e., fellowship or extensive preceptorship, have difficulty making the transition to the laparoscopic approach. This explains why only an estimated 30% of all inguinal hernias are performed by either TAPP or TEP. The financial considerations also play a role certainly. The reimbursement for the laparoscopic technique is no greater for the most part than a conventional open technique, both of which are quite low compared to other procedures. This may contribute to the incentive for a general surgeon to invest the time and dedication needed to reach competency in this procedure. Nowadays, the majority of general surgeons do have quite extensive experience with laparoscopy in cholecystectomy, and this is sufficient to be able to perform a TAPP repair. Recurrence rates are very low with both the open and laparoscopic mesh repairs with randomized studies showing no difference between the two. In these studies, the use of large pieces of mesh seems to help to reduce long-term recurrences. Complications with experience and technical improvements are now minimal in the laparoscopic repair, and studies indicate similar complication rates between open and laparoscopic repairs. Open repairs appear to have a higher rate of groin hematoma and genital edema. One disadvantage of the laparoscopic repair is an increase in cost because of the equipment required [1], but with earlier return to work, this cost is outweighed by the benefits to patient and society. A major advantage of the laparoscopic approach is the ability to detect and repair a contralateral defect at the same operation with only a moderate increase in operating time.

As with laparoscopic cholecystectomy, there is a definite learning curve with the laparoscopic approach to inguinal hernia repair, with the TEP technique requiring more of a learning curve than TAPP but that with general laparoscopic experience the learning curve for hernia repair will become short, thus minimizing the chances of complications seen during the development of this procedure.

Some earlier studies showed increased recurrence rates with the laparoscopic technique and questioned the added cost (8 VA Study). However, over the past several years, more studies have shown that when performed by experienced surgeons with high volume of laparoscopic procedures, there is a clear advantage. The added cost earlier criticized is offset by the quicker return to baseline function and the advantage of exploring and repairing the contralateral side if indicated. Additional techniques avoiding use of costly deposable products (i.e., balloon dissection devices) further bring the cost down.

The relatively newer technique of single incision or single port (SILS and SPA) as well as robotic surgery has introduced the potential for further reducing the number of port sites. There have been reports that these techniques may be on par with conventional laparoscopic methods. The question as to whether these procedures will have significant advantages is currently being evaluated in many centers.

References

1. Kingsley D, Vogt DM, Nelson MT, et al. Laparoscopic intraperitoneal onlay inguinal herniorrhaphy. Am J Surg. 1998;176(6):548–53.
2. Jenkins JT, O'Dwyer PJ. Inguinal hernias. BMJ. 2008;336(7638):269–72.

3. McCormack K, Scott NW, Go PM, Ross S, Grant AM. Laparoscopic techniques versus open techniques for inguinal hernia repair. Cochrane Database Syst Rev. 2003;CD001785
4. Memon MA, Cooper NJ, Memon B, Memon MI, Abrams KR. Meta-analysis of randomized clinical trials comparing open and laparoscopic inguinal hernia repair. Br J Surg. 2003;90(12):1479–92.
5. Rutkow IM. Demographic and socioeconomic aspects of hernia repair in the United States in 2003. Surg Clin North Am. 2003;83(5):1045–51. v-vi.
6. Eklund A, Montgomery A, Bergkvist L, Rudberg C. Chronic pain 5 years after randomized comparison of laparoscopic and Lichtenstein inguinal hernia repair. Br J Surg. 2010;97(4):600–8.
7. Castorina S, Luca T, Privitera G, El-Bernawi H. An evidence-based approach for laparoscopic inguinal hernia repair: lessons learned from over 1,000 repairs. Clin Anat. 2012 Jan 24. [Epub ahead of print]
8. Neumayer L, Giobbie-Hurder A, Jonasson O, Fitzgibbons Jr R, Dunlop D, Gibbs J, Reda D, Henderson W, Veterans Affairs Cooperative Studies Program 456 Investigators. Open mesh versus laparoscopic mesh repair of inguinal hernia. N Engl J Med. 2004;350:1819–27.

11. Outcomes After Transabdominal Preperitoneal Inguinal Hernia Repair

Nicole Fearing and Kimberly Ponnuru

Hernia surgery remains one of the most common general surgical procedures in the United States and Europe today. Surgeons perform approximately 600,000–800,000 inguinal hernia repairs in the United States yearly [1–3]. While most repairs utilize an open technique, laparoscopic hernia surgery comprises 10–15% of all repairs [2, 3]. Several surgeons reported performing the transabdominal preperitoneal in 1992. The first description of a transabdominal preperitoneal repair (TAPP) was by Arregui and his colleagues in 1992 [4]. Laparoscopic TAPP is often compared to the open inguinal hernia repair and the laparoscopic totally extraperitoneal repair (TEP). When discussing methods of hernia repair with a patient, topics such as recurrence, return to work time, cost, pain, neuralgia, and other complications should be reviewed.

Complications

Open repair, TAPP, and TEP repair all carry the risk of infection, groin hematoma, postoperative pain, recurrence, urinary retention, testicular complaints, and mesh-related complications. In addition, laparoscopic repairs have risks unique to laparoscopy such as trocar or Veress needle injuries, port site herniation, and hypercarbia or hypotension secondary to pneumoperitoneum [5].

B.P. Jacob and B. Ramshaw (eds.), *The SAGES Manual of Hernia Repair*,
DOI 10.1007/978-1-4614-4824-2_11,

Bowel Obstruction

TAPP repair can be complicated by bowel obstruction from migration of the intestine beneath the peritoneal flap. This can largely be prevented by careful tacking or suturing of the peritoneal flap over the mesh at the completion of the procedure. Kapiris et al. reported their results of 3,530 repairs in 3,017 patients with the TAPP repair [6]. In their experience, they had a total of seven small bowel obstructions due to bowel herniating into the peritoneum. They changed their technique from reapproximating the peritoneum with staples over the mesh to suturing it closed with a running suture. This change in peritoneal closure decreased the incidence of bowel obstruction from 0.8% with a stapled closure to 0.1% with sutured closure [6]. Obstructive symptoms in the immediate postoperative period require a thorough investigation to exclude the diagnosis of peritoneal herniation. This may be done by physical exam, ultrasound, or CT scan. If missed, peritoneal hernia can lead to adherence of small bowel to mesh with erosion of the mesh or incarceration and eventual strangulation of the bowel. When caught early, repair may be done laparoscopically with little sequelae.

Urological Complications

Urologic complications following TAPP exist but are rare. Most are minor and include scrotal seroma or hematoma, testicular pain, and secondary hydroceles [7, 8]. A few reports of major urologic complications have been reported as both short-term and long-term complications. Bladder injury is a rare but serious complication that can present at the time of surgery or within a few days of surgery. It has been reported to occur in less than 1% of patients [9]. There is no consensus regarding the routine use of urinary catheters at the time of surgery, although some surgeons do routinely place them and others do not. At the time of initial surgery, if a bladder injury is suspected, a urinary catheter may be inserted (if not already present), and methylene blue saline may be infused into the bladder to pinpoint the place of injury. Surgical repair of the bladder and mesh removal are usually required due to concern about mesh infection in this setting.

Erosion of the mesh into the bladder has been reported years after the initial TAPP. Mesh removal and surgical repair of the bladder were required. Mesh removal has been done in a formal open fashion as well as endoscopically [7, 10].

While uncommon, obstructive azoospermia following laparoscopic hernia repair should always be discussed with a patient who is still interested in having children. The reported incidence ranges from 0.3 to 7.2%. The etiology includes transection of the vas deferens, disrupted vascular supply, or obstruction following reaction from the mesh that causes scarring and obstruction of the vas deferens [11].

Debate continues regarding laparoscopic inguinal hernia repair in a patient with a previous radical prostatectomy. Scarring in this area may make opening the peritoneum difficult and dissection of the hernia tedious. The risk of complications may be higher in this setting. Those who tackle inguinal hernias with a TAPP repair should be very experienced in the repair of standard laparoscopic repairs prior to doing these more complicated procedures.

Another issue is the patient who may have the need for a radical prostate surgery in the months or years following a laparoscopic inguinal hernia repair. Laparoscopic or robotic retropubic prostatectomies have been successfully performed on patients who have had a previous laparoscopic inguinal hernia repair [12]. However, the previous preperitoneal dissection leads to scarring that can complicate the exposure during prostatectomy, especially where the bladder takedown is involved. This should be discussed with male patients at the time of the preoperative assessment so that patients can be educated on the risks that laparoscopic hernia surgery has in relation to prostate surgery.

Postoperative Pain

Of all of the complications, postoperative pain, otherwise known as inguinodynia, and recurrence deserve a closer review due to their frequency and impact on the patient. The much publicized Veterans Administration study on open mesh versus laparoscopic mesh repair of inguinal hernia showed that patient-reported outcomes and satisfaction were most negatively impacted by postoperative neuralgia and hernia recurrence [13]. These findings were also reproduced by Hawn and colleagues in their paper in 2006 on patient-reported outcomes after inguinal hernia surgery [5, 14]. Most studies note that patients have less immediate postoperative pain and less chronic postoperative pain following laparoscopic repair compared to open repair. Several large multicentered studies and one meta-analysis confirm less long-term, chronic postoperative pain following laparoscopic hernia repair in comparison with open repair [13, 15–17]. The decreased incidence of postoperative pain following laparoscopic hernia repair is significant when one considers the difficulty in treating chronic postoperative pain and the negative impact that it has on patient satisfaction.

Dickenson et al. demonstrated in a retrospective study that 14% of patients developed chronic (>1 year) postoperative pain following laparoscopic hernia repair. This is greater than the risk of recurrence and is problematic in that chronic postoperative pain often is not easily treated surgically. In this study, the researchers identified preoperative pain, age <50 years old, and recurrent hernia repair as risk factors for the development of postoperative pain [18].

The type of mesh used does not appear to affect the incidence of chronic pain. Bittner et al. reported in 2011 their 1-year results of the use of four difference types of meshes: standard heavyweight mesh, pure middleweight polypropylene, lightweight composite polypropylene, and a titanized lightweight mesh. The end point of incidence of chronic pain at the end of 1 year was examined. Using the TAPP procedure in 600 patients, they found no difference in the rate of chronic pain regardless of the type of mesh used. However, use of the lighter-weight meshes appeared to improve the early postoperative period [19].

Recurrence

Recurrence rates after a laparoscopic TAPP inguinal hernia repair have been reported from 0 to 13%. When comparing laparoscopic to open hernia repair, many single-institution studies are too small to demonstrate statistical significance in terms of recurrence rates. Of the multicentered prospective studies, most demonstrate similar recurrence rates between TAPP and open repair with mesh. Even the much heralded VA study demonstrated similar recurrence rates when the TAPP repair was performed by an experienced surgeon [13]. Experience in the TAPP hernia repair remains a generally accepted requirement in order to achieve similar recurrence rates as observed with an open mesh repair. A study by Johansson et al. randomized 613 patients to TAPP, open preperitoneal hernia repair with mesh, or conventional repair. They report similar recurrence rates between laparoscopic and open inguinal hernia repair [15]. A prospective randomized controlled trial of laparoscopic TAPP versus open inguinal mesh repair was published by Douek et al. in 2003. A total of 403 patients were randomized to either an open repair under local anesthesia or a laparoscopic TAPP repair under general anesthesia. The patients were seen and assessed after a minimum of 5 years from the surgeon by an independent surgeon who was not involved in the original study. 65% of patients from the original study were reviewed, 120 open repair and 122 laparoscopic. Their follow-up showed no difference in the recurrence rate between the two groups [20]. In 2001, a 7-year two-center experience in laparoscopic TAPP was published in by Kapiris et al. They performed 3,530 TAPPs in 3,017 patients. Their overall recurrence rate was 22 recurrences or 0.62% with 17of the 22 being in the first 325 repairs performed prior to their change in technique of using a small mesh. With the change to a larger mesh, their recurrence rate was 0.16% [6]. Finally, the EU Hernia Trialists Collaboration performed a meta-analysis consisting of 41 trials. The results again confirmed the similar recurrence rates for TAPP versus open repair with mesh [16].

Overall, mesh size and surgeon experience remain the most important factors in maintaining similar recurrence rates between open and TAPP hernia repairs.

Mesh Infections

Mesh infection with laparoscopic inguinal hernia is rarely reported in the literature. Kapiris et al. reported four incidences of mesh infection in their large experience with TAPP repair for an overall total of 0.11%. In three of the patients, they were able to determine that the patient had a perioperative focus of infection. They reported having to remove the mesh in one patient laparoscopically, and in the other three, a groin abscess was drained. Of those patients, two did well afterward, and the third developed a groin sinus and eventually had the mesh removed in an open fashion [6]. In all patients with hernia repair, it is important to preoperatively evaluate for any sign of infection and treat appropriately prior to surgery to decrease the mesh infection rate.

TAPP Vs. TEP

There has long been a debate over the best laparoscopic inguinal hernia repair. Proponents of TAPP repair argue that TAPP provides a panoramic view of the myopectineal orifice in comparison to its surroundings and is superior to the narrow view provided during TEP repair.

TEP was advocated as an alternate to the TAPP since TEP did not require intraperitoneal violation and the inherent risk of bowel injury and trocar injury that may come with it [21]. Despite that view, there has only been one randomized controlled trial of TAPP vs. TEP inguinal hernia repair. This was a small study with only 52 patients within it, but it showed there was no difference between the two procedures in time to return to work, hernia recurrence, and complications [22].

With the use of a TEP repair, there is the chance that a surgeon may have to convert to a TAPP repair. In Misra's study of 185 patients who underwent a TEP repair at their center, 10.5% had to undergo a conversion to a TAPP or open repair. Reasons for conversion included peritoneal tearing, irreducible hernia, inadequate space, bleeding, and prolonged operating room time [23].

McCormick et al. performed a systematic review of TAPP vs. TEP articles to determine which method was associated with superior outcomes in terms of major complications including intra-abdominal injuries. While the review produced no prospective randomized studies demonstrating a difference in intra-abdominal injuries, several observational studies suggest an increase in intra-abdominal injuries during TAPP vs. TEP. However, given the rarity of these injuries, the clinical significance of this observation remains undetermined until examined by a sufficiently powered randomized controlled study [9].

TAPP Vs. Open for Recurrent Hernias

Controversy exists as to whether patient outcomes are better with a laparoscopic or open repair for a recurrent inguinal hernia. A meta-analysis of four randomized controlled trials comparing laparoscopic with open mesh repair of recurrent inguinal hernia showed no difference between laparoscopic and open repair in terms of recurrence or chronic pain. As secondary measures were evaluated, the analysis showed that laparoscopic repair whether TAPP or TEP had earlier return to daily activities and less immediate postoperative pain. However, the laparoscopic surgery was associated with increased operative times [24]. A prospective randomized trial by Mahon et al. comparing TAPP vs. open mesh repair for bilateral and recurrent inguinal hernias was not included in this meta-analysis due to the inability to analyze the recurrent hernia group separately. However, in reviewing the study by Mahon, the results are similar to that concluded by the meta-analysis. There was no difference between TAPP and open mesh repair in terms of recurrence. TAPP repair resulted in less postoperative and chronic pain and faster return to normal activities [25].

Cost

Assessing the cost of laparoscopic versus open inguinal hernia repair remains nebulous. The cost analysis changes depending on whether the patient, the surgeon, the hospital, or the employer's costs are considered. For example, the laparoscopic repair results in longer operating room times and often requires more disposable instrumentation than an open repair. This translates into higher hospital costs. From the surgeon's perspective, the extra time spent performing a repair laparoscopically decreases the time he or she has available to generate additional revenue through procedures or office visits. The extra time spent in the operating room during a laparoscopic repair is not rewarded financially by insurers enough to offset the loss in other revenue-producing activities. However, from the employer's standpoint, laparoscopic repairs offer a quicker return to work compared to open. The ability of an employee to return to work results in less cost to an employer. In addition, if an employee's time away from work is unpaid leave, then the longer recovery time is more costly to the employee.

In summary, determining the best hernia repair technique depends on the surgeon's experience as well as the patient's expectations and needs. The outcomes of the transabdominal preperitoneal repair remain similar or better than that of open repair. The key to maintaining equivalent or improved outcomes with TAPP compared to open remains the surgeon's experience with TAPP. Therefore, the surgeon should tailor his surgical approach based on his experience with laparoscopic hernia repair and on the unique clinical scenario for each patient.

References

1. SAGES patient information for laparoscopic inguinal hernia repair. http://www.sages.org/publication/id/PI06. Accessed 30 Aug 2011
2. Fitzgibbons R, Puri V. Invited Commentary-Laparoscopic inguinal hernia repair. Am Surg. 2006;72:197–208.
3. Rutkow IM. Demographic and socioeconomic aspects of hernia repair in the United States in 2003. Surg Clin North Am. 2003;83:1045–51.
4. Arregui ME, Davis CJ, Yucel O. Laparoscopic mesh repair of inguinal hernia using a preperitoneal approach: a preliminary report. Surg Laparosc Endosc. 1992;2:53–8.
5. Takata MC, Duh Q. Laparoscopic inguinal hernia repair. Surg Clin North Am. 2008;88:157–78.

6. Kapiris SA, Brough WA, Royston CMS, O'Boyle C, Sedman PC. Laparoscopic transabdominal preperitoneal TAPP hernia repair. A 7-year two-center experience in 3017 patients. Surg Endosc. 2001;15:972–5.
7. Kocot A, Gerharz EW, Riedmiller H. Urological complications of laparoscopic inguinal hernia repair: a case series. Hernia. 2011;15:583–6.
8. Hume RH, Bour J. Mesh migration following laparoscopic inguinal hernia repair. J Laparoendosc Surg. 1996;6(5):333–5.
9. McCormack K, Wake B, Perez J, et al. Laparoscopic surgery for inguinal hernia repair: systematic review of effectiveness and economic evaluation. Health Technol Assess. 2005;9(14):1–203.
10. Agrawal A, Avill R. Mesh migration following repair of inguinal hernia: a case report and review of literature. Hernia. 2006;10(1):79–82.
11. Shin D, Lipshultz LI, Goldstein M, et al. Herniorrhaphy with polypropylene mesh causing inguinal vasal obstruction. A preventable cause of obstructive azoospermia. Ann Surg. 2005;241(4):553–8.
12. Ming Do H, Turner K, Dietel A, Wedderburn A, Liatsikos E, Stolzenburg J. Previous Laparoscopic inguinal hernia repair does not adversely affect the functional of oncological outcome of endoscopic extraperitoneal radical prostatectomy. Urology. 2011;77:963–8.
13. Neumayer L, Giobbie-Hurder A, Jonasson O, et al. Open mesh versus laparoscopic mesh repair of inguinal hernia. New Engl J Med. 2004;350:1819–27.
14. Hawn MT, Itani KMF, Giobbie-Hurder A, et al. Patient reported outcomes after inguinal herniorrhaphy. Surgery. 2006;140:198–205.
15. Johansson B, Hallerback B, Glise H, et al. Laparoscopic mesh versus open preperitoneal mesh versus conventional technique for inguinal hernia repair: a randomized multicenter trial (SCUR Hernia Repair Study). Ann Surg. 1999;230(2):225–31.
16. Grant AM, EU Hernia Trialists Collaboration. Laparoscopic versus open groin hernia repair: meta-analysis of randomised trials based on individual patient data. Hernia. 2002;6(1):2–10.
17. The MRC Laparoscopic Groin Hernia Trial Group. Laparoscopic versus open repair of groin hernia: a randomized comparison. Lancet. 1999;354:185–90.
18. Dickinson KJ, Thomas M, Fawole AS, Lyndon PJ, White CM. Predicting chronic post-operative pain following laparoscopic inguinal hernia repair. Hernia. 2008;12(6):597–601.
19. Bittner R, Leibl BJ, Kraft B, Schwarz J. One year results of a prospective, randomized, clinical trial comparing four meshes in laparoscopic inguinal hernia repair (TAPP). Hernia. 2011;15:503–10.
20. Douek M, Smith G, Oshowo D, Stoker DL, Wellwood JM. Prospective randomized controlled trial of laparoscopic versus open inguinal hernia mesh repair: five year follow up. BMJ. 2003;326:1012–3.
21. Felix EL, Michas CA, Gonzalez MH. Laparoscopic hernioplasty: Tapp vs TEP. Surg Endosc. 1995;9:984–9.
22. Schrenk P, Woisetschlager R, Reiger R, Wayand W. Prospective randomised trial comparing postoperative pain and return to physical activity after transabdominal

preperitoneal, total preperitoneal or Shouldice technique for inguinal hernia. Br J Surg. 1996;83:1563–6.

23. Misra MC, Bansal VK, Kumar S, Prashant B, Bhattacharjee HK. Total extra-peritoneal repair of groin hernia: prospective evaluation at a tertiary care center. Hernia. 2008;12:65–71.
24. Karthikesalingam A, Markar SR, Holt PJE, Praseedom RK. Meta-analysis of randomized controlled trials comparing laparoscopic with open mesh repair of recurrent inguinal hernia. BJS. 2010;97(1):4–11.
25. Mahon D, Decadt B, Rhodes M. Prospective randomized trial of laparoscopic (transabdominal preperitoneal) vs open (mesh) repair for bilateral and recurrent inguinal hernia. Surg Endosc. 2003;17:1386–90.

12. Cord Structure Complications in Inguinal Hernia Surgery

Aaron M. Lipskar and Mark A. Reiner

Inguinal hernia surgery remains the most common elective general surgical procedure performed in the United States. It is a relatively safe operation, with worldwide morbidity averaging 6%, mortality 0.3%, and a recurrence rate in the range of less than 1–10%. Complications of inguinal herniorrhaphy can occur both intraoperatively and during the postoperative period. This chapter will focus on intraoperative cord structure complications in both open and laparoscopic inguinal herniorrhaphy. The focus of this chapter will be on male patients due to the relative inconsequences of cord injuries in female patients.

In order to understand and avoid cord complications, a thorough review of embryology and anatomy is first required.

Embryology

The gonads form from the mesoderm in the subserous fascia on either side of the vertebral column at the tenth thoracic level and are anchored by the gubernaculum, a suspensory ligament that ultimately anchors the testes to the scrotum. Beginning during the seventh week of gestation, the gubernaculum begins to shorten as the testes begin their descent. During gestation, the gonads begin a retroperitoneal or subserous descent, and if there is male differentiation, this descent continues into the scrotum. After the eighth gestational week, the processus vaginalis forms as a peritoneal evagination, pushing out extensions of the transversalis fascia, the internal oblique muscle, and the external oblique muscle. These fascial and muscular extensions ultimately form the inguinal canal. The everted transversalis fascia forms the deep or internal ring and eventually becomes the internal spermatic fascia. The everted external oblique muscle forms

B.P. Jacob and B. Ramshaw (eds.), *The SAGES Manual of Hernia Repair*, DOI 10.1007/978-1-4614-4824-2_12,

the superficial or external ring and eventually becomes the external spermatic fascia. The internal oblique muscle fibers and fascia develop into the cremasteric muscle fibers and fascia. By the 12th week of gestation, the intra-abdominal phase of gonadal descent is complete, and the testes can be found in the vicinity of the deep inguinal ring. The testes remain in this area until about the seventh month of gestation at which point the inguinal-scrotal phase of the gonadal descent through the processus vaginalis continues in response to further shortening of the gubernaculum and increased abdominal pressure by the growth of the abdominal viscera. Just around the time of normal term delivery, the testes normally have completely entered the scrotal sac, and the remains of the gubernaculum are a small ligamentous band attaching the testes to the scrotal floor. During the first year of life, the proximal end of the processus vaginalis usually obliterates, leaving only a distal remnant sac, known as the tunica vaginalis, which wraps around the testes and normally has a collapsed lumen.

The structures of the spermatic cord come together in their entirety just before the testes begin its final descent through the deep inguinal ring. The testes then drag a string of elongating vessels, nerves, and the vas deferens through the inguinal canal during the inguinal-scrotal phase of the descent. This embryologic journey is critical in understanding the anatomy of the spermatic cord structures and potential cord complications and methods to avoid them during inguinal hernia repair.

Anatomy

As the spermatic cord passes through the inguinal canal, it consists of the tunica vaginalis (the remnant of the processus vaginalis), vas deferens, the pampiniform venous plexus, three arteries with associated veins (testicular artery, deferential artery, and cremasteric artery), three nerves (ilioinguinal nerve, genital branch of the genitofemoral nerve, and sympathetic testicular nerve plexus), and lymphatics. The pampiniform plexus, vas deferens, deferential artery, testicular artery, testicular nerves, and the lymphatics are enveloped in the three layers of spermatic fascia (external spermatic fascia from the external oblique, cremasteric muscle and fascia from the internal oblique, and internal spermatic fascia from the transversalis fascia). The remaining structures course along the superficial surface of the external spermatic fascia.

Vas Deferens

The vas deferens, also known as the ductus deferens, originates from the fetal mesonephric ducts on the testes. During the embryologic time, the testes sit near the deep inguinal ring, and the seminal vesicles develop from the mesonephric ducts near the pelvic urethra. During the testes' final descent, the vas deferens assumes its anatomic course in the spermatic cord connecting the testes to the urethra, functioning to transport sperm from the testes to the urethra. Anatomically, the vas deferens courses cephalad from its insertion in the urethra and crosses the inferior epigastric arteries, eventually entering the spermatic cord inferomedially and coursing posteriorly through the inguinal canal and into the scrotum.

Pampiniform Venous Plexus

The pampiniform venous plexus can be found anteriorly to the vas deferens in the cord and is a network of many small spermatic veins and tributaries from the epididymis. This venous plexus forms the mass of the spermatic cord, and the small veins unite to form 3 to 4 larger veins at the level of the superficial inguinal ring. As they traverse the inguinal canal and enter the abdomen through the deep inguinal ring, they coalesce into first two and eventually one testicular vein ultimately emptying into either the vena cava on the right and renal vein on the left. This venous plexus functions as both venous return and temperature regulation.

Arteries

There are three arteries associated with the spermatic cord. The testicular artery originates from the abdominal aorta and courses obliquely and downward over the ureters until the level of the internal inguinal ring at which point it joins the other cord structures and traverses the inguinal canal. The testicular artery branches and becomes tortuous distally, which may have significant consequence if they are injured. The deferential artery (the artery to the vas deferens) usually arises from the anterior trunk of the superior vesicular artery. It then courses with the vas deferens through the inguinal canal, ultimately uniting with the testicular artery. The cremasteric artery is a branch of the inferior epigastric artery and runs with the spermatic cord but superficial to the spermatic fascia. It supplies the connective tissue of the cord structures and also eventually anastomoses with the testicular artery.

Nerves

There are two nerves that course through the inguinal canal and run superficial to the spermatic fascia. In addition, the sympathetic testicular nerve plexus runs within the spermatic cord. All of these structures are susceptible to injury during inguinal hernia repair. The ilioinguinal nerve arises from the first lumbar nerve and enters the inguinal canal between the internal and external oblique muscles and exits through the superficial inguinal ring, providing sensation to the skin of the upper and medial thigh as well as the penis and upper scrotum. The genital branch of the genitofemoral nerve arises from L1 to L2 and enters the inguinal canal just lateral to the inferior epigastric vessels and enters the inguinal canal either by piercing the transversalis fascia or passing through the deep inguinal ring. It then descends behind the spermatic cord, supplying both the scrotum and cremasteric muscle complex. The sympathetic testicular nerve plexus runs with the spermatic cord structures and innervates the testes.

The Posterior Perspective

Anatomy is most commonly reviewed from an anterior perspective, although one of the unique challenges of laparoscopy is that the cord structure is visualized from a posterior perspective. Whether an intraperitoneal or preperitoneal approach is utilized, the cord structure needs to be relearned from this point of view (Fig. 12.1). The spermatic cord structures can be found superior to the iliopubic tract when looking at the myopectineal orifice defined by the internal oblique muscle and transversus abdominis muscle superiorly, the iliopsoas muscle laterally, and the lateral edge of rectus abdominis and pubis pectin medially. Additionally, from the posterior perspective, there is an anatomic area commonly known as the *triangle of doom* that has been characterized in order to assist surgeons in avoiding cord complication or major vascular bleeding during laparoscopic inguinal hernia repair. The triangle of doom is formed by the vas deferens

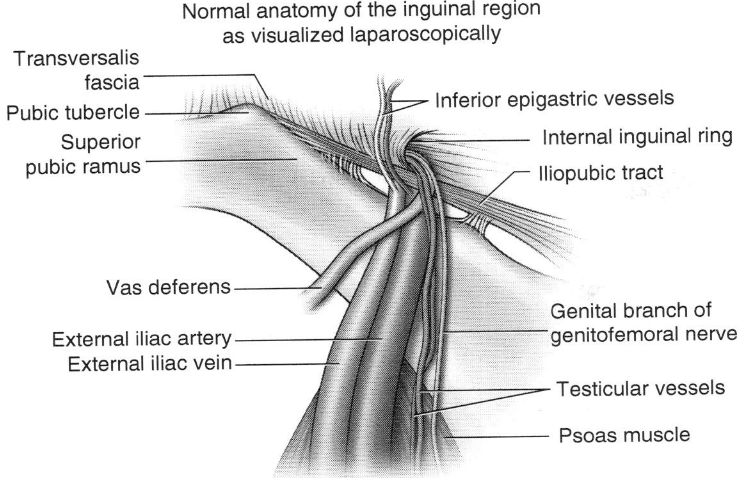

Fig. 12.1. Normal anatomy of the inguinal region as seen at laparoscopy.

medially and the vessels of cord laterally, with the apex pointing superiorly. This space contains the external iliac vessels, deep circumflex iliac vein, femoral nerve, and genital branch of the genitofemoral nerve.

Cord Complications

With a thorough understanding of the anatomy and physiology of the spermatic cord structures, the mechanism and clinical significance of cord structure injuries can be more easily appreciated. As aforementioned, there is no clinically significant effect to injury of the cord structures in a female patient other than nerve injuries, so this section will again focus on primarily male patients.

Complications of Spermatic Cord Injury

Ischemic Orchitis

Ischemic orchitis is best defined as postoperative inflammation of the testicle after inguinal hernia repair. This complication is significantly more common after open repairs. Clinically, ischemic orchitis usually presents 1–3 days following hernia repair as a painful, indurated, and swollen testicle, and it is often associated with a low-grade fever. It occurs in <1% of all hernia repairs, but the incidence increases to ~5% in recurrent hernia repairs due to scar formation. The etiology of ischemic orchitis is almost always due to injury of the pampiniform venous plexus rather than the testicular artery itself. It is most commonly caused by venous congestion of the testicle secondary to thrombosis of veins within the venous plexus and likely occurs during dissection of the hernia sac away from the cord structures. In addition, complete stripping of the cremasteric muscle fibers may cause injury to the pampiniform plexus as well. Testicular sonography will demonstrate decreased testicular blood flow and can aid in determining whether the testicle is simply ischemic or if it is necrotic. In the case of straightforward ischemia, treatment is nonoperative and involves reassurance and analgesia, as this condition usually improves by six weeks postoperative. There is some debate about the role of antibiotics in ischemic orchitis, but we do not routinely treat with antibiotics. Interestingly, testicular ultrasounds performed at 6 months postoperatively have been shown to show resolution of the flow abnormality in the vast majority of cases. Emergent orchiectomy is only necessary in the case of testicular necrosis, which would only be caused by significant injury to the venous plexus and/or the testicular artery.

Testicular Atrophy

Testicular atrophy can be best defined as shrinking of the testicle and associated dysfunction. The inciting injury is to the testicular artery rather than to the pampiniform plexus in cases of testicular atrophy. Testicular atrophy usually occurs over several months and is not always preceded by an immediate postoperative episode of testicular swelling. Whether ischemic orchitis will progress to testicular atrophy is impossible to determine. Testicular atrophy does not require emergent orchiectomy, but the consequences of an atrophic testicle are significant and irreversible, often requiring elective orchiectomy. The Shouldice clinic reported an incidence of testicular atrophy of 0.036% in primary open mesh-free repairs and 0.46% in recurrent hernia repairs. The incidence of testicular atrophy in laparoscopic repairs is quite small, although it has been reported.

Avoidance of these testicular complications is best accomplished by careful and minimal handling of the spermatic cord structures while dissecting the hernia sac. There does not appear to be a benefit of stripping the spermatic cord structures in either open or laparoscopic techniques, and leaving the cord intact should minimize the incidence of these complications.

Ductus (Vas) Deferens Injury

The vas deferens can be inadvertently injured during inguinal hernia repair by either transection or obstruction. Either of these etiologies can ultimately lead to infertility.

Complete transection of the vas deferens is a complication seen more often in open repairs as compared to laparoscopic repairs, as isolation of the vas deferens by digital manipulation is a standard part of the open procedure. This complication is far more common in recurrent hernia repairs due to scar tissue. Complete transection of the vas deferens remains rare, but when it does occur and if it is recognized, the vas deferens should be reanastomosed using 6.0 Prolene suture over a stent, preferably with a urology consult.

Obstruction of the vas deferens cannot only lead to infertility but also result in dysejaculation, an entity defined as pain or burning in the groin just before, during, or immediately after ejaculation. The incidence of dysejaculation syndrome has been quoted to be approximately 0.4%. The symptoms are usually self-limited. The etiology of the obstruction is thought to be crushing or scarring of the vas deferens, which can occur in both the open and laparoscopic approaches with rough instrumentation that causes fibrosis through the muscular wall of the vas deferens. Gentle and minimal handling of the cord structures in laparoscopic repairs and avoidance of using forceps or other instruments to handle the structures in open repairs can minimize the occurrence of this complication.

Testicular Ptosis

Testicular ptosis is a less significant complication defined as sagging of the testicle on the side of a previous inguinal hernia repair. Ptosis will routinely occur if the cord structures are skeletonized, and the cremasteric muscle fibers are divided, either in the open or laparoscopic approach. This complication can be avoided if the cremaster muscle is left intact or by fixing the medial stump of the muscle to the pubic tubercle, as done in the Shouldice technique.

Scrotal Hematoma

Due to the abundant vascularity of the spermatic cord, scrotal hematomas after inguinal hernia repairs are common due to excessive handling of the cord structures and slow bleeding from the vascular cord structures, with an overall incidence of ~5%. This complication is minor and can occur in both open and laparoscopic approaches. Patients present with scrotal swelling and ecchymotic discoloration.

These hematomas are self-limiting and almost always resorb spontaneously. Treatment is usually limited to elevation and tincture of time. Similar to other cord structure complications, this can be minimized with gentle handling of the spermatic cord.

Hydrocele Formation

Hydroceles have been reported to occur in 0.7% of patients after inguinal hernia repair and are thought to be caused by excessive skeletonization of the cord structures with a disruption of lymphatic drainage. Another theory is that an open distal hernia sac causes hydroceles. They are treated the same way primary hydroceles are treated.

Nerves

While not truly cord complications, nerve injuries remain a common problem following both open and laparoscopic hernia repairs, with incidences approaching 15–20%. Nerves can be injured by either transection, injury, or excess retraction. Complete nerve transection generally causes numbness but does not lead to neuralgias. Postoperative neuralgias can be grouped into those that cause symptoms within hours of awakening from anesthesia and those that cause chronic pain symptoms. Patients with acute neuropathic pain immediately after herniorrhaphy will often benefit from immediate reexploration. The mechanism of nerve injury is different depending on operative approach. Injury to the genital branch of the genitofemoral nerve and ilioinguinal nerve can occur during dissection of the cord in open hernia repairs, as these structures run external to the spermatic fascia but alongside the spermatic cord. Some authors therefore advocate the identification and ligation of these nerves with minimal residual effect in order to minimize these complications. In laparoscopic repairs, injury to the genitofemoral nerve usually occurs due to tacking the mesh improperly. A complete discussion of nerve injuries during herniorrhaphy is beyond the scope of this chapter.

Conclusions

Injury to the components of the spermatic cord structures remains one of the more common complications of hernia repair in male patients, sometimes causing severe long-term sequelae. Almost all of the complications can occur during either the open or laparoscopic approach, although most of the cord-specific complications are more common in open repairs and especially in open repairs of recurrent hernias. The best method of avoiding these injuries is obtaining a thorough knowledge of the embryology and anatomy of the inguinal canal and the spermatic cord, handling the tissues gently during the repair and avoiding overskeletonization of the cord.

Suggested Reading

1. Bendavid R. Complications of groin hernia surgery. Surg Clin North Am. 1998;78(6):1089–103.
2. Schoenwolf GC, Larsen WJ. Larsen's human embryology. 4th ed. Philadelphia, PA: Elsevier Livingstone; 2009. p. 525–30.
3. Sherman V, Macho JR, Brunicardi FC. Inguinal hernias, chapter 37. In: Brunicardi FC, Andersen DK, Billiar TR, Dunn DL, Hunter JG, Matthews JB, Pollock RE, editors. Schwartz's principles of surgery. 9th ed. New York: McGraw-Hill; 2010.
4. Shouldice EB. The Shouldice repair for groin hernias. Surg Clin North Am. 2003;83:1163–87.
5. Tetik C, Arregui ME, Dulucq JL, et al. Complications and recurrences associated with laparoscopic repair of groin hernias. Surg Endosc. 1994;8(11):1316–23.

13. Intraoperative Complications During Laparoscopic Hernia Repair

Davide Lomanto and Rajat Goel

Laparoscopic repair for inguinal hernia was first reported in the early 1990s by Ger, Schultz, Corbitt, and Filipi [1–4]. Today, the two most common laparoscopic hernia repairs are transabdominal preperitoneal repair (TAPP) and the total extraperitoneal repair (TEP). Both involve placement of a prosthetic mesh in the preperitoneal space to cover all potential hernia sites in the myopectineal orifice within the inguinal region. TAPP requires an incision in the peritoneum to access the preperitoneal space, where as in TEP, the dissection is done in the preperitoneal space itself. Both laparoscopic hernia techniques require full exposure of the myopectineal orifice, removal of excess preperitoneal fat and cord lipomas, complete assessment of all potential hernia sites, full reduction of direct hernia contents, evaluation to assess a femoral hernia component, complete dissection of the proximal indirect sac from the cord structures, and finally appropriate placement and judicious fixation of mesh in preperitoneal space.

The laparoscopic inguinal hernia repairs (TAPP and TEP) are looked upon as technically demanding procedures. They have a "learning curve," and complication rates have been shown to drop with increased surgical experience [5–7]. Proper training and supervision can shorten the learning curve and reduce the complications and recurrences [8]. The high-volume centers have reported comparable result outcomes, if not better, in terms of recurrence, chronic residual pain, and quality of life [8–10]. This definitely suggests that surgeons who complete the learning curve can deliver results that are not only acceptable but also impressive and significantly better than open repair in bilateral and recurrent inguinal hernias [9–12]. The improved outcomes can be attributed to assimilation of results of published literature and identifying factors that contribute to complications and failure of repair. It is important to critically analyze each of these factors and help postulate surgical techniques that would reap good surgical outcomes.

B.P. Jacob and B. Ramshaw (eds.), *The SAGES Manual of Hernia Repair*,
DOI 10.1007/978-1-4614-4824-2_13,

Table 13.1. Summary of intraoperative complications.

Related to laparoscopic technique	Related to laparoscopic hernia repair
Trocar injury to bowel and bladder[a]	Vascular injury: Femoral, epigastric, gonadal, iliac, and others
Subcutaneous emphysema	Nerve injury: Lateral femoral cutaneous, genitofemoral, ilioinguinal, iliohypogastric, and femoral
Cardiopulmonary complications related to hypercapnia	Visceral injury: Bladder and bowel
	Injury to cord structures: Vas deferens and gonadal vessels

[a]More common in TAPP

The complication rates for laparoscopic repair of inguinal hernia ranges from less than 3% to as high as 20%. [6, 13–15]. A summary of the complications specifically related to TAPP and TEP can be found in Table 13.1.

Laparoscopic Inguinal Complications

Noteworthy *intraoperative complications* specific to laparoscopic inguinal repair are:

Vascular Injury

- This can involve the iliac vessels, femoral vessels, inferior epigastric vessels, gonadal vessels, muscular branches, vessels over the pubic arch (including "corona mortis" vein), or other vessels in the region.

Visceral Injury

- *Bowel injuries* can occur with trocar entry, or during the course of dissection in large irreducible hernias, sliding hernias, or with the use of electrodiathermy. The incidence of bowel injuries is greatly reduced, but not completely eliminated, with TEP as compared to TAPP repair.
- *Urinary tract injuries* are reported in laparoscopic inguinal hernia repair. These include bladder injuries and rarely even urethral rupture.

Nerve Injuries.

The myopectineal orifice of Fruchaud has several nerves coursing in it, viz., ilioinguinal nerve, iliohypogastric nerve, genitofemoral nerve with its medial genital (external spermatic nerve) and lateral femoral (lumboinguinal nerve) branches, femoral nerve, and lateral femoral cutaneous nerve. All these are prone to injury, either during lateral dissection or during mesh fixation. It can result in long-term pain and discomfort [16].

Injury to Cord Structures.

The vas deferens can be damaged or transected, as can the gonadal vessels during the course of dissection.

Complications can occur at every step of the operation even though some of them are occasionally reported. However, it is important to analyze all of them chronologically, so that we can define methods to prevent them, or tackle them once they occur.

Risk Reduction Strategy

A risk reduction strategy is required to improve the clinical outcome of laparoscopic hernia repair, and this must be adopted during the following surgical steps:

1. Placement of the first trocar
2. Placement of the working port
3. Dissection of the preperitoneal space
4. Dissection of the hernia sac
5. Mesh placement and fixation
6. Closure of the port

Placement of the First Trocar

Since the TEP repair involves a preperitoneal placement of a trocar, injuries that can be avoided during the first trocar placement during a laparoscopic inguinal hernia repair are limited to those found during a TAPP inguinal hernia repair. Most, if not all, of these injuries that are expected from the first trocar entry can be attributed to a sharp instrument like a Veress needle or sharp trocar entering the peritoneal cavity and causing potentially vascular or visceral injury [13, 14]. This type of injury

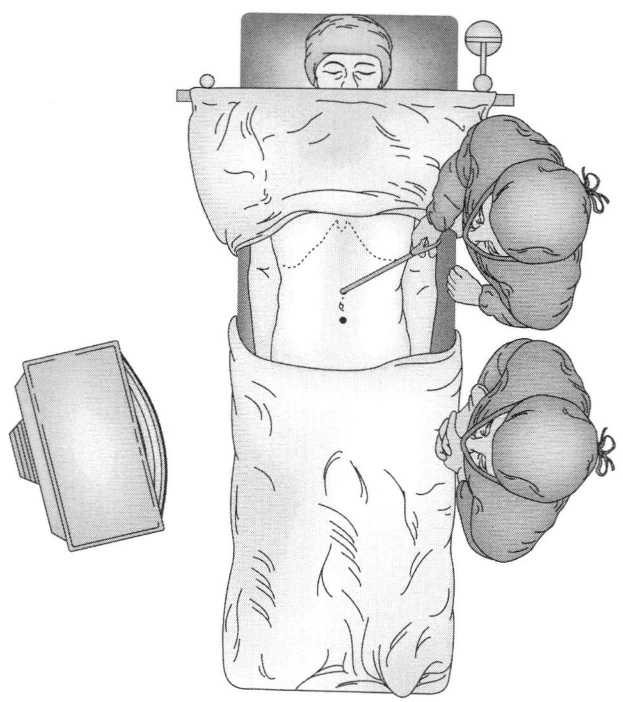

Fig. 13.1. OT setup for right-sided hernia repair.

is not common in a TEP repair in which the preperitoneal space is entered under direct vision and a preperitoneal domain is maintained during the procedure. The surgeon stands on the opposite side of hernia, and the camera setup is on the same side of the hernia on the foot end of the patient (Fig. 13.1). Few authors [17] advocate the use of Veress needle or blind trocar entry in the suprapubic area to create the space, as this maneuver can lead to an inadvertent injury of the bladder or bowel and is simply avoidable with other techniques. Veress needle is also contraindicated when the patient has had a previous laparotomy (especially with an infraumbilical midline incision) as previous incisions often result in scarring with distortion of tissue planes and visceral adhesions to the anterior abdominal wall. Consequently, injury can be minimized by judiciously using an open-entry technique in an area distant from the previous incision. Open entry under direct vision certainly does not eliminate visceral or vascular injury, but its use is certainly more logical in those situations and has been shown to minimize risks.

We strongly recommend an open-entry method for both TAPP and TEP repair, where the skin is incised and subcutaneous fat dissected to bare the anterior rectus sheath. The fascia is then incised and rectus muscle fibers split to expose the posterior rectus sheath, which is then incised in TAPP to introduce the Hasson's trocar under vision and held in place with stay sutures where as in TEP, this preperitoneal plane is maintained and a space is created inferiorly toward the pubic symphysis, using gauze, finger, or balloon specially designed for this purpose. A Hasson's trocar is then introduced in this plane and optics introduced to confirm the plane which is subsequently insufflated with carbon dioxide gas at 8–10 mmHg.

During this step, in TEP repair, the posterior rectus sheath can be inadvertently breached along with the peritoneum which can result in pneumoperitoneum. This pneumoperitoneum can have a pressure effect on the anterior abdominal wall, thereby minimizing the operating space and making further dissection difficult. It is important to identify and repair these tears early to facilitate smooth surgery. In case of previous surgical scarring, extra caution and vigilance is required at every step [18]. In select cases, it may be safer to opt for elective open repair.

Placement of Working Trocars

Two working trocars of 5 mm each is all that is required for the laparoscopic hernia repair in addition to a 10-mm infraumbilical trocar for the camera. These two trocars are usually placed in the midline, one-third and two-thirds (3 fingerbreadths above pubic symphysis) approximately the distance from the umbilicus to pubic symphysis, respectively, in TEP repair (Fig. 13.1), and lateral to rectus sheath approximately on either side, approximately one fingerbreadth below the umbilicus in case of TAPP. The placement of lower trocar 3 fingerbreadths above pubic symphysis in TEP not only helps in prevention of bladder injury but also helps in complete and proper placement of the mesh. Bladder injury can also be prevented by asking patient to void just before being transferred to operation theater and elective catheterization in case of bilateral and large hernias. All trocars must be introduced under direct vision, taking care not to thrust the sharp tip into the bladder, peritoneum, or underlying bowel. The inferior epigastric vessels must be avoided especially if the trocars are not inserted along the midline. These vessels can bleed significantly if damaged (Fig. 13.2). Direct pressure tamponade or electrodiathermy is usually sufficient, or the vessel can be clipped

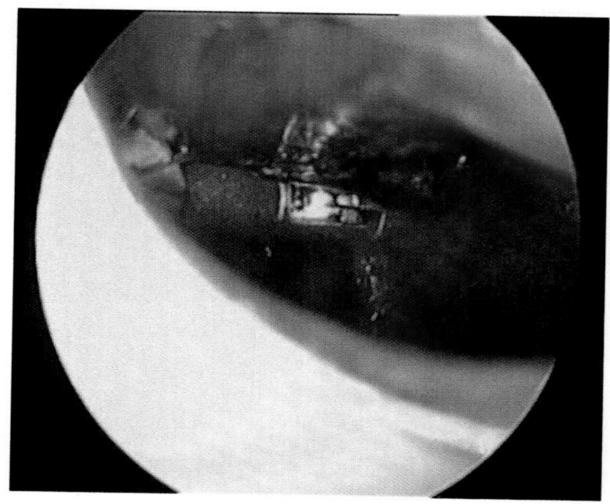

Fig. 13.2 Injury to inferior epigastric vessel.

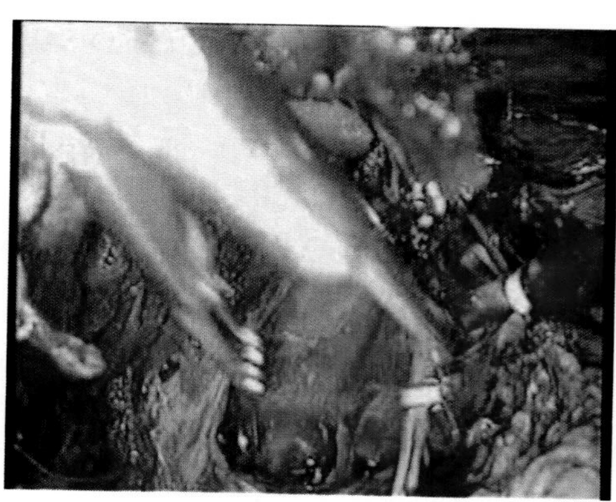

Fig. 13.3 Clipping of inferior epigastric with Hemolock.

with hemolock (Fig. 13.3). Rarely, a transfascial or intracorporeal suture may be necessary. Peritoneal tears are discussed vide infra. Any visceral injury at this stage may require immediate conversion to a laparotomy.

Dissection of the Preperitoneal Space

In TAPP repair, a transverse incision is made from the medial umbilical ligament extending laterally till the anterior superior iliac spine just above the internal ring, and preperitoneal flaps are created, where as dissection of the preperitoneal space in TEP repair is done either with special balloon dissectors mentioned earlier or with blunt dissection using the telescope and the two working trocars. The space must be clearly defined, starting with the pubic arch and symphysis in the midline. The bladder should be gently dissected off the pubis and rectus muscle superolaterally. During the dissection of the bladder from the rectus muscle and pubic symphysis, difficulty may be encountered if the patient has undergone previous surgery involving the prevesical space of Retzius (e.g., previous TEP, prostate surgery). The bladder is particularly vulnerable when it makes up part of the direct sac and also if dissection is carried beyond medial umbilical ligament in case of TAPP repair. Adhesions in this plane can result in bladder injury. It is important for such procedures to be carried out by experienced surgeons with gentle and meticulous dissection, minimizing the use of electrodiathermy. Once injured, it is important to identify the injury on table. The presence of urine in the dissection plane or a sudden decompression of a distended bladder should arouse suspicion. The bladder tear should be sutured in two layers with absorbable material, using additional ports if necessary. The temptation to Endoloop such tears should be resisted. The bladder should be decompressed postoperatively with a urinary catheter. It is helpful to preoperatively catheterize patients undergoing bilateral repair or those in which a lengthy procedure is anticipated, on account of large hernial sacs, irreducibility, previous surgical scarring, or in the early stage of TEP learning curve. Complex bladder injuries, including urethral tears will, more often than not, require laparotomy and urological repair. If a bladder injury is encountered, it is strongly recommended to avoid mesh insertion and therefore prudent to stage the hernia repair using a different method after the patient recovers from the bladder repair.

The medial dissection is done in the zone between the inferior epigastric vessels on either side, allowing adequate contralateral dissection. The ipsilateral set of inferior epigastric vessels is reflected upward (anteriorly) with the help of one 5-mm blunt dissector, while the other dissector opens up the plane laterally. Bleeding from these vessels has been discussed vide supra. The area bound by the vas deferens superomedially and gonadal vessels superolaterally constitutes the so-called triangle of doom. It houses the common iliac vessels. All dissection must stay clear of this zone and be carried out superior to it. Injury to these vessels can be fatal and usually involves laparotomy and vascular repair.

The lateral dissection (Bogros' space) is done beyond the anterior superior iliac spine, all the way up to the psoas muscle inferolaterally, thereby exposing the nerves in the so-called lateral triangle of pain. The musculopectineal orifice of Fruchaud has several nerves coursing it.

These include ilioinguinal nerve, iliohypogastric nerve, genitofemoral nerve with its medial genital (external spermatic nerve) and lateral femoral (lumboinguinal nerve) branches, femoral nerve, and lateral femoral cutaneous nerve. Injury to the nerves at this point can result in postoperative discomfort and chronic groin pain. If an injury occurs inadvertently, the nerve should be infiltrated with a local anesthetic. This, however, does not ensure uneventful sequelae. The only effective management of these nerve injuries is their prevention. Peritoneal tears can also occur during this dissection. Its consequences and management are discussed vide infra.

Dissection of Hernial Sac

This is a vital step of the procedure. It is important to identify all potential hernial sacs in the myopectineal orifice. Failure to recognize a complex hernia intraoperatively accounts for approximately 15% of failed repairs [5, 19]. The iliopubic tract must be completely bared. The thinned out transversalis fascia (commonly referred to the pseudosac) and the peritoneum should be delineated fully, identifying any indirect and direct components to the hernia. A rational blend of predominantly blunt and minimal sharp dissection must be carried out, with sparing use of electrodiathermy. An indirect sac must be carefully separated from the spermatic cord and its contents. If a lipoma is identified accompanying the cord, it must be meticulously dissected out to prevent any recurrence. A sliding hernia or a fully or partially irreducible hernial sac can predispose to visceral injury. Bowel injury merits laparotomy in most cases. The hernia repair may be deferred depending on the amount of contamination. Whenever there is spillage of bowel contents, we recommend laparotomy and repair of bowel only in the primary sitting. The mesh repair should be deferred for another day, after an appropriate interval and recovery.

If the indirect sac is long or complete, it is often wise to circumcise and ligate (using a premade nonabsorbable loop) the sac in the inguinal canal. The distal end must be left open to avoid a hydrocele. Unnecessary dissection can result in lymphatic destruction with seroma or formation, or even bleeding intraoperatively with subsequent hematoma formation in the postoperative period. The seroma or hematoma can occur in the groin, or go down to the scrotum. Extensive cord dissection should be supplemented with a good scrotal compressive dressing in the early postoperative period. Seromas are common after some laparoscopic

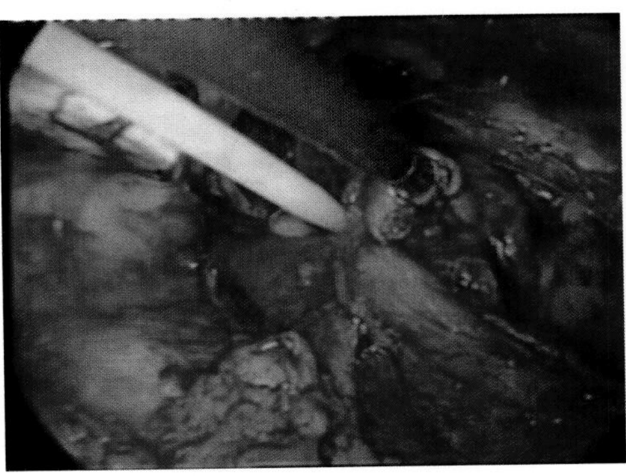
Fig. 13.4 Use of Endoloop for peritoneal tear closure.

inguinal hernia repairs, and while it is not possible to eliminate their occurrence completely, a forewarned patient is forearmed and all patients should be told in advance about them. Seromas should be left untouched as almost 100% of them, even the very large ones, will eventually reabsorb within the first 3–6 months.

Rough handling of the cord structures can also cause bleeding from the testicular and cremasteric vessels. This can also preclude to hematoma formation and potential orchitis or testicular atrophy. Firm pressure usually controls this bleed, and diathermy is sparingly used. The vas deferens can be inadvertently transected during dissection of the cord structures. Unilateral injury may not have any consequence. If recognized, especially in fertile-aged men, all attempts must be made to repair it with an end-to-end anastomosis, with a conversion to open surgery if required. In the elderly, it can be safely ligated or clipped in situ.

Any breech in the peritoneum, including the indirect sac or pseudosac should be avoided at this stage. If a tear does occur, it results in escape of insufflated gas to the intraperitoneal cavity. This not only affects the respiratory dynamics but also results in loss of working domain, making further dissection difficult and possibly dangerous. Pneumoperitoneum can also precipitate postoperative ileus. All such tears should be closed, usually with a vicryl or chromic catgut Endoloop (Fig. 13.4). Larger tears may need multiple nonabsorbable loops or intracorporeal sutures. At times, the pneumoperitoneum may warrant the placement of a Veress needle in the left subcostal position (Palmer's point) to deflate the gas and restore the domain. A missed tear can result in omental or intestinal herniation [20] through the defect, with potential intestinal obstruction, incarceration, strangulation, and delayed fistulization.

Mesh Placement and Fixation

Ample dissection in the extraperitoneal space allows proper placement of an appropriate mesh in a laparoscopic inguinal hernia repair. The choice of mesh may vary, but commonly used is the flat polypropylene mesh. Variants of this mesh, with less content of polypropylene or with partially absorbable components, are also being used, with the rationale of light weight, large pores (less foreign body reaction), better handling, and better long-term comfort. The flat mesh used should be at least 15 cm in width and 10–12 cm in height to cover the entire myopectineal orifice. The correct size of the mesh is important to prevent a late recurrence due to an eventual "shrinkage" of the prosthesis [21]. This necessitates adequate dissection to allow the mesh to fit in, without folding or rolling at the edges.

Irrespective of the prosthesis used, all meshes should be opened and handled with upmost aseptic care, with change of gloves before handling the mesh. They should be delivered in the space through an appropriately sized trocar (usually 10–12 mm), ideally through a reducer sleeve, to avoid any fraying or damage to the mesh. Slitting of the mesh is discouraged, as it is a potential space for recurrences, as reported in the early series of the laparoscopic repair.

While selecting the mesh type and size, it is important to define the hernial defect. The mesh should cover all potential hernial sites apart from the defined defect. This includes the direct hernia in the Hesselbach's triangle, indirect hernia lateral to the inferior epigastric vessels and along the inguinal canal, femoral hernia in the femoral canal inferior to the Cooper's ligament, and obturator hernia in the obturator canal.

A flat mesh in the preperitoneal space is in constant danger of being displaced by intra-abdominal forces, before the fibrosis and scarring allows it to be incorporated as part of the posterior wall of the inguinal canal. During this period, inadequate mesh fixation can result in recurrence. The medial edge of the mesh is particularly prone to being displaced more than the lateral edge. When this displacement is enough to expose the medial part of the inguinal canal, including the Hesselbach's triangle, a recurrence is inevitable. This highlights the need to maintain the mesh in position. Perhaps, the commonest method advocated today is to use an anchorage device like tacks or staples to fix the mesh. It is important to have a good positioning of these anchorage devices, viz., Cooper's ligament, superior and medial to the direct defect so that the mesh overlaps the defect by 4 cm. It is strongly recommended to avoid

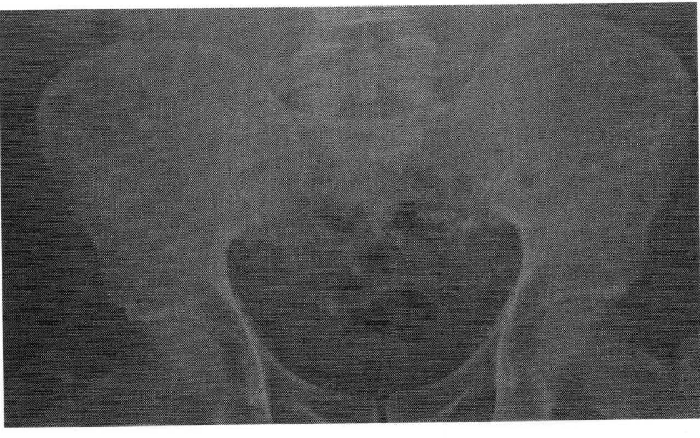

Fig. 13.5 Plain X-ray film of a patient after bilateral TEP hernia repair complaining of postoperative chronic pain.

any tacks or staples below the iliopubic tract, especially avoiding the triangles of doom and pain. No lateral fixation is advocated to avoid inadvertent damage to the nerves (Fig. 13.5). If a nerve is accidentally injured and this is identified on table, the anchorage device should be removed and a local anesthetic infiltrated in the region. Misplaced staple devices can also account for nerve irritation and injury. Postoperative pain and paresthesias can be a menace and haunt both the patient and the surgeon, with no cure guaranteed even with the utmost of corrective measures.

Several studies have recommended no fixation, but have been found wanting [22, 23]. Tissue glues are being used to fix the mesh in place, with encouraging early results [24]. Suturing of the mesh has also been described but requires expertise. Alternatively, anatomical meshes have also been designed for this purpose, which do not require any additional fixation. They conform to the space by virtue of their shape and prevent the mesh from migrating [25]. Self-gripping mesh materials are emerging and may be beneficial and have recently been shown to be safe and effective for all inguinal hernia types by Jacob et al. [26].

Despite the product type, it is clear that proper anatomic dissection and subsequent mesh placement is required to minimize recurrence. The medial edge of the mesh should extend to the midline, and if a bilateral hernia repair is performed, the two mesh pieces should be large enough that the mesh overlap at the midline. This is necessary to minimize recurrences, especially in larger direct hernia defect patients.

Closure of the Port

After the mesh is appropriately placed and fixed, the operating field should be examined to rule out mesh displacement or folding. All hernial sacs and peritoneal folds must be defined. The mesh must be tucked inferior to the pseudosac and peritoneum and the indirect sac must be posterior to the mesh. Peritoneal tears must be looked for and dealt with appropriately, as mentioned earlier. It is strongly advocated to desufflate, wait a few minutes, and then re-insufflate to observe the mesh placement and more importantly to confirm hemostasis. Working trocars should be removed under vision to rule out bleeding from the rectus muscle or vessels in the abdominal wall. Hemostasis must be achieved. The anterior rectus sheath (fascia) should be closed under direct vision. In case of TAPP repair, the camera port site is closed with 2/0 absorbable suture like vicryl to prevent postoperative port site hernias as reported in other laparoscopic procedures [27, 28]. Scrotal or groin compression should be given, if necessary.

Conclusion

Laparoscopic inguinal hernia repairs, TAPP and TEP, are technically demanding procedures due to unfamiliar anatomy and are prone to complications for the beginners. They have a stiff learning curve. Good surgical technique, at every step of the procedure, can be mastered with time. Once the learning curve is through, satisfactory outcomes can be delivered with results comparable and even better than conventional repair. It is important for surgeons in the learning curve to be cautious and ideally supervised by experts so that potentially fatal complications do not put the procedure in disrepute.

References

1. Ger R. The laparoscopic management of groin hernias. Contemp Surg. 1991;39:15–9.
2. Schultz L, Graber J, Pietrafitta J, et al. Laser laparoscopic herniorrhaphy: a clinical trial, preliminary results. J Laparoedosc Surg. 1990;1:41–5.
3. Corbitt J. Laparoscopic herniorrhaphy. Surg Laparosc Endosc. 1991;1:23–5.

4. Filipi C, Fitzgibbons RJ, Salerno GM, et al. Laparoscopic herniorrhaphy. Surg Clin North Am. 1992;72:1109–24.
5. Felix EL, Michas CA, Gonzalez MH. Laparoscopic hernioplasty: why does it work? Surg Endosc. 1997;11:36–41.
6. Frankum CE, Ramshaw BJ, White J, et al. Laparoscopic repair of bilateral and recurrent hernias. Am Surg. 1999;65:839–42.
7. Wright G, O'Dwyer PJ. The learning curve for laparoscopic hernia repair. Semin Laparosc Surg. 1998;5:227–32.
8. Cheah WK, So JBY, Lomanto D. Endoscopic extraperitoneal inguinal hernia repair: a series of 182 repairs. Singapore Med J. 2004;45:267–70.
9. Johansson B, Hallerback B, Glise H, Anesten B, Smedberg S, Roman J. Laparoscopic mesh versus open preperitoneal mesh versus conventional technique for inguinal hernia repair: a randomized multicenter trial (SCUR Hernia Repair Study). Ann Surg. 1999;2:225–31.
10. Liem MS, van der Graaf Y, van Steensel CJ, Boelhouwer RU, Clevers GJ, Meijer WS, Stassen LP, Vente JP, Weidema WF, Schrijvers AJ, van Vroonhoven TJ. Comparison of conventional anterior surgery and laparoscopic surgery for inguinal-hernia repair. N Engl J Med. 1997;22:1541–7.
11. Memon MA, Cooper NJ, Memon B, Memon MI, Abrams KR. Meta-analysis of randomized clinical trials comparing open and laparoscopic inguinal hernia repair. Br J Surg. 2003;12:1479–92.
12. Macintyre IM. Best practice in groin hernia repair. Br J Surg. 2003;2:131–2.
13. Felix E, Habertson N, Varteian S. Laparoscopic hernioplasty: surgical complications. Surg Endosc. 1999;13:328–31.
14. Tetik C, Arregui M, Dulucq J, et al. Complications and recurrences with laparoscopic repair of groin hernias. A multi-institutional retrospective analysis. Surg Endosc. 1994;8:1316–23.
15. Davis CJ, Arregui ME. Laparoscopic repair for groin hernias. Surg Clin N Am. 2003;83:1141–61.
16. Kraus MA. Nerve injury during laparoscopic inguinal hernia repair. Surg Laparosc Endosc. 1993;4:342–5.
17. Dulucq JL. Pre-peritoneal approach in laparoscopic treatment of inguinal hernia. J Chir. 2000;137:285–8.
18. Dulucq JL, Wintringer P, Mahajna A. Totally extraperitoneal (TEP) hernia repair after radical prostatectomy or previous lower abdominal surgery: is it safe? A prospective study. Surg Endosc. 2006;20:473–6.
19. Ryan E. Recurrent hernias: an analysis of 369 consecutive cases of recurrent inguinal and femoral hernias. Surg Gynecol Obstet. 1953;96:343–54.
20. Azurin D, Schuricht A, Stoldt H, Kirkland M, Paskin D, Bar A. Small bowel obstruction following endoscopic extraperitoneal-preperitoneal herniorrhaphy. J Laparoendosc Surg. 1995;5:263–6.
21. Schumpelick V, Klinge U, Welty G, Klosterhalfen B. Meshes within the abdominal wall. Chirurg. 1999;70:876–87.
22. Ferzli GS, Frezza EE, Pecoraro Jr AM, Ahem KD. Prospective randomized study of stapled versus unstapled mesh in laparoscopic preperitoneal inguinal hernia repair. J Am Coll Surg. 1999;5:461–5.

23. Smith AI, Royston CM, Sedman PC. Stapled and nonstapled laparoscopic transabdominal preperitoneal (TAPP) inguinal hernia repair: a prospective randomized trial. Surg Endosc. 1999;8:804–6.
24. Surendra M, Katara A, Cheah WK, Lomanto D. RCT on use of fibrin glue vs stapler fixation in totally endoscopic preperitoneal hernia repair. 93rd congress of the American College of Surgeons, New Orleans 7–11 Oct 2007. Awarded for "Excellence paper of merit"
25. Cu WG, Katara AN, Domino JP, Wong HB, So JB, Lomanto D, Cheah WK. Comparison between anatomic polyesther (Parietex) mesh and polypropylene (Prolene) mesh with fixation in totally endoscopic extraperitoneal inguinal hernia repair. Asian J Endosc Surg. 2010;3:137–9.
26. Laxa B, Reiner M, Jacob BP. Self-gripping mesh for laparoscopic TEP inguinal hernia repair. Interim Results of an Ongoing Prospective Study. AHS Poster and Abstract. 2012
27. Bunting DM. Port-site hernia following laparoscopic cholecystectomy. JSLS. 2010;14:490–7.
28. Owens M, Barry M, Janjua AZ, Winter DC. A systematic review of laparoscopic port site hernias in gastrointestinal surgery. Surgeon. 2011;9:218–24.

14. Urinary Retention After Laparoscopic Inguinal Hernia Repair

David A. McClusky III

Postoperative urinary retention (POUR) has been defined as the inability to void in the presence of a full bladder. A single episode of prolonged retention can lead to bladder overfilling and detrusor damage while increasing the risk of bladder dysmotility or even long-term atony. Treating this condition requires bladder catheterization, with the potential for significant discomfort, urethral trauma, stricture, and catheter-based infection [1]. Urethral catheterization delays hospital discharge and increases the costs of care after inguinal hernia repair [2]. Given its impact, it is imperative that minimally invasive surgeons understand the etiology, potential prevention, and treatment of postoperative urinary retention.

Incidence

POUR most frequently occurs after anorectal, spine, and gynecologic surgery involving the pelvis. It is a known complication after both open and laparoscopic inguinal hernia repair with an incidence ranging between 0.2% and 30% [3]. Such a large range is rarely informative, particularly when attempting to establish benchmarks for performance. Deciphering the impact of single-center studies using a small cohort (where a relatively low occurrence rate can erroneously translate into a large incidence) and in studies where POUR is ill defined can be challenging. Prospective randomized trials and larger retrospective reports that are less susceptible to overestimation can be helpful in this regard (Tables 14.1 and 14.2).

Among the 13 single and multicenter randomized controlled trials listed in Table 14.1, the incidence of urinary retention ranges between

B.P. Jacob and B. Ramshaw (eds.), *The SAGES Manual of Hernia Repair*, DOI 10.1007/978-1-4614-4824-2_14,

Table 14.1. POUR incidence within randomized controlled trials comparing laparoscopic inguinal hernia repair and open inguinal hernia repair.

Investigator	Year	Technique(s)	# Patients	Laparoscopic POUR (%)	Open POUR
Fitzgibbons [21]	1995	TEP/TAPP	686	5.8	[a]
Wright [34]	1996	TEP	60	2	2%
Liem [35]	1997	TEP	482	1	0.4%
Wellwood [36]	1998	TAPP	200	7	3%
Johansson [5]	1999	TAPP	200	2	1.5%
MRC group [6]	1999	TEP/TAPP	352	2.8	2%
Andersson [37]	2003	TEP	81	5.2	2.3%
Bringman [38]	2003	TEP	92	2.2	0%
Neumeyer [7]	2004	TEP/TAPP	989	2.8	2.2%
Winslow [24]	2004	TEP	147	7.9	1.1%
Eklund [4]	2006	TEP	665	4.2	7.5%
Pokorny [23]	2008	TEP/TAPP	119	5	1.8%
Langeveld [39]	2010	TEP	323	1.9	0.3%
Gong [22]	2011	TEP/TAPP	102	6.8	3.2%

[a]This trial was a multicenter trial comparing differing approaches to laparoscopic inguinal hernia repair

Table 14.2. POUR incidence within single-center retrospective reviews of laparoscopic inguinal hernia repair experience.

Investigator	Year	Technique(s)	# Patients	POUR incidence (%)
Ramshaw [40]	1996	TEP	167	2.5
Ramshaw [40]	1996	TAPP	244	5.7
Aeberhard [8]	1999	TEP	1,605	3.1
Moreno-Egea [41]	2000	TEP	131	2.3
Kapiris [10]	2001	TAPP	3,530	2
Ramshaw [28]	2001	TEP/TAPP	955	3.4
Lau [18]	2002	TEP	120	3.3
Garg [42]	2009	TEP	929	5.3
Dulucq [9]	2009	TEP/TAPP	2,356	0.2
Swadia [11]	2011	TEP	1,042	0.38

1% and 7.9%. The highest incidence in those studies including >300 patients in the laparoscopic group is 4.2% [4]. The three multicenter trials report an incidence between 2% and 2.8% [5–7]. The incidence among the group of centers reporting their experience on greater than 500 patients ranges from 0.2% to 5.8% (Table 14.2). POUR rates are consistently less than 3% in series involving over 1,000 patients published after the year 2000 [8–11]. Taking this number in consideration with the incidence noted in the multicenter randomized controls listed above, 2–3% is arguably a reasonable target for performance benchmarks.

Bladder Anatomy and Physiology

Within the lower urinary tract, the bladder can be viewed as a dynamic receptacle for urine that is equipped to both store and empty its contents. It is sufficiently compliant that it can accommodate a socially acceptable volume of urine (normally around 300 mL), with the capability of sending a signal when that volume has been reached. The individual smooth muscles of the bladder detrusor are small spindle-shaped cells with a central nucleus. Smooth muscle within the detrusor lacks the ability to form a fused tetanic contraction—unlike smooth muscle within the GI tract or uterus. This suggests there is poor electrical coupling between cells and prevents synchronous activation of cells during active stretching during urine storage. This is also why contraction of the bladder during micturition requires stimulation by external signals coordinated by a complex neural network. Pharmacologic agents that effect smooth muscle contraction, such as calcium antagonists, and potassium channel agonists have a direct effect on bladder emptying.

Neural control of the lower urinary tract involves integration of three sets of peripheral nerves involving the parasympathetic, sympathetic, and somatic nervous systems. These processes involve afferent activity from myelinated Aδ and unmyelinated C nerves located within the smooth muscle of the detrusor wall and the bladder mucosa with the capability of sensing bladder distention and responding to nociceptive signals. These signals transmit information through the pelvic, hypogastric, and pudendal nerves to the lumbosacral spinal cord to be further processed within the pontine micturition center and the CNS. Centralized input controls both the sympathetic and parasympathetic pathways.

Sympathetic activity induces relaxation of the bladder and contraction of the bladder outlet and urethra. Parasympathetic stimulation induces bladder contraction and relaxation of the external sphincter. Drugs that alter the awareness of bladder sensation (e.g., anesthetic agents) and factors that decrease afferent signaling (including nocioceptive stimuli from the pelvis, bladder, and rectum) can potentially alter micturition reflexes significantly.

Risk Factors

Patient-Specific Factors

A number of studies have identified patients at increased risk for POUR based on preexisting comorbidities. Concurrent neurological disorders that decrease bladder sensation and micturition reflex activities include stroke, polio, cerebral palsy, multiple sclerosis, pathologic lesions in the spine, and neuropathy associated with diabetes or alcohol [12].

The impact of age and gender is controversial. Several studies evaluating POUR in surgical patients, particularly after anorectal surgery, have reported a higher incidence of POUR in men [13, 14] and in patients over age 50 [15]. Age-related progressive neural degeneration and gender-specific pathologies such as benign prostatic hypertrophy may contribute to these increased risks [12, 15–17]. These results, however, have not been widely replicated in the surgical literature, and none have utilized multivariate regression to determine whether age and gender are independent risks [18, 19]. Additionally, no demographic risk factors have been identified in trials evaluating POUR after laparoscopic inguinal hernia repair [18, 20].

Anesthesia

Petros reported a 19% incidence of POUR in patients receiving general anesthesia during open inguinal hernia repair [17]. As noted above, a large number of pharmacologic agents, particularly those used during anesthesia, impact bladder contractility and decrease micturition reflex activity. General anesthesia affects bladder function either by direct action on the detrusor muscle, through inhibition of the autonomic nervous system within the spine and the pontine micturition center, and by decreasing voluntary bladder control within the central nervous system. Specifically, diazepam, pentobarbital, and propofol have been shown to decrease detrusor contraction, while isoflurane, methoxyflurane, and halothane suppress detrusor contraction [15].

Technical Considerations

There are no significant differences in POUR rates when comparing open and laparoscopic inguinal hernia repair among the larger randomized controlled trials designed to study this topic (Table 14.1). Further, when considering the different laparoscopic approaches, Dulucq, Fitzgibbons, Pokorny, and Gong all independently noted that no differences existed between the TEP and TAPP repairs [9, 21–23]. This would suggest that technique rarely factors into the development of POUR after laparoscopic inguinal herniorrhaphy.

Winslow and colleagues posted the only results that suggested that there are differences between the open and laparoscopic approaches. They posited, "Because the TEP repair involves dissection in the preperitoneal space near the bladder, operative manipulation may be a contributory factor [24]." Although they later note that the more likely contributor was the general anesthesia used during laparoscopy, the anatomy encountered during a laparoscopic dissection is worth considering.

Dissection around the bladder within the preperitoneal space of Retzius and down into the retropubic space below the pelvic bone could injure branches of the pelvic plexus that are located along the anterior and lateral aspects of the bladder. Disruption of these branches could impact the parasympathetic signals affecting external sphincter relaxation and bladder contraction. As such, limiting dissection along the anterior aspect of the bladder, particularly under the pubis, may be warranted.

Intravenous Fluid Administration

In their study, evaluating the bladder function after outpatient surgery, Pavlin and colleagues noted there is a correlation between intraoperative intravenous fluid administration and postoperative bladder volume [25]. This may explain how Petros and Toyonaga independently identified fluid administration as a significant risk factor for POUR in patients who received greater than 1,000 mL of fluids during anorectal

[19, 26] and after open inguinal hernia repair [17]. Kozol tested this in a randomized controlled trial restricting patients to 500 mL of intravenous fluids (experimental group) or unlimited intravenous fluid administration (control). Fifteen percent of patients required catheterization in the control group, while 9% required intervention in the experimental group (P=NS) [27]. Both Koch and Lau, however, were unable to replicate these results after laparoscopic inguinal hernia repair [18, 20].

This has led some to look to other strategies involving postoperative fluid administration. Koch, for example, noted a lower incidence of POUR in patients after laparoscopic inguinal hernia repair receiving less than 500 mL of fluid in the postoperative setting [20]. Overall, although limiting intraoperative intravenous fluids to under 1 L and/or postoperative fluids to under 500 mL may limit the risks of POUR, more research is needed. At a minimum, patients who have received a high amount of intravenous fluids should be monitored closely.

Postoperative Pain and Analgesia

The pelvic pain associated with inguinal hernia surgery increases sympathetic tone, stimulating alpha-receptors in the internal ureteral sphincter. This leads to increased pressure on the bladder neck and increases the risk for retention. The most important decision regarding treatment of this pain involves balancing the need to mitigate the sympathetic response with the potential inhibitory effect of analgesics on the nociceptive reflex associated with bladder distention. In this setting, non-opioid analgesics have proven to be the superior choice.

As early as 1988, Stallard and Prescott demonstrated that the use of opioids for postoperative pain management resulted in a higher incidence of POUR in a cohort of 280 general surgical patients (8% vs. 3%) [2]. Koch and colleagues noted similar findings in patients after laparoscopic inguinal hernia repair [20].

In vitro, morphine is a potent presynaptic inhibitor of detrusor acetylcholine. This effect may lower parasympathetic tone and lead to passive filling. In their manuscript, Stallard and colleagues also note, “the most probable reason for painless retention is that the sensory cortex is unaware of impulses reaching it from the bladder stretch receptors … patients may well not feel discomfort from a distended bladder [2].”

Diagnosis and Treatment

POUR will remain a persistent problem after laparoscopic inguinal hernia repair even as the strategies to prevent it continue to evolve. As Ramshaw pointed out in his comments describing the incidence of POUR in his large single-center cohort, "Some minor complications have remained consistent throughout our series, and it is possible that these problems are unavoidable [28]." With this in mind, surgeons should remain vigilant in considering its diagnosis and remain familiar with the evidence supporting its treatment.

The diagnosis of POUR is not always clear. Anesthesia reversal agents, pain medications, and the diminished awareness of bladder sensation in the postoperative setting may mask the traditional signs of bladder overdistention. For example, over 60% of patients with a volume exceeding bladder capacity in an outpatient surgical setting did not experience discomfort or an urgent desire to void [2, 25].

Ultrasound assessment of bladder volume is both sensitive and specific for detecting POUR at volumes that exceed 600 mL [29–31]. Although specific guidelines outlining the use of ultrasound have not been developed, detection within 1–2 h after surgery prevents both the incidence of permanent detrusor damage and the need for additional treatment after the initial catheterization [32]. This, combined with the finding that most patients will void within 75 min after outpatient surgical procedures, suggests that ultrasound assessment seems prudent if patients have not voided within 2 h of their procedure [25, 30]. If ultrasound is not available, Pavlin suggests that patients who have not voided by the time of discharge should have their bladder evacuated with instructions to return for medical evaluation if they have not voided within 8–12 h [25].

Bladder catheterization is the immediate treatment in patients who find that they cannot urinate despite an urgent need, in those whose bladder volumes exceed 600 mL on ultrasound, or in those who have not voided within 8–12 h after discharge. A onetime in-out catheterization is appropriate as long as the patient can be monitored until voiding spontaneously.

If the patient is unable to void within 8–12 h after the initial catheterization, controversy remains as to whether intermittent catheterization is acceptable or the use of an indwelling catheter is required. Lau and Lam studied this question comparing in-out catheterization versus overnight indwelling catheterization in 60 surgical patients after various outpatient surgical procedures. There were no differences between the groups in terms of recatheterization and urinary tract infection. The indwelling catheter group, however, had a nonsignificant increase in the length of stay (2.2 days vs. 3.3 days, $P = 0.18$). The authors noted that a urology consultation is recommended in the rare instance that recatheterization is required beyond 12–24 h [33].

References

1. Hinman F. Postoperative overdistention of the bladder. Editorial. Surg Gynecol Obstet. 1976;142:901–2.
2. Stallard S, Prescott S. Postoperative urinary retention in general surgical patients. Br J Surg. 1988;75:1141–3.
3. Gönüllü NN, Dülger M, Utkan NZ, Cantürk NZ, Alponat A. Prevention of postherniorrhaphy urinary retention with prazosin. Am Surg. 1999;65:55–8.
4. Eklund A, Rudberg C, Smedberg S, et al. Short-term results of a randomized clinical trial comparing Lichtenstein open repair with totally extraperitoneal laparoscopic inguinal hernia repair. Br J Surg. 2006;93:1060–8.
5. Johansson B, Hallerbäck B, Glise H, Anesten B, Smedberg S, Román J. Laparoscopic mesh versus open preperitoneal mesh versus conventional technique for inguinal hernia repair: a randomized multicenter trial (SCUR hernia repair study). Ann Surg. 1999;230:225–31.
6. MRC Laparoscopic Groin Hernia Trial Group. Laparoscopic versus open repair of groin hernia: a randomised comparison. Lancet. 1999;354:185–90.
7. Neumayer L, Giobbie-Hurder A, Jonasson O, et al. Open mesh versus laparoscopic mesh repair of inguinal hernia. N Engl J Med. 2004;350:1819–27.
8. Aeberhard P, Klaiber C, Meyenberg A, Osterwalder A, Tschudi J. Prospective audit of laparoscopic totally extraperitoneal inguinal hernia repair. Surg Endosc. 1999;13:1115–20.
9. Dulucq J-L, Wintringer P, Mahajna A. Laparoscopic totally extraperitoneal inguinal hernia repair: lessons learned from 3,100 hernia repairs over 15 years. Surg Endosc. 2009;23:482–6.
10. Kapiris S, Brough W, Royston C, O'Boyle C, Sedman P. Laparoscopic transabdominal preperitoneal (TAPP) hernia repair. Surg Endosc. 2001;15:972–5.
11. Swadia ND. Laparoscopic totally extra-peritoneal inguinal hernia repair: 9 year's experience. Hernia. 2011;15:273–9.
12. Tammela T, Kontturi M, Lukkarinen O. Postoperative urinary retention. I. Incidence and predisposing factors. Scand J Urol Nephrol. 1986;20:197–201.
13. Prasad M, Abcarian H. Urinary retention following operations for benign anorectal diseases. Dis Colon Rectum. 1978;21:490–2.
14. Zaheer S, Reilly W, Pemberton J, Ilstrup D. Urinary retention after operations for benign anorectal diseases. Dis Colon Rectum. 1998;41:696–704.

15. Baldini G, Bagry H, Aprikian A, Carli F. Postoperative urinary retention: anesthetic and perioperative considerations. Anesthesiology. 2009;110:1139–57.
16. Keita H, Diouf E, Brouwer T, Dahmani S, Mantz J, Desmonts J. Predictive factors of early postoperative urinary retention in the postanesthesia care unit. Anesth Analg. 2005;101:592–6.
17. Petros J, Rimm E, Robillard R, Argy O. Factors influencing postoperative urinary retention in patients undergoing elective inguinal herniorrhaphy. Am J Surg. 1991;161:431–3.
18. Lau H, Patil N, Yuen W, Lee F. Urinary retention following endoscopic totally extraperitoneal inguinal hernioplasty. Surg Endosc. 2002;16:1547–50.
19. Toyonaga T, Matsushima M, Sogawa N, et al. Postoperative urinary retention after surgery for benign anorectal disease: potential risk factors and strategy for prevention. Int J Colorectal Dis. 2006;21:676–82.
20. Koch CA, Grinberg GG, Farley DR. Incidence and risk factors for urinary retention after endoscopic hernia repair. Am J Surg. 2006;191:381–5.
21. Fitzgibbons RJ, Camps J, Cornet DA, Nguyen NX, Litke BS, Annibali R. Laparoscopic inguinal herniorrhaphy: results of a multicenter trial. Ann Surg. 1995;221:3–13.
22. Gong K, Zhang N, Lu Y, et al. Comparison of the open tension-free mesh-plug, transabdominal preperitoneal (TAPP), and totally extraperitoneal (TEP) laparoscopic techniques for primary unilateral inguinal hernia repair: a prospective randomized controlled trial. Surg Endosc. 2011;25:234–9.
23. Pokorny H, Klingler A, Schmid T, et al. Recurrence and complications after laparoscopic versus open inguinal hernia repair: results of a prospective randomized multicenter trial. Hernia. 2008;12:385–9.
24. Winslow ER, Quasebarth M, Brunt LM. Perioperative outcomes and complications of open vs laparoscopic extraperitoneal inguinal hernia repair in a mature surgical practice. Surg Endosc. 2004;18:221–7.
25. Pavlin DJ, Pavlin EG, Fitzgibbon DR, Koerschgen ME, Plitt TM. Management of bladder function after outpatient surgery. Anesthesiology. 1999;91:42–50.
26. Petros J, Bradley T. Factors influencing postoperative urinary retention in patients undergoing surgery for benign anorectal disease. Am J Surg. 1990;159:374–6.
27. Kozol R, Mason K. Post-herniorrhaphy urinary retention: a randomized prospective study. J Surg Res. 1992;52:111–2.
28. Ramshaw B, Shuler F, Jones H, et al. Laparoscopic inguinal hernia repair: lessons learned after 1224 consecutive cases. Surg Endosc. 2001;15:50–4.
29. Griffiths C, Murray A, Ramsden P. Accuracy and repeatability of bladder volume measurement using ultrasonic imaging. J Urol. 1986;136:808–12.
30. Pavlin D, Pavlin E, Gunn H, Taraday J, Koerschgen M. Voiding in patients managed with or without ultrasound monitoring of bladder volume after outpatient surgery. Anesth Analg. 1999;89:90–7.
31. Rosseland L, Stubhaug A, Breivik H. Detecting postoperative urinary retention with an ultrasound scanner. Acta Anaesthesiol Scand. 2002;46:279–82.
32. Kitada S, Wein A, Kato K, Liven R. Effect of acute complete obstruction in the rabbit urinary bladder. J Urol. 1989;141:166–9.

33. Lau H, Lam B. Management of postoperative urinary retention: a randomized trial of in-out versus overnight catheterization. ANZ J Surg. 2004;74:658–61.
34. Wright D, Kennedy A, Baxter J, Fullarton G. Early outcome after open versus extraperitoneal endoscopic tension-free hernioplasty: a randomized clinical trial. Surgery. 1996;119:552–7.
35. Liem M, Graaf Y, van Steensel C, et al. Comparison of conventional anterior surgery and laparoscopic surgery for inguinal hernia repair. Surv Anesthesiol. 1997;41:369.
36. Wellwood J, Sculpher M, Stoker D, et al. Randomised controlled trial of laparoscopic versus open mesh repair for inguinal hernia: outcome and cost. BMJ (Clinical research ed). 1998;317:103.
37. Andersson B, Hallén M, Leveau P, Bergenfelz A, Westerdahl J. Laparoscopic extraperitoneal inguinal hernia repair versus open mesh repair: a prospective randomized controlled trial. Surgery. 2003;133:464–72.
38. Bringman S, Ramel S, Heikkinen T, Englund T, Westman B, Anderberg B. Tension-free inguinal hernia repair: TEP versus mesh-plug versus Lichtenstein: a prospective randomized controlled trial. Ann Surg. 2003;237:142.
39. Langeveld HR, Van't Riet M, Weidema WF, et al. Total extraperitoneal inguinal hernia repair compared with Lichtenstein (the LEVEL-Trial). Ann Surg. 2010;251:819–24.
40. Ramshaw B, Tucker J, Duncan T, et al. Technical considerations of the different approaches to laparoscopic herniorrhaphy: an analysis of 500 cases. Am Surg. 1996;62:69–72.
41. Moreno-Egea A, Aguayo J, Canteras M. Intraoperative and postoperative complications of totally extraperitoneal laparoscopic inguinal hernioplasty. Surg Laparosc Endosc Percutan Tech. 2000;10:30–3.
42. Garg P, Rajagopal M, Varghese V, Ismail M. Laparoscopic total extraperitoneal inguinal hernia repair with nonfixation of the mesh for 1,692 hernias. Surg Endosc. 2009;23:1241–5.

15. Recurrent Inguinal Hernia: The Best Approach

Abe Fingerhut and Mousa Khoursheed

Recurrence is, with chronic pain, among the most challenging complications of inguinal hernia repair. The true incidence of recurrence remains difficult to determine. While many authors tout a low recurrence rate for their technique, their personal series or team results, large series [1, 2], or national registries indicate that as many as one of five hernia operations (17%) are for recurrent hernia [3]. As this is only a surrogate of the true recurrence rate, however, recurrence may be even higher because (a) the definition of recurrence varies considerably from one report to another, (b) follow-up is not always complete [4], (c) not all patients recognize or complain of their recurrence or go back to their surgeon [4], and (d) not all recurrences undergo reoperation.

The best approach to treat recurrent hernia has been a subject of debate for years, both in the open and later, in the endoscopic arenas. By "approach," we mean the overall approach to the problem (technique, use of mesh), not just the anatomic, surgical approach. "Anterior" and "posterior" refer to the anatomic surgery approach, whereas pre- and retrofascial refer to the anatomic placement of mesh. The actual techniques used have been described elsewhere and will not be highlighted in this chapter, which will concentrate on the indications.

Mesh repair has been shown to decrease the re-recurrence rate [5] as compared to suture techniques. Based on the previous experiences of Cheatle in 1920 and Henry in 1936, Nyhus largely popularized the preperitoneal approach, stressing the advantage of going through fresh, unscarred tissue for his mesh repair [6], and especially when dealing with recurrent hernia [7]. Later on, this idea resurfaced when the proponents of laparoscopic hernia repair emphasized that the endoscopic technique also entailed a posterior (retrofascial) preperitoneal mesh. Of note, at that time, the majority of

B.P. Jacob and B. Ramshaw (eds.), *The SAGES Manual of Hernia Repair*, DOI 10.1007/978-1-4614-4824-2_15,

the recurrences were due to failures of anterior, most often tissue, repairs and also, sometimes, after prefascial mesh repair. Today, we face the quandary that recurrence can occur after a posterior as much as an anterior repair and/or after almost any type of mesh repair.

But there is more to the question than choosing the "best anatomic approach," i.e. the surgical technique adapted to the previous route for repair. On one hand, there are the characteristics of the previous repair: was the previous repair tissue only or with mesh, which incision was used, and last, was the postoperative course complicated or not; on the other, there are the characteristics of the recurrence (type, number, site, and size of the defects; the number of previous repairs; and the presence of a sac). Last, it is also important to eliminate risk factors: not only are there factors that may already have been present during the initial or preceding repair and are responsible for the first recurrence (it would not be wise to leave these factors uncorrected for the second operation) but because recurrence itself should now be considered a high risk factor. Every effort should be made to correct or minimize as many of the other risk factors as possible.

Factors Related to the Previous Repair

Whether the Previous Repair Was a Tissue Repair or a Mesh Repair

Primary repairs that place mesh in the preperitoneal space (such as such as Kugel patch, Prolene Hernia System, plug, or endoscopic repair) make subsequent laparoscopic repair more difficult, because of scarring in the preperitoneal space. Recurrence rates after mesh repair differ with the type of repair, ranging from as low as 1.3% for the Lichtenstein onlay repair to more than 27% for the Kugel repair. If one of these techniques is considered for repair of recurrence, the surgeon should be conscious of these recurrence rates when performing subsequent repairs [8].

Site of the Incision

Likewise, it would seem logical to avoid going through the same incision to repair the recurrence. This would avoid the difficulty in dissection of the different planes that have often amalgamated during healing of the previous operation, potentially exposing the cord structures to accidental injury, if this route were anterior. Specific problems can arise in the plug and Kugel techniques as the mesh is placed posterior to the transverse muscles but through an anterior route. If however the operation were meant to remove infected mesh, then this would be the least devastating route. A distinction between the open and laparoscopic repairs is that the incision of most open anterior repairs lies directly or near the repair, while the incision for the open or laparoscopic preperitoneal operations is usually at some distance from the repair (mesh). The probability that the cord structures are exposed to injury when accomplishing an anterior approach in recurrent hernia must therefore be foremost in the minds of the surgeon undertaking the repair of recurrent inguinal hernia to avoid devascularization of the testicle or injury to the nerves and/or the vas deferens, notably often anterior to the other cord structures and particularly vulnerable in this setting.

Postoperative Course of the Previous Repair

Drawbacks of mesh repair are well known. If the mesh must be removed because of intolerance due to chronic pain, sensation of foreign body, or infection, this would most likely be easiest through the same approach as the previous operation. The repair could be performed during the same operation or ulteriorly through a different approach.

Factors Related to the Recurrence

Type

Whether the recurrence is direct or indirect does not influence the repair.

Number of Defects

All potential sites (orifices) have to be covered [9, 10].

Site

Pelissier et al. [11] remind us that all recurrences are through the myopectineal orifice. An oblique external recurrence through the inguinal canal might well be treated as a primary hernia, whereas a small, sclerotic hole near the pubic tubercle would pose problems of purchase if a suture repair was decided and problems of adequate overlap if a mesh repair were entertained. Most recurrent hernias after tissue repair are located in the inguinal canal (insufficiently treated prehernia lipoma or unrecognized sac?) or just above the pubic tubercle. Recurrence after an anterior mesh repair technique (Lichtenstein and plugs) is found either over the pubic tubercle [12] or around or lateral to the internal ring or, sometimes, both medially and laterally (with the plugs). With the use of the larger meshes, whether through the open or endoscopic route, the recurrences can occur almost anywhere as they are usually attributed to poor technique, migration, shrinking, and plicature... [9]. The femoral canal orifice warrants special mention. As nearly 9% of recurrences are in fact femoral hernias, and dissection medial to the inguinal ligament should eliminate this eventuality. In cases where femoral hernias are present, Itani et al. [8] caution against use of a plug and recommend exposure of Cooper's ligament and lateral fixation of the new mesh to Cooper's ligament.

Size

A small orifice might lend itself easily to a plug (either Perfix or PHS) technique, whereas a full-blown destruction of the inguinal wall (truly an incisional hernia) would require some form of onlay mesh opposition or a plasty.

Number of Previous Operations/Recurrences

If both an anterior (tissue or mesh) and posterior repair have already been performed, there is considerable scarring both in front and behind the transverse plane. The choice of technique is difficult and depends on surgeon preference and expertise. To this, we might add that the preperitoneal space might be difficult to access because of previous radiation therapy, a vascular procedure, or surgery on the bladder or the prostate.

The Presence of a Sac

Obviously, a sac left behind during the index operation is an obvious cause of recurrence ("reappearance") of the hernia and must be treated when dealing with the recurrence. Aside from this particular setting, and as long as the sac is treated, there is currently nothing in the literature today to indicate whether a new or old sac, found or not, or whether the sac was excised or inverted in the previous operation, matters much in the next repair.

Techniques Used for Recurrent Inguinal Hernia

The use of the preperitoneal, retrofascial space for hernia repair was first performed by Usher in 1958 [13]. In accordance with the principle to use mesh for recurrent hernia repair [5], prosthetic reinforcement made its entry to the therapeutic armamentarium when Nyhus introduced the "buttress" technique, i.e., a preperitoneal mesh that reinforced a tissue repair for recurrent hernia [7]. The "giant prosthetic reinforcement of the visceral sac" technique, propagated by Stoppa and his followers in France, was one of the first techniques addressing the specific problem of recurrent hernia [7, 14–16] covering the defect, without sutures [15, 16].

Anterior prefascial repairs have its partisans. Both the Lichtenstein [17–19] and the Gilbert [20] repairs have been suggested as suitable for repair of recurrent inguinal hernia.

In 1993, Lichtenstein and coworkers [19] enumerated five principles that should be entertained when repair of recurrent hernia is accomplished through an anterior approach: (1) do not depend on fascial structures to close or reinforce the defect, (2) reinforce the entire inguinal floor irrespective of the type of hernia, (3) avoid all tension on suture lines, (4) avoid use of scarred or devascularized tissue in the repair of recurrent hernias, and (5) use a large prosthetic material to reinforce the entire inguinal floor permanently. Actually, these principles should probably apply to all types of repair of recurrent hernia, irrespective of the approach. The logical consequence of point number 4 would be to use the endoscopic or open posterior route for recurrence that has occurred after an initial open anterior repair and to consider the open anterior route for recurrence of an endoscopic repair.

With the advent of laparoscopic or endoscopic hernia repair, several authors lauded that minimal invasive techniques, also placing a mesh in the preperitoneal space, could be a specific indication for the repair of recurrent hernia. As that time, most hernia repairs (and therefore recurrences) were through the open, anterior route. Among the advantages of the preperitoneal approach is the facility with which all the potential defects can be detected and covered [21, 22].

When the laparoscopic approach is selected (failed anterior repair), the minimal invasive (laparoscopic) route combines satisfactory re-recurrence rates and less pain medication requirements as shown in a randomized controlled trial from Finland [23], but contrasting with the results of an earlier, smaller, controlled randomized trial [24], in which, although the morbidity was lower, the recurrence rate was higher with TAPP compared with GPRVS. However, when one considers the complexity of the operation and the re-recurrence rates, the open preperitoneal prosthetic mesh repair was considered the best repair. This was also confirmed by Itani et al. [8] who found that mesh removal by endoscopic techniques can be difficult if not impossible (instruments are not strong, inadequate cutting and energy).

Of importance as well is to consider the number of recurrences and how badly the anatomy may be distorted; in particular, how well Fruchaud's myopectineal orifice has been covered in the original (or last) repair [9–11] or, more importantly, how well it is, or may be covered at the time of consideration for repair [8].

In a meta-analysis on seven randomized studies comparing two different techniques for recurrent inguinal hernia repair, Dedemadi et al. [25] pooled the effects of outcomes in 1,542 patients enrolled into five randomized controlled trials and seven comparative studies, using classic and modern meta-analytic methods. They found that there were significantly fewer cases of hematoma/seroma formation in the laparoscopic group compared with the Lichtenstein technique; the relative risk of overall recurrence was higher [3, 25] in the transabdominal preperitoneal group compared with the totally extraperitoneal group. Their conclusion was that laparoscopic versus open mesh repair for recurrent inguinal hernia was equivalent in most of the analyzed outcomes. However, they did not analyze the outcome according to the type of index repair or any of the other hernia or recurrence characteristics enumerated above.

Classifications and Therapeutic Deductions

Classifications should describe the anatomic location, include anatomic function (competency of the internal ring, integrity of the direct floor, defect size, and descent of sac), be reproducible for both hernia specialists and general surgeons, be easy to remember, be applicable to anterior as well as posterior approaches, to laparoscopic as well as open repair, [26–28], lead to a tailored overall approach of repair [26] (mesh vs. suture, anterior vs. posterior surgical approach, pre- or retrofascial placement of the mesh), and serve to compare outcomes between different techniques and patients. Several shortcomings, however, plague the cornucopia of existing hernia classifications, including the composite classification by Zollinger [27, 28]: (1) classifications with preoperative descriptions are limited to what the examiner can see or palpate and do not always predict the true intraoperative anatomical conditions (it is known that the preoperative determination of direct or indirect hernia is incorrect in 50% of cases [29], and the EHS [30] stated that any effort for preoperative distinction was "useless"); (2) recurrent hernia, a clinical variable, has been "added" to a list of anatomical variables, usually lumping all types of recurrent hernia into the last "potpourri" category (the most advanced), without much distinctive details. Several other authors have similarly only added a "R" to the anatomic categorization as for primary hernia [27, 28] to designate the recurrent aspect of the hernia; (3) last, when classifications are too simple, a complete description is not possible, and it becomes difficult to "tailor" the repair to the exact type of recurrent hernia.

To the best of our knowledge, only one classification specifically deals with recurrent hernia [31], but is incomplete as well. Certainly, this classification takes into consideration how many recurrences have occurred (first, second, or more), the site (near the internal ring, above the pubic tubercle, whole inguinal wall), the size (> or <2 cm), whether the sac is reducible or not, and patient characteristics such as obesity, and all factors that have been considered as risk factors of further recurrence. However, in this classification, the above-mentioned variables are poorly delineated and compacted into only three grades: R1, R2, and R3 (Table 15.1). The authors give preferential advice according to whether the previous repair was anterior or posterior only in the R2 category. They do not distinguish between previous mesh and suture techniques.

Guarnieri [32] classified recurrent hernia into four categories: (1) high recurrent hernia (1/3 superior, i.e., hernia close to the internal ring and occupying not more than 1/3 of the posterior wall), (2) low recurrent hernia (1/3 inferior, i.e., hernia close to the pubic tubercle and occupying not more than 1/3 of the posterior wall), (3) total recurrent hernia (the entire or nearly the entire posterior wall is involved),and (4) multiple recurrent hernia (more than one hernia opening).

Table 15.1. According the Campanelli classification, recurrent hernias can be divided into three types.

Type R1: first recurrence "high," oblique external, reducible hernia with small (<2 cm) defect in nonobese patients, after pure tissue or mesh repair
Type R2: first recurrence "low," direct, reducible hernia with small (<2 cm) defect in nonobese patients, after pure tissue or mesh repair
Type R3: all the other recurrences – including femoral recurrences; recurrent groin hernia with big defect (inguinal eventration); multirecurrent hernias; non-reducible, linked with a controlateral primitive or recurrent hernia; and situations compromised from aggravating factors (e.g., obesity) or anyway not easily included in R1 or R2, after pure tissue or mesh repair

Recommendations and Indications

It is primordial to carefully review previous operative reports to correctly choose between the available techniques for subsequent recurrent hernia repair according to the above-mentioned variables.

When mesh is chosen, light-weight meshes have some advantages with respect to long-term discomfort and foreign-body sensation in open hernia repair, but are possibly associated with an increased risk for hernia re-recurrence (possibly due to inadequate fixation and/or overlap).

The European [30] recommendations for recurrent hernia are the following: if the previous repair was through an anterior route, consider open preperitoneal mesh or endoscopic approach (if expertise is present, and preferably TEP rather than TAPP), and if the previous repair was through a posterior route, consider an anterior mesh (Lichtenstein). After conventional open repair, endoscopic inguinal hernia techniques result in less postoperative pain and faster convalescence than the Lichtenstein technique. Itani et al. [8] based their decision on whether the index repair was a tissue or mesh repair. If the initial repair was a tissue (anterior) repair, then either the anterior or posterior approaches can be used to repair the recurrent hernia [8]. If the initial repair was a mesh repair, then the recurrence repair should preferably employ an approach in the space in which the tissue planes have not been violated previously [8]. An anterior approach is clearly the best choice after failed posterior repair, no matter if it was performed open or laparoscopically.

The International Hernia Society [10] recommends not to try to remove preperitoneal mesh endoscopically, but to place a second mesh over the first. If the original mesh was a plug, the prominent part of the plug should be divided, better by electrocautery than by scissors, so that a flat mesh can be applied.

In patients with an R1 recurrence, according to Campanelli [31], most authors [26, 30, 31, 33–35] prefer a Gilbert's plug repair through an anterior approach, under local anesthesia.

In patients with an R2 recurrence, Campanelli [31] and Miserez [26] perform a preperitoneal modified Wantz repair [15] under local anesthesia. If R2 recurrence is secondary to a previous preperitoneal mesh repair, an anterior approach with a Lichtenstein, Gilbert, or Trabucco repair is preferable. In both cases, only local anesthesia is used, and the patient is discharged immediately.

In patients with an R3 recurrence, Campanelli [31] and Miserez [26] prefer a Stoppa operation by preperitoneal approach, the Wantz technique, or the laparoscopic technique for either the uni- or bilateral hernia.

There are two groups of patients in whom a second preperitoneal dissection might be considered [36]:

1. Those with multiple recurrent hernias where both spaces have already been dissected [37].
2. Those who insist on an endoscopic reoperative approach. The latter most commonly occurs when the herniorrhaphy on the recurrent side was laparoscopic and the patient has had a previous open repair on the opposite side [38].

In patients for whom previous mesh was used, special caution is warranted. The mesh may be tightly adherent, and sometimes, heavy fibrosis envelopes the cord structures, making it particularly difficult to distinguish between these structures and surrounding tissues. Careful and cautious dissection to clearly identify the cord structures is mandatory to avoid inadvertent division or injury to the vas deferens or nerves or, worse, devascularization of the testicle, often ending in orchiectomy [21]. Certainly, these patients should be informed of the (remote but not zero) possibility of orchiectomy.

Indications for mesh removal are ill defined, but most authors overlay mesh unless there is infection [10]. Complete removal of the mesh is most often impossible, and careful delineation of the anatomy and myopectineal orifice is most important. When complete removal is impossible or hazardous, placement of an additional, overlapping mesh avoids the necessity of further dissection and damage to the underlying structures, especially through the endoscopic route where the bladder and iliac vessels are at risk [10]. The second mesh should overlap the first in the area of recurrence and be solidly anchoring to healthy fascia and inguinal ligament, as well as to the previous mesh in areas where the mesh is well incorporated to the inguinal ligament laterally and rectus

Table 15.2. Summary of recommendations according to the initial anatomic approach.

Previous repair route	Mesh	Itani	EHS	Campanelli		Schwab	
Anterior	Yes	A[a], P, E	A, P, E	R1: G		Need to remove mesh	A (R)
				R3: St, W, E		No need	P, E
	No	A,P, E			R2: W		
Posterior	Yes	A	L		R2: L, GT	Need to remove mesh	P (W, St)
						No need	A (L)

A open anterior mesh repair (Lichtenstein (L), Gilbert (G), Rutkow, Trabucco (T)), *P* open posterior mesh repair (Stoppa (St), Nyhus, Wantz (W), Read, Rives (R), Kugel), *E* endoscopic posterior preperitoneal repair (by TEP or TAPP)

[a]Second mesh

fascia medially. Additional dissection and damage to underlying structures will thus be avoided. Among the risk factors for recurrence, some if not most are amenable to preoperative correction. These include technical factors such as the use of short-term absorbable sutures for rraphy or mesh fixation [39] and insufficient coverage when mesh is used [9, 11], and patient-related factors including smoking and to a certain degree, obesity.

Schwab and Klinge [40] proposed the following algorithm for the treatment of recurrent mesh repair according to whether or not the previous operation was complicated or not and whether prosthetic material should be removed or not. If the postoperative course of the preceding operation was uneventful, these authors propose an endoscopic or open posterior repair when the initial route was anterior and the Lichtenstein anterior repair when the initial operation was a posterior repair. If, however, the previous operation was followed by a complication, the authors advise an anterior or posterior transinguinal revision. If the endoscopic route is chosen, practically only the TAPP technique is possible, the TEP is reputed to be too difficult [41]. If the prior operation was an anterior mesh (Lichtenstein) repair, then an open posterior repair (Wantz or Stoppa) seems appropriate.

The use of local anesthesia for recurrent hernia is not well studied. Obviously, endoscopic repairs are always performed under general anesthesia. Theoretically, all other procedures can be done under local anesthesia. However, the increased complexity and longer dissection times are characteristics that might preclude the use of local anesthesia. Table 15.2 summarizes the therapeutic potentials according the recommendations of the authors who have tried to systematize repair.

Conclusion

In conclusion, we recommend the following: when faced with *recurrence after tissue repair*, the surgeon can choose between an open anterior (Lichtenstein plug, or plug and patch, or Prolene Hernia System) repair, an open posterior (Read, Rives, Stoppa, Kugel, Nyhus, Wantz) repair, and a laparoscopic (TAPP or TEP) repair, essentially based on the size of the hernia defect and surgeon preference and/or expertise [3].

If dealing with a *recurrence after a mesh repair*, the technique of repair will depend on surgeon experience and on which anatomic approach was used for the previous operation (anterior or posterior). For *recurrence after mesh placed through an open anterior approach*, then a Read, Rives, Stoppa, Nyhus, Wantz, Kugel, or a laparoscopic (TEP OR TAPP) approach may be used.

For *recurrence after mesh placed through a posterior* (laparoscopic for example) *approach*, the recommendation is to perform a laparoscopic TAPP (if experienced in laparoscopy) or an open Lichtenstein, Prolene Hernia System, or plug and patch technique if experienced in open techniques. Decisions may be based on the size of the hernia defect and surgeon preference and/or expertise [3].

If mesh removal is needed, it is most likely best removed through an open anterior approach, while some isolated plugs can be removed safely laparoscopically. *If a second mesh repair is envisioned* in the same operation, we propose an endoscopic or open posterior repair when the initial route was anterior and the Lichtenstein anterior repair when the initial operation was a posterior repair.

References

1. Liem MS, van Vroonhoven TJ. Laparoscopic inguinal hernia repair. Br J Surg. 1996;83:1197–204.
2. Neumayer L, Giobbie-Hurder A, Jonasson O, Fitzgibbons Jr R, Dunlop D, Gibbs J, et al. Open mesh versus laparoscopic mesh repair of inguinal hernia. N Engl J Med. 2004;350:1819–27.
3. Bisgaard T, Bay-Nielsen M, Kehlet H. Re-recurrence after operation for recurrent inguinal hernia. A nationwide 8 year follow-up study on the role and type of repair. Ann Surg. 2008;248:347–8.
4. Hay JM, Boudet MJ, Fingerhut A, Pourcher J, Hennet H, Habib E, Veryières M, Flamant Y. Shouldice inguinal hernia repair in the male adult. Ann Surg. 1995;222:719–27.
5. Sevonbius D, Gunnarsson U, Nordin R, Nilsson E, Sandblom G. Repeated groin hernia recurrences. Ann Surg. 2009;249:516–8.
6. Nyhus LM, Stevenson JK, Listerud MB, Harkins HN. Preperitoneal herniorrhaphy: a preliminary report in fifty patients. West J Surg Obstet Gynecol. 1959;67:48–54.
7. Nyhus LM, Pollak R, Bombeck T, Donahue PE. The preperitoneal approach and prosthetic buttress repair for recurrent hernia. The evolution of a technique. Ann Surg. 1988;208:733–7.
8. Itani KMF, Fitzgibbons R, Awad SS, Duh Q-Y, Ferzli GS. Management of recurrent inguinal hernias. J Am Coll Surg. 2009;209:653–8.
9. Kukleta JF. Causes of recurrence in laparoscopic inguinal hernia repair. J Minim Access Surg. 2006;3:187–91.

10. Bittner R, Arregui ME, Bisgaard T, Dudai M, Ferzli GS, Fitzgibbons RJ, Fortelny RH, Klinge U, Kockerling F, Kuhry E, Kukleta J, Lomanto D, Misra MC, Montgomery A, Morales-Conde S, Reinpold W, Rosenberg J, Sauerland S, Schug-Pass C, Singh K, Timoney M, Weyhe D, Chowbey P. Guidelines for laparoscopic (TAPP) and endoscopic (TEP) treatment of inguinal hernia [International Endohernia Society (IEHS)]. Surg Endosc. 2011;25:2773–843.
11. Pelissier E. Inguinal hernia: the size of the mesh. Hernia. 2002;5:169–71.
12. Bay-Nielsen M, Nordin P, Nilsson E, Kehlet H. Operative findings in recurrent hernia after a Lichtenstein procedure. Am J Surg. 2001;182:134–6.
13. Usher FC, Oschsner J, Tuttle Jr LL. Use of Marlex mesh in the repair of incisional hernias. Am Surg. 1958;24:969–74.
14. Stoppa RE, Rives JL, Warlaumont CR, Palot JP, Verhaeghe PJ, Dellatre JF. The use of Dacron in the repair of hernias of the groin. Surg Clin North Am. 1984;64:269–85.
15. Wantz GE. Giant prosthetic reinforcement of the visceral sac. Surg Gynecol Obstet. 1989;169:408–17.
16. Stoppa R, Petit J, Henry X. Unsutured Dacron prosthesis in groin hernias. Int Surg. 1975;60:411–2.
17. Gilbert AI. An anatomic and functional classification for the diagnosis and treatment of inguinal hernia. Am J Surg. 1989;157:331–3.
18. Kark AE, Kurzer M, Waters KJ. Tension-free mesh hernia repair: review of 1098 cases using local anaesthesia in a day unit. Ann R Coll Surg Engl. 1995;77:299–304.
19. Lichtenstein IL, Shulman AG, Amid PK. The cause, prevention, and treatment of recurrent groin hernia. Surg Clin North Am. 1993;73:529–44.
20. Wilson MS, Deans GT, Brough WA. Prospective trial comparing Lichtenstein with laparoscopic tension-free mesh repair of inguinal hernia. Br J Surg. 1995;82:274–7.
21. Wantz GE. Testicular atrophy and chronic residual neuralgia as risks of inguinal hernioplasty. Surg Clin North Am. 1993;73:571–81.
22. Kurzer M, Belsham PA, Kark AE. Prospective study of open preperitoneal mesh repair for recurrent inguinal hernia. Br J Surg. 2002;89:90–3.
23. Kouhia ST, Huttunen R, Silvasti SO, Heiskanen JT, Ahtola H, Uotila-Nieminen M, Kiviniemi VV, Hakala T. Lichtenstein hernioplasty versus totally extraperitoneal laparoscopic hernioplasty in treatment of recurrent inguinal hernia–a prospective randomized trial. Ann Surg. 2009;249:384–7.
24. Beets GL, Dirksen CD, Go PM, Geisler FE, Baeten CG, Kootstra G. Open or laparoscopic preperitoneal mesh surgical repair for recurrent inguinal hernia? A randomized controlled trial. Surg Endosc. 1999;13:323–7.
25. Dedemadi G, Sgourakis G, Radtke A, Dounavis A, Gockel I, Fouzas I, Karaliotas C, Anagnostou E. Laparoscopic versus open mesh repair for recurrent inguinal hernia: a meta-analysis of outcomes. Am J Surg. 2010;200:291–7.
26. Miserez M, Alexandre JH, Campanelli G, Corrcione F, Cuccurullo D, Pascual MH, Hoeferlin A, Kingsnorth AN, Mandala V, Palot JP, Schumpelick V, Simmermacher RK, Stoppa R, Flament JB. The European hernia society hernia classification: simple and easy to remember. Hernia. 2007;11:113–6.
27. Zollinger RM. Classification systems for groin hernias. Surg Clin North Am. 2003;83:1053–63.

28. Zollinger Jr RM. An updated traditional classification of inguinal hernias. Hernia. 2004;8:318–22.
29. Kraft BM, Kolb H, Kuckuk B, Haaga S, Leibl BJ, Kraft K, Bittner R. Diagnosis and classification of inguinal hernias. Surg Endosc. 2003;17:2021–4.
30. Simons MP, Aufenacker T, Bay-Nielsen M, Bouillot JL, Campanelli G, Conze J, de Lange D, Fortelny R, Heikkinen T, Kingsnorth A, Kukleta J, Morales-Conde S, Nordin P, Schumpelick V, Smedberg S, Smietanski M, Weber G, Miserez M. European Hernia Society guidelines on the treatment of inguinal hernia in adult patients. Hernia. 2009;13:343–403.
31. Campanelli G, Pettinari D, Cavalli M, Avesani ED. Inguinal hernia recurrence: classification and approach. J Minim Access Surg. 2006;3:147–50.
32. Guarnieri F, Franco M, Nwamba C, Smaldone W, http://www.guarnieriherniacenter.com/pages/Congresses/Orlando_Poster_2.pdf.
33. Shulman AG, Amid PK, Lichtenstein IL. The "plug" repair of 1402 recurrent inguinal hernias: 20-year experience. Arch Surg. 1990;125:265–7.
34. Stoppa R, Warlaumont C, Marrasse E, Verhaeghe P. Pathogenesis of inguinal hernias. Minerva Chir. 1989;44:737–44.
35. Trabucco EE. The office hernioplasty and the Trabucco repair. Ann Ital Chir. 1993;64:127–49.
36. Pokorny H, Klingler A, Schmid T, Fortelny R, Hollinsky C, Kawji R, Steiner E, Pernthaler H, Függer R, Scheyer M. Recurrence and complications after laparoscopic versus open inguinal hernia repair: results of a prospective randomized multicenter trial. Hernia. 2008;12:385–9.
37. Rutkow IM, Robbins AW. Demographic, classification, and socioeconomic aspects of hernia repair in the United States. Surg Clin North Am. 1993;73:413–26.
38. Knook MTT, Weidema WF, Stassen LPS, van Steensel CJ. Laparoscopic repair of recurrent inguinal hernias after endoscopic herniorrhaphy. Surg Endosc. 1999;13:1145–7.
39. Novik B, Nordin P, Skullman S, Dalenbäck J, Enochsson L. More recurrences after hernia mesh fixation with short-term absorbable sutures: a registry study of 82 015 Lichtenstein repairs. Arch Surg. 2011;146:12–7.
40. Schwab R, Klinge U. Principle actions for re-recurrences. In: Schumelick V, Fitzgibbons RJ, editors. Recurrent hernia: prevention and treatment. Heidelberg: Springer; 2007. p. 339–44.
41. Andersson B, Hallen M, Leveau P, Bergenfelz A, Westerdahl J. Laparoscopic extraperitoneal inguinal hernia repair versus open mesh repair: a prospective randomized controlled trial. Surgery. 2003;133:464–72.

16. Athletic Groin Pain and Sports Hernia

Nathaniel Stoikes and L. Michael Brunt

Sports hernia has become a topic of increasing interest in both the sports and surgical communities as a number of high-profile athletes have been treated for this condition. This condition is not a true hernia and, as such, the term "sports hernia" is not anatomically correct; rather, the condition is better designated as "athletic pubalgia" given the variations clinical presentations and underlying pathophysiology. Nonetheless, as sports hernia is firmly ingrained in the lexicon of the medical and lay literature, it will be used interchangeably with athletic pubalgia in this review. Although sports hernia has garnered the most attention, most athletic groin injuries do not evolve into a sports hernia type pubalgia and are successfully managed with conservative measures. These injuries can be challenging both from a diagnostic and clinical management standpoint for many reasons including the extensive differential diagnosis, anatomic complexity of the groin region, unpredictability regarding time to return to sport, risk of chronicity, and the variety of management options. This chapter will discuss basic considerations in athletic groin injuries, describe the clinical entity of sports hernia in detail, and review the various surgical approaches to its management.

Background

Groin injuries are common in sports with repetitive, high speed cutting, turning, twisting, and kicking motions, such as soccer, football, and ice hockey. The reported incidence of groin injuries in elite level athletes has ranged from 5 to 28% in soccer players [1] to 6–15% in hockey players [2, 3] but is not exclusive to these sports. In contrast to most sports injuries, these typically are soft tissue injuries (i.e., not skeletal) that do not

B.P. Jacob and B. Ramshaw (eds.), *The SAGES Manual of Hernia Repair*, DOI 10.1007/978-1-4614-4824-2_16,

necessarily arise from direct physical contact. Various risk factors for the development of groin injuries have been described: [4] these include a prior history of groin injury, older player status, and lack of off-season sports-specific conditioning activity (e.g., ice skating for hockey players). In one prospective study of NHL players, reduced adductor muscle strength was significantly associated with an increased risk of adductor strain injury [5]. More importantly, implementation of an adductor strengthening program reduced the injury incidence by almost 80%.

Presentation

Establishing a diagnosis of a sports hernia can be challenging as the findings are often subtle, and patients can have a varied presentation. It should be considered in part a diagnosis of exclusion, but the differential diagnosis can be vast as there are many components to the dynamic abdominal and pelvic region that must be ruled out.

A typical scenario is that of an athlete who presents with complaints of moderately intense pain and discomfort in the region of the superior pubis and in the lower abdominal/inguinal region associated with exertion. In some cases, the pain may be more vague and radiate to the upper thigh or across the lower abdomen. These symptoms are most pronounced with explosive movements and usually abate with rest. Pain may also be noted with sneezing and coughing. Pain along the upper adductor muscle group, principally the adductor longus and its attachment to the inferior pubis, is not unusual.

A detailed history including location of pain, quality and intensity of pain, onset, duration, and inciting factors should be noted. Other important details include how the athlete has managed these symptoms since the injury, including rest and treatments that he or she has undergone. It is key to note how long the patient has truly rested or decreased activity as most athletic groin injuries eventually resolve with conservative management

On physical exam, symptoms can be reproduced through a series of maneuvers involving an evaluation of the abdominal core. Thorough examination should include assessment for inguinal hernia, palpation of the inguinal floor, pubis, rectus abdominis, adductor muscles, and hips. Pain may be elicited in these regions during a resisted sit-up, trunk rotation, and resisted hip and thigh movements including hip flexion and adduction. True inguinal hernia pathology is rarely found, but the inguinal floor may feel weak or have a slight bulging effect on Valsalva coupled with tenderness in the inguinal floor. In our series at Washington University, we identified the following in patients who subsequently underwent surgery for a sports hernia: 90.7% weak inguinal floor; 80.2% tenderness in medial inguinal floor; 63.8% pain with resisted sit-up, floor; 63.8% pain with resisted sit-up; 73.3% pain with trunk rotation; and 56.7% pain with resisted adduction [6].

Differential Diagnosis

The differential diagnosis and clinical presentation of various athletic groin injuries (Table 16.1) has been extensively reviewed elsewhere [7–9]. The most common causes of groin pain in athletes are muscle strains of the musculature of the lower abdominal wall, hip flexors, and adductor muscles of the upper thigh. Other causes include:

1. Osteitis pubis
2. Pubic stress fracture
3. Inguinal hernia
4. Sports hernia/athletic pubalgia
5. Hip joint injury (labral tears, femoral-acetabular impingement, other hip pathology)

Table 16.1. Differential diagnosis of athletic groin injuries.

- Pelvis
  - Traumatic fracture or contusions
  - Stress-related fractures
  - Osteitis pubis
- Muscular strains
  - Abdominal: rectus abdominis, obliques
  - Hip flexors/iliopsoas
  - Adductor group (longus, brevis, magnus, pectineus, obturator externus)
- Hip Injuries
  - Labral tears
  - Femoral-acetabular impingement
  - Osteoarthritis
  - Stress fractures
- Sports hernia/athletic pubalgia
- Inguinal hernia
- Nonathletic causes (endometriosis, ovarian pathology, inflammatory bowel disease, etc.)

Imaging

Since the diagnosis of sports hernia pubalgia can be elusive, various imaging modalities can be used to provide more objective evidence for diagnosis and to assist in excluding other potential causes. Plain x-rays of the hip and pelvis are low yield but should be done in selected athletes to identify any gross structural abnormalities or stress fractures. Pelvic MRI provides more detailed structural information of the pelvis and soft tissues (muscles and tendons) and is the preferred imaging modality for evaluation of chronic athletic groin pain in our center. The pelvic MRI should include both axial, coronal, and sagittal oblique sequences. Common MRI findings can be divided into two main subtypes: bony and soft tissue. Bony pathology includes edema and stress reaction in the parasymphyseal pubis and a secondary cleft sign in the pubis which is an abnormal extension of the central symphyseal cleft at the anterior and inferior margin of the pubis (Fig. 16.1). Soft tissue findings include muscle tears or edema of the adductor muscle groups, lower rectus abdominis muscle, or at the common insertion site of rectus-adductor complex on the pubis (Fig. 16.2).

Though not commonly used in North America, ultrasound of the groin has been utilized preferentially by some groups [10]. The advantage of this modality is the ability to view the dynamic movements of the inguinal floor during a Valsalva maneuver, but it is operator dependent.

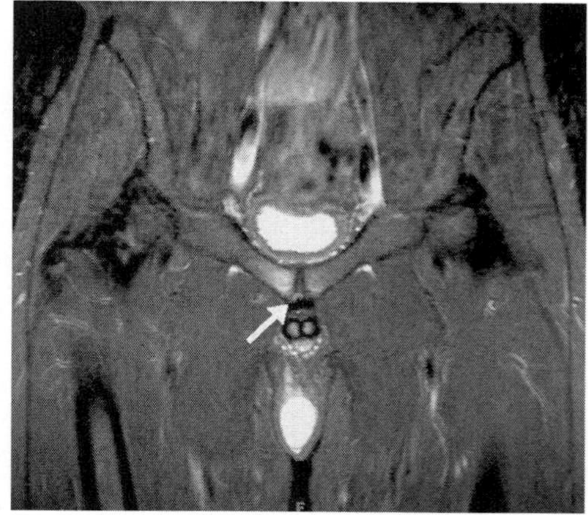

Fig. 16.1. Coronal STIR (short T1 inversion recovery) MRI sequence that shows a symphyseal cleft and parasymphyseal edema seen commonly in athletic pubalgia. *Arrow* indicates the "cleft" (*white* signal) between the pubis and the aponeurosis (*black* structure). Note also the marrow edema in the pubis which is more pronounced on the right (symptomatic) side.

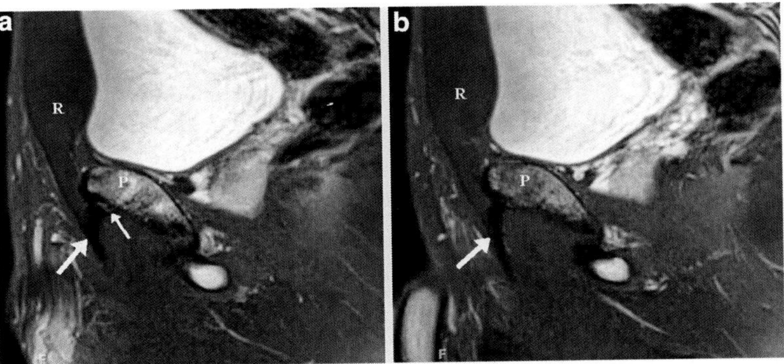

Fig. 16.2 Sagittal T2-weighted MRI images with fat suppression just off the midline sequences that show a tear or disruption in the rectus-adductor complex at the pubis. The *large arrow* points to the tendon origin of the adductor longus (dark structure) as it goes down the thigh. (**a**) Abnormal side which shows a partial separation of the common aponeurosis formed at the junction of the rectus muscle and adductor origin from the periosteum of the anteroinferior pubic bone. *R* rectus, *P* pubis. (**b**) Normal side.

Pathophysiology

As evidenced by the pathology found on imaging modalities and at surgical exploration, the groin is a dynamic area with a fixation point located at the pubis. The theory of a "pubic joint" originates from Meyers [11, 12] wherein the pubis is the fulcrum between the abdominal muscles and upper thigh muscles. As with any point of fixation carrying stress loads, unequal distribution of or imbalance of forces can lead to excessive stress on the focal point (the pubis) and the opposing muscle units (rectus abdominis, hip flexors, or adductors), leading to further weakness of the region. The end result of this process is pubalgia type pain and weakening or disruption of the rectus-adductor complex where it attaches at the pubis.

Other mechanisms include weakening in the inguinal floor and canal that is caused again by excessive force transmitted across the pubis from the powerful thigh musculature. The bowing of the inguinal floor and resultant widening of the inguinal canal causes the rectus to retract medically and superiorly which creates increased tension, and, thereby, pain across the pubis [10]. These observations are consistent with our experience in which common findings at operation (Figs. 16.3 and 16.4) have been an attenuated external oblique aponeurosis (96.7%), weak inguinal floor (100%), torn internal oblique (63.9%), and rectus abnormalities (80.3%).

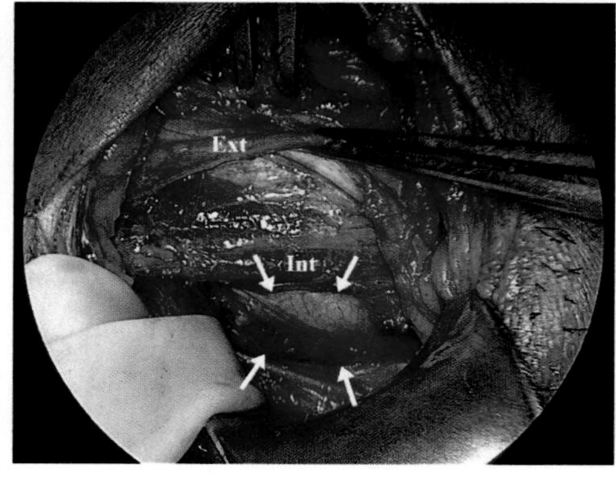

Fig. 16.3. Disrupted posterior inguinal floor in an athlete undergoing repair of sports hernia pubalgia. *Ext* external oblique, *Int* internal oblique. *Arrows* point to the weakened posterior floor.

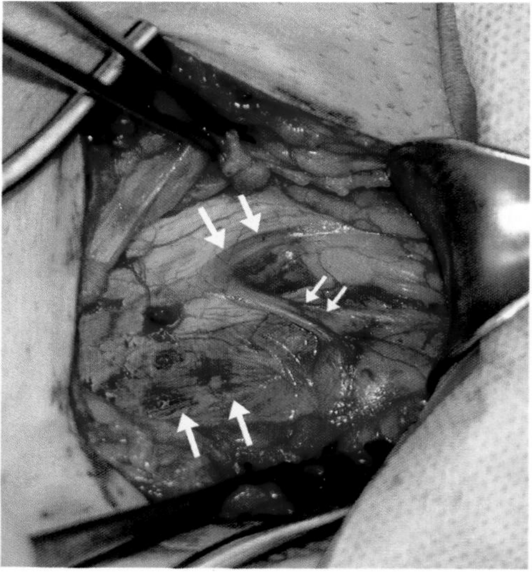

Fig. 16.4. Attenuated external oblique (*large arrows*) found at operation for sports hernia pubalgia. Note the ilioinguinal nerve exiting a slit in the external oblique at a sharp angle (*small arrows*).

Regardless, the common mechanism is likely a combination of overuse and imbalance of forces acting across the pelvis [13].

Muschawek has also postulated that bulging of the posterior inguinal floor may compress the genital nerve which can produce pain during Valsalva [10]. As a result, selective resection of the genital nerve is performed in some of her athletes [14]. Finally, some groups have suggested that defects within the external oblique, which may be coupled with entrapment and compression of the ilioinguinal and iliohypogastric nerves, are the primary mechanisms of injury and pain [15].

Likely, there is no one mechanism that leads to sports hernia pubalgia, and a combination of these mechanisms, which all focus on different aspects of the physiology and anatomy of the groin, is grounded in the fundamental principle that high-performance athletes stress their bodies to maximum levels, which results in the accentuation of dynamic processes in the lower body, thereby, stressing inherently weak regions such as the groin. Factors which could impact the development of this condition but which are as yet unproven might include the following: increased weight/strength training, year-round training with no time off, single-sport focus at a young age, and lack of strength and balance in the abdominal core.

Management Options

In the early phase of the clinical presentation, rest and other standard conservative management measures as described below are indicated. In selected cases, a combination of steroid and local anesthetic injection can provide some symptomatic relief and may facilitate a return to play or assist in differentiating the source of the pain. It is also important to note the scope of the problem for the patient, which may also impact the management approach. For example, the aggressiveness of the approach and progression to surgical intervention may be different for a recreational athlete versus a scholarship college athlete or professional athlete. In a sense, the latter's livelihood depends upon a quick return to top performance, which thereby makes the risk to benefit ratio for surgery more acceptable. Also, the recreational athlete does not have access to professional trainers and other resources, which can lead to a delay in the diagnosis and a prolonged time period in which the patient is neither resting nor able to resume full athletic activity.

In all cases, first-line management of an athletic groin injury should be conservative with rest. Activities that produce symptoms, especially explosive or torquing maneuvers, are to be avoided. Nonsteroidal anti-inflammatory medications, ice, and physiotherapy should be incorporated into the regimen as well. Light lower body activities such as jogging or stationary biking can begin as symptoms improve, and sports-specific activities can be added in an incremental fashion. Explosive maneuvers and intense gamelike conditions should be delayed until full lower abdominal and lower body exercises can be performed. If conservative measures have failed after 8–10 weeks, and the clinical presentation suggests a more chronic sports hernia type pubalgia, then surgical intervention should be considered.

Surgical Technique

There is no consensus on the preferred surgical technique for the treatment of sports hernia. The techniques reported can be broadly grouped: open primary tissue repair, open tension-free mesh reinforcement, and laparoscopic mesh repair. Adjuncts to these procedures include neurectomy and adductor tendon release.

1. *Open primary repairs*

   (a) *Meyer's technique*: Goals of this technique include realigning the infero-lateral rectus to the pubis and inguinal ligament using a primary sutured repair.

   (b) Muschawek technique: This approach is also known as the "minimal repair" technique [13, 14]. It involves repair of the posterior inguinal floor using two sequential imbricating running sutures. The genital nerve is resected in select cases, and the internal ring is buttressed with a cuff of internal oblique muscle.

2. *Open tension-free mesh repair*: This is the preferred approach by the authors and utilizes the principles of the Lichtenstein tension-free hernioplasty. The primary goal is to reinforce the posterior inguinal floor rather than to reconstruct the internal inguinal ring as one would do for an indirect hernia. Technical points include resection of the ilioinguinal nerve if it is entrapped by within a slit in the external oblique aponeurosis or if it will be tethered by the mesh. Damaged internal oblique/tranversus abdominis muscle fibers are debrided as needed. Lightweight polypropylene mesh is secured with nonabsorbable sutures to the inguinal ligament laterally and to the transversus abdominis/conjoined tendon medially (Fig. 16.5). The mesh is split, and the tails are secured around the cord structures in a standard fashion. Importantly, additional interrupted sutures are placed medially to anchor the mesh to the distal rectus to further stabilize the rectus and pubis. The external oblique aponeurosis is reapproximated with absorbable suture such that the attenuated portion is excluded. The Montreal group [16] also uses a tension-free mesh approach but places the mesh just beneath the external oblique aponeurosis rather than on the posterior floor, and in most cases, ilioinguinal and/or iliohypogastric neurectomy is also performed.

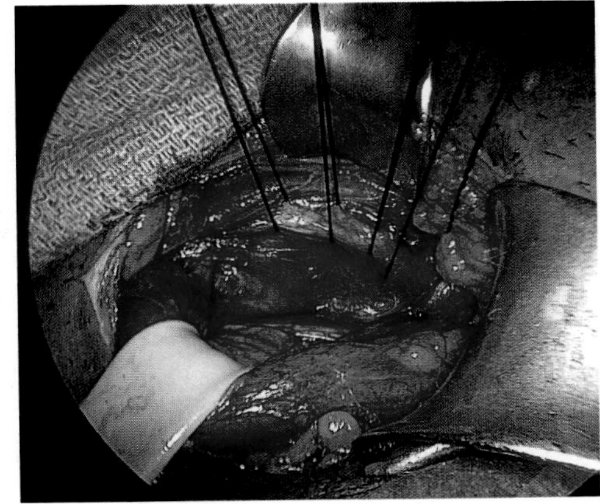

Fig. 16.5. Sutures anchoring the medial side of the repair of the right inguinal floor. The sutures are placed in a mattress fashion through lightweight tension-free polypropylene mesh.

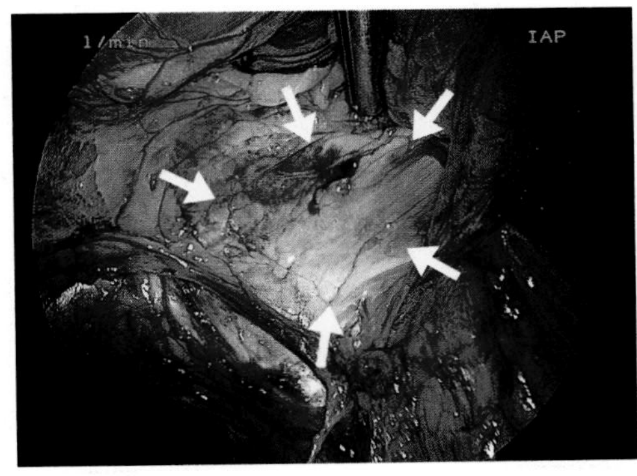

Fig. 16.6. Posterior laparoscopic view of weakened posterior inguinal floor (*arrows*).

3. *Laparoscopic mesh repair*: Laparoscopic mesh repair is favored by some groups [17–19]. This approach also provides support for the weakened posterior inguinal floor (Fig. 16.6) but anecdotally has been associated with a somewhat higher rate of incomplete relief of symptoms, although good results have been reported in several case series. The advantage is that it may allow faster return to play compared to some other approaches. It is typically done via the totally extraperitoneal approach.

Adjunct procedures: An adductor release as described by Meyers [20] entails releasing the epimysial fibers of the adductor longus approximately 2–3 cm from its attachment to the pubis. The actual tendon is not transected but instead "decompressed" with relaxing incisions to soften the adductor compartment and to relieve it of pressure, tension, and edema.

Surgical Outcomes

Outcomes of surgical management are listed in Table 16.2. Overall results in terms of return to full athletic activity range from 60% to 90%, with most series reporting greater than 90% of patients returning to their sport. Follow-up is variable and not reported in some instances. Also, the interval return to play is variable or not reported, which may be multifactorial secondary to both the procedure and varied time pressures for rehabilitation (in season vs. off-season). In the Washington University Medical Center experience, we have done repairs is over 150 elite and recreational athletes [21]. The majority (63%) were professional or college athletes. Follow-up regarding symptoms at 13.6 months found successful return to sport in 91% of athletes. Initially, adductor release was not a part of the management algorithm, and, as a result, five athletes have subsequently required adductor releases for recalcitrant adductor symptoms. Currently, adductor release as described by Meyers [20] is done in selected patients that have significant adductor pathology at the time of inguinal floor reinforcement.

Postoperative Care and Rehabilitation

Operative repair of a sports hernia/athletic pubalgia is only one component to the treatment of the disease process and, equally important in the athlete's full return to competition, in our view, is the use of a

Table 16.2. Reported outcomes of repair of sports hernia pubalgia.

Author	Type repair	No. of cases	Length of follow-up	Return to sport
Polglase [23]	Primary	64	8 months	63%
Gilmore [24]	Primary	300	–	97%
Steele [25]	Primary	47	–	77%
Meyers [20]	Primary "pelvic floor repair"	5,218	24 months	95.3%
Muschawek [14]	Primary "minimal repair"	129	–	
Joesting [26]	Open mesh	45	12 months	90%
Brown [26]	Open mesh	98	–	97%
Brunt [22]	Open mesh	132	13.6 months	91%
Van Veen [18]	Laparoscopic mesh	55	24 weeks	91%
Ziprin [19]	Laparoscopic mesh	17	–	94%
Evan [27]	Laparoscopic mesh	287	3 months–4 years	90%
Paajanen [28]	Laparoscopic mesh	30	3 months	90%

Table 16.3. Postoperative rehabilitation program after sports hernia repair.

Phase 1 week 1
Walking, starting with short distances, and progressing up to 45–60-min walks once per day
Light stretching (hamstring, quadriceps, calf and low back as tolerated)
Phase 2 week 2
Active hip range of motion exercises
Walking on inclined treadmill, backward walking
Begin bike workouts with slow continuous progression to interval sprint work
Wall sits with Swiss ball
Phase 3 week 3
Continue exercises from phase 2
Active release technique/deep tissue massage of hip and leg musculature
Pool walking
Monitored sports-specific skill development activities
Phase 4 week 4
Continue exercises from phase 3
Advance hip flexor stretching with progression into resistance strengthening, progressive resistive exercises
Lower abdominal strengthening and lower extremity strengthening exercises to include body weight squats, step-ups, etc.
Begin increasing sport-specific activities (more intense skating, running sprints, limited contact drills)
Phase 5 weeks 5–6
Continue exercises from phase 4
Transition to weight room and strength and conditioning program
Full practice, scrimmage with team
End-stage exercises with an emphasis on maintaining proper muscles length and abdominal strength through adherence of a core stabilization program

For a more detailed description of rehab exercises, see [22]

structured postoperative rehabilitation program. The program that we have utilized consists of a set of exercises that focus on strengthening the core and lower body (Table 16.3) [22]. Attention to adductor flexibility and strength is essential and involves an incremental increase in activity over a period of 5–8 weeks (five phases).

Summary

Sports hernia/athletic pubalgia is a complex entity that requires a systematic approach to the diagnostic evaluation and treatment. Surgeons who treat these athletes must understand the broader differential diagnosis of groin pain in athletes and the fact that this is not a true inguinal hernia. Treatment is based on a spectrum of management options that requires a multidisciplinary approach, and careful patient selection for surgery is a key component of the management algorithm. Multiple surgical techniques exist that may achieve a successful outcome, and regardless of the approach, the rehabilitation after surgery is integral to return of the athlete to competition.

References

1. Ekstrand J, Hilding J. The incidence and differential diagnosis of acute groin injuries in male soccer players. Scand J Med Sci Sports. 1999;9:98–103.
2. Pettersson R, Lorenzton R. Ice hockey injuries: a 4 year prospective study of a Swedish elite ice hockey team. Br J Sports Med. 1993;27:251–4.
3. Stuart MJ, Smith A. Injuries in Junior A ice hockey: a 3 year prospective study. Am J Sports Med. 1995;23:458–61.
4. Emery C, Meeuwisse W. Risk factors for groin injuries in hockey. Med Sci Sports Exerc. 2001;33:1423–33.
5. Tyler T, Nicholas S, Campbell R, McHugh M. The association of hip strength and flexibility with the incidence of adductor muscle strains in professional ice hockey players. Am J Sports Med. 2001;29:124–8.
6. Brunt L, Quasebarth M, Bradshaw J, Barile R. Outcomes of a standardized approach to surgical repair and postoperative rehabilitation of athletic hernia. AOSSM Annual Meeting 2007:Calgary 2007.
7. Nam A, Brody F. Management and therapy for sports hernia. J Am Coll Surg. 2008;206:154–64.
8. Anderson K, Strickland AM, Warren R. Hip and groin injuries in athletes. Am J Sports Med. 2001;29:521–33.
9. Caudill P, Nyland J, Smith C, Yerasimides J, Lach J. Sports hernias: a systematic literature review. Br J Sports Med. 2008;42:954–64.
10. Muschawek U, Berger LM. Sportsmen's groin - diagnostic approach and treatment with the minimal repair technique. Sports Health. 2010;2:216–21.
11. Meyers WC, Yoo E, Devon ON, et al. Understanding "sports hernia" (athletic pubalgia): the anatomic and pathophysiologic basis for abdominal and groin pain in athletes. Oper Tech Sports Med. 2007;15:165–77.
12. Meyers WC, Greenleaf R, Saad A. Anatomic basis for evaluation of abdominal and groin pain in athletes. Oper Tech Sports Med. 2005;13:55–61.
13. Minnich JM, Hanks JB, Muschawek U, Brunt LM, Diduch DR. Sports hernia: diagnosis and treatment highlighting a minimal repair technique. Am J Sports Med. 2011;39:1341–9.
14. Muschawek U, Berger L. Minimal repair technique of sportsmen's groin: an innovative open-suture repair to treat chronic groin pain. Hernia. 2010;14:27–33.

15. Irshad K, Feldman L, Lavoie C, Lacroix V, Mulder D, Brown R. Operative management of "hockey groin syndrome": 12 years experience in national hockey league players. Surgery. 2001;130:759–66.
16. Brown R, Mascia A, Kinnear DG, Lacroix VJ, Feldman L, Mulder DS. An 18 year review of sports groin injuries in the elite hockey player: clinical presentation, new diagnostic imaging, treatment, and results. Clin J Sport Med. 2008;2008:221–6.
17. Paajanen H, Syvähuoko I, Airo I. Totally extraperitoneal endoscopic (TEP) treatment of sportsman's hernia. Surg Laparosc Endosc Percutan Tech. 2004;14:215–8.
18. van Veen RN, de Baat P, Heijboer MP, et al. Successful endoscopic treatment of chronic groin pain in athletes. Surg Endosc. 2007;21:189–93.
19. Ziprin P, Prabhudesai DG, Abrahams S, Chadwick SJ. Transabdominal preperitoneal laparoscopic approach for the treatment of sportsman's hernia. J Laparoendosc Adv Surg Tech A. 2008;18:669–772.
20. Meyers WC, McKechnie A, Philippon MJ, Homer MA, Zoga AC, Devon ON. Experience with "sports hernia" spanning two decades. Ann Surg. 2008;248:656–65.
21. Brunt LM. Management of sports hernia and athletic pubalgia. In: Kingsnorth A, LeBlanc K, editors. Management of abdominal wall hernias. New York: Springer; 2012 (in press).
22. Brunt LM, Barile R. My approach to athletic pubalgia. In: Byrd TW, ed. Operative Hip Arthroscopy. 3rd ed: Springer; 2012; pp. 57–67.
23. Polglase AL, Frydman GM, Farmer KC. Inguinal surgery for debilitating chronic groin pain in athletes. Med J Aust. 1991;155:674–7.
24. Gilmore J. Groin pain in the soccer athlete: fact, fiction, treatment. Clin Sports Med. 1998;17:787–92.
25. Steele P, Annear P, Grove JR. Surgery for posterior inguinal wall deficiency in athletes. J Sci Med Sport. 2004;7:415–21.
26. Joesting DR. Diagnosis and treatment of sportsman's hernia. Curr Sports Med Rep. 2002;1:121–4.
27. Evans DS. Laparoscopic transabdominal pre-peritoneal (TAPP) repair of groin hernia: one surgeons's experience of a developing technique. Ann R Coll Surg Engl. 2002;84:393–8.
28. Paajanen H, Brinck T, Hermunen H, Airo H. Laparoscopic surgery for chronic groin pain in athletes is more effective than nonoperative treatment: a randomized clinical trial with magnetic resonance imaging of 60 patients with sportsman's hernia (athletic pubalgia). Surgery. 2011;150:99–107.

Part IV
Current Debates in Inguinal Hernia Repair

17. TAPP vs. TEP

Alfredo M. Carbonell II

The two most common techniques for laparoscopic inguinal hernia repair are the transabdominal preperitoneal (TAPP) technique and the totally extraperitoneal (TEP) technique. Although in the end both techniques are used to place mesh in the preperitoneal space to cover the entire myopectineal orifice, they differ in how access to that space is obtained.

With the TAPP approach, the peritoneal cavity is entered, the peritoneum is incised horizontally, and the preperitoneal space is developed, gaining access to the space of Retzius and Bogros. Mesh is placed to cover the entire myopectineal orifice, and the peritoneal flap is then closed with either suture, staples, or tacks. Conversely, with the TEP repair, a dissecting balloon is placed into the preperitoneal space at the level of the umbilicus. The balloon is inflated, which potentiates the preperitoneal space. The surgeon then works within the confines of this space to place the mesh, similar to the TAPP approach. At the conclusion, the preperitoneal space is desufflated and it collapses upon itself.

The Arguments for TAPP or TEP

Since, ultimately, the hernia recurrence rates are the same, the debate as to which approach is best is largely predicated upon notions of differences in cost, operative time, intraoperative complications, and postoperative pain. There have been three prospective, randomized, controlled trials comparing TAPP and TEP; thus, the majority of the data are from prospective, nonrandomized, comparative trials of the two techniques. The following section will explore some of the arguments made in favor of one technique or the other and investigate what the available literature shows.

B.P. Jacob and B. Ramshaw (eds.), *The SAGES Manual of Hernia Repair*,
DOI 10.1007/978-1-4614-4824-2_17,

Learning Curve

Argument: TAPP Is Easier to Learn than TEP

The learning curve for any surgical procedure is surgeon specific. Historically, most have learned the TAPP technique first, and then transitioned to the TEP repair after some experience. In one study of TAPP repairs, complications and recurrences decreased after the first 50 patients [1]. Another group performing TEP saw their complication and recurrence rate drop dramatically after their first 100 cases, while their conversion rate only decreased after 700 cases, and operative times were halved after the first 1,000 cases [2]. If we assume that operative time is a surrogate marker for technical mastery, a Cochrane database review summarized that inexperienced operators (up to 20 procedures) had an operative time of 70 min for TAPP and 95 for TEP. With experience (30–100 procedures), the estimated duration was 40 min for TAPP and 55 min for TEP [3]. These data suggest that TAPP is in fact easier to learn. Perhaps, this is due to the fact that the surgeon has a much wider field of view during TAPP and can see both inside the preperitoneal and intraperitoneal space maintaining orientation. This may allow for easier manipulation of the hernia sac and the intraperitoneal contents, compared to the tight working space and trocar configuration constraints of the TEP repair.

Operative Time

Argument: TEP is quicker to perform since the balloon dissector does the dissection, and in the end, there is no peritoneal flap requiring closure.

In an early randomized controlled trial of TEP ($n=24$) versus TAPP ($n=28$), there was an insignificant 6-min time advantage in favor of TAPP [4]. Other nonrandomized studies appear to show a slight time advantage in favor of the TAPP repair as well [3]. Two more recent prospective trials did not demonstrate a time difference whatsoever [5, 6].

Conversion

Argument: TEP often requires conversion to TAPP.

Due to the nature of the techniques, a TEP is typically converted to TAPP or open, while a TAPP is converted to open. Conversion with TEP will occur when too large a tear is created in the peritoneum and in TAPP when there is an inability to adequately develop or prepare the preperitoneal space for mesh placement. Patients with prior preperitoneal space surgery, particularly prior mesh repairs, may have a higher conversion rate, and consideration should be given to performing the hernia repair in a TAPP fashion from the outset. In historical prospective randomized trials, TEP has been associated with a higher conversion rate [7–9]. A more recent randomized trial showed no conversions in any of their TAPP or TEP cases [5]. Conversion is clearly a matter of experience and likely decreases as a surgeon becomes more facile with one or both techniques.

Cost

Argument: TEP is associated with higher supplies costs since it requires an expensive pneumatic balloon dissector to create the preperitoneal space.

The interpretation of cost data is unreliable, as the figures are country-specific and unique to each institution performing the surgery. The need for a balloon dissector is not absolute with TEP, and the dissection can be performed manually. In one single randomized trial, balloon dissection was compared to CO_2-supported trocar dissection, and there appeared to be no difference in morbidity or recurrence rate, although balloon dissection was associated with a lower need for conversion to TAPP and a mean 8-min time advantage [10]. With reusable trocars and balloon-less manual dissection, the cost of a TEP repair can be significantly reduced. Another factor to consider is the use of a fixation construct such as a stapler, tacking device (metallic or absorbable), or fibrin sealant. At least one of these products is often used in laparoscopic inguinal hernia repair and is associated with a significant cost regardless of TAPP or TEP approach. Two recent randomized trials of TAPP versus TEP failed to demonstrate a cost difference between the techniques [5, 6].

Intraoperative Complications

Argument: TAPP is associated with higher rates of vascular and visceral injuries and port-site hernias.

To date, three studies have reported vascular injuries, one actually demonstrated a higher injury rate in TEP [11] while the other two showed no difference [12, 13]. Two comparative trials reported a higher rate of visceral injury with TAPP compared to TEP, albeit the incidence was less than 1% in both series [7, 8]. Several studies have reported on port-site hernia rate, and it appears that TAPP has a higher incidence, upward of 3.7% [7].

In a large study on bowel obstruction after inguinal hernia repair, multivariate analysis demonstrated that TAPP had a relative risk of 2.79 compared to 0.57 with TEP [14]. Although the study was unable to determine the etiology of the bowel obstruction (hernia vs. adhesive), the data is compelling, nevertheless. Knowledge of adhesions of the omentum or bowel to metallic tacks or staples, as well as sutures is well-known. It is more likely that patients undergoing TAPP repair have their peritoneal flap closed with a fixation construct, predisposing TAPP patients to the potential sequelae of adhesions, such as bowel obstruction, or worse, construct-bowel erosion. Newer absorbable fixation constructs have become available, yet it is too early to determine whether there is an adhesion advantage to their use and the associated cost may make them prohibitive for routine use.

TEP is associated with peritoneal tears which collapse the preperitoneal space, making the operation lengthier, more laborious, and possibly requiring conversion to TAPP for completion. Peritoneal tears during TEP are commonplace, particularly with reoperative inguinal hernia repair. Although they are related to surgeon experience, they are easily managed by ligation of the tear or placement of an intraperitoneal Veress needle to decompress the pneumoperitoneum. This complication does in fact increase operative time by a mean of 20 min and is associated with an eightfold increase in the rate of conversion to TAPP [15]. Whether the tear should be closed at all due to the potential for bowel obstruction or mesh adhesion bears mention. To that effect, two studies have reported no complications after 16-month [16] and 4-year [15] follow-up in patients in whom peritoneal tears were not closed.

Pain

Argument: TAPP is associated with higher rates of vascular and visceral injuries and port-site hernias. TEP is associated with less pain since no peritoneal flap is opened and hence the only fixation constructs needed are the ones placed into the mesh if any are used at all.

Fixation constructs may or may not have an impact on symptoms of pain after the repair, as the data are conflicting. One recent prospective randomized trial found no difference in pain between TAPP and TEP. The TAPP group had tack mesh fixation and sutured peritoneal closure, while the TEP group had no mesh fixation [6]. Another randomized trial avoided the use of mesh fixation in both groups, and the TAPP group's peritoneal flap was sutured closed. This study found TAPP to be more painful at 1 h, 24 h, and 3 months postoperative [5]. If there is a slight pain difference, it may be transient, as one prospective study demonstrated a higher incidence of postoperative pain with TAPP compared to TEP at 1 month, but not at 6 months or 1 year. In that study, 18.1% of TAPP patients had >10 tacks placed, while 2.3% of the TEP patients had >10 tacks placed. Additionally, a subgroup analysis demonstrated less pain at all time points in TAPP patients with <10 tacks compared to those with >10 tacks [17].

If number of tacks used is proportional to the degree of pain then perhaps avoiding tacks or staples altogether can help eliminate pain. The current data suggest that nonmesh fixation in TEP, although not associated with a decrease in pain, is safe, cheaper, and does not result in an increased rate of recurrence [18]. Nonmesh fixation studies in TAPP are lacking; however, one randomized trial compared fibrin sealant versus staples for mesh fixation during TAPP while the peritoneal flap was sutured closed. No difference in recurrence rate or postoperative pain was noted between the two fixation methods [19].

Summary

In summary, the TAPP technique is easier to learn, yet is associated with an overall low but higher risk of visceral injury and port-site hernia compared to TEP. Surgeon preference will always drive technique choice, as both are equally effective at treating hernia disease.

References

1. Voitk AJ. The learning curve in laparoscopic inguinal hernia repair for the community general surgeon. Can J Surg. 1998;41(6):446–50.
2. Feliu-Pala X, Martín-Gómez M, Morales-Conde S, Fernández-Sallent E. The impact of the surgeon's experience on the results of laparoscopic hernia repair. Surg Endosc. 2001;15(12):1467–70.
3. Wake BL, McCormack K, Fraser C, et al. Transabdominal pre-peritoneal (TAPP) vs totally extraperitoneal (TEP) laparoscopic techniques for inguinal hernia repair. Cochrane Database Syst Rev. 2005;(1):CD004703
4. McCormack K, Wake BL, Fraser C, et al. Transabdominal pre-peritoneal (TAPP) versus totally extraperitoneal (TEP) laparoscopic techniques for inguinal hernia repair: a systematic review. Hernia. 2005;9(2):109–14.
5. Krishna A, Misra MC, Bansal VK, et al. Laparoscopic inguinal hernia repair: transabdominal preperitoneal (TAPP) versus totally extraperitoneal (TEP) approach: a prospective randomized controlled trial. Surg Endosc. 2012;26(3):639–49.
6. Gong K, Zhang N, Lu Y, et al. Comparison of the open tension-free mesh-plug,

transabdominal preperitoneal (TAPP), and totally extraperitoneal (TEP) laparoscopic techniques for primary unilateral inguinal hernia repair: a prospective randomized controlled trial. Surg Endosc. 2011;25(1):234–9.

7. Cohen RV, Alvarez G, Roll S, et al. Transabdominal or totally extraperitoneal laparoscopic hernia repair? Surg Laparosc Endosc. 1998;8(4):264–8.
8. Felix EL, Michas CA, Gonzalez MH. Laparoscopic hernioplasty. TAPP vs TEP. Surg Endosc. 1995;9(9):984–9.
9. Van Hee R, Goverde P, Hendrickx L, Van der Schelling G, Totté E. Laparoscopic transperitoneal versus extraperitoneal inguinal hernia repair: a prospective clinical trial. Acta Chir Belg. 1998;98(3):132–5.
10. Bringman S, Ek A, Haglind E, et al. Is a dissection balloon beneficial in totally extraperitoneal endoscopic hernioplasty (TEP)? A randomized prospective multicenter study. Surg Endosc. 2001;15(3):266–70.
11. Khoury N. A comparative study of laparoscopic extraperitoneal and transabdominal preperitoneal herniorrhaphy. J Laparoendosc Surg. 1995;5(6):349–55.
12. Tamme C, Scheidbach H, Hampe C, Schneider C, Köckerling F. Totally extraperitoneal endoscopic inguinal hernia repair (TEP). Surg Endosc. 2003;17(2):190–5.
13. Lepere M, Benchetrit S, Debaert M, et al. A multicentric comparison of transabdominal versus totally extraperitoneal laparoscopic hernia repair using PARIETEX meshes. JSLS. 2000;4(2):147–53.
14. Bringman S, Blomqvist P. Intestinal obstruction after inguinal and femoral hernia repair: a study of 33,275 operations during 1992–2000 in Sweden. Hernia. 2005;9(2):178–83.
15. Muzio G, Bernard K, Polliand C, Rizk N, Champault G. Impact of peritoneal tears on the outcome and late results (4 years) of endoscopic totally extra-peritoneal inguinal hernioplasty. Hernia. 2006;10(5):426–9.
16. Shpitz B, Lansberg L, Bugayev N, Tiomkin V, Klein E. Should peritoneal tears be routinely closed during laparoscopic total extraperitoneal repair of inguinal hernias? A reappraisal. Surg Endosc. 2004;18(12):1771–3.
17. Belyansky I, Tsirline VB, Klima DA, et al. Prospective, comparative study of postoperative quality of life in TEP, TAPP, and modified Lichtenstein repairs. Ann Surg. 2011;254(5):709–15.
18. Tam K-W, Liang H-H, Chai C-Y. Outcomes of staple fixation of mesh versus nonfixation in laparoscopic total extraperitoneal inguinal repair: a meta-analysis of randomized controlled trials. World J Surg. 2010;34(12):3065–74.
19. Fortelny RH, Petter-Puchner AH, May C, et al. The impact of atraumatic fibrin sealant vs. staple mesh fixation in TAPP hernia repair on chronic pain and quality of life: results of a randomized controlled study. Surg Endosc. 2012;26(1):249–54.

18. Fixation Versus No Fixation in Laparoscopic TEP and TAPP

Viney K. Mathavan and Maurice E. Arregui

Hernias have been a subject of interest since the dawn of surgical history. The treatment has evolved through several stages. Bassini revolutionized the treatment of inguinal hernia by the introduction of the technique to restore the conditions which exist under normal circumstances. The concept of the tension-free repair was introduced by Lichtenstein. Nyhus and Stoppa have described the inguinal hernioplasty through the posterior approach. Nyhus used small piece of mesh to reinforce the primary repair, but Stoppa used giant prosthesis for the repair. The mesh used by Nyhus was small and required suture fixation. The approach by Stoppa used a giant prosthesis (mesh) requiring single suture fixation in the midline. Laparoscopic inguinal hernia was first reported by Ger and Colleagues in 1990 [1]. They repaired the hernia in dogs by stapling the abdominal opening of patent processus vaginalis. The other minimally invasive techniques which have been described include plug and patch repair and intraperitoneal onlay mesh repair. These two techniques are not commonly used. Currently, laparoscopic inguinal hernia repairs are performed mostly with placement of synthetic mesh into the preperitoneal space. It can be done either by transabdominal preperitoneal (TAPP) approach or the totally extraperitoneal (TEP) approach. The TAPP approach was first described by Arregui et al. [2] in 1992. It requires laparoscopic access into the peritoneal cavity and placement of mesh in the preperitoneal space after reducing the hernia sac. The first TEP inguinal hernia repair was described by McKernan and Laws [3] in 1993. This approach involves preperitoneal dissection and placement of mesh in the preperitoneal space without entering into the abdominal cavity. Laparoscopic approach has been refined into an attractive alternative to open hernia repair for many patients and surgeons. There is abundant literature which supports that the laparoscopic inguinal

B.P. Jacob and B. Ramshaw (eds.), *The SAGES Manual of Hernia Repair*,
DOI 10.1007/978-1-4614-4824-2_18,

hernia repair can be performed with excellent results. The results of open mesh repairs are also good and the learning curve for laparoscopic technique is long. In the United States, about 15–20% of all inguinal hernias are repaired laparoscopically. With most laparoscopic approaches, mesh is fixed to the abdominal wall with spiral tacks, clips, or sutures. The need for fixation of mesh, however, is controversial. Some have suggested that fixation of the mesh is necessary to prevent hernia recurrence. However, fixation of mesh is thought to contribute to increased postoperative pain and the risk of nerve injury. The purpose of this chapter is to describe the TAPP and TEP repair and then discuss the literature with and without fixation of the mesh.

Indications and Contraindications

For the patients with a straightforward, unilateral, first-time hernia, both open mesh and laparoscopic mesh repairs offer excellent results and the choice depends upon surgeon experience and patient preference. A Cochrane meta-analysis found no significant difference in hernia recurrence rates between laparoscopic and open mesh techniques [4]. Laparoscopy offers advantages for recurrent inguinal hernias previously repaired by open technique. It bypasses the need to dissect in scarred tissue planes, thereby avoiding the risk of orchitis, testicular atrophy, and chronic inguinodynia. Laparoscopy also makes it possible to see the myopectineal orifice and identify the femoral hernias. The mesh can be placed over the entire myopectineal orifice. It avoids the groin incision and subsequent risk of wound complication [5–8]. Laparoscopic approach is a major benefit for patients who present with bilateral inguinal hernias. Studies show a significant advantage over the open repair in terms of less postoperative pain and an earlier return to work, without finding any difference in recurrence rates or complications [9–11]. When the diagnosis of an inguinal hernia is uncertain, diagnostic laparoscopy provides a definitive diagnosis and an opportunity to repair the hernia at the same time. Some surgeons also think that women should undergo laparoscopic repair of all inguinal hernias as synchronous femoral hernias are common and can be missed. Laparoscopy is also better in patients who engage in intense physical activity as it avoids dividing the aponeurosis of the external oblique and minimizes scar tissue between muscle planes. Contraindications for laparoscopic hernia repair include patients, for whom general anesthesia is risky due to their comorbidities.

Patients with prior pelvic operations and irradiation, or who have had a recurrence from a prior laparoscopic approach, should undergo an open inguinal hernia repair.

Operative Technique

The operative steps to perform TEP and TAPP repairs are similar [12, 13] and are described below.

Operative Steps for Transabdominal Preperitoneal Repair

The operative steps are well standardized. After transperitoneal incision, wide dissection is done laterally, across the midline, and parietalization of the cord is necessary to prepare the inguinal space for placement of a large mesh. Prosthetic mesh is used for repair. A 6×6-in. or 6×5-in. sheet of nonabsorbable mesh is cut to fit the preperitoneal space. A larger mesh may be used but a smaller mesh is not advised. A preformed, contoured mesh can also be used for coverage. Some surgeons prefer to slit the mesh with the tails wrapped around the cord. We do not recommend this. The mesh should cover the myopectineal orifices, including the direct, indirect, and femoral hernia spaces. When the mesh is smoothed out, it overlaps the pubic bone and crosses the midline. It is important to examine the mesh carefully to eliminate any wrinkles or folds. Recently, some surgeons have reported using biological mesh that becomes a scaffold for the patient's own collagen and is eventually absorbed. Long-term results of this are not yet known.

Operative Steps for Totally Extraperitoneal Repair

The initial creation of the preperitoneal space can be done bluntly or with a balloon. We prefer to use blunt dissection [14]. It is important to perform a wide dissection especially laterally and posteriorly with parietalization of the cord and identification and removal of herniated preperitoneal fat (lipoma of the cord). This is necessary for placement of a large mesh in the method of Stoppa [15]. We use a piece of 6-in. by 5-in. (15×12.5 cm) polypropylene lightweight mesh or Mersilene mesh. We do not slit it. We then use two blunt graspers to lay the mesh so that

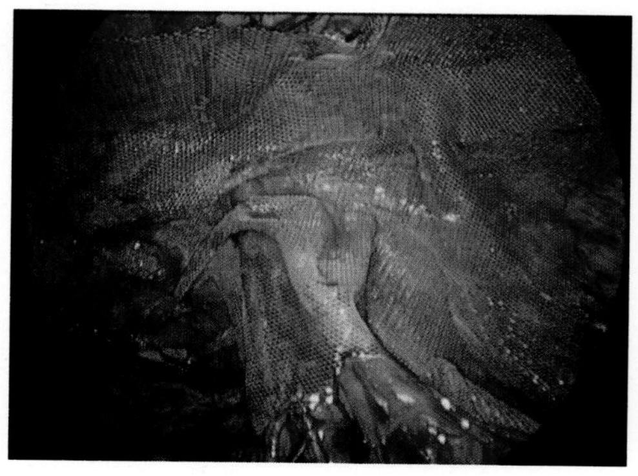

Fig. 18.1. Mesh without staples.

medially it crosses the midline and covers the direct, femoral, and indirect inguinal spaces. Laterally, it covers the lateral inguinal space (Fig. 18.1).

Fixation of the Mesh

The mesh is anchored to the posterior wall of the groin by the majority of surgeons. Mesh fixation theoretically ensures that it will remain where it was placed long after the operation. Such fixation is safe in most patients. Since the nerves at risk for injury are below the iliopubic tract, injury or entrapment of the nerves (genitofemoral nerve, lateral femoral cutaneous nerve, and femoral nerve) can be avoided by placing all mesh anchors into or above the iliopubic tract. The ilioinguinal and iliohypogastric nerves are above the iliopubic tract and can be compromised by fixation in thin patients. The landmarks must be identified when placing fixation. To avoid nerve injury, some authors suggest that the surgeon should be able to feel the stapler by pushing against it from anteriorly with the opposite hand. No staples should be placed unless the stapling device can be felt with the opposite hand. It also helps in placing the staples more perpendicular. Fitzgibbons has pointed out, however, that the ilioinguinal and iliohypogastric nerves travel laterally and anteriorly and can be potentially injured with this approach. The first staples are placed into the Cooper's ligament. This stabilizes the mesh and allows the surgeon to fan the mesh out in a lateral direction. The staples are then subsequently placed into the transversalis fascia medial to the inferior epigastric vessels. The lateral staples are placed by using the bimanual technique to prevent any damage to the nerves below the iliopubic tract. The purpose of the staples is to hold the mesh in place until the body's own inflammatory response takes place and not to provide any strength to the repair. Many surgeons, including us, do not use the staples. There are various descriptions of where and how to place staples or tacks and methods to avoid nerve injury. Some only fix medially.

Fixation Versus No Fixation

Several investigators have questioned the need for mesh fixation, which has been implicated as a source of chronic inguinodynia. Mesh fixation is believed to prevent hernia recurrence as it is an important measurable outcome. The mechanisms of recurrence have been studied by many investigators and are mostly related to technique [16–19]. One of the most common reasons for recurrence is incomplete dissection of the myopectineal orifice. Incomplete dissection is more often associated with inadequate reduction of the hernia sac, missed hernias, missed lipomas or preperitoneal fat, insufficient exposure for adequate mesh size, or rolling of the mesh edges. The mesh rolling usually occurs laterally and inferiorly in an area where fixation is contraindicated. Another common reason for hernia recurrence is inadequate overlap of the hernia defect from placement of a small mesh. The average mesh size in patients who had a recurrence was 6.0 cm × 9.2 cm in the trial by Fitzgibbons and colleagues [17]. It is now generally believed that the mesh size should be at least 10 cm × 15 cm to cover all of the potential hernia sites, to provide at least 4-cm overlap with the hernia, and to avoid problems with mesh migration, shrinkage, and rolling.

Felix et al. [18] reported too small a mesh to be the cause of hernia recurrence in 29% recurrences and 90% of these occurred in TAPP repairs. Inadequate lateral fixation was one of the major causes of failure in their review—36% of TAPP and 22% of TEP repairs. In TEP repair, there may be a tendency not to dissect far enough off the cord structures to allow the mesh lay under the peritoneum. In TAPP repairs, as the peritoneum is closed, the cord structures may be tented, lifting the mesh, and may lead to lateral recurrence. To prevent lateral recurrences, some surgeons have utilized a keyhole, but that may lead to recurrence itself. Phillips et al. [19] in a multicenter review of recurrence following laparoscopic hernia repair found too small a mesh in 60% cases and nonfixation of the mesh in 20% cases. Avoiding mesh fixation prevents nerve entrapment. Kraus

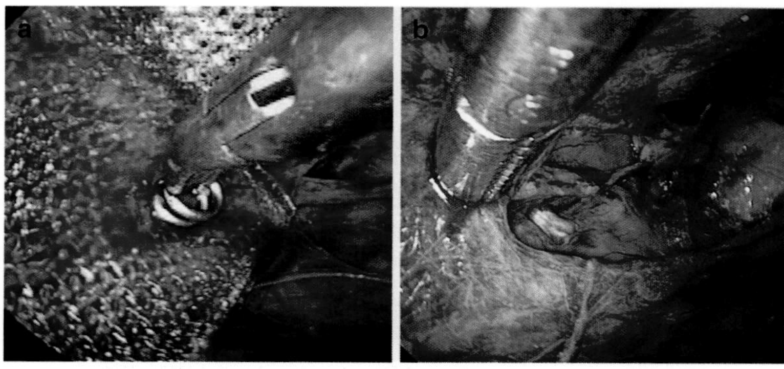

Fig. 18.2. (**a** and **b**) Fixation tack on the nerve.

first reported [20] damage to the lateral femoral cutaneous nerve of the thigh and subsequently noted injury to the femoral branch of the genitofemoral nerve [21]. The cause of injury was misplacement of staples, and he concluded that more accurate positioning would decrease the incidence of nerve injuries. There are numerous anecdotal reports of new groin pain that is well localized, corresponds with the location of a fixation tack, and is ameliorated by its removal (Fig. 18.2a, b). There are several prospective randomized studies comparing stapled versus unstapled mesh in laparoscopic preperitoneal inguinal hernia repair. Ferzli et al. [22] in a prospective randomized study reported no difference in the hernia recurrence rate between the stapled and unstapled groups over 12-month follow-up period in 92 patients. Taylor et al. [23] conducted a large prospective multicenter double-blinded randomized trial for 500 hernias repaired with TEP. They found no difference in recurrence between stapled and unstapled group. They also looked at pain after hernia repair. Moderate to severe pain was reported in 2% of fixated repairs and none in patients with unfixated mesh. There are several other randomized studies comparing fixation versus nonfixation with similar results [24–27, 28]. Most of these studies involve TEP repair and with small hernias. TEP without fixation may not be appropriate for everyone. Whether larger defects can be repaired without mesh fixation has not been adequately answered. Some suggest that mesh fixation should be used in patients with large hernial defects. Hollinsky et al. [29] did a cadaver experiment in nonfixed mesh. They recommended minimum mesh overlap of 2 cm for small hernias. For a hernia size 2 cm and larger, the distance between the margin of the prosthesis and the hernial opening should be equal to the diameter of the hernia. From 4 cm and larger, they recommended that the prosthesis should be secured with a stapler. Based on this experiment, Lau et al. [30] did selective nonfixation of hernias for the size smaller than 4 cm and recommended fixation of mesh for hernias more than 4 cm. The original open GPRVS repair by Stoppa was designed for the complicated or recurrent hernia using a very large mesh. In theory, even a defect greater than 4 cm could be repaired with this approach without fixation but with a greater sized mesh. One study found [25] decreased incidence of postoperative urinary retention in nonfixation group. Cost containment is also a consideration during stapling the mesh in laparoscopic hernia repair. The elimination of the disposable stapling device, either an endostapler or a helical tacker, can reduce the operative cost by $150–$300. The helical tacker costs about $293 at our hospital. The markup by the hospital is likely three times or greater. Persistent groin pain has also encouraged the use of alternative methods of fixation that avoid the use of tacks including fibrin glues, acrylate adhesives, self-gripping mesh, and absorbable sutures.

Fibrin glue has been proposed as an alternative, atraumatic method for mesh fixation based on its effective adhesive and wound- healing properties. It is a biodegradable preparation combining human plasma-derived fibrinogen and thrombin. Chevrel and Rath [31] first proposed fibrin sealant as an alternate means of mesh fixation in hernia repair, with the aim of reducing the rate of hernia recurrence. Katkhouda et al. [32] have since employed a pig model using a TEP technique to evaluate the tensile strength of mesh fixation 12 days after the use of fibrin sealant, demonstrating equal strength to staples. In a randomized trial between fibrin glue versus staples in TAPP repair, Lovisetto et al. [33] found lower incidence of postoperative neuralgia. The results of these studies have encouraged surgeons to use fibrin sealant as an alternative to mechanical mesh fixation. With the results of nonfixation being the equivalent to fixation, fibrin glue seems redundant and an added expense.

Self-Gripping Mesh Without Additional Fixation in TAPP and TEP

Recently a new material became available that may preclude the need for additional fixation as the mesh itself is self-gripping to muscle and adipose tissue. Made of a monofilament polyester weave with polylactic acid microhooks on one surface, and shown to be beneficial in open Lichtenstein hernia repairs, this material may have applications in TAPP and TEP repair. As reported at the American Hernia Society meeting in 2012 held in New York City, Jacob et al. presented early data from a prospective study. Self-gripping mesh was implanted in 64 hernias repaired by TEP technique. Follow-up with Carolinas Comfort Scale™ showed that only 7.7% of the patients were considered symptomatic at the first 2-week postoperative visit, and 0 patients were symptomatic at the second visit held between 3 and 6 months after surgery. Patients took an average of five tablets of narcotic and returned to full unrestricted activity within 5 days. The mean direct defect size was 2.5 cm, and no additional fixation was used in any case. To date, there are no reported recurrences or chronic pain.

Conclusion

The decision to fix the mesh in laparoscopic hernia repair depends upon the size of the hernia and the size of mesh used. For small hernia, the mesh can be safely placed without fixation. But for large hernias, the fixation may be required to prevent recurrence, though there is risk of nerve entrapment and cost considerations.

References

1. Ger R, Monroe K, Duvivier R, et al. Management of indirect inguinal hernias by laparoscopic closure of the neck of the sac. Am J Surg. 1990;159:370–3.
2. Arregui ME, Davis CJ, Yucel O. Laparoscopic mesh repair of inguinal hernia using a preperitoneal approach: a preliminary report. Surg Laparosc Endosc. 1992;2:53–8.
3. McKernan JB, Laws HL. Laparoscopic repair of inguinal hernias using a totally extraperitoneal prosthetic approach. Surg Endosc. 1993;7:26–8.
4. McCormack K, Scott N, Go P, et al. Laparoscopic techniques versus open techniques for inguinal hernia repair. Cochrane Database Syst Rev. 2003;(1):CD001785.
5. Eklund A, Rudberg C, Leijonmarck CE, et al. Recurrent inguinal hernia: randomized multicenter trial comparing laparoscopic and Lichtenstein repair. Surg Endosc. 2007;21:634–40.
6. Feliu X, Jaurrieta E, Vinas X, et al. Recurrent inguinal hernia: a ten-year review. J Laparoendosc Adv Surg Tech A. 2004;14:362–7.
7. Kouhia ST, Huttunen R, Silvasti SO, et al. Lichtenstein hernioplasty versus totally extraperitoneal laparoscopic hernioplasty in treatment of recurrent inguinal hernia-a prospective randomized trial. Ann Surg. 2009;249:384–7.

8. Itani KM, Fitzgibbons Jr R, Awad SS, et al. Management of recurrent inguinal hernias. J Am Coll Surg. 2009;209(5):653–8.
9. Mahon D, Decadt M, Rhodes M. Prospective randomized trial of laparoscopic (transabdominal preperitoneal) vs open (mesh) repair for bilateral and recurrent inguinal hernia. Surg Endosc. 2003;17:1386–90.
10. Wauschkuhn C, Schwarz J, Boekeler U, et al. Laparoscopic inguinal hernia repair: gold standard in bilateral hernia repair? Results of more than 2800 patients in comparison to the literature. Surg Endosc. 2010;24(12):3026–30.
11. Feliu X, Claveria R, Besora P. Bilateral inguinal hernia repair: laparoscopic or open approach? Hernia. 2011;15(1):15–8.
12. Takata MC, Duh QY. Laparoscopic inguinal hernia repair. Surg Clin North Am. 2008;88:157–78.
13. Felix EL, Swanstrom, L, Eubanks, S. Laparoscopic inguinal hernia repair. In: Soper NJ, editor. Mastery of endoscopic and laparoscopic surgery. 3rd ed. Philadelphia, PA: Lippincott Williams and Wilkins. 2008; 523–37.
14. Spitz JD, Arregui ME. Sutureless laparoscopic extraperitoneal inguinal herniorrhaphy using reuseable instruments: two hundred three repairs without recurrence. Surg Laparosc Endosc Percutan Tech. 2000;10:24–9.
15. Stoppa RE, Rives JL, Warlaumont CR, et al. The use of Dacron in the repair of hernias of the groin. Surg Clin North Am. 1984;64:269–85.
16. Lowham AS, Filipi CJ, Fitzgibbons RJ, et al. Mechanisms of hernia recurrence after preperitoneal mesh repair. Ann Surg. 1997;225:4211–431.
17. Fitzgibbons RJ, Camps J, Cornet DA, et al. Laparoscopic inguinal herniorrhaphy: results of a multicenter trial. Ann Surg. 1995;221:3–13.
18. Felix E, Scott S, Crafton B, et al. Causes of recurrence after laparoscopic hernioplasty. Surg Endosc. 1998;12:226–31.
19. Phillips EH, Rosenthal R, Fallas M, et al. Reasons for early recurrence following laparoscopic hernioplasty. Surg Endosc. 1995;9:140–5.
20. Kraus MA. Nerve injury during laparoscopic inguinal hernia repair. Surg Laparosc Endosc. 1993;3:342–5.
21. Kraus MA. Laparoscopic identification of preperitoneal nerve anatomy in the inguinal area. Surg Endosc. 1994;8:377–80.
22. Ferzli GS, Frezza EE, Pecararo Jr AM, Ahern KD. Prospective randomized study of stapled versus unstapled mesh in a laparoscopic preperitoneal inguinal hernia repair. J Am Coll Surg. 1999;188(5):461–5.
23. Taylor C, Layani L, Liew V, et al. Laparoscopic inguinal hernia repair without mesh fixation, early results of a large randomized clinical trial. Surg Endosc. 2008;22:757–62.
24. Moreno-Egea A, Torralba Martinez JA, Morales Cuenca G, Aguayo Albasini JL. Randomized clinical trial of fixation vs nonfixation of mesh in total extraperitoneal inguinal hernioplasty. Arch Surg. 2004;139(12):1376–9.
25. Koch CA, Greenlee SM, Larson DR, Harrington JR, Farley DR. Randomized prospective study of totally extraperitoneal inguinal hernia repair: fixation versus no fixation of mesh. JSLS. 2006;10(4):457–60.

26. Messaris E, Nicastri G, Dudrick S. Total extraperitoneal laparoscopic inguinal hernia repair without mesh fixation. Prospective study with 1-year follow-up results. Arch Surg. 2010;145(4):334–8.
27. Khajanchee YS, Urbach DR, Swanstrom LL, Hansen PD. Outcomes of laparoscopic herniorrhaphy without fixation of mesh to the abdominal wall. Surg Endosc. 2001;15:1102–7.
28. Smith AI, Rayston MS, Sedman PC. Stapled and nonstapled laparoscopic transabdominal preperitoneal (TAPP) inguinal hernia repair. A prospective randomized trial. Surg Endosc. 1999;13:804–6.
29. Hollinsky C, Hollinsky KH. Static calculations for mesh fixation by intraabdominal pressure in laparoscopic extraperitoneal herniorrhaphy. Surg Laparosc Endosc Percutan Tech. 1999;9(2):106–9.
30. Lau H, Patil NG. Selective non-stapling of mesh during unilateral endoscopic total extraperitoneal inguinal hernioplasty: a case control study. Arch Surg. 2003;138(12):1352–5.
31. Chevral JP, Rath AM. The use of fibrin glues in the surgical treatment of incisional hernias. Hernia. 1997;1:9–14.
32. Katkhouda N, Mavor E, Friedlander MH, et al. Use of fibrin sealant for prosthetic mesh fixation in laparoscopic extraperitoneal inguinal hernia repair. Ann Surg. 2001;233:18–25.
33. Lovisetto F, Zonta S, Rota E, et al. Use of human fibrin glue (Tissucol) versus staples for mesh fixation in laparoscopic Transabdominal preperitoneal hernioplasty. Ann Surg. 2007;245:222–31.

19. Laparoscopic Versus Open Repair for the Uncomplicated Unilateral Inguinal Hernia

Pradeep Pallati and Robert J. Fitzgibbons Jr.

Inguinal hernias are common; 27% of men and 3% of women will develop one in their lifetime. In the United States, according to the National Hospital Discharge Survey, approximately 720,000 inguinal hernia repairs were performed in the year 2005 [1]. Descriptions of Inguinal hernia repairs have appeared in medical writings as far back as 1500 B.C. [2]. However, the modern era of inguinal herniorrhaphy is generally felt to have begun in the late 1800s, thanks to the revolutionary procedure developed by Bassini. His prototype tissue repair was based on sound anatomical principles and incorporated the developing disciplines of anesthesia and antisepsis. The steps he recommended to prepare the groin for the eventual approximation of his famous "triple layer" (transversalis fascia, transversus abdominis muscle, and internal oblique muscle) to the inguinal ligament are still used in almost all conventional open repairs, both tissue- and tension-free. Although this operation was associated with results unheard of in Bassini's time, population-based studies in the twentieth century consistently revealed a recurrence rate in the 10–15% range when performed in general practice. The late 1980s and early 1990s saw two parallel developments, which would profoundly affect the way inguinal hernia surgery was performed. The first was the widespread acceptance of the routine use of prosthetic material for all adult inguinal hernias, complicated or uncomplicated. The second was the development of laparoscopic inguinal herniorrhaphy, which quickly followed the laparoscopic revolution spawned by the need to retrain surgeons in the laparoscopic method, so they could continue to perform cholecystectomy. Now, most surgeons agree that the laparoscopic method is the procedure of choice for recurrent hernias after a failed

B.P. Jacob and B. Ramshaw (eds.), *The SAGES Manual of Hernia Repair*,
DOI 10.1007/978-1-4614-4824-2_19,

open procedure because the repair can be performed in an undissected space and for bilateral inguinal hernias as both hernias can be repaired through the same minimal access sites.

A more contentious issue is the application of laparoscopy to the uncomplicated unilateral inguinal hernia. It is now clear that in experienced hands, either operation can be associated with low recurrence rates (i.e., <2%). Because of this fact, recurrence rates as an outcome metric may be less significant than some others. So, a discussion comparing laparoscopic inguinal herniorrhaphy (LIH) with a conventional open tension-free approach (TFR), the subject of this chapter, has to be based on other factors such as short- and long-term pain, risk/benefit ratio as it relates to complications, cost, and return to normal activities. The purpose of this chapter is to explore these other factors to allow the reader to make state of the art decisions for his or her patient.

Laparoscopic Inguinal Hernia Repair

Ger described the first LIH repair in 1982 [3]. He used a clip-applying device to close the internal ring in beagle dogs with congenital indirect inguinal hernias. His approach did not include reconstruction of the inguinal floor, so would have only been applicable to Nyhus type 1 inguinal hernias. Technical problems with the clip applier could never be solved, and thus it was never used in humans on a large-scale basis. Schulz and colleagues tried to capitalize on Ger's idea by packing hernia defects with bulky mesh material. In the end, this approach failed because it did not address the need to reinforce the entire myopectineal orifice to minimize the chance of recurrence. But this did lead to the development of the *intraperitoneal onlay mesh repair* (IPOM), which will be described briefly below.

The most commonly performed laparoscopic repairs today do not attempt to solve the problem intra-abdominally. Rather, they are performed in the preperitoneal space in a manner similar to conventional open preperitoneal inguinal hernia repairs. The principal is to expose all critical anatomical elements in the preperitoneal space and then to use prosthetic material to cover the entire myopectineal orifice. The preperitoneal space can be accessed laparoscopically in two ways:

1. One can perform a laparoscopy, incise the peritoneum from the abdominal cavity, dissect the preperitoneal space, and then cover the entire dissected area, the myopectineal orifice, with a

widely overlapping prosthesis. This is known as the *transabdominal preperitoneal repair* (TAPP) repair.

2. The preperitoneal space can also be entered by dissecting in the space between the posterior rectus sheath and the rectus muscle to enter the preperitoneal space without ever purposely breaching the peritoneal cavity. Once the space is entered, the operation proceeds in an identical fashion as the TAPP. This is known as the *totally extraperitoneal repair* (TEP).

The *intraperitoneal onlay mesh repair* (IPOM) is the only truly minimally invasive laparoscopic hernia repair because a radical dissection of the preperitoneal space is avoided. The principle is that by placing a large overlapping prosthesis as in the TAPP and TEP one layer deeper, that is, directly on the peritoneum, a dissection of the preperitoneal space can be avoided. The IPOM however never became popular because of the reluctance of surgeons to place prosthetic material in the abdominal cavity in contact with intra-abdominal viscera. However, with the IPOM technique now being used routinely for ventral hernias and because of the development of better prosthetic materials, interest in the technique has been renewed especially in TAPP or TEP operations when it is determined that adequate peritoneal coverage of prosthesis is not possible.

Detailed descriptions of these procedures are provided elsewhere in this manual. What follows though is an abbreviated discussion of the technical aspects of the two commonly performed laparoscopic herniorrhaphies as well as the conventional open inguinal herniorrhaphies in order to better place our comparison of the two approaches into perspective.

Transabdominal Preperitoneal (TAPP) Repair

After obtaining peritoneal access at the umbilicus, diagnostic laparoscopy is performed to rule out any unrelated pathology, and both myopectineal orifices are inspected. Two additional trocar sleeves are placed on either side of the umbilicus. The peritoneum is incised transversely to a point medial to the anterior superior iliac spine, staying approximately 2 cm above the internal inguinal ring on the side of the hernia defect. A combination of blunt and sharp dissection is performed in the preperitoneal space to expose the critical anatomical landmarks with the judicious use of electrocautery. Both pubic tubercles, the inferior epigastric vessels, Cooper's ligament, and the iliopubic tract are identified. The spermatic cord structures are mobilized and the peritoneal flap is dissected well proximal to the bifurcation of the vas deferens and the internal spermatic vessels. A direct hernia sac easily reduces during the preperitoneal dissection. A small indirect hernia sac can be dissected away from the cord structures and reduced. A large prosthesis (at least 15 × 10 cm) is placed to generously cover the entire myopectineal orifice, including the site of potential weakness for a femoral hernia. Slitting of the mesh laterally to create a new deep ring is optional. If mesh fixation is chosen, it is begun at the contralateral pubic tubercle medially extending onto the anterior abdominal wall at least 4 cm superior to the hernia defect, to the anterior superior iliac spine laterally, and to the tissue just above Cooper's ligament inferiorly. The most common prosthetic mesh devices are made from polypropylene or polyester, materials known to erode into intra-abdominal viscera on occasion. Therefore, meticulous peritoneal coverage of the prosthesis is essential. The goal is isolation of the prosthesis from the viscera.

Totally Extraperitoneal (TEP) Repair

A three-trocar approach for the TEP repair is used. An infraumbilical incision is performed and either the ipsilateral or contralateral anterior rectus sheath is entered vertically, depending upon the preference of the surgeon. The posterior sheath is visualized after retraction of the rectus muscle, and blunt dissection develops the space between the rectus muscle and the posterior rectus sheath, to allow placement of a trocar sleeve to begin gas insufflation. Additional trocar sleeves are then placed into this space, either in the midline or laterally. A popular adjunct for creating the preperitoneal space is to use a dissecting balloon. Once the preperitoneal space has been completely developed, the operation proceeds in a fashion identical to the TAPP repair. Unlike the TAPP repair, closure of a peritoneal flap is not necessary.

Open Inguinal Hernia Repair

Conventional open tissue repairs were the mainstay for inguinal hernias for most of the twentieth century. Indeed, there have been at least 70 different named tissue repairs described in the literature since the time of Bassini [4]. However, in the late 1990s, Lichtenstein and colleagues [5] revolutionized the approach to inguinal hernia repair by popularizing the routine use of prosthetic material to bridge the hernia defect rather than approximate tissue structures that were not normally in apposition as is performed in the tissue repairs. Many techniques for placement of a prosthesis are described in the literature, which are grouped under the heading of tension-free repairs or TFR. Numerous randomized controlled clinical trials as well as systematic reviews of the same have unequivocally shown that the TFR procedures are superior to the tissue repairs for most parameters analyzed. The only exception might be the Shouldice tissue repair but only when performed in a specialty center such as the Shouldice clinic. Therefore, for the purposes of our comparison, only the TFR approach will be considered.

The procedure as described by Lichtenstein is considered the gold standard TFR. In this technique, the groin is initially prepared by dividing the external oblique aponeurosis through the external inguinal ring followed by mobilization of the cord structures from the inguinal floor. Next, the indirect or direct hernia sac and its contents are reduced into the preperitoneal space after being dissected away from surrounding structures. Instead of approximating anatomical structures as in tissue repairs, a large space is created beneath the aponeurosis of the external oblique from a point at least 2 cm medial to the pubic tubercle to the anterior superior iliac spine laterally which allows the placement of a large flat mesh prosthesis widely overlapping the areas where direct and indirect hernias occur. The mesh is sutured to the anterior rectus sheath 2 cm *medial* to the pubic tubercle, and this suture is then continued laterally in a running fashion, securing the caudal edge of the prosthesis to either side of the pubic tubercle and the inguinal ligament to the level of the internal ring. The mesh is then slit to accommodate the cord structures and the tails thus created are passed beneath the external oblique to the anterior superior iliac spine with the superior tail overlapping the inferior. A so-called shutter valve stitch approximates the inferior surface of the superior tail to the inferior surface of the inferior tail and the inguinal ligament. The mesh is then trimmed in situ and fixed to the rectus sheath medially and the internal oblique muscle cranially with a few interrupted sutures. The external oblique aponeurosis is again closed over the cord structures and the skin is approximated.

Multiple other mesh-based TFR techniques have now been described in the literature, most notable of which is the plug and patch mesh hernioplasty [6], which remains a popular alternative to the classic Lichtenstein. The preperitoneal space can also be accessed using an open approach as originally described by Stoppa [7] but now adapted to a more minimally invasive open technique such as the Kugel [8]. The Prolene Hernia System [9] exploits both the conventional anterior space and the preperitoneal by using a bilayer prosthesis consisting of two flat pieces of mesh connected by a polypropylene cylinder. For the purpose of the comparison in this chapter, all of these mesh-based procedures will be considered equivalent when performed by a surgeon experienced in a particular operation.

LIH Versus TFR

The Veterans Affairs Cooperative Studies Program 456: "Open Mesh Versus Laparoscopic Mesh Repair of Inguinal Hernia" [10]

This landmark study was published in 2004 in the New England Journal of Medicine. This was a well-funded study, which was carefully developed with clear-cut methods. The study surgeons were experienced with both techniques but for the most part did not have a specialty interest in inguinal hernia repair. This was by design because the goal of the study was to compare LIH to TFR in a setting of general practice rather than a specialty hernia center. The primary outcome was recurrence at 2 years. The results were unfavorable for LIH not only in terms of recurrence but also in many other parameters studied when compared to other randomized controlled trials especially those performed in laparoscopic centers of excellence. It has been criticized by LIH proponents that the surgeons were less skilled. The study certainly cannot be completely discounted though and may indeed be more reflective of how these procedures are performed in general practice. Because of the large number of patients involved (2,164), the study can dominate meta-analysis, and this will be pointed out as we contrast and compare TFR to LIH.

Repair or No Repair?

The initial question to be answered is whether an inguinal hernia needs to be repaired at all? For a patient presenting with significant symptoms, the answer is obviously yes. For patient presenting with minimal or no symptoms, the answer is not clear. A multicenter, prospective, randomized controlled trial of watchful waiting versus elective repair published in JAMA in 2006 [11] has shown that "a strategy of watchful waiting is a safe and acceptable option for men with asymptomatic or minimally symptomatic inguinal hernias." In this study, hernia accidents (defined as a strangulation or a bowel obstruction) were uncommon at a rate of 1.8 per 1,000 patient years, which translates into a cumulative risk of one fifth of 1% per year. At 2 years, 23% of the watchful waiting patients had crossed over to receive surgical repair, but that still left the majority that had avoided an operation. Further analysis of the data in this study showed that watchful waiting approach was cost effective [12] and that patients who ultimately cross over to operation because of symptoms do as well as those who proceed with immediate repair [13]. Longer-term results are pending. O'Dwyer [14] performed a similar randomized controlled trial but at a single specialized institution in Scotland and did not report as favorable results. At 1 year, there was a trend, which suggested that operating on asymptomatic patients might improve quality of life and reduce potentially serious morbidity. In a second publication, using Kaplan–Meier estimates, these investigators predict a conversion rate from observation to operation of 84% at 7.5 years. They concluded "there seems little point in watchful waiting because the majority of patients will require an operation in the foreseeable future." This study was limited to patients older than 55 years of age who had to have a visible bulge to qualify for watchful waiting. Thus, the population was older and had more advanced hernias than in the former study, there were significantly smaller number of patients (160), and revised calculations were needed after the study had been initiated due to slow accrual to achieve 80% power. (The percentage of asymptomatic patients who were expected to develop pain was changed from 15% to 20%.) As a result of these trials, many surgeons and patients opt for watchful waiting approach for minimally symptomatic inguinal hernias. The recent guidelines published by the European Hernia Society recommend that watchful waiting is an acceptable option for men with minimally symptomatic or asymptomatic inguinal hernia [15]. Of note, these studies recruited only men with inguinal hernias. This is because the natural history of a groin hernia is worse in women than in men [16], and hence, all women should be offered repair regardless of symptoms.

What Repair, Laparoscopic or Open?

Anesthesia

Laparoscopic repair of inguinal hernia almost always requires general anesthesia, while open repair can be easily performed under local or regional anesthesia. The use of local anesthesia has been shown to result in shorter duration of admission, less postoperative pain, and fewer micturition difficulties [17]. The patient satisfaction rates are also high. Despite the powerful argument in favor of local anesthesia for a conventional inguinal herniorrhaphy, it is underutilized as it is used in only 6–18% open repairs [18]. Thus, the importance of this argument for conventional surgery is greatly diminished.

Early Complications

There is a higher rate of rare but serious intraoperative complications with the laparoscopic approach. Major vascular and visceral (especially bladder) injury has been reported and is seen more commonly with the TAPP procedure (0.65% versus 0–0.17% for TEP and open mesh repair). Trocar sleeve site hernias and intestinal obstruction due to inadequate peritoneal closure or adhesions are also theoretically more likely with the TAPP procedure. Other local complications including hematoma and wound infection are more often seen with open approach, while seroma formation is common with laparoscopic approach.

In the Veterans Affairs (VA) cooperative trial discussed above [10], the overall incidence of intraoperative and immediate postoperative complications was higher in the laparoscopic group including life-threatening events. However, in a meta-analysis performed by Schmedt et al. [19], a significantly higher total morbidity was found for the Lichtenstein repair compared to laparoscopic repair when the VA trial was excluded.

Late Complications

Recurrence

Recurrence of the hernia remains the most import parameter to measure the efficacy of an inguinal hernia repair. Since 1996, a number of randomized trials have compared laparoscopic and open mesh repairs of inguinal hernias (Table 19.1). In the VA trial, the recurrence rate was significantly higher among patients with unilateral inguinal hernia in the laparoscopic group than in the open group (10.1% versus 4.0%; OR 2.9; 95% CI, 1.8–4.5). However, the study also has shown that in the hands of highly experienced surgeons (>250 laparoscopic hernia repairs), the recurrence rate was comparable between laparoscopic and open repairs (5.1% versus 4.1%; OR 1.3; 95% CI, 0.6–2.7). Similarly, Langeveld

Table 19.1. Comparative trials of laparoscopic and open inguinal hernia repair using mesh.

Author, year	Hernias (n) LH vs. OH	Intervention	Recurrence rate (%)	Salient results
Horeyseck et al. 1996	100 vs. 100	TAPP vs. Lichtenstein	8 vs. 0	Higher recurrence, higher cost
Zieren et al. 1996	86 vs. 105	TAPP vs. PP	2.3 vs. 0	Higher recurrence, higher cost, similar complications
Sarli et al. 1997	64 vs. 66	TAPP vs. Lichtenstein	0 vs. 0	Similar complications, missed contralateral hernias in OH group
Champault et al. 1997	50 vs. 50	TAPP vs. Stoppa	6 vs. 2	Lower morbidity, higher patient comfort, higher recurrence rate
Khoury et al. 1998	169 vs. 146	TAPP vs. MP	2.5 vs. 3	Similar recurrence rates, earlier return to normal activity, fewer nerve complications
Paganini et al. 1998	52 vs. 56	TAPP vs. Lichtenstein	2 vs. 0	Similar return to normal activity, higher cost
Aitola et al. 1998	24 vs. 25	TAPP vs. Lichtenstein	13 vs. 8	Similar return to work, higher recurrences
Picehio et al. 1998	53 vs. 52	TAPP vs. Lichtenstein	Not mentioned	Higher pain scores, similar recovery periods
Kumar et al. 1999	25 vs. 25	TEP vs. Lichtenstein	4 vs. 8	Lower pain score, fewer local complications
Johansson et al. 1999	613 total	TAFP vs. preperitoneal mesh vs. conventional	2 vs. 5.5 vs. 2	Earlier resumption of normal activity and return to work, higher cost
MRC group 1994	468 vs. 460	TEP vs. mainly tension free	1.9 vs. 0	Earlier resumption of normal activity, less long-term pain, higher recurrence rate
Beets et al. 1999	56 vs. 52	TAPP vs. Stoppa	12.5 vs.1.9	Lesser pain, fewer early complications
Sarli et al. 2000	40 vs. 46	TAPP vs. Lichtenstein	0 vs. 4.3	Lesser pain, earlier return to work

(continued)

Table 19.1. (continued)

Author, year	Hernias (n) LH vs. OH	Intervention	Recurrence rate (%)	Salient results
Writiht et al. 2002	145 vs. 151	TEP vs. mostly Lichtenstein	2 vs. 2	Similar recurrences, similar missed contralateral hernias
Pikoulis et al. 2002	309 vs. 234	TAPP vs. MP	1.9 vs. 0.4	Higher cost, higher recurrence rate
Mahon et al. 2003	60 vs. 60 (all bilateral or recurrent)	TAPP vs. Lichtenstein	6.7 vs. 1.7	Shorter operative lime, less pain, earlier return to work
Andersson et al. 2003	81 vs. 87	TEP vs. Lichtenstein	2.5 vs. 0	Similar complications, earlier return to work, less pain, higher recurrence rate
Douek et al. 2003	122 vs. 120	TAPP vs. Lichtenstein	1.6 vs. 2.5	Less groin pain, less frequent paresthesias
Bringman et al. 20O3	Total no – 298	TEP vs. MP vs. Lichtenstein	1.3 vs. 1.3	Shorter sick-leave period, less time to full recovery
Lal et al. 2003	25 vs. 25	TEP vs. Lichtenstein	0 vs. 0	Earlier return to work, better cosmesis, similar recurrence rate
Colak et al. 2003	67 vs. 67	TEP vs. Lichtenstein	2.9 vs. 5.9	Short follow-up
Heikkinen et al. 2004	62 vs. 61	TAPP vs. Lichtenstein	8 vs.3.2	Similar recurrence rate, less long-term groin pain
Neumayer et al. 2004	862 vs. 834	TAPP/TEP vs. Lichtenstein	10.1 vs. 4	Less pain, higher recurrence rate for primary hernias
Lau et al. 2006	100 vs. 100	TEP vs. Lichtenstein	0 vs. 0	1-year data only, increased chronic pain
Eklund 2007	73 vs. 74	TAPP vs. Lichtenstein	19 vs. 18	Recurrent hernias, less postoperative pain and sick leave
Butters et al. 2007	81 vs. 76 vs. 74	TAPP vs. Lichtenstein vs. Shouldice	1.2 vs. 1.3 vs. 8.1	Open repair associated with nerve injury

Hallen 2008	73 vs. 81	TEP vs. Lichtenstein	4.3 vs. 5.1	Increased testicular pain in TEP group, long-term follow-up of old data
Pokorny et al. 2008	Total no – 365	TEP vs. TAPP vs. Bassini vs. Shouldice vs. Lichtenstein	5.9 vs. 4.7 vs. 3.4 vs. 4.7 vs. 0.0	Small number of patients
Eklund et al. 2009	665 vs. 705	TEP vs. Lichtenstein	3.5 vs. 1.2	Three surgeons in the TEP group were responsible for 57% (12/21) of all recurrences, less chronic pain
Langeveld et al. 2010	336 vs. 324	TEP vs. Lichtenstein	3.8 vs. 3.0	Higher intraoperative complications, similar pain

LH laparoscopic hernia repair, *OH* open inguinal hernia repair, *TAPP* transabdominal preperitoneal hernia repair, *PP* patch plug repair, *MP* mesh plug repair, *TEP* totally extraperitoneal repair et al. [20] have shown that experience decreases the incidence of recurrence with laparoscopic approach.

On further meta-analysis performed by the European Hernia Society working group on data with a minimum of 4 years follow-up, the Lichtenstein technique performs slightly but not significantly better concerning the recurrence, OR of 1.16 (95% CI, 0.63–2.16).

The literature considering recurrence after TAPP versus TEP is not elaborate. At the time of a meta-analysis published in 2005, there was only one randomized controlled study [21], and it included a small number of patients. The meta-analysis [22] showed that there were no differences between the two groups, but confidence intervals were all very wide, and hence, it does not rule out clinically important differences.

Chronic Pain

Early literature which discussed the incidence of chronic pain such as the VA trial [10] or a meta-analysis performed by the respected European hernia trialist group [23] showed little difference between the laparoscopic and open repair. However, Table 19.2 is a representative collection of relatively recent studies, which consistently show that LIH performs better than TFR in this regard. Aasvang and colleagues [24] studied 464 patients from Denmark and Germany using sophisticated tools designed to identify risk factors for postoperative pain. They determined that TFR was a risk factor for chronic pain at 6 months. Based on this literature, the European Hernia Society guidelines [15] state, "When only considering chronic pain, endoscopic surgery is superior to open mesh."

Most of the literature dealing with chronic groin pain is relatively short term. However, Eklund et al. [25] published a randomized controlled trial comparing TEP LIH with a Lichtenstein TFR, which showed that the frequency of any degree of chronic pain up to 5 years after operation was twice as high in the Lichtenstein group as in the TEP group. Moderate to severe pain occurred in 1.9% patients in the TEP group versus 3.5% in the Lichtenstein group at 5 years. They conclude, "the present study demonstrated an advantage of TEP over Lichtenstein hernia repair with respect to chronic postoperative pain at long-term follow-up."

Contralateral Hernia

The ability to easily explore the opposite groin at the time of LIH has resulted in an incidence of contralateral hernia much higher than one

Table 19.2. Studies comparing chronic groin pain after open versus laparoscopic inguinal hernia repair.

Author, year	Study design	Intervention	Incidence of pain (%)	Salient features
Macintyre et al. 2002	Questionnaire study	TEP vs. Lichtenstein	22.5 vs. 38.3	Mean follow-up of 21 months
Grant et al. 2004	Prospective randomized study	TEP vs. Lichtenstein	18.1 vs. 20.1	Questionnaire study of a randomized trial
Gunnarson et al. 2006	Retrospective study	TEP/TAPP vs. Lichtenstein	25 vs. 32	Study from Swedish Hernia registry
Berndsen et al. 2007	Prospective randomized study	TAPP vs. Shouldice	8.5 vs. 11.4	Non-mesh open technique
Beldi et al. 2008	Retrospective study	Laparoscopic vs. open non-mesh vs. open mesh	16.6 vs. 17.5 vs. 25	Small number of patients
Eklund et al. 2010	Prospective randomized study	TEP vs. Lichtenstein	1.9 vs. 3.5	Chronic pain diminishes with long-term follow-up
Kehlet et al. 2010	Prospective non-randomized study	TAPP vs. Lichtenstein	14.6 vs. 30.3	Light-weight mesh in laparoscopy compared to heavy-weight mesh in open group
Bright 2010	Retrospective study	TAPP vs. TEP vs. Open	1.5 vs. 3 vs. 0.7	Attendance to chronic pain clinic. Open is better than laparoscopic repair.

TAPP transabdominal preperitoneal hernia repair, *TEP* totally extraperitoneal repair

Table 19.3. Studies reporting incidence of contralateral hernia.

Author, year	Intervention	Total number of patients	Incidence of contralateral hernia (%)
Phillips et al. 1998	Diagnostic laparoscopy followed by TEP	73	50
Evans et al. 2000	TAPP	2,000	22
Ferzli et al. 2000	TEP	552	11.2
Koehler et al. 2002	Diagnostic laparoscopy followed by TEP	69	13
Singhal et al. 2005	TAPP procedure	377	18.8
Oleynikov et al. 2007	TEP	100	22

TEP totally extraperitoneal hernia repair, *TAPP* transabdominal preperitoneal hernia repair

would have predicted in the prelaparoscopic era. Table 19.3 is a listing of LIH publications where the contralateral hernia incidence was recorded. One can appreciate a rate between 11% and 50%. These incidentally found hernias can easily be repaired through the same access ports as the index hernia, and the morbidity has been shown to be similar in both unilateral and bilateral laparoscopic repairs [26]. Not surprisingly, LIH enthusiasts have used this fact as an argument to support LIH. However, there are two problems with routine repair of a contralateral hernia. The first is that a consistent definition of an incidental hernia does not exist, and therefore, what one surgeon calls a normal variant, another might call a hernia. The second problem revolves around the issue discussed above, chronic groin pain. Since the vast majority of these patients are asymptomatic, a strong argument can be made for doing nothing and take a "watchful waiting" approach. The rationale for this is to avoid a chronic postherniorrhaphy groin pain syndrome in a patient who was previously asymptomatic. For these reasons, debate continues whether there is a role for treatment on the contralateral side, if the patient is asymptomatic. Surgeons who favor the TEP approach using a balloon dissector to create the preperitoneal space tend to have the lowest threshold for contralateral repair because invariably the contralateral preperitoneal space is at least partially developed which makes subsequent TEP repair more difficult. In addition, this partial dissection is thought to increase the occurrence of a contralateral hernia.

Cost-Effectiveness

From a hospital standpoint, the laparoscopic approach is associated with higher costs compared to the open approach. However, from a socioeconomic perspective, laparoscopic approach is more cost effective. McCormack et al. [27] reviewed the cost-effectiveness in 2005 and at that time showed that when productivity costs and quality of life are included in the analyses, laparoscopic approach was advantageous. However, this study based primarily on randomized trials performed in the late 1990s, and at that time, the operative times were longer for the laparoscopic approach compared to open. With increasing expertise, the operative times are equal if not better, and hence, the cost analysis would probably favor laparoscopic approach. The problem with this analysis is that the funding for the direct medical costs and socioeconomic costs does not come from the same "pot." Although there have been studies showing equivalent financial expenditure when a concerted effort is made to minimize items such as disposables for LIH, these tend to be flawed because a concerted effort to control the TFR costs is not included. Just as any gambler knows that in the end, the house is always going to win based on basic mathematics; it is impossible to take an operation which can be performed even without an anesthesiologist which only requires a few instruments, some suture, and a relatively cheap prosthesis (TFR) and try to argue cost equivalence for an operation which must be performed under general anesthesia and has expensive high-tech equipment needs which must be amortized (LIH). Depending upon the final form of health care reform, which is now inevitable, this could represent a severe threat to LIH.

Future Pelvic Surgery

An advantage of the TFR procedure is that it does not enter the preperitoneal space and, therefore, does not affect future operations such as prostatectomy, which might need to be performed later in life. The laparoscopic approach, on the other hand, enters the retropubic preperitoneal space and, with placement of mesh, results in scarring. Although recent literature suggests that prostatectomy is technically possible, it is more difficult [28]. The general consensus at present is to avoid LIH in patients with a strong family history of prostate cancer and to perform prostate cancer screening in elderly male patients undergoing laparoscopic inguinal hernia repair.

Recommendations

Watchful Waiting

Adult male with minimal or asymptomatic unilateral inguinal hernia

Open Repair

Large scrotal hernia
Patient who cannot tolerate general anesthesia
Recurrent hernia when original was performed in the preperitoneal space
↑ risk for prostate cancer

Laparoscopic Repair

Recurrent hernia when original was performed in the conventional anterior space
Bilateral hernias
Women with groin hernia
Sports hernia

Laparoscopic or Open Repair

Choice for the uncomplicated unilateral hernias should depend on the surgeon's expertise.

References

1. DeFrances CJ, Cullen KA, Kozak LJ. National hospital discharge survey: 2005 annual summary with detailed diagnosis and procedure data. Vital Health Stat. 2007;13(165):1–209.
2. Lyons AS, Pertrucelli II RJ. Medicine: an illustrated history. New York: Harry N. Abrams Publishers; 1987.

3. Ger R. The management of certain abdominal herniae by intraabdominal closure of the neck of the sac. Ann R Coll Surg Engl. 1982;64:342–4.
4. Amid PK. Groin hernia repair: open techniques. World J Surg. 2005;29(8):1046–51.
5. Lichtenstein IL, Shulman AG, Amid PK, et al. The tension free hernioplasty. Am J Surg. 1989;157:188–93.
6. Rutkow IM, Robbins AW. Mesh plug hernia repair: a follow-up report. Surgery. 1995;117:597.
7. Stoppa RE. The treatment of complicated groin and incisional hernias. World J Surg. 1989;13:545–54.
8. Kugel RD. Minimally invasive, nonlaparoscopic, pre- peritoneal, and sutureless, inguinal herniorrhaphy. Am J Surg. 1999;178:298–302.
9. Vironen J, Nieminen J, Eklund A, et al. Randomized clinical trial of Lichtenstein patch or Prolene Hernia System for inguinal hernia repair. Br J Surg. 2006;93(1):33–9.
10. Neumayer L, Giobbie-Hurder A, Jonasson O, et al. Open vs. laparoscopic mesh repair of inguinal hernias. N Engl J Med. 2004;350(18):1819–27.
11. Fitzgibbons RJ, Giobbie-Hurder A, Gibbs JO, et al. Watchful waiting vs. repair of inguinal hernia in minimally symptomatic men. JAMA. 2006;295(3):285–92.
12. Stroupe KT, Manheim LM, Luo P, et al. Tension-free repair versus watchful waiting for men with asymptomatic or minimally symptomatic inguinal hernias: a cost effectiveness analysis. J Am Coll Surg. 2006;203(4):458–68.
13. Thompson JS, Gibbs JO, Reda DJ, et al. Does delaying repair of an asymptomatic hernia have a penalty? Am J Surg. 2008;195(1):89–93.
14. Chung L, Norrie J, O'Dwyer PJ. Long-term follow-up of patients with a painless inguinal hernia from a randomized clinical trial. Br J Surg. 2011;98:596–9.
15. Simons MP, Aufenacker T, Bay-Nielsen M, et al. European Hernia Society guidelines on the treatment of inguinal hernia in adult patients. Hernia. 2009;13:343–403.
16. Koch A, Edwards A, Haapaniemi S, Nordin P, Kald A. Prospective evaluation of 6895 groin hernia repairs in women. Br J Surg. 2005;92(12):1553–8.
17. Nordin P, Zetterström H, Gunnarsson U, Nilsson E. Local, regional or general anaesthesia in groin hernia repair: multicentre randomized trial. Lancet. 2003;362:853–8.
18. Sanjay P, Woodward A. Inguinal hernia repair: local or general anaesthesia? Ann R Coll Surg Engl. 2007;89(5):497–503.
19. Schmedt CG, Sauerland S, Bittner R. Comparison of endoscopic procedures vs. Lichtenstein and other open mesh techniques for inguinal hernia repair: a meta-analysis of randomized controlled trials. Surg Endosc. 2005;19:188–99.
20. Langeveld HR, van't Riet M, Weidema WF, Stassen LP, Steyerberg EW, Lange J, Bonjer HJ, Jeekel J. Total extraperitoneal inguinal hernia repair compared with Lichtenstein (the LEVEL-Trial): a randomized controlled trial. Ann Surg. 2010;251(5):819–24.
21. Schrenk P, Woisetschlager R, Rieger R, et al. Prospective randomised trial comparing postoperative pain and return to physical activity after transabdominal preperitoneal, total preperitoneal or Shouldice technique for inguinal hernia repair. Br J Surg. 1996;83:1563–6.
22. McCormack K, Wake BL, Fraser C, Vale L, Perez J, Grant A. Transabdominal pre-peritoneal (TAPP) versus totally extraperitoneal (TEP) laparoscopic techniques for inguinal hernia repair: a systematic review. Hernia. 2005;9:109–14.

23. Grant AM, Scott NW, O'Dwyer PJ, MRC Laparoscopic Groin Hernia Trial Group. Five-year follow-up of a randomized trial to assess pain and numbness after laparoscopic or open repair of groin hernia. Br J Surg. 2004;91:1570–4.
24. Aasvang EK, Gmaehle E, Hansen JB, Gmaehle B, Forman JL, Schwarz J, Bittner R, Kehlet H. Predictive risk factors for persistent postherniotomy pain. Anesthesiology. 2010;112(4):957–69.
25. Eklund A, Montgomery A, Bergkvist L, Rudberg C, Swedish Multicentre Trial of Inguinal Hernia Repair by Laparoscopy (SMIL) study group. Chronic pain 5 years after randomized comparison of laparoscopic and Lichtenstein inguinal hernia repair. Br J Surg. 2010;97(4):600–8. PubMed PMID: 20186889.
26. Wauschkuhn CA, Schwarz J, Boekeler U, Bittner R. Laparoscopic inguinal hernia repair: gold standard in bilateral hernia repair? Results of more than 2800 patients in comparison to literature. Surg Endosc. 2010;24(12):3026–30.
27. McCormack K, Wake B, Perez J, Fraser C, Cook J, McIntosh E, Vale L, Grant A. Laparoscopic surgery for inguinal hernia repair: systematic review of effectiveness and economic evaluation. Health Technol Assess. 2005;9:1–203. iii–iv.
28. Erdogru T, Teber D, Frede T, Marrero R, Hammady A, Rassweiler J. The effect of previous transperitoneal laparoscopic inguinal herniorrhaphy on transperitoneal laparoscopic radical prostatectomy. J Urol. 2005;173(3):769–72.

20. Polyester, Polypropylene, ePTFE for Inguinal Hernias: Does It Really Matter?

Dmitry Oleynikov and Matthew Goede

For over 20 years, following studies demonstrating the Lichtenstein technique, inguinal hernia repair has been routinely performed with the use of a prosthetic mesh device. The closure of inguinal hernias with mesh without tension has become the new standard of care for hernia repair. It is clear that tension-free hernia repair with mesh is superior to tissue repair alone, especially when considering the risk of recurrence. However, early studies did not differentiate between different mesh products, because at that time, few meshes were commercially available for surgeons to use. For instance, all original data demonstrating the effectiveness of the Lichtenstein repair is limited to the utilization of heavyweight polypropylene mesh [1].

Ever since the use of polypropylene mesh was described by Usher in 1959 for the repair of inguinal hernias [2], surgeons have been in search of the perfect mesh. Prior to the use of polypropylene, which has been the predominant mesh used in the repair of the inguinal hernia for the last 50 years, Koontz described the use of tantalum wire mesh in 1951 [3]. Numerous other materials have been described in the repair of inguinal hernias, including those comprised of nylon and stainless steel.

The ideal mesh needs to be strong enough to resist bursting pressures generated by the abdomen. It should be chemically inert, so as not to cause an inflammatory or foreign-body reaction, be noncarcinogenic, and lack properties that would cause allergic or hypersensitivity reactions. Mesh must have specific mechanical properties so that it can be easily and inexpensively fabricated, modified, or cut without unraveling or losing its shape. Mesh needs to have good handling features intraoperatively, be sterilizable, and be resistant to infection. Most

B.P. Jacob and B. Ramshaw (eds.), *The SAGES Manual of Hernia Repair*, DOI 10.1007/978-1-4614-4824-2_20,

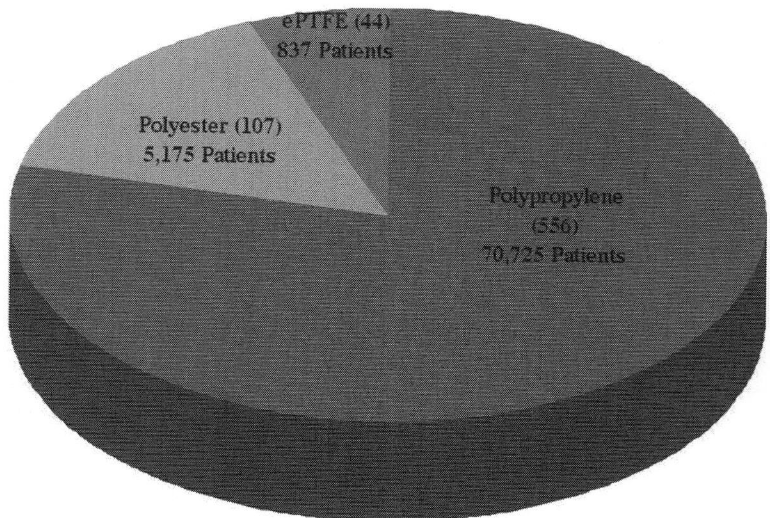

Fig. 20.1. Number of published studies based on mesh type. See Table 20.1 for details.

Table 20.1. Number of published studies based on mesh type.

	Polyester (107)	ePTFE (44)	Polypropylene (556)
# of patients	5,175	837	70,725
Recurrence (%)	0.7–3	1–4	1–9
Infection (%)	0–1	0–2	0–1
Chronic pain (%)	0.5–3	2–7	2–10

See Fig. 20.1

importantly, mesh must be able to be easily incorporated into the surrounding tissues and allow for long-term reinforcement of the tissues.

Recently, as new mesh options have become available and long-term follow-up has been performed, mesh material has been studied for its relative advantages, disadvantages, costs, and rates of recurrences (Fig. 20.1 and Table 20.1). Initially, studies only reviewed recurrence rates for a number of mesh products. As evidence was reported related to the likelihood of heavyweight polypropylene shrinkage while in the host body due to a severe reaction, new materials that were less likely to shrink began to be introduced. Shrinkage was not the only problem noted with traditional mesh use; rates of infection were also reviewed. Authors found that certain meshes were more likely to be colonized by bacteria, and clearance of bacteria was impossible in certain mesh types. Weight of the mesh contributed to chronic pelvic discomfort and pain, which was also noted in recent studies as a factor for choosing the proper mesh. Careful strength analysis of different types of mesh demonstrated that meshes were overengineered, and their relative thickness and constitutions were far heavier than the typical forces they were experiencing while implanted in the groin region. Finally, cost has recently become a determining factor in many institutions related to mesh choice, be it for contracting or other preferences. Only certain meshes are now available at hospitals, thus further limiting the choice of physicians in those institutions. New surgical techniques of mesh placement, such as using a plug in the indirect hernia space or placing the mesh in the preperitoneal space, has further complicated the best-mesh question as the performance of these meshes differ in the performance of traditionally anterior mesh patches as described by Lichtenstein.

Tissue Repair Versus Mesh Repair

Although some centers claim recurrence rates with primary tissue repairs that are equivalent to that of tension-free mesh repairs, large studies have shown inferior results with tissue repair. Proponents of tissue repairs cite the multiple but rare complications associated with mesh-like chronic pain or infection. However, a meta-analysis of over 11,000 patients showed that the use of mesh, placed either open or laparoscopically, decreased both the recurrence rate and the incidence of chronic pain [4]. And while it may be true that implantation of a foreign body might introduce some new complications like infection or migration of the mesh, it appears that these are rare events and occur in less than 1% of cases in which they are used. Since most tissue repairs are performed with suture made of the same material most mesh is made of, even tissue repairs have some degree of foreign-body reaction. It appears that in mesh repairs, the inflammatory reaction is short and self-limiting. In a study by Di Vita [5], inflammatory markers were measured following Bassini and Lichtenstein hernia repairs. They found a significant increase in leukocytosis 6 and 24 h after a Lichtenstein repair, but not in a Bassini repair. After Lichtenstein repair, the fibrinogen levels were significantly increased at 24 and 48 h, and the alpha-1 antitrypsin levels were significantly increased at 6, 24, and 48 h, without a corresponding increase seen in the Bassini repairs. Interleukin-6 (IL-6) and C-reactive protein (CRP) increased in both repairs but was significantly higher in the Lichtenstein group. Interestingly though, by postoperative day 7, the markers had returned to their baselines in both groups. Despite the increases in inflammatory markers, the patients in the Lichtenstein group had significantly less postoperative pain.

Choice of Mesh Repair

The choice of mesh is largely based on the technique being performed. The requirements for an intraperitoneal onlay mesh (IPOM) are significantly different than those for a recurrent hernia being repaired in an open Lichtenstein technique. All of the commercially available mesh products have literature to support their use and acceptable complication and recurrence rates. However, there is very little comparative data between the different mesh products. The three materials currently used in the majority of inguinal hernia repairs have more than a 40-year track record. Usher described the use of polypropylene in 1959, Calne described the use of polyester in 1967 [6], and Copello described the use of Teflon (PTFE) in 1968 [7]. However, polypropylene has approximately four times as many articles published about it than does polyester or ePTFE [8].

All of the current commercially available meshes have foreign-body reactions. Insertion of a prosthetic starts a biochemical cascade that leads to the eventual incorporation of the prosthetic. Fibrinogen, immunoglobulins, and albumin begin to coat the material after it is implanted. Cellular elements, including platelets, macrophages, and neutrophils, followed by fibroblasts and smooth muscle cells, then migrate into the prosthetic. However, the degree of this response and the overall result is significantly different between materials. While this inflammatory response may or may not benefit the strength of an inguinal repair, it has significantly different repercussions when it is placed in the vicinity of other tissue, for example, the iliac vessels, spermatic cord, or bowel.

In an attempt to optimize this inflammatory reaction, manufacturers have begun to coat the base mesh with several substances that would improve some characteristics of the mesh: fluoropolymers, titanium, D-glucan, silicone, and omega-3 fatty acids have all been used to try to decrease the inflammatory response to a mesh polymer, usually polypropylene.

When contact with the abdominal viscera is anticipated, be it from the rarely performed IPOM or during a preperitoneal open or laparoscopic repair in which the peritoneum is significantly torn and total coverage of the mesh is no longer possible, a mesh that does not react with the bowel is necessary. Until recently, microporous ePTFE was the only acceptable option. However, there are now multiple meshes that have a polypropylene or polyester base with some kind of anti-adhesion barrier (e.g., collagen, hyaluronic acid, omega-3 fatty acids, or cellulose) to prevent integration with the bowel. ePTFE is known for its relative inertness. It was initially developed as a vascular conduit because of this feature, but its use was soon expanded to tissue reinforcement. While inertness is a useful feature when near abdominal viscera, its inability to incorporate into surrounding tissues makes the repair rely heavily on the mesh fixation for durability.

In laparoscopic preperitoneal repairs, a major determinant of mesh selection is the handling properties of the material. Because of the limited space, especially in a total extraperitoneal (TEP) repair, a mesh with some memory favors deployment, retention, and fixation. However, with traditional polypropylene mesh, as memory is increased, the compliance decreases, which leads to an increase in foreign-body sensation. Several designs have been developed, be it anatomic or 3-dimensional shapes, which allow the mesh to rest in the myopectineal orifice, thereby allowing a lighter-weight polypropylene mesh to be used. Polyester mesh has good memory and increased compliance, which makes its use in TEP repairs appealing. Shah retrospectively compared polypropylene and polyester mesh used in laparoscopic repairs [9]. The authors conclude that polyester had a significantly lower incidence of chronic pain and foreign-body sensation as well as the sensation of a mass in the groin compared with polypropylene.

While mesh infection in inguinal hernia repair is uncommon, mesh that would be completely resistant to infection would be ideal [10]. There are several characteristics of a mesh that affect its resistance to infection. Microporous meshes which have pores less than 10 μ m cannot accommodate macrophages but can allow the passage and presence of bacteria, leading them to be more susceptible to infection. This is the reason that infected ePTFE requires removal to clear the infection. Also, the construction of the mesh can provide interstices in which bacteria can "hide" and lead to persistent infection. Multifilament, woven, or knitted meshes like Dacron and some other polyester and polypropylene meshes have been reported to have this bacterial harboring effect. The use of monofilament polypropylene in infected fields has been described, with successful outcomes at times. It appears that with the development of biologic prosthetics, the use of synthetic prosthetics in infected fields will become more of historical interest.

The overall result in hernia repair is to obliterate the defect and relieve the symptoms of the patient. The cure cannot be worse than the disease. Therefore, in an attempt to decrease the symptoms of the repair, namely, pain and foreign-body sensation, lightweight meshes have gained popularity recently. The density of a mesh seems to have a role in how a prosthetic behaves once it is implanted. Less dense mesh can minimize contracture and pain; however, the optimal density and pore size are yet to be determined. In an innovative study by Agarwal [11], patients with bilateral inguinal hernias underwent TEP repairs with heavyweight polypropylene mesh implanted in one groin and reduced-polypropylene large-pore lightweight mesh implanted in the other groin, thereby serving as the control. All the patients reported a difference between the two sides, and there was less foreign-body sensation in the lightweight polypropylene side in the short term. At 1 year, the incidence of pain was similar for both heavyweight and lightweight polypropylene. In a meta-analysis that evaluated heavyweight, lightweight, and partially absorbable meshes performed by Markar, they found that prolonged pain and foreign-body sensation was almost double in the heavyweight mesh group, while the recurrence rates were the same between all the classes of mesh [4].

While it seems logical that strength would be a major determinant in mesh choice, the breaking strength of most of the commercially available meshes far exceeds the forces generated by the abdominal cavity. However, with the transition toward more lightweight meshes, there are several meshes available today that are equal to or slightly less than the burst strength of the abdominal wall. A comprehensive study by Deeken [12] was performed looking at nine different FDA-approved meshes. Suture retention exceeded 20 N, the tear strength of the abdominal wall, in all of the meshes except for the polypropylene-poliglecaprone mesh. Tear resistance was less than 20 N in woven PTFE, two configurations of lightweight polypropylene, and polypropylene-poliglecaprone. To further complicate the issue, for some meshes, the suture retention strength, tensile testing, and tear resistance were different based on the orientation of the mesh. However, strength alone cannot be the determinate for an appropriate mesh. Mesh that is overly stiff can lead to the sensation of a foreign body. Tantalum and stainless steel wire meshes were some of the initially described hernia meshes, but they were rapidly abandoned,

Table 20.2. Cost of mesh per cm^2[a].

Company	Weight	Dominant material	Design	Cost per cm^2
Covidien	Medium	Polyester	Multifilament	$0.44
	Light	Polyester	Monofilament	$0.46
	Light	Polyester	Self-fixating	$1.54
	Heavy	Polypropylene	Mono/multi	$0.68
	Heavy	Polypropylene	Open weave	$0.98
Ethicon	Light	Polypropylene	Monofilament	$0.53
	Heavy	Polypropylene	Knitted	$0.31
	Light	Polyester	Knitted	$0.51
Bard Davol	Light	Polypropylene	Monofilament	$0.24
	Heavy	Polypropylene	Monofilament	$0.38
	Medium	Polypropylene	Knitted monofilament	$1.42
	Light	Polypropylene	Knitted monofilament	$1.69
Columnar	Heavy	Polyester	Mosquito net	<$0.01
Gore	Medium/heavy	PTFE (teflon)	Knitted monofilament	$0.86

[a]All costs are approximate retail catalog prices

partially due to their rigidity and the chronic discomfort they imposed on the patient. The development of biologic prosthetics opens a new area of research into inguinal repairs. The proponents of biologics state that the use of mesh combines the benefits of both tissue and mesh repairs. The use of the biologic prosthetic allows for a tension-free repair. The mesh leaves no foreign body behind as the biologic is replaced with native collagen. When new collagen is produced in a wound, it has a strength of approximately 75% of the native connective tissue, which would seem to favor the use of prosthetic mesh for the foreseeable future. It may be that the selection of mesh is more of an academic problem. There have been multiple studies showing successful and durable repairs with minimal complications using such low-cost materials like nylon or polyethylene mosquito netting [13]. The use of mosquito netting sheds light on an important but frequently overlooked concept in mesh repairs—cost. As newer mesh is developed with features such as self-adhering cleats, partially absorbable mesh, and impregnated mesh, one needs to weigh the improvement in performance and intraoperative handling over the increase in cost (Table 20.2). There is also data that seems to suggest that choice of mesh may outweigh the operative technique. Champault looked at both laparoscopic and open Lichtenstein repairs that used either polypropylene or beta-D-glucan-coated lightweight polypropylene mesh. While the incidence of chronic pain was the same between the two techniques, the incidence of chronic pain was less in patients with the D-glucan-coated mesh independent of the technique [14].

Conclusion

Considering that factors such as the fibril size, pore size, and pliability within the same material all play into the behavior of a prosthetic, it quickly becomes near impossible to fully elucidate a comparison between different prosthetics. Even though multiple prosthetics are made from the same material, there are other factors, such as geometry of the weave and size of the fibers, that will cause two meshes made of the same material to behave very differently once implanted into a patient. The majority of the inguinal hernia literature as it pertains to mesh is between different manufacturing techniques within the same material (heavyweight vs. lightweight mesh). In the short term, it appears that lightweight mesh may be less symptomatic, but long-term benefits seem to be less apparent as many implanted heavyweight products have led to terrific results when used by experienced hands.

Differences in mesh material, technique, and location of mesh all contribute to the difficulty in deciding what specific mesh product to use. In conclusion, the surgical technique and the overall size of the mesh placed during a laparoscopic inguinal hernia repair matter more so than the actual mesh material.

References

1. Lichtenstein IL, Shulman AG, Amid PK. Use of mesh to prevent recurrence of hernias. Postgrad Med. 1990;87(1):155–8. 160.
2. Usher FC, Hill JR, Ochsner JL. Hernia repair with Marlex mesh. A comparison of techniques. Surgery. 1959;46:718–24.
3. Koontz AR. The use of tantalum mesh in inguinal hernia repair. Surg Gynecol Obstet. 1951;92(1):101–4.
4. Markar SR, Karthikesalingam A, Alam F, Tang TY, Walsh SR, Sadat U. Partially or completely absorbable versus nonabsorbable mesh repair for inguinal hernia: a systematic review and meta-analysis. Surg Laparosc Endosc Percutan Tech. 2010;20(4):213–9.

5. Di Vita G, Milano S, Frazzetta M, et al. Tension-free hernia repair is associated with an increase in inflammatory response markers against the mesh. Am J Surg. 2000;180(3):203–7.
6. Calne RY. Repair of bilateral hernia. A technique using mersilene mesh behind the rectus abdominus. Br J Surg. 1967;54(11):917–20.
7. Copello AJ. Technique and results of teflon mesh repair of complicated re-recurrent groin hernias. Rev Surg. 1968;25(2):95–100.
8. Earle DB, Mark LA. Prosthetic material in inguinal hernia repair: how do I choose? Surg Clin North Am. 2008;88(1):179–201. x.
9. Shah BC, Goede MR, Bayer R, et al. Does type of mesh used have an impact on outcomes in laparoscopic inguinal hernia? Am J Surg. 2009;198(6):759–64.
10. Gilbert AI, Felton LL. Infection in inguinal hernia repair considering biomaterials and antibiotics. Surg Gynecol Obstet. 1993;177(2):126–30.
11. Agarwal BB, Agarwal KA, Mahajan KC. Prospective double-blind randomized controlled study comparing heavy- and lightweight polypropylene mesh in totally extraperitoneal repair of inguinal hernia: early results. Surg Endosc. 2009;23(2):242–7.
12. Deeken CR, Abdo MS, Frisella MM, Matthews BD. Physicomechanical evaluation of polypropylene, polyester, and polytetrafluoroethylene meshes for inguinal hernia repair. J Am Coll Surg. 2011;212(1):68–79.
13. Yang J, Papandria D, Rhee D, Perry H, Abdullah F. Low-cost mesh for inguinal hernia repair in resource-limited settings. Hernia. 2011;15:485–9.
14. Champault G, Bernard C, Rizk N, Polliand C. Inguinal hernia repair: the choice of prosthesis outweighs that of technique. Hernia. 2007;11(2):125–8.

Part V
Essentials of Ventral and Incisional Hernia Repair

21. Evolution of Incisional and Ventral Hernia Repair

Malini D. Sur and L. Brian Katz

> *The difficulties of obtaining a "radical cure" in the large ventral hernia are well known, and from time to time various new principles have been suggested.*
>
> H.C. Wardleworth Nuttall, FRCS, 1926

Despite numerous advances in surgical techniques over the last century, successful long-term treatment of ventral hernias remains a challenge for general surgeons. With a reported incidence between 9 and 20% after laparotomy, incisional hernias occur when there is a protrusion of intra-abdominal contents through a postoperative abdominal wall defect. They range from small, isolated fascial defects to large, complex recurrent hernias with visceral involvement. Laparoscopy has helped limit the need for laparotomy, but incisional hernias from prior midline and transverse incisions as well as trocar and extraction sites continue to pose a risk of life-threatening bowel obstruction and ischemia. Some 100,000–200,000 incisional hernia repairs are performed annually in the United States with estimated rates of reoperation within 5 years of 12% following the first repair and 23% following the second repair [1]. Methods of repair have changed over time and continue to vary across institutions. In the last three decades, several randomized controlled trials (RCTs) helped to compare surgical techniques and support standardized approaches to treating patients with incisional hernias. The aim of this chapter is to review the evolving management of ventral and incisional hernias over the last 100 years with an emphasis on evidence-based literature.

B.P. Jacob and B. Ramshaw (eds.), *The SAGES Manual of Hernia Repair*,
DOI 10.1007/978-1-4614-4824-2_21,

Prevention

A number of patient risk factors have been implicated in incisional hernia formation, including obesity, chronic obstructive pulmonary disease, immunosuppression, and steroid use. The development of postoperative wound infection is also a particularly important predictor of subsequent hernia formation. While many of these patient factors are unavoidable, technical aspects of wound closure are important to consider in hernia prevention. Surgical residents of past and present have been lectured on the value of meticulous fascial closure technique in the prevention of subsequent dehiscence. Taking wide tissue bites, maintaining short intervals between stitches, and placing nonstrangulating tension on sutures while knot-tying are thought to keep sutures from tearing through fascial edges [2]. Early descriptions of midline laparotomy closure included continuous and interrupted suturing with either rapidly or slowly absorbable suture material. In 2010, a meta-analysis of 14 RCTs evaluating techniques of elective midline laparotomy closure in 6,752 aggregated patients definitively concluded that an elective primary or secondary midline laparotomy has the lowest chance of progressing to an incisional hernia when the fascia is closed in a continuous technique using slowly absorbable suture [3].

In addition to closure technique, incisional direction has been suggested as a risk factor for hernia formation. Some surgeons argue that the closure of a transverse incision allows sutures to be placed perpendicular to the dominant fascial collagen bundles, thus theoretically reducing the risk of sutures tearing through fascia. Transverse incisions are also more often closed in two layers, offering greater wound strength. The latest Cochrane review examining pooled data from 7 RCTs comparing transverse and midline incisions for various abdominal operations suggested a lower incidence of incisional hernia following transverse laparotomy. However, the length and location of the incisions varied across studies and follow-up ranged from 4 months to 4 years. Long-term data on these patients would help support the notion that risk of hernia formation should be considered when planning the direction of a laparotomy incision [4].

Finally, the concept of prophylactic use of mesh during laparotomy closure in clean cases has become popularized over the last decade. Data from a RCT comparing primary versus mesh closure in 85 patients undergoing open abdominal aortic aneurysm repair between 2003 and 2007 found a significantly lower rate of incisional hernia formation over 3 years without mesh infections when a prophylactic mesh was used [5].

Manual Reduction

The emergency department often requests surgical consultation for suspected incarcerated ventral hernias. Patients typically present with pain centered over a new and persistent bulge in the abdominal wall. Obstructive symptoms are often present. Rarely, patients with a delayed presentation may be floridly septic from strangulated bowel. Fever, tachycardia, and leukocytosis with neutrophil predominance must be noted. Abdominal scars should correspond to the given surgical history. A tender, irreducible mass associated with a surgical scar suggests an incarcerated incisional hernia. In the patient with a known chronically incarcerated hernia, significant tenderness in other areas of the abdomen should raise suspicion for other diagnoses.

For centuries, manual reduction or "taxis" was the only treatment for incarcerated ventral hernias. In the late 1800s and early 1900s, surgeons began to warn against the risk of returning compromised bowel to the abdomen. Today, the question of when reduction is safe persists. Erythema and crepitus over the hernia with associated peritonitis indicate bowel ischemia, and immediate operative repair is usually indicated without attempts at reduction. However, a delayed surgical approach without reduction of herniated contents, when the patient is severely dehydrated, has severe obesity and/or loss of abdominal domain, and other extenuating circumstances may be appropriate if there is no suspicion of strangulation. When overt stigmata of strangulation are absent, successful reduction with delayed repair may avoid the increased risks of emergent surgery in a patient with multiple comorbidities. Harissis et al. followed 101 patients with incarcerated anterior abdominal wall hernias after attempted reduction. In 60% of cases, the hernia was successfully reduced, and the patient showed no signs of occult bowel ischemia during 24-h observation. Although most underwent elective repair within 30 days, some patients were lost to follow-up. In patients with anticipated noncompliance with follow-up instructions, strong consideration should be given to inpatient repair after hernia reduction and medical optimization [6].

Primary Suture Repair

For much of the twentieth century, ventral and incisional hernia repairs were repaired primarily using suture alone. Primary incisional hernia repair involves incising the skin through the prior scar and dissecting down to the defect. The hernia sac is isolated and excised. Healthy fascial edges are identified and joined together using nonabsorbable or slowly absorbable sutures. It is now believed that more than half of all primary ventral hernia repairs eventually fail, but the technique remains an option in grossly contaminated cases where nonabsorbable mesh is contraindicated or regions where mesh is unavailable. Many surgeons believe that small defects less than 2 cm may be amenable to primary suture repair without a long-term increase in recurrence risk compared to a mesh repair, but data supporting this conclusion is lacking.

Component Separation

By the early 1900s, surgeons had recognized the challenges in obtaining a lasting ventral hernia repair. The introduction of relaxing aponeurotic incisions was an important step toward reducing tension in primary suture repairs. In 1926, Nuttall described a method of "rectus transplantation" in which the inferior edge of the rectus muscle was detached from the pubic symphysis and transposed to the contralateral side as an adjunct to a primary suture repair. The method of component separation used today, however, is adapted from the technique described by Ramirez et al. in 1990. This method initially requires dissection of skin and subcutaneous fat away from the anterior rectus sheath and the external oblique aponeurosis. The latter is then incised longitudinally about 2 cm lateral to the rectus sheath and extended in either direction as needed. Taking advantage of a relatively avascular plane, the external oblique is then separated from the internal oblique muscle. For further tension release, the posterior rectus sheath can be divided from the rectal muscle. Recent descriptions of endoscopic and laparoscopic approaches to component separation remain to be tested in high numbers. Despite these advances in surgical technique, primary ventral hernia repairs continue to be associated with high recurrence rates [7, 8].

Mesh-Based Repair

In the late 1800s, Billroth foresaw the development of prosthetic mesh when he wrote, "If we could artificially produce tissues of the density and toughness of fascia and tendon the secret of the radical cure of hernia would be discovered." Over the next century, surgeons came to envision an "ideal" mesh that would have several additional qualities. In a concise summary, Shankaran et al. described this ideal prosthesis as noncarcinogenic; capable of being sterilized; chemically inert; unlikely to produce a significant host immune response; resistant to mechanical forces, infection, and visceral adhesions; and amenable to mass fabrication in an affordable manner [10, 11].

The first prosthetic mesh was developed in 1900 when Witzel and Goepel made silver filigrees by hand in Germany. Silver was thought to be bacteriocidal, but its rigidity, slow disintegration, and propensity toward sinus tract formation were problematic. Tantalum and stainless steel meshes were introduced in the 1940s and 1950s, respectively, but their stiffness caused patient discomfort. The development of flexible plastic-based prostheses in the mid-1900s was a major advance in hernia repair. Nylon mesh was used in inguinal hernia repairs during World War II, but its susceptibility to weakening from denaturation and hydrolysis was a disadvantage. In the late 1950s, Usher first described the use of a knitted, polypropylene mesh for incisional hernia based on animal studies. Polypropylene would go on to become the most widely utilized mesh for ventral hernia repair today. Flexible and relatively affordable, polypropylene mesh could be easily placed as an "overlay" to buttress a primary fascial repair anteriorly. With their description of mesh placement in the "preperitoneal" plane immediately posterior to the rectus muscle, Rives and Stoppa, using a polyester mesh, independently helped to popularize mesh repair. The creation of composite prostheses combining polypropylene with adhesion-resistant coatings further expanded its versatility as an "underlay" beneath the fascia within the peritoneum or as an "inlay" to bridge a fascial defect. Polyester and expanded polytetrafluoroethylene prostheses have become increasingly popular in recent years [9, 10, 11].

During the 1990s, Luijendkil et al. conducted the first multicenter RCT comparing outcomes of suture versus underlay polypropylene mesh repair of primary and first-time recurrent incisional hernia in 181 elective surgical patients. The 3-year recurrence rate was 46% for suture repair and 23% for mesh repair. In a follow-up study, the authors found a 10-year recurrence rate of 63% for suture repair and 32% for mesh repair with no significant difference in complications. Aside from suture repair, wound infection and history of abdominal aortic aneurysm were independent risk factors for recurrence. Hernia size did not affect the recurrence rate. Based on this data, surgeons were encouraged to "abandon" primary suture repair of incisional hernias, even for small defects [12, 13].

In a retrospective analysis of incisional hernia repairs at 16 Veterans Affairs Medical Centers (VAMC) between 1997 and 2002, Hawn et al. found that the underlay mesh position, whether laparoscopic or open, was specifically associated with a significantly reduced risk of recurrence compared to suture repairs. On the other hand, onlay or inlay mesh placement, which comprised 30% of the repairs, did not appear to reduce the recurrence risk when compared to suture repairs. There was no data suggesting that mesh placement affected rates of enterocutaneous fistula development [14].

Interestingly, despite strong evidence supporting the utilization of mesh in incisional hernia repairs, significant variability in the practice still existed across the United States at the turn of the century. Using the same VAMC data, Gray et al. showed that mesh was used in only 70% of cases. The strongest predictor of mesh use was the hospital where the operation was performed, with rates varying from 40% at one facility to 90% at another. Long-term facility-level analysis of this data showed that the rate of mesh use at the hospital level was significantly associated with the 5-year hospital recurrence rate for all cases. Specifically, a 3% decrease in the recurrence rate was associated with every 10% increase in the rate of mesh use. Other complications and patient satisfaction was not correlated with the hospital rate of mesh placement [15, 16].

Advent of Laparoscopy

After the first laparoscopic cholecystectomy by Muhe in 1985, minimally invasive surgery was rapidly expanded to other common operations in general surgery with the hopes of reducing postoperative pain and length of stay. Leblanc is credited for having described the first laparoscopic ventral hernia repair in 1992. After pneumoperitoneum is achieved and trocars are inserted, the fascial defect is visualized. Any omental and intestinal adhesions are lysed to clear an approximately 4-cm circumferential margin of healthy fascia. The mesh is tailored to the size and shape of the defect, and sutures may be placed for transfascial fixation. The mesh is inserted into the abdomen, and sutures are passed through fascia using a suture passer. Circumferential fixation is achieved using tacks or additional transfascial sutures. A specific advantage of the laparoscopic approach is the ability to view the fascial defect and identify visceral involvement while avoiding the pitfalls of a tedious anterior dissection. Additionally, contact between the mesh and skin flora is theoretically substantially reduced as the mesh is inserted into the abdomen through a trocar. On the other hand, achieving laparoscopic access involves inherent risks of inadvertent vascular or visceral injury. An extensive lysis of adhesions, which is often required in complex incisional hernias, is also considerably more challenging with the physical constraints of laparoscopy.

Although some early voices called for widespread adoption of laparoscopic ventral hernia repair, it was not until recently that randomized studies demonstrated its efficacy. Between 2004 and 2007, Itani et al. performed an RCT across 4 VAMCs, assigning 146 patients with ventral hernias to an open or laparoscopic repair. The laparoscopic group had significantly lower pain scores, a shorter return to work activities, and fewer complications such as wound infections and seroma formation at 8 weeks. The authors noted, however, serious complications such as bowel injury, sepsis, and anesthesia-related problems only occurred in the laparoscopic group. Overall rates of recurrence were similar in the 2 groups at 2-year follow-up [17].

Questions remain regarding technical aspects of laparoscopic ventral hernia repair, particularly with respect to the method of mesh fixation to the abdominal wall. In a recent study by Bansal et al., 68 patients with ventral hernias were randomized to laparoscopic repair with tacker fixation after placement of four transfacial sutures or laparoscopic repair with suture fixation alone. Use of sutures alone was associated with significantly longer operative time but less postoperative pain. No recurrences were found in the short 3-month follow-up period. In an observational study comparing 27 patients who underwent suture repairs to 21 patients who had tack repairs, the recurrence rate was 14% at 18-month follow-up, but no association with repair method was identified [18, 19].

Evidence suggests that as experience with laparoscopic abdominal wall hernia repair grows, long-term outcomes will improve. LeBlanc et al. compared their first 100 and second 100 laparoscopic ventral hernia repairs and found that the later group had a lower recurrence rate, despite older mean age and higher number of comorbidities. Traditional support for an open approach to incarcerated hernias has also been challenged as some studies suggest acceptable outcomes when emergent laparoscopic repair is performed in experienced hands. Further studies are needed to evaluate the long-term outcomes of laparoscopic repair methods [20, 21].

Strategies for Contaminated Cases

Ventral hernia repair in a contaminated setting is a uniquely challenging problem for the general surgeon. Mesh infection is a feared postoperative complication often requiring emergency mesh removal. The usual culprit is *Staphylococcus aureus*, often methicillin resistant. Mesh infection is of special concern in contaminated cases. Contamination may be present at the outset from a coexisting ostomy, an enterocutaneous fistula, a chronically infected wound, an infected mesh from a previous repair, or strangulated bowel. Additionally, any clean case may become contaminated after inadvertent bowel injury or concomitant bowel resection. The traditional approach to ventral hernia repair in the presence of contamination was limited to primary repair with or without component separation. Over the last decade, however, surgeons have increasingly utilized biologic mesh derived from bovine or human acellular dermal matrix (HADM) in these repairs. The use of biologic mesh for ventral hernia repair is discussed in detail elsewhere in this manual. One ongoing concern is the significant cost of biologic mesh products, and this remains a potential barrier to widespread use [22].

Conclusion

Ventral hernia repair has considerably evolved over the last 100 years. Use of synthetic mesh has become widespread and is associated with a lower long-term recurrence rate. Familiarity with laparoscopic repair methods is growing across academic and community settings. Continuous advances in mesh technology may help to achieve improved mesh prostheses. Many challenges remain, however. Standardized descriptions of hernias and repair methods are needed so that prospective data analysis is more accurate. Additional well-designed studies are needed to understand long-term outcomes of various repair methods. Finally, as improved mesh prostheses are developed, the overall value to the patient and system must be taken into consideration to allow general utilization. It will become increasingly important to understand the value of the mesh and the entire treatment regimen, rather than focusing on costs alone.

References

1. Flum DR, Horvath K, Koepsell T. Have outcomes of incisional hernia repair improved with time? A population-based analysis. Ann Surg. 2003;237(1):129–35.
2. Harth K, Rosen MJ. Repair of ventral abdominal wall hernias. In: Souba WW, Fink MP, Jurkovich GJ, Kaiser KR, Pearce WH, Pemberton JH, Soper NJ, editors. ACS surgery: principles and practice. New York: WebMD Professional Publishing; 2007.
3. Diener MK, Voss S, Jensen K, Büchler MW, Seiler CM. Elective midline laparotomy closure: the INLINE systematic review and meta-analysis. Ann Surg. 2010;251(5):843–56.
4. Brown SR, Tiernan J. Transverse versus midline incisions for abdominal surgery. Cochrane Database of Syst Rev. 2005;(4):CD005199. DOI: 10.1002/14651858.CD005199.pub2.
5. Bevis PM, Windhaber RA, Lear PA, Poskitt KR, Earnshaw JJ, Mitchell DC. Randomized clinical trial of mesh versus sutured wound closure after open abdominal aortic aneurysm surgery. Br J Surg. 2010;97(10):1497–502.
6. Harissis HV, Douitsis E, Fatouros M. Incarcerated hernia: to reduce or not to reduce? Hernia. 2009;13(3):263–6.
7. Nuttall HCW. Rectus transplantation in the treatment of ventral herniae. Br Med J. 1926;1(3395):138–39.
8. Ramirez OM, Ruas E, Dellon AL. "Components separation" method for closure of abdominal-wall defects: an anatomic and clinical study. Plast Reconstr Surg. 1990;86(3):519–26.
9. Usher FC, Fries JG, Ochsner JL, Tuttle Jr LL. Marlex mesh, a new plastic mesh for replacing tissue defects. II. Clinical studies. AMA Arch Surg. 1959;78:138–45.
10. Shankaran V, Weber DJ, Reed 2nd RL, Luchette FA. A review of available prosthetics for ventral hernia repair. Ann Surg. 2011;253(1):16–26.
11. Read RC. Milestones in the history of hernia surgery: prosthetic repair. Hernia. 2004;8:8–14.
12. Luijendijk RW, Hop WC, van den Tol MP, de Lange DC, Braaksma MM, IJzermans JN, Boelhouwer RU, de Vries BC, Salu MK, Wereldsma JC, Bruijninckx CM, Jeekel J. A comparison of suture repair with mesh repair for incisional hernia. N Engl J Med. 2000;343(6):392–8.
13. Burger JW, Luijendijk RW, Hop WC, Halm JA, Verdaasdonk EG, Jeekel J. Long-term follow-up of a randomized controlled trial of suture versus mesh repair of incisional hernia. Ann Surg. 2004;240(4):578–83. discussion 583–5.
14. Hawn MT, Snyder CW, Graham LA, Gray SH, Finan KR, Vick CC. Long-term follow-up of technical outcomes for incisional hernia repair. J Am Coll Surg. 2010;210(5):648–55. 655–7.
15. Gray SH, Vick CC, Graham LA, Finan KR, Neumayer LA, Hawn MT. Variation in mesh placement for ventral hernia repair: an opportunity for process improvement? Am J Surg. 2008;196(2):201–6. Epub 2008 May 29.
16. Hawn MT, Snyder CW, Graham LA, Gray SH, Finan KR, Vick CC. Hospital-level variability in incisional hernia repair technique affects patient outcomes. Surgery. 2011;149(2):185–91.

17. Itani KMF, Hur K, Kim LT, Anthony T, Berger DH, Reda D, Neumayer L, for the Veterans Affairs Ventral Incisional Hernia Investigators. Comparison of laparoscopic and open repair with mesh for the treatment of ventral incisional hernia: a randomized trial. Arch Surg. 2010;145(4):322–8.
18. Bansal VK, Misra MC, Kumar S, Rao YK, Singhal P, Goswami A, Guleria S, Arora MK, Chabra A. A prospective randomized study comparing suture mesh fixation versus tacker mesh fixation for laparoscopic repair of incisional and ventral hernias. Surg Endosc. 2011;25(5):1431–8.
19. Greenstein AJ, Nguyen SQ, Buch KE, Chin EH, Weber KJ, Divino CM. Recurrence after laparoscopic ventral hernia repair: a prospective pilot study of suture versus tack fixation. Am Surg. 2008;74(3):227–31.
20. LeBlanc KA, Whitaker JM, Bellanger DE, Rhynes VK. Laparoscopic incisional and ventral hernioplasty: lessons learned from 200 patients. Hernia. 2003;7(3):118–24.
21. Shah RH, Sharma A, Khullar R, Soni V, Baijal M, Chowbey PK. Laparoscopic repair of incarcerated ventral abdominal wall hernias. Hernia. 2008;12(5):457–63.
22. Candage R, Jones K, Luchette FA, Sinacore JM, Vandevender D, Reed 2nd RL. Use of human acellular dermal matrix for hernia repair: friend or foe? Surgery. 2008;144(4): 703–9. discussion 709–11.

22. Tissue Ingrowth: The Mesh–Tissue Interface: What Do We Know So Far?

Gregory J. Mancini and A. Mariah Alexander

For any given hernia patient, the primary challenge is for the surgeon to utilize a technique and a prosthetic choice (given the anatomy, intraoperative findings, and defect size) that combined will provide the best overlap and optimize the surface area of the mesh/tissue interface. Due to the importance of tissue ingrowth at this mesh/tissue interface (MTI) in preventing recurrence, the MTI may very well be the most important aspect involved with a hernia repair. Examining the prosthetics used in hernia surgery has only recently garnered attention in the literature. The title itself infers a challenge to a long-held axiom that the mesh materials are inert in the human body. Any general surgeon who has had the opportunity to operate in a mesh-occupied surgical field can validate that the material explanted often has little in common with the original material implanted. Questions persist about what is happening at the mesh–tissue interface after the material is surgically placed. This chapter will focus in the interactions of prosthetic mesh material with the host tissues in the dynamics of hernia surgery.

Background: History of Mesh Implants

Early modern records of hernia repair show Witzel and Geopel utilizing gold and silver wires interwoven in a filigree pattern and implanted as a prosthetic mesh. Gold and silver filigree materials gave way to stainless steel mesh in the 1940s. The plastics revolution of the 1950s and 1960s provided the early building block for mesh materials still widely used today: polypropylene, polyester, and polytetrafluoroethylene (PTFE) mesh. Polyester was knitted into braided mesh fabric in the 1950s and become the first multifilament, macroporous, nonmetallic mesh to be

B.P. Jacob and B. Ramshaw (eds.), *The SAGES Manual of Hernia Repair*,
DOI 10.1007/978-1-4614-4824-2_22,

widely adopted in hernia repair. Dr. Francis Usher is widely credited with the development of surgical polypropylene. He published his findings in *JAMA* in 1962 regarding a new synthetic, nonabsorbable, monofilament mesh used to close contaminated wounds [1]. This polypropylene monofilament was later woven for mesh production. W.L. Gore developed the process of expanding PTFE (ePTFE) to create a soft, flexible, and durable microporous sheet mesh that gained broad application in laparoscopic ventral hernia repair in the 1990s. These three mesh materials account for over 90% of the mesh market worldwide.

The Ideal Situation

Hernias occur because of a mismatch between the regional strength of the abdominal wall fascia and the tensile forces generated during active living. Ideally, any material or technique used in hernia repair would shift the balance in favor of abdominal wall integrity. The high recurrence rates observed in primary suture repair techniques motivated surgeons to look into permanent implantable material. The material would have optimal tensile strength to bolster the integrity of the abdominal wall and withstand the stressors of vigorous physical activities. Yet it would remain as soft, flexible, compliant, and as dynamic as the muscles and fascia that the material supports. Additionally the material would be inexpensive, easily sterilized, chemically inert, noncarcinogenic, and hypoallergenic. Creating the ideal hernia material poses a tremendous challenge to our biomedical engineers and industry partners. Options include synthetic nonabsorbable materials, synthetic absorbable materials, and nonsynthetic or biologic materials.

Current State of the Art

Realistically, the ideal mesh has yet to be created. Many of the synthetic mesh materials available today fulfill much of the requirements outlined, so much so that prosthetic mesh is used in the vast majority hernia repairs worldwide. The widespread utilization of mesh combined with the prevalence of hernia disease has allowed surgeons to observe the shortcomings of these materials. Hernia recurrence became an accepted consequence of primary suture repair herniorrhaphy. The mesh era introduced lower hernia recurrence rates along with unforeseen and

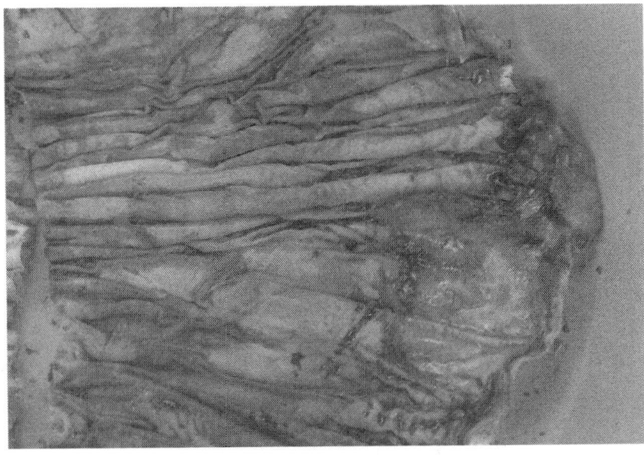

Fig. 22.1. Explanted ePTFE/polypropylene composite mesh after failed hernia repair shows mesh contraction.

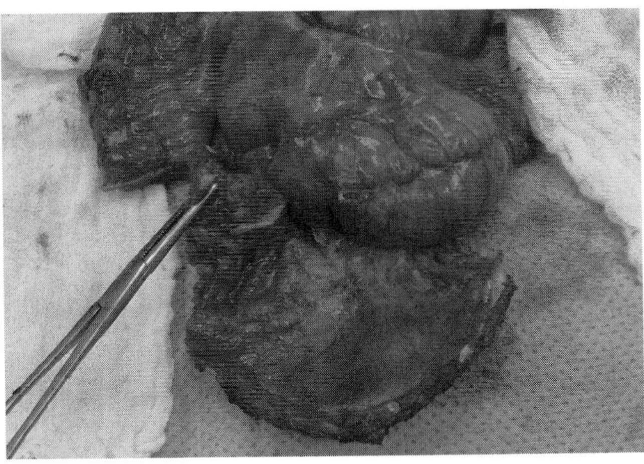

Fig. 22.2. Explanted intra-abdominal mesh material with erosion into the small bowel visceral.

unexpected new problems. Mesh infections, erosions, migration, and loss of biocompliance, though rare occurrences, have been seen with nearly every type of prosthetic material used in hernia surgery (Figs. 22.1, 22.2, 22.3, and 22.4). Recent mesh explant studies by Ramshaw et al. have begun to characterize the chemical and mechanical alterations that

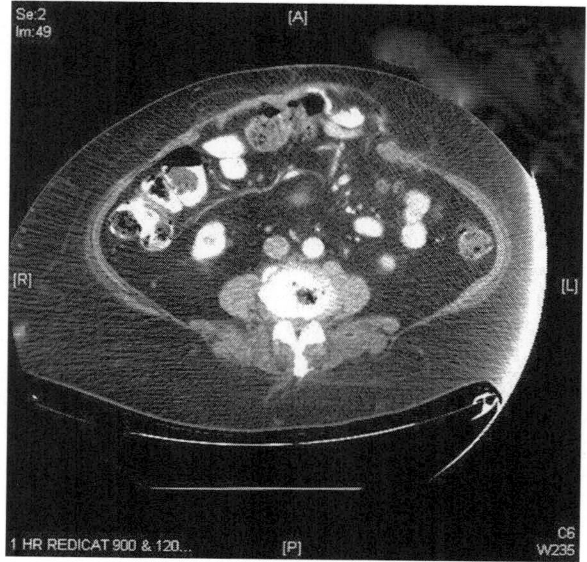

Fig. 22.3. CT scan of the abdomen shows retraction of the mesh implant from the left rectus muscle of abdominal wall allowing hernia recurrence.

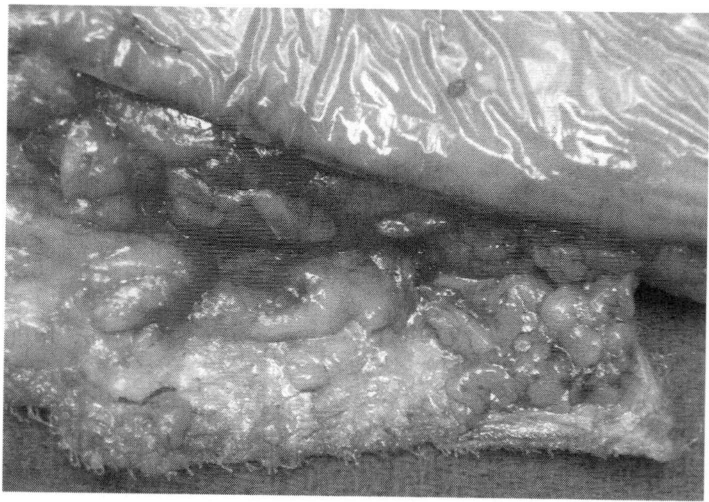

Fig. 22.4. Explanted polypropylene mesh material that shows dense fibrosis within the surrounding soft tissue.

the mesh undergoes in vivo [2]. There is a puzzling disconnect between the millions of well-healed mesh hernia repairs and the poorly tolerated but well-documented mesh repair complications.

Host Response to Foreign Material

A fundamental principle of prosthetic implant use in hernia surgery is that the host response to the material has a common inflammatory pathway. The phases of normal wound healing, hemostasis, inflammation, proliferation, and remodeling, are well understood. What is less well understood is how wound healing is affected by the presence of a prosthetic mesh implant. Assertions that synthetic materials have inert characteristics have been shown to be less than true [3–5]. The implant undergoes an assault by the host immune response, first, as a bystander in the acute phase and then chronically as it is recognized as nonself.

Incorporation begins at the time of implantation. Tissue trauma occurs during the process of hernia repair, such that acute phase reactants are recruited to the injury site. The implant is subjected to the neutrophil and macrophage oxidative stress that can begin the chemical alteration of the implant. It is unlikely, due to the short duration, that the mesh experiences significant chemical or mechanical alterations occurring in this phase of wound healing.

As the tissues begin to heal, the normal transition to fibroblast recruitment and collagen deposition is disrupted by a chronic foreign body response. A cell-mediated chronic inflammatory reaction to the implant chemo-attracts T cells and more macrophages. At this phase, the macrophages assume an activated morphology producing abundant amounts of hydrolytic enzymes that further chemically alter the mesh material [6–8].

The chronic immune response to the mesh is focused at the implant–host interface. This is only part of the healing process underway in at the surgical site. Around the implant, normal revascularization occurs with development of granulation tissue and collagen remodeling. The amount of chemical alteration of the mesh and the degree of collagen disruption seen at the implant–host interface depends both on the properties of the mesh implant and the individual host immune system. The variety of mesh products combined with wide variance in the host immune response may account for the broad spectrum of observations seen in clinical practice [9–11].

In summary, at the host–implant interface, two major processes are taking place. The host reaction to the prosthetic causes a chemical change in the material that can lead to mechanical changes such as mesh shrinkage, stiffening, and fracture. Likewise, the prosthetic causes a chronic host response that disrupts collagen deposition and remodeling process that may lead to tissue scarification, contracture, or encapsulation. The subsequent sections of this chapter will look at how different prosthetic materials, different surgical techniques, and different patient characteristics may alter this common inflammatory pathway.

Material Basics

Polypropylene mesh begins as monofilament that synthesized through a controlled polymerization of propylene chains. The monofilament is then woven in to a mesh implant. Different proprietary weave techniques account for the wide variety of commercial products in the marketplace. Inspection of the macrostructure of the mesh reveals polypropylene implants with different material weight, pore size, tensile strength, and flexibility. At a molecular level, all polypropylene meshes share a common morphology. The propylene chains are carbon backbone with hydrogen and methyl side chains. Degradation occurs when free radicals and oxygen attack the methyl groups creating chain fractures and cross-links [12]. Additionally, aldehydes and carboxylic acid are produced as chemical by-products. Evidence of this happening in vivo comes from Cozad et al. explant study. The materials were harvested and then tested utilizing spectral and thermal analysis [2].

Polyethylene terephthalate (PET) is a synthetic polyester polymer created by combining ethylglycol and terephthalic acid. Like polypropylene, polyester is a created by polymerization of a base monomer into long chains. Similarly, polyester has a carbon backbone. The ester side chains of polyester confirm differently the surface interactions as compared to polypropylene materials. Polyester has hydrophilic properties that attract water molecules to its surface. In biologic systems, polyester's hydrophilic properties may insulate the implant from the oxidative stresses generated in the host immune response. Cozar's synthetic mesh explant study showed that polyester mesh experiences both chemical and mechanical degradation in vivo. Concerns that the braided and woven pattern of polyester mesh may provide a greater surface area for bacterial colonization have been disproven. An animal study in which polyester mesh was intentionally inoculated with bioluminescent staphylococcus at the time of implantation showed significant clearance by postoperative day one [13].

PTFE is essentially a long-carbon chain backbone with fluoride atoms as side groups. The carbon–carbon and carbon–fluoride covalent bonds of this compound provide chemical and mechanical stability. Expanded polytetrafluoroethylene (ePTFE) used in implants is made in a proprietary process by combining PTFE nodes that are interconnected by PTFE fibrils. ePTFE's synthetic manufacturing process yields a microporous sheet of material that has air spaces between the PTFE nodes allowing for air flow but hydrophobic making it waterproof. Though chemically stable, in vivo studies have shown mechanical changes in ePTFE. Schoenmaeckers et al. looked at ePTFE shrinkage after laparoscopic ventral hernia repair in 40 patients. Surface area shrinkage rates observed ranged from 0 to 24%, with a mean of 7.5% after an average 17.9 months after implantation [14].

Mesh Weight (Density)

The concept of mesh weight or density has mainly pertained to discussions about polypropylene mesh. Hernia recurrence with this material appeared to be related to mesh contraction or shrinkage allowing separation from the fascial edge. The early heavyweight polypropylene mesh contains 80 g/m^2 of polypropylene and provided tensile strengths of 90 N/cm. Tensiometry studies showed that this mesh product had tensile strengths logarithmically greater than that of healthy fascia (12–16 N/cm). Conversely, newly designed lightweight mesh contains 30 g/m^2 of polypropylene and provides 30–40 N/cm of tensile strength. As data emerged about chronic host response causing mechanical changes in the mesh, a new concept evolved. Less synthetic material would elicit less host inflammation, a thereby reduced mesh contraction [15, 16]. This concept of the impact of mesh weight on mesh contraction has not been applied to PET of ePTFE.

Mesh Pore Size

Good integration into the host tissue is a desired quality of a hernia material. The pores within the mesh allow for host collagen deposition, thereby strengthening the integration of the mesh to the abdominal wall.

This concept is why most all hernia implants utilize a woven mesh design. Early polypropylene and polyester mesh materials were often constructed by large fibers interlocked by tight weaves, making small pore sizes of less than 1 mm (1,000 microns). Despite this small pore size, early polypropylene and polyester meshes are still considered macroporous. Newer polyester and polypropylene materials are woven with smaller fibers or monofilaments and use a looser weave patterns that provide larger pore sizes [17, 18].

This contrasts with ePTFE that has an average pore size of 3 microns, making it microporous. In comparison, the average size of a platelet is 3 microns, a water droplet is 10 microns, a macrophage is 21 microns, and a fibroblast is 30 microns. The microporous structure of ePTFE limits the depth of cellular infiltration within the material and thereby limits the degree of tissue incorporation. This attribute can be favorable when the mesh is implanted near anatomic structures, like intestinal serosa, where tissue ingrowth is not desired. The chronic foreign body response is limited to the ePTFE surface which produces a dense, collagen-rich fibrous capsule. Studies on larger pore (30–90 micron) ePTFE implants are in progress to assess if mesh encapsulation can be converted to mesh integration [19].

Animal Experimentation of Mesh–Tissue Interface

While there may not be one "best" product, animal experiments at the very least have proven that the products indeed are NOT created equal. Animal studies have helped show that the tissue ingrowth begins early and increases in strength over time. In a porcine laparoscopic ventral hernia model, Majercik et al. [20] demonstrated that the bulk of tissue ingrowth occurs during the first 2 weeks after inserting a polypropylene mesh, and by 4 weeks, the strength of the ingrowth had already reached a strength equivalent to 95% of the peak strength seen at 12 weeks. By fixing sheets of polypropylene and ePTFE composite mesh to the abdominal walls and then harvesting them at different time intervals (2, 4, 6, and 12 weeks), the authors were able to demonstrate a peel strength of 0.83 pounds at 2 weeks, of 1.06 pounds at 4 weeks, and 1.13 pounds at 12 weeks (5 N). Histologic examination of specimens showed complete cellular infiltration into and through the entire layer of the polypropylene up to the ePTFE layer. This study, which looked at the peel strength of the polypropylene layer used in a heavyweight polypropylene/ePTFE composite mesh, concluded that the bulk of tissue ingrowth happens during the first 2 weeks after implantation. At 4 weeks, the strength then increases to a value that is equivalent to 94% of the peak strength measured at 12 weeks postimplantation. [20]

Interestingly, not all biomaterials are incorporated into native tissue by this cellular phenomenon equally. As early as 1995, Bellón et al. published results that compared the cellular response to, and subsequent tissue integration of, two different mesh prostheses in a rabbit model [21]. At the time, products were made of only one material, either heavyweight polypropylene or ePTFE. The authors suspected the two materials incited different levels of inflammation and therefore implanted these two meshes into the anterior abdominal wall of rabbits, ensuring that each mesh was exposed to the peritoneal cavity. Necropsy was performed at 14, 30, 60, and 90 days. Microscopically, the host tissue response differed between the ePTFE and the polypropylene. At the 2-week point, the ePTFE formed a fibrous capsule without cellular infiltration. Conversely, the polypropylene was integrated throughout with loose collagen fibers and had cellular infiltration consisting of macrophages and myofibroblasts. Collagen fibers and neovascular capillaries were not readily visible on the ePTFE until 2 months after implantation. By 3 months postimplantation, the capsule tissue was substantial, and the cell population had stabilized consisting of mostly fibroblasts. In contrast, the polypropylene mesh demonstrated early and complete integration into the host tissue. The process of angiogenesis began within the first 2 weeks and cells were distributed within the pores of the mesh. They concluded that polypropylene incited a more intense inflammatory foreign body reaction and that polypropylene had superior tissue integration. Therefore, ePTFE was more suitable for implantation intraperitoneally where it would be exposed to the viscera and that polypropylene would be better suited for tissue integration.

The evolution of laparoscopic hernia repair pushed mesh development to meet the unique needs of the peritoneal cavity. Two different surface were required, one surface that optimized tissue integration at the abdominal wall (macroporous) and another to limit visceral adhesions and ingrowth (microporous). The first of this kind paired heavyweight polypropylene/ePTFE in a composite mesh. Ianatti et al. studied the differences in the strength of tissue attachment to the two different materials in a porcine model. Again, the meshes were evaluated at different time intervals (2, 4, 6, and 12 weeks). The results showed that the strength of tissue ingrowth was significantly higher for the polypropylene composite graft relative to the strength of ingrowth into the pure ePTFE material at each time point. For example, at 2, 4, and 12 weeks, the mean peel strength for the ePTFE was 0.50 pounds, 0.53 pounds, and 0.51 pounds, respectively (0.51 pounds equals 2.27 N). This was significantly less than the peel strength of the polypropylene at 2, 4, and 12 weeks respectively being 0.825, 1.06, and 1.12 pounds ($p<0.05$) (equivalent to 3.68, 4.70, and 5.0 N) [22].

The authors then looked at histology slides and found at 2 weeks, the macroporous polypropylene component of the composite mesh was entirely infiltrated with fibroblasts and inflammatory cells with collagen deposition occurring throughout the polypropylene. The microporous surface of the ePTFE, however, showed no cellular penetration through the ePTFE at 2 weeks. There were obvious differences in the histologic reaction and peel strengths between the different biomaterials suggesting that tissue ingrowth and peel strength was superior for the polypropylene layer of the polypropylene/ePTFE composite mesh compared to a pure ePTFE material against the peritoneum. The tissue ingrowth maturation process for the polypropylene seems to reach 74% of its max by 2 weeks and 95% of its maximum by 4 weeks. The strength then plateaus after a 12-week period of time in animal studies; however, there may be evidence that cellular turnover continues for up to a year, and the severity of the continuing process may be dependent on the type of mesh implanted.

This degree of inflammation produced in response to various mesh products was recently studied using immunohistochemical testing for Ki-67, which is an accepted and established marker of cell proliferation and turnover. In a rabbit study that compared tissue ingrowth analysis between a control of polypropylene and three mesh products: a heavyweight polypropylene/ePTFE composite mesh (hPP), pure ePTFE (ePTFE), and a reduced weight polypropylene/oxidized regenerated cellulose composite mesh (rPP), the authors looked at results at both 4 and 12 months postimplantation. The authors found that the hPP mesh had significantly higher Ki-67 levels than the rPP and the ePTFE groups at 4 months. At 12 months, a significant decrease in Ki-67 scores from the 4-month point was found in the rPP group only, while the hPP group maintained elevated levels of Ki-67. This interesting finding suggests that the heavyweight polypropylene-based mesh material incites an ongoing inflammatory process and scar remodeling that lasts even 1 year later. This finding was not seen with the lightweight polypropylene product or with the pure ePTFE. The translation of this finding into a human clinical setting remains unknown but may suggest that heavyweight polypropylene may have poor long-term biocompatibility compared to lightweight polypropylene and ePTFE. This poor biocompatibility may lead to poor mesh compliance and [23].

The compliance of the mesh implants may change over time for two reasons. First, a thicker scar plate may form as a result of chronic inflammation and collagen turnover. Second, the chronic inflammatory process may cause chemical alterations to the material structure. Both likely impact the long-term loss of mesh compliance in the mesh seen in human explant studies. With loss of mesh compliance, the abdominal wall becomes less pliable resulting in physical discomfort, limitations in daily activities, and overall dissatisfaction. The group from Charlotte, North Carolina, performed a rabbit comparison study, and within that study, they reported on mesh compliance 1 year after implant. Using a differentiated variable reluctance transducer (DVRT) that provided measurements of the axial forces required to stretch the mesh, the group reported compliance data on pure polypropylene, a composite mesh of polypropylene and ePTFE, pure ePTFE, and a composite of lightweight polypropylene and an oxidized cellulose layer. At 1 year, they showed that the compliance of the pure two-sided ePTFE mesh was superior to the other three meshes [24].

Interestingly, using the same DVRT method to then analyze the peel strength of the mesh products, the group did not demonstrate a significant difference in peel strengths between those four materials, although the heavyweight polypropylene/ePTFE composite trended toward having the greatest peel strength. Having no significant differences in the tissue ingrowth to ePTFE, lightweight polypropylene composite mesh, and heavyweight polypropylene composite mesh has been shown in a number of rabbit studies published by the same group [24–26]. This finding is not consistent with other published rabbit and porcine studies that compared the same products [22, 27] and may be related to factors that include the type of animal model used and the method of obtaining and calculating the peel strength. In conclusion, while the polypropylene-based mesh materials show superior tissue ingrowth and superior peel strengths, the long-term loss of material compliance may result in increased mesh failures at the mesh–tissue interface.

In a porcine adhesiogenic laparoscopic ventral hernia model, McGinty et al. compared the 3D polyester/anti-adhesive collagen composite mesh to the pure, two-layered ePTFE mesh (DualMesh®, Gore, Arizona) and used heavyweight polypropylene as a control. After laparoscopic insertion and survival for 4 weeks, the peel strength of the mesh from the abdominal wall was analyzed using a digital tensiometer and found to be significantly less for the pure ePTFE than for the polyester/anti-adhesive collagen composite mesh or the pure polypropylene control (1.3 N/cm vs. 2.8 N/cm, $p=0.001$ vs. 2.1 N/cm, $p=0.05$, respectively). Histologically, there was excellent fibrous growth into and through the polypropylene and the polyester component of the composite mesh. There was no tissue growth through the ePTFE. This finding supports the notion that complete tissue ingrowth can be found in a 3D polyester mesh and that this leads to superior adherence strength when compared to the peel strength seen with pure two-sided ePTFE [28].

In another study, the 3D polyester/anti-adhesive collagen composite mesh was compared to a heavyweight polypropylene/ePTFE composite mesh (heavyweight polypropylene parietal layer) [29]. The same porcine model was used. A pure polypropylene mesh was used as a control. While the study reported on a number of variables, regarding the issue of tissue ingrowth as measured by the peel strength of the mesh from the abdominal wall, the authors concluded that the polyester composite product and the polypropylene composite product had no significant difference in abdominal wall adherence. This result suggests that in this study, a 3D polyester mesh has similar fibrous ingrowth properties as the polypropylene mesh [29].

In another prospective animal study using the same adhesiogenic porcine model, polyester/anti-adhesive collagen composite mesh was compared to a composite mesh made of lightweight, polydioxanone polymer-encapsulated polypropylene on the peritoneal surface and oxidized regenerated cellulose as the anti-adhesive barrier on the visceral surface [30]. A regular polypropylene was inserted as a control. After 1 month, the mesh was harvested and as part of the evaluation, peak peel strength was measured using a digital force gage tensiometer (Omega DFG51-10 microprocessor-based digital force gage, http://www.omega.com). The results showed that in this study, the peel strength was significantly higher for the 3D polyester composite mesh than for the encapsulated lightweight polypropylene composite mesh (17.2 N vs. 10.7 N), respectively ($p<0.002$) [30]. The bottom line conclusion is that the synthetic mesh materials are not equal, and in any given scenario, each of the mesh materials will behave differently.

Clinical Observations and Explant Findings

The base chemical composition, the material density, and the woven macrostructure design of a have an interrelated impact on how the mesh will be received by the host immune system. The overall trend in mesh design is to create an implant that has a more physiologic biocompatibility with the host. This means that the mesh can withstand the physiologic stress experience by the abdominal wall and can remain minimally altered by the host immune response over the life span of the host. The market response to this trend has been the development of monofilament materials woven into lightweight (<30 g/m^2) mesh with wide pore spaces [31, 32]. More data is needed to determine whether the newer lightweight and large pore macroporous materials will deliver the desired result.

Does the Patient Matter?

To date, the primary focus on improving hernia outcomes has been on the surgical technique. Though evolving surgical technique is crucial to improved outcomes, the patient's individual physiology is major factor that must be considered. Knowing our patients unique social habits, genetic constitution, current medical comorbidities, and past surgical history is just the beginning of the hernia planning process. With imperfect techniques, imperfect materials, and imperfect patients, successful hernia surgery requires the surgeon to choose an individualized "best-fit" scenario. This contrasts to usual surgical thinking that tries to define a single standard surgical technique and apply it to all patients.

The lifestyle choices that patients make often play a significant role in hernia occurrence or recurrence after surgery. The most detrimental choice is that of smoking tobacco. Aside from the pulmonary function compromise that increases perioperative morbidity and mortality, smoking has a direct impact on wound healing and tissue remodeling. Smokers have twice the inguinal hernia recurrence rates and four times ventral hernia recurrence rates compare to nonsmokers. Basic science studies show that type I and III collagen synthesis rates are negatively affected. Also, matrix metalloproteinases, enzymes responsible for collagen degradation, are expressed in higher levels [33]. Together, the biologic imbalance induced by smoking shifts the wound healing toward low-quality collagen with decreased tensile strength. In the case of a primary hernia, the fascial integrity weakens over time. In the case of hernia recurrence after mesh implantation, poor collagen integration may allow failure at the tissue–mesh interface.

Genetic constitution plays a significant role in hernia development. Rare but well-documented collagen synthesis disorders such as Marfan and Ehlers–Danlos syndromes have high incidence of hernia. Inherited disorders such as homocystinuria, elastosis, and congenital hip dislocation have also shown to have an elevated incidence of hernia. Common histologic findings of all these conditions are poorly organized collagen macrostructure. Altered cross-linking within between collagen fibers as well as altered ratios of type I and III collagen content is seen. Similarly, genetic causes of poor tissue remodeling, as observed in aortic aneurysmal disease, have increased hernia incidence. Genetic overexpression of tissue matrix metalloproteinases leads to excessive destruction the extracellular matrix and tissue growth factors. Altering the cell signaling for local fibroblasts and removing critical tissue scaffolding impair collagen synthesis and remodeling [34, 35].

The classic predictors for poor wound healing such as malnutrition, obesity, diabetes mellitus, corticosteroid use, immunosuppression, and active infection effect hernia outcomes. Malnutrition and corticosteroids suppress immune function thereby reducing collagen deposition. Obesity generates elevated tensile forces that may overwhelm fixation techniques at the tissue–host interface and is associated with increased surgical site infections. Diabetes impairs macrophage function and fibroblast migration and alters the balance between the accumulation of ECM components and their remodeling by MMPs [36].

Summary

Mesh implants require sufficient integration within the host tissue to prevent dislocation and reduce recurrences, and knowledge regarding tissue ingrowth at the mesh–tissue interface is still evolving. Successful outcomes from a hernia operation are dependent on optimizing for each individual patient the choice of the surgical technique and the implant materials. We know that the prosthetic materials we implant in patients during a hernia repair are not inert to the body's immune response and, on the contrary, are likely to dictate the final strength of the MTI ingrowth. The base material composition and three-dimensional macrostructure of the mesh impact the body's response. We know that an individual's immune response to the implant is highly variable and poorly understood, and genetic variance in the immune response may have a significant role in modulating the foreign body response. We know that mesh materials are implanted in a wide variety of locations in the body and applied with different surgical techniques. Further human basic science and clinical research is needed in this area.

References

1. Usher FC, Allen JE, Crothswait RW, Cogan JE. Polypropylene monofilament: new, biologically inert suture for closing contaminated wounds. JAMA. 1962;179(10):780–2.
2. Cozad MJ, Grant DA, Bachman SL, Grant DN, Ramshaw BJ, Grant SA. Materials characterization of explanted polypropylene, polyethylene terephthalate, and expanded polytetrafluoroethylene composites: spectral and thermal analysis. J Biomed Mater Res B Appl Biomater. 2010;94(2):455–62.
3. Junge K, Binnebosel M, Rosch R, Jansen M, Kammer D, Otto J, Schumpelick V, Klinge U. Adhesion formation of a polyvinylidenfluoride/polypropylene mesh for intra-abdominal placement in a rodent animal model. Surg Endosc. 2009;23:327–33.
4. Beets GL, van Mameren H, Go PMNYH. Long-term foreign-body reaction to preperitoneal polypropylene mesh in the pig. Hernia. 1998;2:153–5.
5. Klinge U, Klosterhalfen B, Muller M, OttingerA P, Schumpelick V. Shrinking of polypropylene mesh in vivo: an experimental study in dogs. Eur J Surg. 1998;164:965–9.
6. Binnebosel M, Klinge U, Rosch R, Junge K, Lynen-Jansen P, Schumpelick V. Morphology, quality, and composition in mature human peritoneal adhesions. Arch Surg. 2006;393:59–66.
7. Binnebosel M, Rosch R, Junge K, Lynen-Jansen P, Schumpelick V, Klinge U. Macrophage and T-lymphocyte infiltrates in human peritoneal adhesions indicate a chronic inflammatory disease. World J Surg. 2007;32:296–304.
8. Bhardwaj RS, Henze U, Klein B, Zwadlo-Klarwasser G, Klinge U, Mittermayer CH, Klosterhalfen B. Monocyte-biomaterial interaction inducing phenotypic dynamics of monocytes: a possible role of monocyte subsets in biocompatibility. J Mater Sci Mater Med. 1997;8:737–42.
9. Klinge U, Junge K, Stump F, Ottinger AP, Klosterhalfen B. Functional and morphological evaluation of a low-weight, monofilament polypropylene mesh for hernia repair. J Biomed Mater Res. 2002;63(2):129–36.
10. Klinge U, Klosterhalfen B, Birkenhauer V, Junge K, Conze J, Schumpelick V. Impact of polymer pore size on the interface scar formation in a rat model. J Surg Res. 2002;103:208–14.
11. Junge K, Klinge U, Klosterhalfen B, Mertens PR, Rosch R, Schachtrupp A, Ulmer F, Schumpelick V. Influence of mesh materials on collagen deposition in a rat model. J Invest Surg. 2002;15:319–28.
12. Costello CR, Bachman SL, Ramshaw BJ, Grant SA. Materials characterization of explanted polypropylene hernia meshes. J Biomed Mater Res B Appl Biomater. 2007;83(1):44–9.
13. Engelsman AF, van Dam GM, van der Mei HC, Busscher HJ, Ploeg RJ. In vivo evaluation of bacterial infection involving morphologically different surgical meshes. Ann Surg. 2010;251(1):133–7.
14. Schoenmaeckers E, van der Valk S, van den Hout H, et al. Computed tomographic measurements of mesh shrinkage after laparoscopic ventral incisional hernia repair with an expanded polytetrafluoroethylene mesh. Surg Endosc. 2009;23:1620–3.

15. Klosterhalfen B, Junge K, Klinge U. The lightweight and large porous mesh concept for hernia repair. Expert Rev Med Devices. 2005;2(1):103–17.
16. Klostergalfen B, Klinge U, Schumpelick V. Functional and morphological evaluation of different polypropylene-mesh modifications for abdominal wall repair. Biomaterials. 1998;19:2235–46.
17. Conze J, Rosch R, Klinge U, Weiss C, Anurov M, Titkowa S, Oetinger A, Schumpelick V. Polypropylene in the intra-abdominal position: influence of pore size and surface area. Hernia. 2004;8:365–72.
18. Conze J, Junge K, Weib C, Anurov M, Oettinger A, Klinge U, Schumpelick V. New polymer for intra-abdominal meshes- PVDF copolymer. J Biomed Mater Res B Appl Biomater. 2008;87(2):321–8.
19. Zhang Z, Wang Z, Liu S, Kodama M. Pore size, tissue ingrowth, and endothelialization of small-diameter microporous polyurethane vascular prostheses. Biomaterials. 2004;25(1):177–87.
20. Majercik S, Tsikitis V, Iannitti DA. Strength of tissue attachment to mesh after ventral hernia repair with synthetic composite mesh in a porcine model. Surg Endosc. 2006;20(11):1671–4.
21. Bellón JM, Contreras LA, Buján J, Carrera-San Martin A, Jorge-Herrero E, Campo C, Hernando A. A new type of polytetrafluoroethylene prosthesis (Mycro Mesh): an experimental study. J Mater Sci Mater Med. 1996;7(8):475–8.
22. Iannitti DA, Hope WW, Tsikitis V. Strength of tissue attachment to composite and ePTFE grafts after ventral hernia repair. JSLS. 2007;11(4):415–21.
23. Novitsky YW, Cristiano JA, Harrell AG, Newcomb W, Norton JH, Kercher KW, Heniford BT. Immunohistochemical analysis of host reaction to heavyweight-, reduced-weight-, and expanded polytetrafluoroethylene (ePTFE)-based meshes after short- and long-term intraabdominal implantations. Surg Endosc. 2008;22(4):1070–6.
24. Novitsky YW, Harrell AG, Cristiano JA, Paton BL, Norton HJ, Peindl RD, Kercher KW, Heniford BT. Comparative evaluation of adhesion formation, strength of ingrowth, and textile properties of prosthetic meshes after long-term intra-abdominal implantation in a rabbit. J Surg Res. 2007;140(1):6–11.
25. Matthews BD. Absorbable and nonabsorbable barriers on prosthetic biomaterials for adhesion prevention after intraperitoneal placement of mesh. Int Surg. 2005;90 (3 Suppl):S30–S4.
26. Harrell AG, Novitsky YW, Cristiano JA, Gersin KS, Norton HJ, Kercher KW, Heniford BT. Prospective histologic evaluation of intra-abdominal prosthetics four months after implantation in a rabbit model. Surg Endosc. 2007;21(7):1170–4.
27. Greenawalt KE, Butler TJ, Rowe EA, Finneral AC, Garlick DS, Burns JW. Evaluation of sepramesh biosurgical composite in a rabbit hernia repair model. J Surg Res. 2000;94(2):92–8.
28. McGinty JJ, Hogle NJ, McCarthy H, Fowler DL. A comparative study of adhesion formation and abdominal wall ingrowth after laparoscopic ventral hernia repair in a porcine model using multiple types of mesh. Surg Endosc. 2005;19(6):786–90.
29. Duffy AJ, Hogle NJ, LaPerle KM, Fowler DL. Comparison of two composite meshes using two fixation devices in a porcine laparoscopic ventral hernia repair model. Hernia. 2004;8(4):358–64.

30. Jacob BP, Hogle NJ, Durak E, Kim T, Fowler DL. Tissue ingrowth and bowel adhesion formation in an animal comparative study: polypropylene versus Proceed versus Parietex Composite. Surg Endosc. 2007;21(4):629–33.
31. Klinge U, Klosterhalfen B, Conze J, Limberg W, Obolenski B, Ottiner AP, Schumelick V. Modified mesh for hernia repair that is adapted to the physiology of the abdominal wall. Eur J Surg. 1998;164:951–60.
32. Junge K, Klinge U, Prescher A, Giboni P. Elasticity of the anterior abdominal wall and impact for reparation of incisional hernias using mesh implants. Hernia. 2001;5:113–8.
33. Knuutinen A, Kokkonen N, Risteli J, Vähäkangas K, Kallioinen M, Salo T, Sorsa T, Oikarinen A. Smoking affects collagen synthesis and extracellular matrix turnover in human skin. Br J Dermatol. 2002;146(4):588–94.
34. Klein T, Bischoff R. Physiology and pathophysiology of matrix metalloproteases. Amino Acids. 2011;41(2):271–90.
35. Antoniou GA, Georgiadis GS, Antoniou SA, Granderath FA, Giannoukas AD, Lazarides MK. Abdominal aortic aneurysm and abdominal wall hernia as manifestations of a connective tissue disorder. J Vasc Surg. 2011;54(4):1175–81.
36. Brem H, Tomic-Canic M. Cellular and molecular basis of wound healing in diabetes. J Clin Invest. 2007;117(5):1219–22.

23. Patient Comorbidities Complicating a Hernia Repair: The Preoperative Workup and Postoperative Planning

Scott Philipp

Abdominal wall hernias are a common problem encountered by medical practitioners. Their contribution to chronic pain and loss of form and function are reasons why they often come to the attention of the hernia surgeon. Hernia surgery continues to evolve at a frantic pace, with many differing techniques and products available, and better results being reported. However, complications from hernia surgery still abound and recurrence rates, especially in certain patient populations, leave the surgical community looking for better answers. As we continue to learn and improve, several comorbid conditions need to be considered prior to embarking on the surgical treatment of an abdominal wall hernia. Recognizing the presence of these potentially complicating factors and optimizing them prior to surgery will ideally increase the success of the surgery and the positive impact on the patient's quality of life.

Comorbid Conditions and Considerations

Surgical History

It is of primary importance to elicit a complete history of any previous abdominal surgery prior to proceeding with repair of an abdominal wall hernia. If previous operations were performed at outside institutions, then efforts should be made to obtain those operative reports to assist in preoperative planning. The presence of intra-abdominal scar tissue cannot be evaluated preoperatively although it should always be considered and

B.P. Jacob and B. Ramshaw (eds.), *The SAGES Manual of Hernia Repair*,
DOI 10.1007/978-1-4614-4824-2_23,

appropriate preparations be made. This includes the possibility of dense adhesions with involvement of omentum, small and large bowel, and other intra-abdominal structures. This risk is potentially increased if the patient has a previous history of serious intra-abdominal infection. Taking down adhesions is usually necessary for the successful completion of a ventral hernia repair and can significantly increase operative times and operative risk. If one or more previous attempts at hernia repair have already been made, then this risk is amplified. The previous placement of mesh can also add complexity and risk. It is potentially helpful to discover the material, size, and position of all previously placed pieces of foreign materials, and this information should be considered during operative planning. The possibility of mesh migration, contraction, erosion, eventration, and dense adhesion to intra-abdominal organs should be anticipated.

Morbid Obesity

The incidence of morbid obesity in our communities is growing. The impact of obesity on hernia surgery is still being investigated although it is known to be associated with increased hernia recurrence rates [1]. There are now several retrospective reviews investigating the impact of morbid obesity on hernia repair outcomes. The largest study looking at patients undergoing laparoscopic ventral hernia repair found that a preoperative BMI greater than 40 imparted an increased risk of recurrence without increased perioperative morbidity [2]. The results of several other smaller studies are divided [3–6]. Morbid obesity increases risk for recurrence and postoperative complications after inguinal hernia repair as well [7]. Current expert opinion considers morbid obesity a potentially correctable risk factor for postoperative complications, and hernia recurrence and efforts should be made for patients to lose weight prior to proceeding with an elective hernia repair, ideally to a BMI less than 35. A recent survey found morbid obesity to be the number one cited contraindication to ventral hernia repair among surgeons [8].

Smoking

The physiologic impact of tobacco smoking has been well-defined. In addition to its effects on the cardiovascular, pulmonary, and nervous systems, it can prevent appropriate wound healing and impairs the immune system. Effects include impaired tissue oxygenation, peripheral vasoconstriction, hyperglycemia, insulin resistance, impairment of growth factors, and immune modulators, among others. In clinical studies, smoking has been shown to significantly increase perioperative morbidity, particularly wound infection and hernia recurrence, after ventral and inguinal hernia repair [9, 10]. It is also a risk factor for development of an incisional hernia after other operations [11]. Smoking is a modifiable risk factor, and therefore, all efforts should be made to help a patient quit smoking prior to elective surgery. It should not delay surgery that is urgent or emergent, although patients should be informed of the impact it could have on their recovery and outcome. For elective hernia repair in patients at high risk for perioperative morbidity, preoperative smoking cessation is mandatory in my opinion, and patient noncompliance should prompt rescheduling at a later time. Smoking cessation should be for at least 1 month prior to surgery to avoid increased pulmonary complications [12]. Compliance can be verified by performing a test for urine cotinine, a metabolite of nicotine.

Age

There is no contraindication to elective hernia repair based on age alone. As the population continues to live longer, more patients will present with hernias later in life. Surgical repair should be considered if the expected improvement in patient quality of life exceeds the potential risks based on other factors.

Diabetes

Hyperglycemia can adversely affect wound healing and the immune response which increases perioperative morbidity. Patients should have optimal control of their blood glucose levels before proceeding with an elective hernia repair. Strict postoperative glycemic control is also important, especially for more complex hernia repairs. Aggressive therapy should target blood glucose levels to a range of 80–150 mg/dL [13].

Pulmonary Disease

There are two things that need to be considered regarding pulmonary function prior to proceeding with a hernia repair: first, the impact of anesthesia—general versus spinal versus local—on the lungs; and second, the potential impact of the hernia repair on pulmonary function. Patients with physical limitations due to their disease or those on supplemental oxygen should avoid general anesthesia if possible. In the case of large symptomatic abdominal wall hernias in which there is no feasible anesthetic alternative, the potential risks should be discussed with the patient and weighed against the expected benefits of the operation. Operative time should be minimized, and local anesthetic should be used to reduce narcotic requirements. For large hernias with loss of abdominal domain, it is important to consider the impact of hernia repair, with restoration of abdominal contents into the true abdominal cavity, on the diaphragm. Pulmonary peak inspiratory pressures should be measured both before and after abdominal wall closure when increased abdominal pressure due to hernia repair is suspected. A significant increase in pressure should prompt reevaluation of the closure technique by the surgeon as this patient is potentially at risk for post-op pulmonary failure.

Cardiac Disease

Estimation of cardiac risk prior to surgery should be performed based on current American College of Cardiology (ACC) and American Heart Association (AHA) guidelines which emphasize three elements: patient-specific clinical variables, exercise capacity, and surgery-specific risk. A detailed history and physical examination is necessary to determine need for further cardiac testing. Elective surgery should be delayed in patients with active or unstable cardiac disease. Emergent surgery (e.g., strangulated hernia) should not be delayed for further cardiac testing as risk assessment would not alter management.

Chronic Constipation and Urologic Conditions

Ongoing conditions that chronically increase intra-abdominal pressure should be identified and treatment initiated prior to elective hernia repair. Patients with chronic constipation should be counseled to increase their dietary fiber intake and prescribed fiber supplementation and stool softeners. Colonoscopy should be considered in the appropriate clinical situations. Those with urinary retention or overflow incontinence should be started on appropriate treatment such that urinary symptoms of frequency and straining are resolved. Dysuria should be investigated with urinalysis and hematuria with urologic consultation and cystoscopy prior to elective hernia repair.

Surgeon Experience and Institutional Capabilities

Hernia surgeons are confronted with a wide spectrum of disease, from simple low-risk operations in young, healthy patients, to technically complicated operations in patients with multiple comorbid conditions. There are several approaches to surgical treatment, including open and laparoscopic techniques, and many options for mesh materials. Surgeon experience and institutional capabilities are important factors to consider prior to proceeding with surgical treatment. Mesh materials of appropriate size should be confirmed available prior to starting surgery. Complications need to be anticipated and plans available should they occur. During laparoscopic surgery, conversion to open should never be considered failure if it is done for the benefit of the patient. Hernia surgery can be very complicated and difficult—calling for assistance should be considered during difficult situations.

Summary

There are many comorbid conditions and other issues to consider when preparing for a hernia repair. It is important to optimize the patient's medical condition(s), nutrition, and overall health prior to proceeding with repair. Patients should be given realistic expectations regarding surgical outcomes and have a clear understanding of the goals of surgical treatment. This is especially important for patients with complex or recurrent hernias. This will allow for a shared decision process to occur between the patient, family, and care team.

Preoperative Workup

At the initial surgical consultation, a complete history and physical examination should be performed. This will elicit the potential complexity of the hernia repair and expose patient risk factors for perioperative morbidity and mortality. Also, a clear understanding of symptoms caused by the hernia and the impact on quality of life can be established. Risks and benefits of surgery can then be discussed and identified risk factors worked up further with noninvasive cardiac studies, laboratory testing, and radiographic imaging.

Cardiac Testing

Patients with cardiac risk factors and those undergoing intermediate and high risk surgical procedures based on ACC/AHA guidelines should be sent for noninvasive cardiac testing. Patients with severe or unstable heart disease should have elective surgery delayed until appropriate cardiac intervention is performed.

Laboratory Studies

Blood testing should be performed based on identifiable risk factors found during initial history and physical examination. Complete blood count and coagulation factors should be tested to evaluate for occult infections, anemia, platelet disorders, and coagulopathy. Chemistry testing should be performed to evaluate for hepatic and renal disease, electrolyte imbalance, hyperglycemia, and thyroid function. A hemoglobin A1c can evaluate long-term glycemic control. Urine cotinine testing is useful for evaluating compliance with smoking cessation.

Radiographic Imaging

Radiographic imaging should not be routinely used for diagnosis and planning of surgical repair of hernias. Pelvic ultrasound can sometimes be useful in the diagnosis of occult inguinal hernia when patient history is convincing for a hernia, but physical examination is unrevealing. Abdominopelvic computed tomography is a useful adjunct in certain patient populations, particularly those with recurrent and/or complex hernias, multiple hernias, hernias in challenging or uncommon locations, and when physical examination is limited or unrevealing.

Table 23.1. Informed consent for **ventral** hernia repair.

Bleeding
Infection
Visceral organ injury
Intestinal injury
Enterocutaneous fistula
Nerve damage
Chronic pain
Seroma
Hernia recurrence
Myocardial infarction
Stroke
Pulmonary failure
Ventilator dependence
Renal failure
Deep venous thrombosis
Pulmonary embolism
Need for further treatments and/or operations

Informed Consent

Appropriately preparing a patient for their upcoming hernia surgery is such a complex and important task that it deserves its own section to adequately discuss it (Tables 23.1 and 23.2). Most patients will come to this discussion with some preconceived notions, either from research, experience shared from a friend or relative, or personal experience. In general, hernia surgery is regarded as routine, low-risk, and easy from which to recover. However, hernias come in all shapes and sizes and carry significantly different degrees of risk and expected outcomes. It is important to have a detailed discussion regarding indications for surgery, preoperative risk factors, surgical plans and contingencies, operative and postoperative risks, and realistic expectations for recovery and long-term outcome. It is equally important to involve the patient and their preferences and wishes in the surgical planning as much as possible.

Perioperative Considerations

The identity of the patient should be confirmed, and informed consent should be reviewed with all questions answered prior to anesthesia induction. NPO status and medications should be confirmed. If a bowel

Table 23.2. Informed consent for **inguinal** hernia repair.

Bleeding
Infection
Visceral organ injury
Bladder injury
Intestinal injury
Injury to vas deferens
Injury to testicular vasculature
Ischemic orchitis
Nerve damage
Chronic pain
Seroma
Hernia recurrence
Myocardial infarction
Stroke
Pulmonary failure
Ventilator dependence
Renal failure
Deep venous thrombosis
Pulmonary embolism
Need for further treatments and/or operations

prep has been performed, then appropriate completion should be verified. Preoperative studies and labs should be reviewed. Type and crossmatch should be sent and blood products confirmed available for selected patients. For diabetic patients, a blood glucose level should be checked and insulin treatment given if necessary. For patients who recently quit smoking, a urine cotinine test should be performed to verify compliance. Preoperative subcutaneous heparin should be administered, and lower extremity intermittent pneumatic compression devices should be initiated based on the 2008 Chest guidelines for DVT prophylaxis [14]. Perioperative antibiotics should be initiated within 1 h of surgical start time. Prior to moving the patient to the operating room, the surgical plan, perioperative considerations, and potential concerns should be discussed with the anesthesiologist. For large abdominal wall reconstructions, preoperative placement of an epidural catheter for pain management after surgery should be considered. If need for an ICU bed is anticipated, this should be confirmed prior to surgery. Also, necessary suture and mesh materials should be confirmed available.

Intraoperative considerations include surgical technique and choice of suture and mesh materials. This will be discussed in detail throughout other sections of this text. Regardless of the operation performed, an emphasis on good surgical technique, strict adherence to sterility, meticulous hemostasis, and avoidance of complications is ideal. Changing the surgical plan and/or asking for assistance should never be considered a failure if done in the best interest of the patient. It is necessary to maintain good communication with the anesthesiologist and surgical team, keeping them informed of progress and problems when they arise. Whenever possible, local anesthetic should be used to decrease intraoperative anesthetic requirements and initial postoperative narcotic requirements. Antibiotics should be redosed during surgery as necessary.

Postoperative Planning

The vast majority of umbilical hernia, inguinal hernia, and small ventral hernia repairs are performed in the outpatient setting. Patients are discharged from the recovery room after appropriate criteria are met. For most ventral hernia repairs patients, an abdominal binder is placed to be worn for comfort as needed. Activity is restricted based on the procedure performed and the preference of the surgeon. In general, laparoscopic procedures allow for a faster return to full activity than open procedures. Oral narcotics should be given for expected incisional pain and stool softeners for constipation. Patients with urinary retention should have a Foley catheter placed and be started on alpha blockers. The catheter can be removed and a postvoid residual checked in 1 week. Persistent urinary retention or an elevated postvoid residual should prompt referral to a urologist for further evaluation. Patients should be evaluated once at 1–4 weeks after surgery to verify successful hernia repair and appropriate patient recovery.

Those patients with significant comorbidities and/or complex hernia repairs will require inpatient admission. Close monitoring for complications and initiation of preventive measures are essential.

Abdominal Compartment Syndrome

Abdominal distension, pulmonary failure, and oliguria are manifestations of abdominal compartment syndrome and should prompt measurement of bladder pressure. Routine bladder pressures should be measured for patients at high risk for abdominal compartment syndrome.

Surgical abdominal decompression should be considered in patients with bladder pressures above 25 mmHg and associated end-organ failure.

Atelectasis/Pneumonia

Preventative measures for atelectasis and pneumonia include early initiation of incentive spirometry, keeping the head of the bed elevated above 30°, early patient mobilization, and use of chlorhexidine mouthwash [15].

Deep Venous Thrombosis and Pulmonary Embolism

Preoperative administration of heparin, intraoperative use of intermittent pneumatic compression devices, and post-op need for unfractionated heparin or low molecular weight heparin are based on 2008 chest guidelines for DVT prophylaxis [14]. All patients should be mobilized quickly and physical therapist assistance used early as needed by the patient.

Enterotomy

A missed or delayed enterotomy is the number one cause for perioperative mortality after ventral hernia repair [16]. Making this diagnosis requires a high index of suspicion and demands prompt surgical intervention.

Paralytic Ileus

This is relatively common after complex hernia repairs that involve extensive intra-abdominal adhesiolysis and can be a source of frustration for patients. Several things can be done to facilitate the return of bowel function including frequent ambulation, adequate intravenous fluid hydration, aggressive correction of electrolyte imbalance, and use of nonnarcotic medications for pain control, among others. Alvimopan, a selective opioid receptor antagonist, has been shown to reduce hospital length of stay and time to GI recovery after abdominal surgery and may be of benefit in post-op hernia patients although this has not been studied [17]. A paralytic ileus lasting longer than 7 days should prompt further workup to rule out other causes such as a mechanical bowel obstruction or intra-abdominal source of infection.

Pain Management

Selected patients should be offered an epidural catheter that can be placed prior to surgery and then used afterward for pain management. Intraoperative usage of local anesthetic should be liberal. Local anesthetic infusion pumps are available and can provide effective pain relief when used by experienced surgeons in selected situations. Otherwise, pain should be controlled using narcotics and nonsteroidal anti-inflammatory drugs.

Summary

Abdominal wall hernias are found in all patient populations and involve a wide spectrum of complexity. An understanding of how comorbid conditions will impact the surgical repair of hernias is critical to achieving successful outcomes. This includes thorough identification of comorbid conditions and other potential risk factors followed by medical optimization and maximal risk reduction prior to surgery. It also includes meticulous preparation including consideration of surgical technique, availability of materials, and understanding of institutional capabilities, good intraoperative communication and surgical judgment, and optimal postoperative prophylaxis and identification of complications. Most important is the emphasis on good communication with the patient. It is critical to have a thorough discussion of the risks and benefits of surgery and set realistic expectations for recovery and long-term results.

References

1. Heniford BT, Park A, Ramshaw BJ, Voeller G. Laparoscopic repair of ventral hernias: nine years' experience with 850 consecutive hernias. Ann Surg. 2003;238(3):391–9.
2. Tsereteli Z, Pryor BA, Heniford BT, Park A, Voeller G, Ramshaw BJ. Laparoscopic ventral hernia repair (LVHR) in morbidly obese patients. Hernia. 2008;12(3):233–8.

3. Ching SS, Sarela AI, Dexter SP, Hayden JD, McMahon MJ. Comparison of early outcomes for laparoscopic ventral hernia repair between nonobese and morbidly obese patient populations. Surg Endosc. 2008;22(10):2244–50.
4. Raftopoulos I, Courcoulas AP. Outcome of laparoscopic ventral hernia repair in morbidly obese patients with a body mass index exceeding 35 kg/m^2. Surg Endosc. 2007;21(12):2293–7.
5. Novitsky YW, Cobb WS, Kercher KW, Matthews BD, Sing RF, Heniford BT. Laparoscopic ventral hernia repair in obese patients: a new standard of care. Arch Surg. 2006;141(1):57–61.
6. Langer C, Schaper A, Liersch T, Lulle B, Flosman M, Fuzesi L, Becker H. Prognosis factors in incisional hernia surgery: 25 years of experience. Hernia. 2005;9(1):16–21.
7. Rosemar A, Angeras U, Rosengren A, Nordin P. Effect of body mass index on groin hernia surgery. Ann Surg. 2010;252(2):397–401.
8. Evans KK, Chim H, Patel KM, Salgado CJ, Mardini S. Survey on ventral hernias: surgeon indications, contraindications, and management of large ventral hernias. Am Surg. 2012;78(4):388–97.
9. Finan KR, Vick CC, Fiefe CI, Neumayer L, Hawn MT. Predictors of wound infection in ventral hernia repair. Am J Surg. 2005;190(5):676–81.
10. Sorensen LT, Friis E, Jorgensen T, Vennits B, Andersen BR, Rasmussen GI, et al. Smoking is a risk factor for recurrence of groin hernia. World J Surg. 2002;26(4):397–400.
11. Sorensen LT, Hemmingsen UB, Kirkeby LT, Kallehave F, Jorgensen LN. Smoking is a risk factor for incisional hernia. Arch Surg. 2005;140(2):119–23.
12. Lindstrom D, Sadr Azodi O, Wladis A, Tonnesen H, Linder S, Nasell H, et al. Effects of a perioperative smoking cessation intervention on postoperative complications: a randomized trial. Ann Surg. 2008;248(5):739–45.
13. Ramos M, Khalpey Z, Lipsitz S, Steinberg J, Panizales MT, Zinner M, et al. Relationship of perioperative hyperglycemia and postoperative infections in patients who undergo general and vascular surgery. Ann Surg. 2008;248(4):585–91.
14. Geerts WH, Bergqvist D, Pineo GF, Heit JA, Samama CM, Lassen MR, et al. Prevention of venous thromboembolism: American college of chest physicians evidence-based clinical practice guidelines (8th edition). Chest. 2008;133(6):381S–453S.
15. Wren SM, Martin M, Yoon JK, Bech F. Postoperative pneumonia-prevention program for the inpatient surgical ward. J Am Coll Surg. 2010;210:491–5.
16. LeBlanc KA, Elieson MJ, Corder JM. Enterotomy and mortality rates of laparoscopic incisional and ventral hernia repair: a review of the literature. JSLS. 2007;11:408–14.
17. Vaughan-Shaw PG, Fecher IC, Harris S, Knight JS. A meta-analysis of the effectiveness of the opioid receptor antagonist alvimopan in reducing hospital length of stay and time to GI recovery in patients enrolled in a standardized accelerated recovery program after abdominal surgery. Dis Colon Rectum. 2012;55(5):611–20.

24. What Is a Complex Abdominal Wall?

Mickey M. Ott and Jose J. Diaz Jr.

The term *complex abdominal wall* has a number of interpretations but generally refers to a patient's abdomen that contains a ventral or an incisional hernia or defect plus one or more of the following characteristics (Fig. 24.1):

(a) Any additional condition that would be classified as a clean contaminated or a contaminated field (including but not limited to stomas)
(b) An enterocutaneous fistula
(c) A history of, or an ongoing, mesh or wound infection
(d) A large-sized defect (often defined as >10 cm in diameter)
(e) Loss of domain
(f) One or more recurrences

Patients with complex abdominal walls will seek surgical repair for a variety of reasons. A surgeon who wishes to approach the repair of a complex abdominal wall should be trained in and ready to employ a variety of techniques as needed to achieve a good outcome. One technique will not be appropriate for every patient, and outcomes will depend on the choice of technique as well as mesh implant for each individual scenario.

Techniques employed, and thus outcomes achieved, will vary depending on the patient and the comorbid conditions, the type of hernia, and on the skill set of the surgeon. Procedures that may be needed include, but are not limited to, the ability to perform extensive adhesiolysis, open component releases, endoscopic component releases, small and large bowel resections, enterostomies, advancement flaps, skin grafts, staged repairs, and laparoscopy. Surgeons must be familiar with a variety of implantable prosthetic materials, as the appropriate implantable mesh

B.P. Jacob and B. Ramshaw (eds.), *The SAGES Manual of Hernia Repair*,
DOI 10.1007/978-1-4614-4824-2_24,

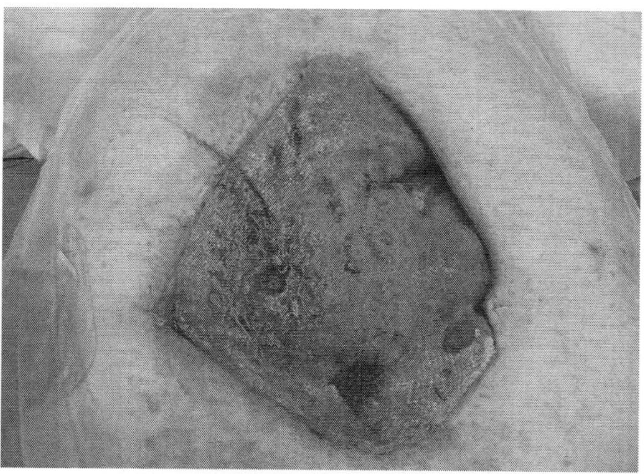

Fig. 24.1. The complex abdominal wall.

may vary depending on the patient. Materials for complex abdominal wall repairs include choosing between the synthetics, the biologics, the absorbable materials, or opting to use no mesh at the time. Finally, anticipating the aftercare is paramount. Taking on a patient with a complex abdomen requires that there be an experienced intensive care unit available that is familiar with these patients and their postoperative management.

The Evolution of Damage Control Surgery

To better understand the complex abdominal wall, it is important to identify some of the etiologies (Table 24.1). One of the primary reasons why surgeons may be seeing an increased number of these complex patients is the increasing frequency with which surgeons are using the open abdomen technique. The term *open abdomen technique* refers to an abbreviated operation, leaving the abdominal fascia open, and creating a temporizing abdominal closure.

In the late 1970s and early 1980s, reports of improved outcomes in coagulopathic trauma patients who had abdominal packing and abbreviated laparotomy began to be published [1, 2]. Dr. Harlan Stone et al. described this strategy, "…This technique of initial abortion of laparotomy, establishment of intra-abdominal pack tamponade, and then completion of the surgical procedure once coagulation has returned to an acceptable level has proven to be lifesaving in previously non-salvageable

Table 24.1. Conditions contributing to the complex abdominal wall hernia.

Condition
Intra-abdominal
Trauma—damage control
Emergency general and vascular surgery
Abdominal compartment syndrome
Visceral edema
Pancreatitis
Intra-abdominal sepsis/lack of source control
Intestinal fistulas, ostomies
Abdominal wall
Loss of domain
Necrotizing fasciitis/loss of abdominal wall tissue
Multiple hernia repair and resultant abdominal wall compromise
Chronic prosthetic mesh infection
Patient comorbidities
Smoking
Malnutrition
COPD
Cardiac/PVD
Diabetes mellitus
Steroid use

situations" [3]. The technique was further refined in the 1990s and was eventually coined "damage control" [4–8]. This concept recognized that critically ill patients can only tolerate a certain level of insult before reaching physiologic exhaustion. In an effort to definitively repair a patient's injury, longer operative procedures only contributed to the development of the deadly triad of hypothermia, acidosis, and coagulopathy. Damage control surgery is characterized by three distinct phases: (1) an abbreviated laparotomy that controls bleeding and intestinal contamination, (2) leaving the OR with the abdomen "open" and continuing resuscitation with correction of coagulopathy in the ICU, and (3) returning to the OR for completion of the definitive operation and staged abdominal wall repair [7–10]. Although this approach has clearly demonstrated improved outcomes, it has resulted in unexpected consequences. These patients who previously had not survived now have a complex abdominal wall defined as those patients with a planned ventral hernia with or without a skin graft, intestinal stomas, fistulas, and complicated infections. This can also include loss of domain, loss of abdominal wall tissue, and/or infected prosthetic mesh.

Intra-abdominal Hypertension and Abdominal Compartment Syndrome

Another clinical situation seen with increasing frequency is the use of the open abdomen technique for the management of intra-abdominal hypertension (IAH) and the prevention and treatment of abdominal compartment syndrome (ACS) (Fig. 24.2). IAH and ACS lie on a continuum of disease process and refer to increasing pressure in the peritoneal space that is subsequently transferred to the abdominal viscera. The presence of IAH has been shown to be independently associated with an increase in mortality [11–14]. This clinical situation is often seen in those patients requiring massive resuscitation after significant trauma and/or hemorrhage. IAH and ACS are relatively new terms that began to be reported in the 1980s and 1990s. In 1984, Kron et al. described four patients after AAA repair who developed abdominal distension, oliguria, and increasing airway pressures [15]. These symptoms were relieved with abdominal decompression. Since that time, the understanding and management of IAH and ACS has continued to evolve and in 2005; the World Society of Abdominal Compartment Syndrome met to establish a set of treatment guidelines [16, 17]. These focused on (1) the need for early serial intra-abdominal pressure (IAP) monitoring when IAH/ACS risk factors are present; (2) improving abdominal wall compliance through sedation, analgesia, and/or pharmacologic paralysis; (3) evacuating intraluminal contents through nasogastric or rectal decompression; (4) evacuating abdominal fluid collections via

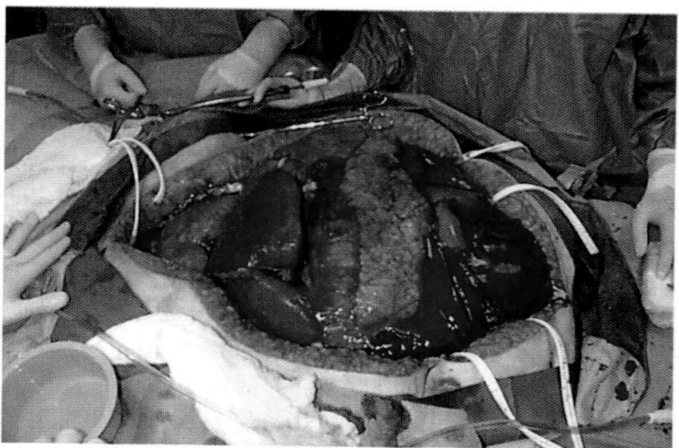

Fig. 24.2. Abdominal compartment syndrome.

percutaneous drainage; (5) correcting positive fluid balance through the use of hypertonic fluids, colloids, and careful diuresis; (6) supporting organ function with vasopressors and judicious goal-directed fluid resuscitation to maintain an abdominal perfusion pressure [calculated as mean arterial pressure (MAP—IAP)] of greater than 60 mmHg; and (7) early surgical intervention when IAP exceeds 25 mmHg. These guidelines highlight the importance of both nonoperative strategies to prevent and reduce elevated IAP, as well as early operative intervention for progressive organ failure. The treatment for ACS is abdominal decompression, but again, these patients are then faced with the morbidity of the open abdomen and the possibility of failure to close the fascia in the midline.

Other Indications for the Open Abdomen

The open abdomen technique has been employed not only for trauma but for general surgery patients as well [18, 19]. In 1981, John H. Duff et al. described 18 patients with severe abdominal sepsis treated by leaving the abdomen open. The technique allowed for wide abdominal drainage, easy access to the abdomen without re-laparotomy, and avoided the complications associated with closing an infected wound. Severe pancreatitis has also been treated in a similar fashion. In 1986, Dr. Michael Wertheimer described his experience with ten patients with necrotizing pancreatitis [20]. Use of the open abdomen technique allowed for optimum wound toilet, prevented recurrent episodes of sepsis, was able to be performed at bedside in the ICU and was associated with improved outcomes.

Intestinal Fistulae, Presence of a Stoma, and Infected Mesh

Frequently, those patients undergoing damage control in the setting of trauma or emergency general surgery develop complications, and one of the more morbid is the development of an enterocutaneous or enteroatmospheric fistula. The treatment of the patient with an enteric fistula is associated with a significant resource burden, increasing both intensive care unit and hospital length of stay, and significantly increasing hospital charges [21]. More importantly, they become a significant

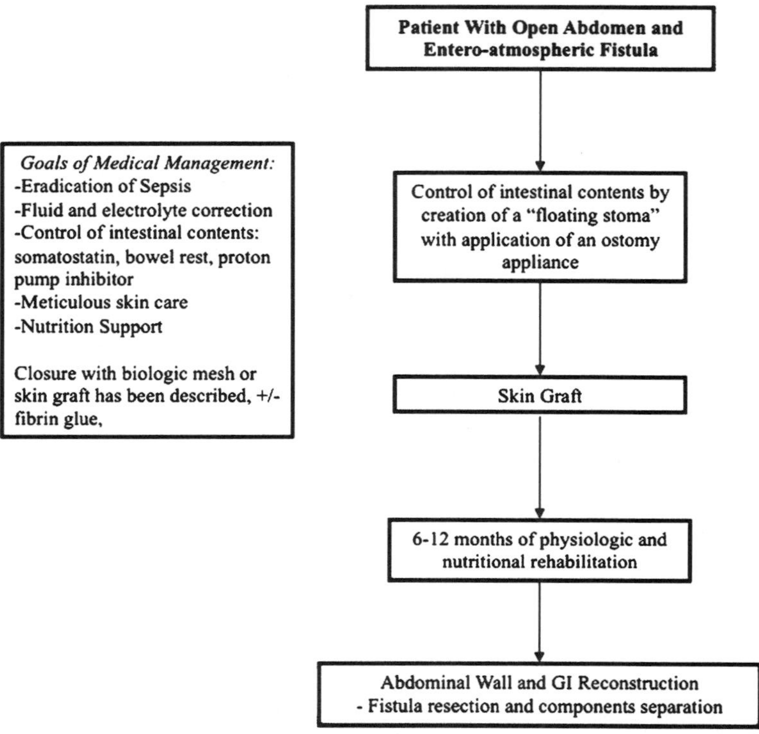

Fig. 24.3. Intestinal fistula complicating the open abdomen flow diagram.

burden to the patient who likely requires tedious wound care, long-term parenteral nutrition, and frequent bouts of sepsis.

The operation to repair an intestinal fistula is associated with an increased risk of infection, risk of recurrent fistulae, and the increased risk of hernia recurrence. The key management issues are the eradication of sepsis, drainage of any intra-abdominal abscess, local wound control of intestinal contents, optimizing nutrition status, and delayed reconstruction (Fig. 24.3) [22, 23]. Achieving these goals is no easy task, and many novel techniques have been developed to aid in the management of a fistula (Fig. 24.4). Restoration of abdominal continuity at the time of abdominal wall reconstruction has been demonstrated to be safe and is the preferred treatment for enterocutaneous fistulas [24, 25].

Not unlike an enteric fistula, just the presence of an ileostomy or colostomy can increase operative morbidity during ventral hernia repair.

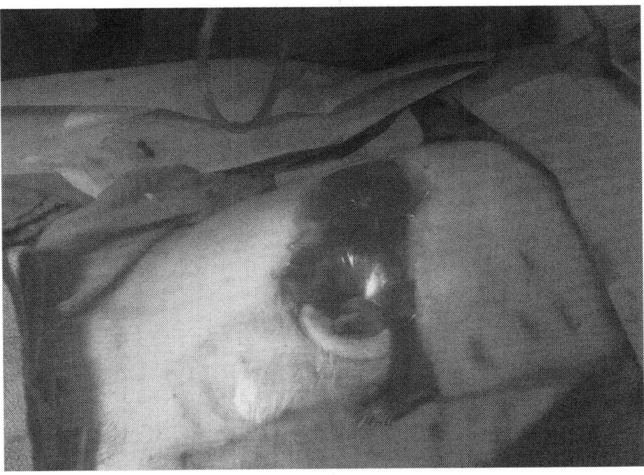

Fig. 24.4. A "floating stoma" has been created using multiple ostomy wafers to create a cylinder around the fistula opening and then surrounding the "stoma" with a VAC dressing. The VAC will control any spillage and assist with wound healing, and an ostomy bag can be placed on the floating stoma to collect intestinal contents by dependent drainage.

In 2009, a multi-institutional trial was undertaken, examining 240 patients with a complex ventral hernia repair [26]. The authors demonstrated that although ostomy takedown and/or fistula takedown can be performed at the same time as ventral hernia repair, this was associated with an increased risk of hernia recurrence and wound infection. The group concluded that if the microbiologic burden is too high, the surgeon can consider a staged procedure, performing the ostomy takedown, but repairing the ventral hernia at a later date. The use of mesh in this clinical situation is controversial as there is a high probability of chronic mesh infection (discussed in Chap. 44).

Patient Comorbidities

Smoking has been shown to increase the risk of hernia recurrence significantly [27]. It is imperative that surgeons insist on abstinence prior to undergoing a complex abdominal wall reconstruction. Obesity causes increased tension on the abdominal wall, both externally from a large panus, and internally from a large visceral mass. This too has been associated with increased risk of wound infection and hernia recurrence [26]. Malnutrition significantly increases overall patient morbidity and mortality, and every effort should be made to optimize a patient's nutritional status prior to tackling their complex abdominal wall [28]. If the patient has a proximal fistula or proximal diverting ostomy, this may require long-term parenteral nutrition. Chronic obstructive pulmonary disease (COPD) and diabetes mellitus (DM) have also been identified as risk factors for hernia development and recurrence [28]. Medications such as corticosteroids or chemotherapeutic agents may also inhibit wound healing [27].

Treatment Options: The Open Abdomen

Figure 24.5 refers to a treatment algorithm for closure of the open abdomen.

Early definitive abdominal closure (EDAC) refers to those techniques that result in a definitive repair during the initial hospitalization. Three techniques have been described to achieve EDAC: (1) delayed pimary fascial closure, (2) fascial bridge closure, and (3) acute components separation.

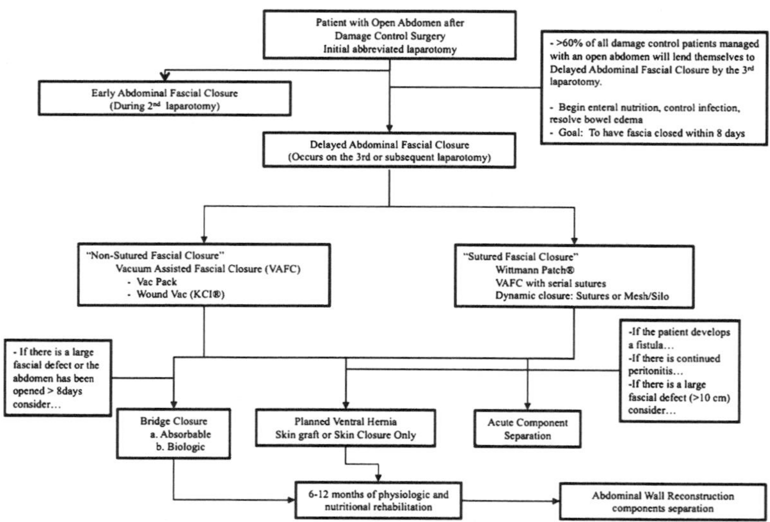

Fig. 24.5. The closure of the open abdomen in trauma, emergency general, and vascular surgery flow diagram.

Delayed Primary Fascial Closure

Delayed primary fascial closure refers to the bringing together of the patient's native fascia by maintaining tension on the fascia until visceral edema resolves or serially tightening the abdominal wall until closure is achieved. Three major techniques to achieve delayed primary fascial closure have shown to be safe and effective including vacuum-assisted closure devices (VACD), the Wittmann Patch (WP), and dynamic/serial fascial tightening with or without the use of temporary mesh. Greater than 80% of patient's will achieve fascial closure using these techniques [9, 29–32]. Ideally, this is achieved within the first week after the initial operation, as the risk of complications dramatically increases after 1 week [32].

Fascial Bridge Closure

When delayed primary fascial closure fails, bridging the fascia with biologic mesh can be considered [9, 26]. Occasionally, this type of repair will be "definitive," and the patient will never need another operation. However, recent data suggests that the likelihood of abdominal wall laxity and recurrent hernia is high [33, 34].

Acute Components Separation

Performing component separation procedure in the acute setting of failed primary fascial closure has been described [35]. However, in the setting of ongoing peritonitis, or systemic inflammatory response syndrome (SIRS), this is not recommended. Moreover, if this procedure fails, the surgeon has now lost the chance to perhaps achieve fascial closure at a later time when conditions are more optimal.

Treatment Options: Planned Ventral Hernia

Once it has been determined that the EDAC cannot be performed due to either massive visceral edema, loss of domain, and/or loss of abdominal wall tissue, the only option left is a planned ventral hernia (Fig. 24.6).

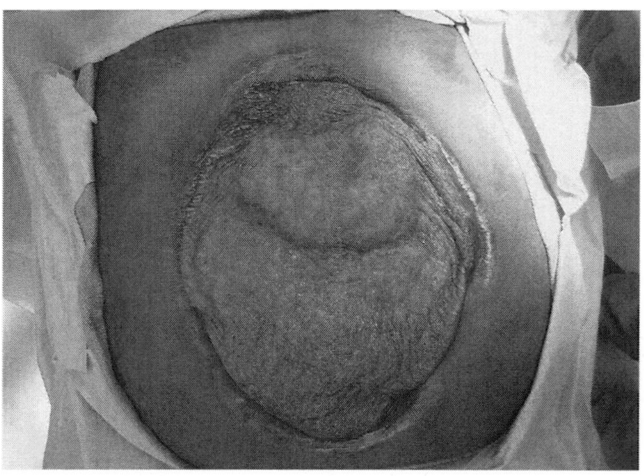

Fig. 24.6. Planned ventral hernia.

This technique, described by Fabian et al., involves achieving visceral coverage with STSG or skin only closure and returning at a later date to fix the abdominal wall defect [36]. Ideally, the abdominal wall reconstruction is not performed until 3–12 months after the original operation to allow for the development of a "neo-peritoneum" and a softening of intra-abdominal adhesions.

Treatment Options: Abdominal Wall Reconstruction

Abdominal wall reconstruction in the patient with a complex abdominal wall requires significant preoperative planning (Fig. 24.7). As discussed previously, optimizing nutritional status, smoking cessation, adequate blood glucose control, and pulmonary and cardiac clearance are essential prior to undergoing this complex operation. Patients need to be counseled that they may require time in the intensive care unit, may require mechanical ventilation postoperatively, and are at significant risk for perioperative complications [37, 38].

An important step to remember prior to attempting abdominal wall reconstruction is reducing the bio-burden in the operative field. If fistula or ostomy output is poorly controlled, or there is a chronically infected wound or mesh, a staged procedure may be preferable, or the procedure

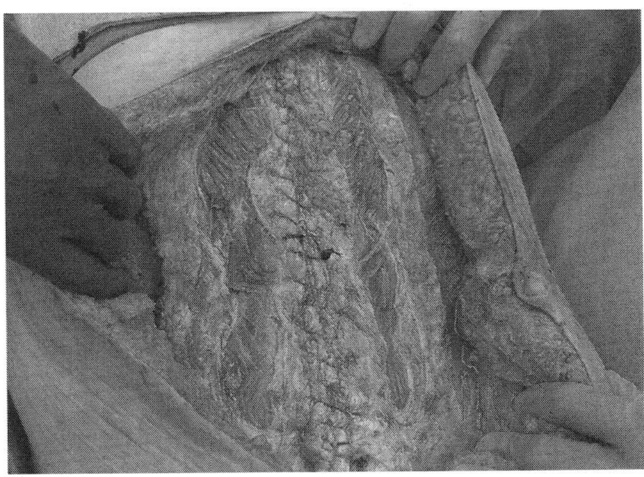

Fig. 24.7 Abdominal wall reconstruction.

should be delayed. The Ventral Hernia Working Group has helped develop a hernia grading system that can assist the surgeon in evaluating a patient's risk for complications [39].

(a) Grade 1 = low risk. These patients are at low risk for complications, having had no history of wound infection and an uncomplicated past medical history. By definition, almost none of the patients with a complex abdominal wall fall under this category.
(b) Grade 2 = comorbid. Includes patients who smoke; are obese, diabetic, immunosuppressed, and malnourished; and have COPD or other factors associated with poor wound healing.
(c) Grade 3 = potentially contaminated. Includes patients who have had a previous wound infection, have a stoma or fistula present, or have violation of the GI tract during their procedure.
(d) Grade 4 = infected. These patients have had gross contamination and/or active infection.

Although, this grading system still requires validation, it provides a resource for surgeons to assist their clinical decision making and counsel their patients.

The primary goal in reconstructing the complex abdominal wall is reapproximating the midline to the greatest extent possible. This should be accomplished using component separation when appropriate

[33, 39–41]. Our group favors component separation with the use of a biologic mesh underlay or onlay to maximize support. The reasoning behind the choice of a biologic mesh is that the majority of these patients will have multiple risk factors for recurrence and/or surgical site infection. Technical details of component separation and other techniques for repair of the complex abdominal wall are discussed elsewhere in this book.

Conclusion

The complex abdominal wall provides a unique challenge for a surgeon. Understanding the etiology of this clinical entity, meticulous perioperative planning, management of patient risk factors, and a systematic approach to the management of these patients will lead the best outcomes.

References

1. Lucas CE, Ledgerwood AM. Prospective evaluation of hemostatic techniques for liver injuries. J Trauma. 1976;16:442–51.
2. Feliciano DV, Mattox KL, Jordan Jr GL. Intra-abdominal packing for control of hepatic hemorrhage: a reappraisal. J Trauma. 1981;21:285–90.
3. Stone HH, Strom PR, Mullins RJ. Management of the major coagulopathy with onset during laparotomy. Ann Surg. 1983;197:532–5.
4. Cue JI, Cryer HG, Miller FB, Richardson JD, Polk Jr HC. Packing and planned reexploration for hepatic and retroperitoneal hemorrhage: critical refinements of a useful technique. J Trauma. 1990;30:1007–11.
5. Burch JM, Ortiz VB, Richardson RJ, Martin RR, Mattox KL, Jordan Jr GL. Abbreviated laparotomy and planned reoperation for critically injured patients. Ann Surg. 1992;215:476–83.
6. Talbert S, Trooskin SZ, Scalea T, et al. Packing and re-exploration for patients with nonhepatic injuries. J Trauma. 1992;33:121–4.
7. Morris Jr JA, Eddy VA, Blinman TA, Rutherford EJ, Sharp KW. The staged celiotomy for trauma. Issues in unpacking and reconstruction. Ann Surg. 1993;217:576–84.
8. Rotondo MF, Schwab CW, McGonigal MD, et al. 'Damage control': an approach for improved survival in exsanguinating penetrating abdominal injury. J Trauma. 1993;35:375–82.
9. Diaz Jr JJ, Cullinane DC, Dutton WD, et al. The management of the open abdomen in trauma and emergency general surgery: part 1-damage control. J Trauma. 2010;68:1425–38.

10. Ott MM, Norris PR, Diaz JJ, et al. Colon anastomosis after damage control laparotomy: recommendations from 174 trauma colectomies. J Trauma. 2011;70:595–602.
11. Cheatham ML, Safcsak K. Is the evolving management of intra-abdominal hypertension and abdominal compartment syndrome improving survival? Crit Care Med. 2010;38:402–7.
12. Mentula P, Hienonen P, Kemppainen E, Puolakkainen P, Leppaniemi A. Surgical decompression for abdominal compartment syndrome in severe acute pancreatitis. Arch Surg. 2010;145:764–9.
13. Balogh ZJ, Martin A, van Wessem KP, King KL, Mackay P, Havill K. Mission to eliminate postinjury abdominal compartment syndrome. Arch Surg. 2011;146(8):938–43.
14. Eddy VA, Key SP, Morris Jr JA. Abdominal compartment syndrome: etiology, detection, and management. J Tenn Med Assoc. 1994;87:55–7.
15. Kron IL, Harman PK, Nolan SP. The measurement of intra-abdominal pressure as a criterion for abdominal re-exploration. Ann Surg. 1984;199:28–30.
16. Cheatham ML, Malbrain ML, Kirkpatrick A, et al. Results from the international conference of experts on intra-abdominal hypertension and abdominal compartment syndrome. II. Recommendations. Intensive Care Med. 2007;33:951–62.
17. Malbrain ML, Cheatham ML, Kirkpatrick A, et al. Results from the international conference of experts on intra-abdominal hypertension and abdominal compartment syndrome. I. Definitions. Intensive Care Med. 2006;32:1722–32.
18. Duff JH, Moffat J. Abdominal sepsis managed by leaving abdomen open. Surgery. 1981;90:774–8.
19. Maetani S, Tobe T. Open peritoneal drainage as effective treatment of advanced peritonitis. Surgery. 1981;90:804–9.
20. Wertheimer MD, Norris CS. Surgical management of necrotizing pancreatitis. Arch Surg. 1986;121:484–7.
21. Teixeira PG, Inaba K, Dubose J, et al. Enterocutaneous fistula complicating trauma laparotomy: a major resource burden. Am Surg. 2009;75:30–2.
22. Draus Jr JM, Huss SA, Harty NJ, Cheadle WG, Larson GM. Enterocutaneous fistula: are treatments improving? Surgery. 2006;140:570–6.
23. Ramsay PT, Mejia VA. Management of enteroatmospheric fistulae in the open abdomen. Am Surg. 2010;76:637–9.
24. Sleeman D, Sosa JL, Gonzalez A, et al. Reclosure of the open abdomen. J Am Coll Surg. 1995;180:200–4.
25. Wind J, van Koperen PJ, Slors JF, Bemelman WA. Single-stage closure of enterocutaneous fistula and stomas in the presence of large abdominal wall defects using the components separation technique. Am J Surg. 2009;197:24–9.
26. Diaz Jr JJ, Conquest AM, Ferzoco SJ, et al. Multi-institutional experience using human acellular dermal matrix for ventral hernia repair in a compromised surgical field. Arch Surg. 2009;144:209–15.
27. Finan KR, Vick CC, Kiefe CI, Neumayer L, Hawn MT. Predictors of wound infection in ventral hernia repair. Am J Surg. 2005;190:676–81.
28. Dunne JR, Malone DL, Tracy JK, Napolitano LM. Abdominal wall hernias: risk factors for infection and resource utilization. J Surg Res. 2003;111:78–84.

29. van Boele HP, Wind J, Dijkgraaf MG, Busch OR, Carel GJ. Temporary closure of the open abdomen: a systematic review on delayed primary fascial closure in patients with an open abdomen. World J Surg. 2009;33:199–207.
30. Ghazi B, Deigni O, Yezhelyev M, Losken A. Current options in the management of complex abdominal wall defects. Ann Plast Surg. 2011;66(5):488–92.
31. Miller PR, Meredith JW, Johnson JC, Chang MC. Prospective evaluation of vacuum-assisted fascial closure after open abdomen: planned ventral hernia rate is substantially reduced. Ann Surg. 2004;239:608–14.
32. Miller RS, Morris Jr JA, Diaz Jr JJ, Herring MB, May AK. Complications after 344 damage-control open celiotomies. J Trauma. 2005;59:1365–71.
33. Ko JH, Wang EC, Salvay DM, Paul BC, Dumanian GA. Abdominal wall reconstruction: lessons learned from 200 "components separation" procedures. Arch Surg. 2009;144:1047–55.
34. Candage R, Jones K, Luchette FA, Sinacore JM, Vandevender D, Reed RL. Use of human acellular dermal matrix for hernia repair: friend or foe? Surgery. 2008;144:703–9.
35. Howdieshell TR, Proctor CD, Sternberg E, Cue JI, Mondy JS, Hawkins ML. Temporary abdominal closure followed by definitive abdominal wall reconstruction of the open abdomen. Am J Surg. 2004;188:301–6.
36. Fabian TC, Croce MA, Pritchard FE, et al. Planned ventral hernia. Staged management for acute abdominal wall defects. Ann Surg. 1994;219:643–50.
37. DiCocco JM, Magnotti LJ, Emmett KP, et al. Long-term follow-up of abdominal wall reconstruction after planned ventral hernia: a 15-year experience. J Am Coll Surg. 2010;210:686–8.
38. Zarzaur BL, DiCocco JM, Shahan CP, et al. Quality of life after abdominal wall reconstruction following open abdomen. J Trauma. 2011;70:285–91.
39. Breuing K, Butler CE, Ferzoco S, et al. Incisional ventral hernias: review of the literature and recommendations regarding the grading and technique of repair. Surgery. 2010;148:544–58.
40. de Vries Reilingh TS, van Goor H, Charbon JA, et al. Repair of giant midline abdominal wall hernias: "components separation technique" versus prosthetic repair: interim analysis of a randomized controlled trial. World J Surg. 2007;31:756–63.
41. Shabatian H, Lee DJ, Abbas MA. Components separation: a solution to complex abdominal wall defects. Am Surg. 2008;74:912–6.

Part VI
Techniques for Ventral and Incisional Hernia Repair

25. Synthetic Prosthetic Choices in Ventral Hernia Repair

Sheila A. Grant

Background on Hernia Mesh for Ventral Repair

Ventral hernia repair is a common procedure with over 250,000 repairs each year in the United States [1]. Most ventral hernias are repaired using tension-free type of repair, but prior to 1970, tension (primary suture) repair was common. Due to the high tension and stress placed on either side of the defect, this tension-type repair led to many complications, such as pain, discomfort, and recurrence [2–8]. To reduce complications, a mesh that could bridge the defect and/or reinforce the abdominal wall was introduced that led to a tension-free type of repair. In 1959, Usher and colleagues are credited with the first modern tension-free repair when they utilized a synthetic polymeric material, a polypropylene monofilament mesh known then as Marlex. However, this need for reinforcement materials was noted as far back as the 1900s. Much earlier, mesh material designs were investigated such as silver mesh (1900 and 1940s), tantalum (1948), and stainless steel (1950s) [8]. The problems stemming from these metallic meshes were disintegration of the metal, metallic fatigue, and fracture, and thus, metallic meshes were discontinued.

The utilization of mesh to bridge the hernia defect led to the reduction of recurrences and alleviated some complications. Many studies have been performed detailing the ability of hernia mesh to reduce complications and recurrences [9–13]. For example, in a study from the Netherlands, hernia recurrence with a sutured tissue repair resulted in a 63% recurrence rate, as opposed to a 32% recurrence rate using a prosthetic [13]. Unfortunately, even with a mesh scaffold, the recurrence rates are still very high with the standard ventral hernia repair. For example, Luijendijk et al. performed a prospective clinical study that

B.P. Jacob and B. Ramshaw (eds.), *The SAGES Manual of Hernia Repair*, DOI 10.1007/978-1-4614-4824-2_25,

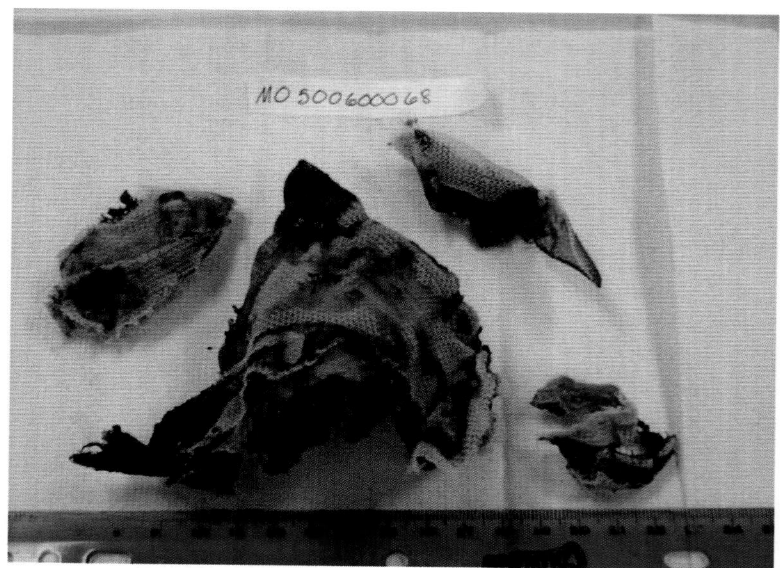

Fig. 25.1. Explanted polypropylene mesh.

demonstrated an approximate 25% recurrence rate of ventral hernias repaired with synthetic mesh within 3 years [14]. Another study showed reoperation rates of 12.3% at 5 years and 23% at 13 years when using hernia mesh for ventral repair [15].

Many of the complications that result when synthetic mesh is used are potentially due to the body's foreign body response. Initially, an aggressive foreign body response was touted as necessary since it resulted in scar plate formation that, for all intents and purposes, reinforced the abdominal wall. However, it has since been discovered that this response may also lead to mesh degradation and other complications. Numerous studies have shown shrinkage, contraction, and distortion of the hernia mesh that have led to pain and recurrence [16–20]. The use of mesh in ventral hernia repair also presented such complications as visceral adhesions, erosion into the bowel, extrusion of the repair materials, and infection [1]. Figure 25.1 displays an explanted hernia mesh. Scar tissue, contraction, and distortion of the mesh are apparent, which may be due to excess foreign body response, mismatch of material-tissue properties, and/or non-inertness of the mesh (oxidation, hydrolysis, etc.), which all could be enhanced by particular patient demographics [16, 17].

Surgeons are faced with controversies and a general lack of consensus on what type of repair should be reinforced, what type of mesh material to use (synthetic vs. biologic), and what type of technique to use for repair. To improve the outcome of ventral hernia repair, Breuing and colleagues [1] developed an algorithm, which provided flowcharts for treatment considerations for incisional ventral hernia repair. Their algorithm took into account the surgical technique (laparascopic vs. open), the size of the defect (less than or greater than 2 cm), and patient assessment for risk of surgical-site occurrence or hernia recurrence. Their group, the Ventral Hernia Working Group, was established to evaluate new technologies and techniques in ventral hernia repair. While the group did mention mesh materials in a broad sense, detailed algorithms are also needed for choosing the "best" hernia mesh for the patient.

Today's mesh can be broadly classified as synthetic, biologic, or resorbable. This chapter will not address the biologic hernia mesh but will investigate the state of the current permanent synthetic and resorbable synthetic mesh.

Current Mesh Materials

An ideal mesh for laparoscopic ventral hernia repair would elicit the correct physiological response such as no adhesion formation on the visceral side, no infection, no allergic or hypersensitivity reaction, limited foreign body reaction, and adequate biocompatibility to recapitulate tissue. But the mesh material would ideally also possess certain engineering properties such as strength, ease of handling, proper mechanical strains (similar to the abdominal wall), be sterilizable, be inert to body and tissue fluids, and be capable to be fabricated in different forms (knits, monofilaments, etc.). Unfortunately, there will never be an ideal mesh because of the complex and variable interactions between the various types of mesh and the complex characteristics and responses presented by different groups of patients. However, using the principles of complexity science, it should be possible over time to make better and better mesh decisions for various techniques and patient groups (clusters).

The three main types of hernia mesh materials are polypropylene, polyethylene terephthalate, and expanded polytetrafluoroethylene (ePTFE). Polypropylene is a semicrystalline material with hydrophobic tendency. Typically polypropylene fibers are extruded and then are woven or knitted into particular monofilament or multifilament designs. These designs dictate the overall mechanical strength and strain of the mesh. Initially, most polypropylene hernia mesh utilized a small, dense pore design. These "heavyweight mesh" had small pores and a surface area greater than 90 g/m^2 area of material, which resulted in an intense foreign body response. The resulting rigid scar plate formed due to granuloma bridging between the small pores. Numerous clinical problems such as mesh extrusion and bowel fistulas, which have occurred with heavyweight polypropylene, have been well documented in literature [21].

To reduce the foreign body response and granuloma bridging [22], mid- and lightweight polypropylene mesh with larger pores (>1 mm), and smaller filaments were designed that still could withstand the intra-abdominal pressures but also would have less material per square meter. While clinical evidence has demonstrated that the efficacy of most lightweight meshes are an improvement over the heavyweight mesh in some patient groups and clinical uses, granulomas and scar tissue formation may still occur [23]. Additionally, lighter weight mesh with larger, open pore design may suffer from premature failure due to mesh displacement or rupture [24].

Polyethylene terephthalate, commonly known as PET or polyester, is another popular hernia mesh. Like polypropylene, PET can also be extruded into synthetic fibers wherein it can be woven into a variety of mesh designs; PET is also less hydrophobic than polypropylene. Clinical evidence has also shown a considerable inflammatory reaction with gross tissue ingrowth into the macroporous interstices of the mesh, causing variable degrees of scar formation. To mitigate some of the inflammatory response and ingrowth potential when placed in contact with the viscera, coated PET mesh became available (Table 25.1).

Polytetrafluoroethylene (PTFE) is a fluorocarbon-based polymer and is a commonly utilized mesh material. Unlike polypropylene and PET, PTFE is extremely hydrophobic and one of the most chemically inert polymers. Also utilized as a hernia mesh material is ePTFE, which is produced by stretching a sheet of PTFE, creating micropores. Unfortunately, clinical data has shown that the microporous structure results in poor integration and scar tissue formation, resulting in mesh contraction and shrinkage [25]. To allow better tissue integration, PTFE mesh is available in an open macroporous, monofilament design (Infinit® by W.L. Gore and Associates). Another macroporous PTFE mesh is

Table 25.1. A partial list of commercially available coated mesh.

Brand	Coating/mesh
C-Qur (atrium)	Omega-3 fatty acid over lightweight polypropylene
Parietex composite (covidien)	Collagen-polyethylene glycol-glycerol over PET
Proceed (ethicon)	Oxidized regenerated cellulose over polypropylene encapsulated by polydioxanone
Sepramesh IP composite (Bard)	Hydrogel layer (sodium hyaluronate, carboxymethylcellulose, polyethylene glycol) over polypropylene co-knitted with polyglycolic acid fibers
Ti-Mesh (Biomet, Inc.)	Covalently bonded titanized surface over polypropylene (light- to medium weight)
PolyPro Mesh (STS)	Polyether urethane urea over polypropylene

It should be noted that some have microporous coatings which are designed for intra-abdominal placement and others (Ti-Mesh and PolyPro Mesh) are macroporous and could induce bowel erosion if place in the peritoneal cavity

MotifMESH™ (Proxy Biomedical). Because these mesh are macroporous, neither of these products are designed for intraperitoneal use.

Coatings

Because of the adverse effects noted clinically with some of the uncoated mesh materials, newer designs have incorporated coatings. These meshes are sometimes noted as barrier mesh and are considered the "second-generation" mesh, with the goal of providing a protective layer to prevent adhesion to the intraperitoneal contents. There are many meshes on the market that have been coated with absorbable or permanent coatings in order to reduce the severity of the inflammatory response, reduce adhesions, and lead to less fibrosis and contraction of the mesh [26]. Table 25.1 provides a partial list of some of the currently available coated mesh.

Studies have shown that these coatings help reduce adhesions and the severity of the inflammatory response. While the short-term outcome is promising, clinical evidence has also shown that some of the coatings are unstable over time and disintegrate, thus potentially leaving the underlying material susceptible to adhesion formation and materials degradation [27]. Durable, longer-lasting coatings are needed for better long-term clinical outcomes.

Resorbable Mesh Materials

An alternative to permanent synthetic mesh are the resorbable mesh. Resorbable mesh is attractive due to their reduce risks of adhesion formations and absence of long-term foreign body responses. The resorbable mesh is typically composed of copolymerized forms of polylactic acid, polyglycolic acid, polyglactin, and/or polycaprolactone. The challenge for absorbable mesh is the degradation rate; too fast of degradation could result in loss of mesh strength, resulting in recurrences. Too slow of degradation could result in long-term foreign body responses. While the number of resorbable mesh on the market is few, a new mesh currently on the market is TIGR Matrix surgical mesh (Novus Scientific). TIGR mesh knits two polymers with different resorbable rates, a fast and a slow degradation rate, so that that strength and integrity of the mesh is secured while reducing inflammatory response. Another recently available resorbable mesh is GORE BIO-A (W.L. Gore). This resorbable synthetic has a faster resorption profile and is microporous compared with TIGR matrix mesh. While resorbable mesh may not be applicable to every hernia procedure, there may be some procedures where resorbable mesh will be the mesh of choice.

Choosing the Best Mesh

While polypropylene, PET, and PTFE make up the majority of current hernia mesh materials, there are over 80 different types of hernia mesh available [1]. Given that the properties of the mesh can vary considerably, choosing the best mesh for a particular patient population and/or procedure can be confusing. Thus, it is not surprising that investigators have performed controlled prospective and retrospective case studies in order to formulate different algorithms and suggestions of mesh usage [28]. Unfortunately, there are some inherent concerns with these studies in that there is usually not enough patient data to support the given recommendations [1].

Since not all hernias are alike and they can differ significantly in size and complexity, the choice of mesh should be based on risk of adhesions, risk of infections, surgeon familiarity, cost, and patient characteristics. In particular, patient characteristics such as BMI, diabetes, tobacco use, second surgeries, previous hernias need to be considered. For example, in an unpublished study performed by our group, polypropylene mesh explanted from high BMI patients have shown more adverse foreign body reaction than mesh explanted from low BMI patients. Studies that take into account patient demographics need to be performed in order to fully characterize patient-material effects and eventually be utilized to develop algorithms that match the best mesh for a particular patient population.

From a materials point of view, the best mesh would be one where the engineering properties of the mesh matches the engineering properties of the abdominal wall. For example, the tensile strength and strain of the mesh material should be equivalent to that of the abdominal wall. Excessive tensile strength or overengineered mesh materials may decrease mesh flexibility and compliance, which can result in excessive inflammation and scarring. A mesh that is too rigid and is implanted in compliant abdominal tissue, for example, could incite severe inflammatory responses. Thus, the abdominal wall biomechanics need to be well understood as well as the mechanics of the mesh materials in order to design optimal mesh implants for hernia repair.

Many studies have investigated the abdominal wall biomechanics [29]. For example, force-elongation response of human abdominal wall was recently determined using tensile tests [29]. When applying an approximately 20 kPa of abdominal pressure, a corresponding biaxial force of about 3.4 N/mm in the transverse and 1.5 N/mm in the longitudinal direction occurs along with a compliance ratio of about 2:1 between the longitudinal and transversal directions. When applying a transverse and longitudinal strains both in the order of 6%, the authors also determined that Young's modulus in the transversal direction was about 50 kPa while the Young's modulus was about 20 kPa in longitudinal direction. Studies like these can help develop mathematical models of the abdominal wall which will assist in optimal mesh design.

There have been many studies that have investigated mesh material properties [30]. A recent study by Deeken et al. [30] investigated physicomechanical properties of polypropylene, PET, and PTFE hernia mesh. While most of the mesh materials are overengineered, significant differences in mechanical properties were found in relation to orientation of the mesh, which highlights the need to understand mesh design,

Table 25.2. Mesh-tissue response.

Mesh physical characteristics	Noted tissue responses
Interstices greater than 75 μm	Allows passage of macrophages, fibroblasts, blood vessels; reduces risk of infection
Interstices less than 10 μm	Leads to rigid scar plate formation due to granuloma bridging; restricts passages of macrophages that may lead to infection
Interstices less than 1.00 mm	Leads to rigid scar plate formation
Density (heavyweight vs. lightweight)	A more severe foreign body reaction (FBR) is noted with heavyweight mesh
Tensile strengths of synthetic mesh	Almost all mesh are overengineered, causing compliance mismatch between the mesh and tissue that can result in enhanced FBR
Strains at physiological loads	Mesh with less strain than tissue can result in enhanced FBR
Coating or composite type of coating	Initial FBR is reduced, adhesions reduced, but long-term performance needs to be characterized
Filament diameter (smaller diameter filaments have more compliance, flexibility)	Less FBR with smaller diameter filaments but too small of filaments may lead to breakage
Isotropic or anisotropic behavior of mesh (based on weave)	Tissue response of different mesh designs has yet to be investigated
Pore design (hexagonal pores, square pores, etc.)	Tissue response of different mesh designs has yet to be investigated

particularly the weave of the mesh. The design of the weave will dictate the shape of the interstices and thus influence the overall mechanical properties and ultimately, the foreign body response. While there are numerous weave designs for hernia mesh that display hexagonal pores, square pores, irregular pores, triangulated pores, etc., there has been surprisingly little scientific evidence in predicting which mesh weave would elicit better clinical results. The lack of studies has resulted in a plethora of mesh designs. In addition, the weave design will impart either isotropic or anisotropic properties of the mesh. Isotropic mesh designs display equal mechanical properties in any direction of applied stress, while anisotropic mesh display different mechanical properties depending upon the direction of applied stress. Anisotropic mesh design results in a mesh that is stronger in one direction than in the other so that it may be possible to initiate different complexities of the foreign body response. In addition, when stress is applied to mesh (such as coughing, jumping), the mesh can change shape dramatically depending upon the weave, which can lead to enhanced inflammatory and foreign body response. Modeling of weave designs in conjunction with the biomechanics of the abdominal wall could possibility lead to better mesh designs and thus better clinical outcomes. Table 25.2 summarizes some of the engineered mesh materials factors that may influence tissue response.

Future of Hernia Mesh Materials

For all intents and purposes, the goal of hernia mesh is to bridge the hernia defect while providing the mechanical strength and fixation which is important for repair. An ideal mesh would match the mesh material properties to that of the tissue while eliciting favorable tissue responses and avoiding any material changes/degradation (shrinkage, oxidation, etc.). Unfortunately, such a mesh does not currently exist. Added to the challenge of designing an optimal mesh is patient response to mesh materials may be different. Implementing continuous quality improvement projects would help in deciphering the optimal mesh design parameters as well as targeting particular patient populations. Until an optimal mesh can be designed, surgeons will have to rely on their own clinical experiences in choosing the best mesh for their patients.

References

1. Brueing NK, Butler CE, Ferzoco S, Franz M, Hultman CS, Kilbridge JF, Rosen M, Silverman RP, Vargo D. Incisional ventral hernias: review of the literature and recommendations regarding the grading and technique of repair. Surgery. 2010;148(3): 544–58.
2. Bendavid R. Recurrences: the fault of the surgeon. In: Schumpelick V, Nyhus LM, editors. Meshes: benefits and risks. New York: Springer; 2004. p. 55.
3. Arroyo A, Garcia P, Perez F, Andreu J, Candela F, Calpena R. Randomized clinical trial comparing suture and mesh repair of umbilical hernia in adults. Br J Surg. 2001; 88:1321–3.
4. Anthony T, Bergen PC, Kim LT, et al. Factors affecting recurrence following incisional herniorrhaphy. World J Surg. 2000;24:95–100.
5. Tentes A, Xanthoulis AI, Mirelis CG, et al. Nuttall technique: a method for subumbilical incisional hernia repair revised. Langenbecks Arch Surg. 2008;393:191–4.

6. Hadad I, Small W, Dumanian GA. Repair of massive ventral hernias with the separation of parts technique: reversal of the lost domain. Am Surg. 2009;75:301–6.
7. Milikan KW. Incisional hernia repair. Surg Clin North Am. 2003;83:1223–34.
8. Shankaran V, Weber DJ, Reed RL, Luchette FA. A review of available prosthetics for ventral hernia repair. Ann Surg. 2011;253(1):16–26.
9. Alkhoury F, Helton S, Ippolito RJ. Cost and clinical outcomes of laparoscopic ventral hernia repair using intraperitoneal nonheavyweight polypropylene mesh. Surg Laparosc Endosc Percutan Tech. 2011;21(2):82–5.
10. Sailes FC, Walls J, Guelig D, Mirzabeigi M, Long WD, Crawford A, Moore JH, Copit SE, Tuma GA, Fox J. Synthetic and biological mesh in component separations: a 10-year single institution review. Ann Plast Surg. 2010;64(5):696–8.
11. Van't RM, Vrijland WW, Lange JF, Hop WC, Jeekel J, Bonjer HJ. Mesh repair of incisional hernia: comparison of laparoscopic and open repair. Eur J Surg. 2002; 168(12):684–9.
12. Yavuz N, Ipek T, As A, Kapan M, Eyuboglu E, Erguney S. Laparoscopic repair of ventral and incisional hernias: our experience in 150 patients. J Laparoendosc Adv Surg Tech A. 2005;6:601–5.
13. Burger JWA, Luijendijk RW, Hop WCJ, Halm JA, Verdaasdonk EGG, Jeekel J. Long-term follow-up of a randomized control trial of suture versus mesh repair of incisional hernia. Ann Surg. 2004;240(4):578–85.
14. Luijendijk RW, Hop WC, van den Tol MP, de Lange DC, Braaksma MM, Ijzermans JN. A comparison of suture repair with mesh repair for incisional hernia. N Engl J Med. 2000;343:392–8.
15. Flum DR, Horvath K, Koepsell T. Have outcomes of incisional hernia repair improved with time? A population-based analysis. Ann Surg. 2003;237:129–35.
16. Cozad M, Ramshaw BR, Grant DN, Bachman SL, Grant DA, Grant SA. Materials characterization of explanted polypropylene, polyethylene terephthalate, and expanded polytetrafluoroethylene composites: spectral and thermal analysis. J Biomed Mater Res B Appl Biomater. 2010;94:455–62.
17. Costello CR, Bachman SL, Ramshaw BR, Grant SA. Materials characterization of explanted heavyweight polypropylene hernia meshes. J Biomed Mater Res B Appl Biomater. 2007;83B:44–9.
18. Klinge U, Klosterhalfen B, Muller M, Ottinger AP, Schumpelick V. Shrinking of polypropylene mesh in vivo: an experimental study in dogs. Eur J Surg. 1998;164: 965–9.
19. Gonzalez R, et al. Relationship between tissue ingrowth and mesh contraction. World J Surg. 2005;29(8):1038–43.
20. Pierce RA, Perrone JM, Nimeri A, Sexton JA, Walcutt J, Frisella MM, Matthews BD. 120-day comparative analysis of adhesion grade and quantity, mesh contraction, and tissue response to a novel omega-3 fatty acid bioabsorbable barrier macroporous mesh after intraperitoneal placement. Surg Innov. 2009;16:46–54.
21. Schmidbauer S, Ladurner R, Hallfeldt KK, Mussack T. Heavy-weight versus low-weight polypropylene meshes for open sublay mesh repair of incisional hernia. Eur J Med Res. 2005;10(6):247–53.

22. Brown CN, Finch JG. Which mesh for hernia repair? Ann R Coll Surg Engl. 2010;92:272–8.
23. Weyhe D, Schmitz I, Belyaev O, Grabs R, Müller K-M, Uhl W, Zumtobel V. Experimental comparison of monofile light and heavy polypropylene meshes: less weight does not mean less biological response. World J Surg. 2006;30(8):1586–91.
24. Gemma Pascual G, Rodrıguez M, Gomez-Giln V, Garcıa-Honduvilla N, Bujan J, Bello JM. Early tissue incorporation and collagen deposition in lightweight polypropylene meshes: bioassay in an experimental model of ventral hernia. Surgery. 2008;144(3): 427–35.
25. Burger JWA, Halm JA, Wijsmuller AR, Raa J, Jeekal ST. Evaluation of new prosthetic meshes for ventral hernia repair. Surg Endosc. 2006;20(8):1320–5.
26. Scheidback H, Tamme C, Tannapfel A, Lippert H, Kockerling F. In vivo studies comparing the biocompatibility of various polypropylene meshes and their handling properties during endoscopic total extraperitoneal (TEP) patchplasty: an experimental study in pigs. Surg Endosc. 2004;18(2):211–20.
27. Sehreinemacher MHF, Emans PJ, Gijbels MJJ, Greve J-WM, Beets GL, Bouvy ND. Degradation of mesh coatings and intraperitoneal adhesion formation in an experimental model. Br J Surg. 2009;96(3):305–13.
28. Eriksen JR, Gogenur I, Rosenberg J. Choice of mesh for laparoscopic ventral hernia repair. Hernia. 2007;11:481–92.
29. Forstemann T, Trzewik J, Holste J, Batke B, Konerding MA, Wolloscheck T, Hartung C. Forces and deformations of the abdominal wall: a mechanical and geometrical approach to the linea alba. J Biomech. 2011;44:600–6.
30. Deeken CR, Abdo MS, Frisella MM, Matthews BD. Physicomechanical evaluation of polypropylene, polyester, and polytetrafluoroethylene meshes for inguinal hernia repair. J Am Coll Surg. 2011;212(1):68–79.

26. Biologic Prosthetics: What Are They and How Do They Interact with the Body?

Gina L. Adrales and Elizabeth Honigsberg

Biologic mesh was developed to address the shortcomings of permanent synthetic mesh, such as chronic inflammation and foreign body reaction, stiffness, and mesh infection. Since the introduction of biologic prosthetics, the market has been rife with new biologic materials attached to largely unsupported claims of superiority and safety. Although the status of literature on biologic mesh is improving, the current data are comprised mainly from animal studies and level III evidence. Over the last decade, surgeons have utilized biologic mesh in a variety of cases including primary and recurrent hernia repair, hernia prophylaxis, and the most widely used application, hernia repair in the contaminated field. The following chapter reviews the origin, structure, and mechanics of biologic mesh and concludes with the current indications and shortcomings of biologic prosthetics.

Biologic Prosthetics

Material Source

First introduced in 1999, biologic prosthetics have been implemented broadly by the surgical community, particularly for complex abdominal wall hernia repair. Bioprosthetics are designed to be acellular, absorbable, three-dimensional extracellular matrices of largely type I collagen, elastin, proteoglycans, and growth factors [1]. Biologic meshes are

B.P. Jacob and B. Ramshaw (eds.), *The SAGES Manual of Hernia Repair*,
DOI 10.1007/978-1-4614-4824-2_26,

derived from a variety of collagen-rich sources that differ by donor (human, porcine, bovine) and by site (dermis, intestinal submucosa, and pericardium). Biologic meshes are characterized broadly as allografts (human cadaver source) or heterografts/xenografts (bovine and porcine sources). Xenografts are regulated by the Food and Drug Administration (FDA), whereas allografts are largely regulated by tissue banks [2]. Thirteen FDA-approved products currently are available for use and are classified according to source material and processing (Table 26.1).

Material Processing

Although the basic construct of biologic mesh as a collagen scaffold is shared by various brands of biologic mesh, the processing of the mesh varies widely. Generally, allografts are minimally processed whereas xenografts require additional processing to inhibit immunogenicity [3]. Mesh manufacturing is a largely proprietary process, and as such, specific details regarding methods for decellularization, cross-linking, and sterilization are often unclear (except what is contained in published patents). Additionally, the sources of human dermis, in terms of donor age and body part, are uncertain. However, each company may have different criteria for acceptable tissue.

The tissues are procured and treated to remove cellular elements, leaving the biologic mesh collagen scaffold. The cells are removed from the grafts by various methods: physical means such as desiccation, chemical processes, or enzymatic reactions. Some of the products are terminally sterilized while others are not, resulting in variations in storage and pre-use hydration requirements. Sterilization options include gamma radiation, ethylene oxide, or hydrogen peroxide.

Natural cross-links of hydrogen bonds stabilize the triple helix collagen structure present in bioprosthetics against enzymatic degradation by collagenase. These natural cross-links weaken with time, permitting binding of the collagenase at the receptor level and breakdown of the collagen. This allows for remodeling and repair of the tissue. Ideally, the collagen scaffold of the biomaterial should not degrade fully before the host can adequately remodel the site with ingrowth of host cells. To address the major shortcoming of biologic mesh, namely, premature degradation and subsequent weakness and laxity, some manufacturers elect to intentionally crosslink the mesh through chemical processing to prevent collagenase binding at the enzyme receptor. This results in supraphysiologic levels of covalent collagen cross-linked bonds with the

Table 26.1. Commercially available biologic grafts.

Trade name	Manufacturer	Source	Processing	Terminal sterilization	Cross-linked	Handling
Allografts						
AlloDerm	LifeCell (Branchburg, NJ)	Human dermis	Freeze-dried, NaCl, sodium deoxycholate	None	No	2-year shelf life requires refrigeration, 20–30-min rehydration
AlloMax	Davol, C.R. Bard (Cranston, RI)	Human dermis	Acetone, hyper-/hypotonic baths, H_2O_2, NaOH	Gamma radiation	No	
FlexHD	Musculoskeletal Tissue Foundation (Edison, NJ, Ethicon (Somerville, NJ))	Human dermis	Hypertonic bath	Detergents, disinfectant, ETOH	No	No need for rehydration
Heterografts						
Surgisis	Cook medical (Bloomington, IN)	Porcine intestine submucosa	Peracetic acid	Ethylene oxide	No	No need for rehydration
Strattice	LifeCell (Branchburg, NJ)	Porcine dermis		E beam radiation	No	2-min rehydration
FortaGen	Organogenesis, Inc, (Canton, MA)	Porcine intestine submucosa			Yes	No need for rehydration

(continued)

Table 26.1. (continued)

Trade name	Manufacturer	Source	Processing	Terminal sterilization	Cross-linked	Handling
XenMatrix	Davol, C.R. Bard (Cranston, RI)	Porcine dermis		E beam radiation	No	No need for rehydration
TutoPatch	Tutogen medical. RTI biologics (Alachua, FL)	Bovine pericardium	Osmotic contrast bathing, hydrogen peroxide, sodium oxide	Gamma radiation	No	No need for rehydration
Veritas	Synovis surgical (St. Paul, MN)	Bovine pericardium	Hydrogen peroxide, ethanol, propylene oxide		No	No need for rehydration
Permacol	Covidien (Norwalk, CT)	Porcine dermis	Hexamethylene diisocyanate	Gamma radiation	Yes	No need for rehydration
CollaMend	Davol, C.R. Bard (Cranston, RI)	Porcine dermis	Sodium sulfide, sodium hypochlorite, hydrocholoric acid, hydrogen peroxide		Yes	3-min rehydration
PeriGuard	Synovis surgical	Bovine pericardium	Glutaraldehyde		Yes	2-min rehydration
SurgiMend	TEI bioscience (Boston, MA)	Bovine fetal dermis		Ethylene oxide	Yes	1-min rehydration

goal of creating a more durable biomaterial [3]. Whereas un-cross-linked biologic mesh may degrade within months, highly cross-linked mesh may persist for years [4–6]. In a rodent model of ventral hernias, Gaertner demonstrated the durability of cross-linked biologics compared to non-cross-linked bioprosthetics [7]. At 6 months, the cross-linked meshes were grossly intact, whereas the non-cross-linked mesh was absent. This correlated with significantly decreased tensile strength of the non-cross-linked meshes.

Intentional cross-linking may decrease mesh degradation and fibroblast encapsulation but could also adversely alter the extracellular matrix structure to limit cell infiltration and negatively impact the remodeling process and reduce ingrowth [3, 8]. Liang et al. demonstrated that a higher degree of cross-linking in bovine pericardium was associated with persistence at 1 year after implantation but also limited cell infiltration with tissue regeneration restricted to the periphery of the mesh [9]. Decreased cell infiltration may have negative consequences such as reducing angiogenesis, mesh incorporation, and resistance to infection [9]. It is important to note that these effects will vary between various patient clusters and cannot yet be predicted for each individual patient.

The Biology of Biologic Mesh

The structure of biologic mesh is meant to favor prosthetic incorporation. Biologic meshes demonstrate superior biocompatibility as compared to synthetic meshes [10]. Native tissue growth into the bioprosthesis theoretically contributes to the strength of the biomaterial. Unlike synthetic mesh, the acellular scaffold of collagen, elastin, and extracellular matrix contains residual growth factors that ideally will attract host endothelial cells and fibroblasts. The porosity of the biologic graft permits migration of host cells and adherence, promotes angiogenesis, and allows collagen deposition and remodeling to replace the graft with host tissue. As described by Melman et al., remodeling is characterized by six factors: cellular infiltrate, individual cell types, neovascularization, extracellular matrix deposition, scaffold degradation, and fibrous encapsulation [10]. Graft degeneration must be balanced with native tissue ingrowth as the host response to the biologic graft can either result in integration of the mesh or a disproportionate inflammatory response leading to excessive fibrosis and scarring, mesh encapsulation, and excessive mesh degradation, all of which ultimately leads to mesh failure [11].

Inflammation and wound healing are critical to the integration of biologic prostheses with host tissue [12]. Monocytes and macrophages are the key cells in this process. Various cytokines are involved including IL-1β that stimulates fibroblast proliferation, IL-8 that stimulate both neutrophils and endothelial proliferation, and VEGF that promotes angiogenesis. Cytokine expression varies depending on the implanted bioprosthesis. Biologic mesh is designed to elicit a minimal chronic inflammatory response. Animal studies have shown, however, that the inflammatory infiltrate and subsequent adhesion formation to the biomaterial vary from mesh to mesh [13]. Orenstein et al. demonstrated that AlloMax (CR Bard) induced the greatest expression of VEGF, IL-8, and IL-6 compared to AlloDerm (LifeCell), FlexHD (MTF), and Gore BioA (W.L. Gore) in an in vitro study. Interestingly, AlloDerm was the lowest inducer of cytokines [12]. The difference in immunologic response is most likely related to differences in the processing and/or sterilization of the different biologic grafts. The inconsistent host inflammatory response to individual bioprostheses has clinical implications, as other authors have demonstrated variable levels of mesh degradation in animal models, with durability of some materials at 9 months postimplantation, while others undergo significant degradation [14]. Mesh degradation ultimately correlates with mesh strength, critical in the setting of abdominal wall defect repair.

As previously noted, cross-linking also affects the remodeling process. Animal models of abdominal wall hernias have demonstrated that in the short-term, non-cross-linked biologic grafts stimulate more favorable remodeling factors with significantly increased earlier cellular infiltration, extracellular matrix deposition, and neovascularization [3, 15]. However, over time, cross-linked biologic meshes showed similar histological results as compared to the non-cross-linked materials. Additionally, these early histologic differences did not correlate with significant differences in the tensile strength of the mesh repair, regardless of cross-linking.

Biologic prostheses are thought to be resistant to infection due to neovascularization during the remodeling process. However, the ability to clear bacteria is variable among biologic prostheses. In a rodent model of infected hernia repair, non-cross-linked biomeshes demonstrated significantly higher rates of bacterial clearance than cross-linked meshes [16]. Cross-linking may prevent fibroblast infiltration and tissue ingrowth, thus retarding the host's ability to clear bacteria. This finding was supported in a retrospective review of patients undergoing complex ventral hernia repair: cross-linked porcine biomeshes showed relatively higher rates of infection and subsequent explantation compared to non-cross-linked meshes [17]. This contradicts the widely held belief that all biologic grafts do not need to be removed if infected.

Current Indications

The theoretical advantage of biologic mesh over synthetic mesh in certain clinical situations has appealed to surgeons, mostly in the United States. These meshes are not yet widely favored in Europe and elsewhere in part due to the high cost of the biologic mesh over its cheaper and more widely applicable synthetic mesh counterpart. Biologic prostheses have been utilized as biologic dressings, maxillofacial reconstruction, breast reconstruction, and in various challenging surgical scenarios, including complex abdominal wall reconstruction and management of enterocutaneous fistulas [1].

The use of biologic mesh in primary or recurrent ventral or inguinal hernia repair in the uncontaminated and previously uninfected field is difficult to justify due to the high material cost without obvious added benefit. There is very little data regarding the performance of biologic mesh in these settings. The poor performance of the mesh in terms of laxity in a bridging repair makes this an unacceptable repair in the uncontaminated setting. Blatnik et al. documented a recurrence rate of 80% for bridging repair with acellular dermal matrix at an average cost of $5,100 per patient, comparing the repair to an "expensive hernia sac." [18] The laxity associated with biologic mesh has been documented in other series [19].

The use of allograft or xenograft as reinforcement of a primary ventral hernia repair is felt to be a more sound approach. This fits with what we know of the science of biologic meshes in that placement in well-vascularized tissue is favorable for the ingrowth and remodeling process. Rosen's group at Case Western investigated this and found a reduction in ventral hernia recurrence rate with a components separation midline repair reinforced with acellular dermal matrix (20%) compared to the 80% recurrence after bridging allograft repair [20].

The presence of contamination may limit the applicability of permanent synthetic mesh in some hernia repairs. Biologic mesh may be acceptable for this purpose or for placement in open wounds as a staged closure in complex abdominal wall reconstruction. There is limited data in both of these areas, with some noting a high risk of hernia recurrence and associated infection. The data is mostly limited to animal models and case series [21, 22]. However, the lack of suitable alternatives has made biologic mesh attractive for contaminated field hernia repair.

The role of biologic mesh has been explored in prevention of parastomal hernias with promising results [23]. Biologic mesh has also been used in the treatment of parastomal hernias where infection is a concern [24]. With increasing reports of prophylactic synthetic mesh placement at the time of ostomy construction, the use of biologic mesh in this preventative setting may decline [25, 26].

Biologic mesh has been utilized in the reinforcement of paraesophageal hernia repair. The randomized controlled trial of mesh repair for paraesophageal hernia lead by Oelschlager is one of the only level I human studies of biologic mesh [27]. This study showed a decreased risk of hernia recurrence with mesh repair, from 24 to 9%. The recommendation for mesh reinforced hiatal repair is made with some caution; significant mesh complications, ranging from mesh erosion to esophageal stenosis and fibrosis as well as a recurrence rate closer to that of the non-mesh group, were documented in a follow-up study [28].

Limitations

Biologic mesh materials have not escaped the complications often associated with synthetic mesh, such as infection and hernia recurrence [2, 28–30]. There are also additional limitations unique to this group of prosthetics. Concern exists over the potential for disease transmission with the use of biologic mesh [1]. Although these materials are processed and often sterilized, there are reported cases of transmission of prion-related disease from allografts. There are no reported cases of HIV transmission, although the risk of HIV transmission is estimated at one in 1.67 million [1, 31]. Despite processing to decellularize biologic mesh, DNA fragments have been shown to remain in tested samples [32]. This could have other implications regarding heterografts and the host immune response.

Another disadvantage is the significant cost of biologic mesh materials. In general, these grafts cost ten times more than the synthetic equivalent, although heterografts on average cost 20% less than allografts [1, 2].

Finally, an often overlooked consideration is the impact of cultural or religious beliefs on patients' acceptance of biologic grafts. The source and processing of the biologic mesh should be considered and discussed with the patient in the process of informed consent [33].

Conclusion

In summary, biologic grafts represent a major advancement in complex hernia repair. Further investigation regarding the appropriate indications and performance of the grafts based on individual properties such as cross-linking is needed. Given the high cost of most of these materials and the limited available data, biologic mesh should be used judiciously and only when permanent synthetic mesh is deemed inappropriate, such as in the contaminated field. The FDA reported complications of these materials, such as visceral erosion, warrant caution, and sound surgical judgment [2, 29, 30].

References

1. Peppas G, Gkegkes ID, Makris MC, Falagas ME. Biological mesh in hernia repair, abdominal wall defects, and reconstruction and treatment of pelvic organ prolapse: a review of the clinical evidence. Am Surg. 2010;76(11):1290–9.
2. Rosen MJ. Biologic mesh for abdominal wall reconstruction: a critical appraisal. Am Surg. 2010;76(1):1–6.
3. Butler CE, Burns NK, Campbell KT, Mathur AB, Jaffari MV, Rios CN. Comparison of cross-linked and non-cross-linked porcine acellular dermal matrices for ventral hernia repair. J Am Coll Surg. 2010;211(3):368–76.
4. Bachman S, Ramshaw B. Prosthetic material in ventral hernia repair: how do I choose? Surg Clin North Am. 2008;88(1):101–12. ix.
5. Courtman DW, Errett BF, Wilson GJ. The role of crosslinking in modification of the immune response elicited against xenogenic vascular acellular matrices. J Biomed Mater Res. 2001;55(4):576–86.
6. Abolhoda A, Yu S, Oyarzun JR, McCormick JR, Bogden JD, Gabbay S. Calcification of bovine pericardium: glutaraldehyde versus no-react biomodification. Ann Thorac Surg. 1996;62(1):169–74.
7. Gaertner WB, Bonsack ME, Delaney JP. Experimental evaluation of four biologic prostheses for ventral hernia repair. J Gastrointest Surg. 2007;11(10):1275–85.
8. Jarman-Smith ML, Bodamyali T, Stevens C, Howell JA, Horrocks M, Chaudhuri JB. Porcine collagen crosslinking, degradation and its capability for fibroblast adhesion and proliferation. J Mater Sci Mater Med. 2004;15(8):925–32.
9. Liang HC, Chang Y, Hsu CK, Lee MH, Sung HW. Effects of crosslinking degree of an acellular biological tissue on its tissue regeneration pattern. Biomaterials. 2004;25(17):3541–52.
10. Melman L, Jenkins ED, Hamilton NA, et al. Early biocompatibility of crosslinked and non-crosslinked biologic meshes in a porcine model of ventral hernia repair. Hernia. 2011;15(2):157–64.

11. Mulier KE, Nguyen AH, Delaney JP, Marquez S. Comparison of Permacol and Strattice for the repair of abdominal wall defects. Hernia. 2011;15(3):315–9.
12. Orenstein SB, Qiao Y, Kaur M, Klueh U, Kreutzer DL, Novitsky YW. Human monocyte activation by biologic and biodegradable meshes in vitro. Surg Endosc. 2010;24(4):805–11.
13. Stanwix MG, Nam AJ, Hui-Chou HG, et al. Abdominal ventral hernia repair with current biological prostheses: an experimental large animal model. Ann Plast Surg. 2011;66(4):403–9.
14. Pierce LM, Grunlan MA, Hou Y, Baumann SS, Kuehl TJ, Muir TW. Biomechanical properties of synthetic and biologic graft materials following long-term implantation in the rabbit abdomen and vagina. Am J Obstet Gynecol. 2009;200(5):549 e541–48.
15. Deeken CR, Melman L, Jenkins ED, Greco SC, Frisella MM, Matthews BD. Histologic and biomechanical evaluation of crosslinked and non-crosslinked biologic meshes in a porcine model of ventral incisional hernia repair. J Am Coll Surg. 2011;212(5):880–8.
16. Harth KC, Broome AM, Jacobs MR, et al. Bacterial clearance of biologic grafts used in hernia repair: an experimental study. Surg Endosc. 2011;25(7):2224–9.
17. Shah BC, Tiwari MM, Goede MR, et al. Not all biologics are equal! Hernia. 2011;15(2):165–71.
18. Blatnik J, Jin J, Rosen M. Abdominal hernia repair with bridging acellular dermal matrix–an expensive hernia sac. Am J Surg. 2008;196(1):47–50.
19. Bluebond-Langner R, Keifa ES, Mithani S, Bochicchio GV, Scalea T, Rodriguez ED. Recurrent abdominal laxity following interpositional human acellular dermal matrix. Ann Plast Surg. 2008;60(1):76–80.
20. Jin J, Rosen MJ, Blatnik J, et al. Use of acellular dermal matrix for complicated ventral hernia repair: does technique affect outcomes? J Am Coll Surg. 2007;205(5):654–60.
21. Saettele TM, Bachman SL, Costello CR, et al. Use of porcine dermal collagen as a prosthetic mesh in a contaminated field for ventral hernia repair: a case report. Hernia. 2007;11(3):279–85.
22. Candage R, Jones K, Luchette FA, Sinacore JM, Vandevender D, Reed 2nd RL. Use of human acellular dermal matrix for hernia repair: friend or foe? Surgery. 2008;144(4):703–9. discussion 709–711.
23. Wijeyekoon SP, Gurusamy K, El-Gendy K, Chan CL. Prevention of parastomal herniation with biologic/composite prosthetic mesh: a systematic review and meta-analysis of randomized controlled trials. J Am Coll Surg. 2010;211(5):637–45.
24. Lo Menzo E, Martinez JM, Spector SA, Iglesias A, Degennaro V, Cappellani A. Use of biologic mesh for a complicated paracolostomy hernia. Am J Surg. 2008;196(5):715–9.
25. Janson AR, Janes A, Israelsson LA. Laparoscopic stoma formation with a prophylactic prosthetic mesh. Hernia. 2010;14(5):495–8.
26. Janes A, Cengiz Y, Israelsson LA. Experiences with a prophylactic mesh in 93 consecutive ostomies. World J Surg. 2010;34(7):1637–40.
27. Oelschlager BK, Pellegrini CA, Hunter J, et al. Biologic prosthesis reduces recurrence after laparoscopic paraesophageal hernia repair: a multicenter, prospective, randomized trial. Ann Surg. 2006;244(4):481–90.

28. Stadlhuber RJ, Sherif AE, Mittal SK, et al. Mesh complications after prosthetic reinforcement of hiatal closure: a 28-case series. Surg Endosc. 2009;23(6):1219–26.
29. Robinson TN, Clarke JH, Schoen J, Walsh MD. Major mesh-related complications following hernia repair: events reported to the Food and Drug Administration. Surg Endosc. 2005;19(12):1556–60.
30. Harth KC, Rosen MJ. Major complications associated with xenograft biologic mesh implantation in abdominal wall reconstruction. Surg Innov. 2009;16(4):324–9.
31. Simonds RJ, Holmberg SD, Hurwitz RL, et al. Transmission of human immunodeficiency virus type 1 from a seronegative organ and tissue donor. N Engl J Med. 1992;326(11):726–32.
32. Gilbert TW, Freund JM, Badylak SF. Quantification of DNA in biologic scaffold materials. J Surg Res. 2009;152(1):135–9.
33. Jenkins ED, Yip M, Melman L, Frisella MM, Matthews BD. Informed consent: cultural and religious issues associated with the use of allogeneic and xenogeneic mesh products. J Am Coll Surg. 2010;210(4):402–10.

27. Open Component Separation for Abdominal Wall Reconstruction

David Earle

The occurrence of ventral hernia as a sequence of abdominal section is so common that it should command our thoughtful consideration. B. Brindley Eads, M.D. 1901

Reconstructive surgery has been defined as trying to make something abnormal normal. This is in contrast to cosmetic surgery, the goal of which is to make something normal, better—at least in the eyes of the beholder. It is important to note that there is no consensus on a single definition of abdominal wall reconstruction, although many use this term to refer to complex abdominal wall hernia repairs that involve some sort of component separation technique as part of the procedure. Complex ventral hernia repair has been an underestimated disease by surgeons and patients alike for years, unless you happen to be the patient or surgeon facing such a daunting task. This sentiment was specifically noted in the closing remarks of the discussion of an article about incisional hernia repair in 1978 by Dr. Harold Harrower from Providence, Rhode Island, who stated, "Junior house officers tend to underestimate the complexity of incisional hernia repairs. Supervision by senior surgeons improves their understanding of the problem and the results" [1]. Local abdominal wall musculoaponeurotic flaps have been utilized as far back as 1894 when Gerseny of Vienna described splitting the rectus fascia [2]. Charles Gibson suggested that these local flaps are only intended for difficult cases that "would have been denied operative relief or subjected to some procedure of doubtful value, such as the implantation of a filigree" [3]. Ramirez described "separation of components" in 1990 as a potential solution to repairing large ventral hernias [4]. His primary goal was to be able to mobilize flaps of the musculoaponeurotic abdominal wall such that they could possibly be reapproximated, or reconstructed. What he did not take in to account in his manuscript were the short and long term

B.P. Jacob and B. Ramshaw (eds.), *The SAGES Manual of Hernia Repair*, DOI 10.1007/978-1-4614-4824-2_27,

physiologic issues associated with this. The anterior fibers of the external oblique muscles, acting bilaterally, are responsible for trunk flexion. This action pulls the midline from both sides, in essence pulling the linea alba "apart." After an external oblique "release," at least in the short term, the absence of the force of the external oblique muscles creating tension on the midline closure may serve as one mechanism for successful healing of the midline repair.

In addition, there is no mutually agreed upon definition of "component separation" save for the fact that some of the aponeuroses, muscles, or overlying sheathes of the abdominal wall are in some way divided and/or mobilized to enable closure of the defect. All muscles and aponeurosis have been mobilized in some way, and many series do not even have a single method of reconstruction, variably utilizing a variety of prosthetics in a variety of locations within the abdominal wall, making comparisons of outcomes nearly impossible [5, 6].

Additionally, it appears that the external oblique is the least important of the flank muscles in terms of respiratory assistance based on electromyography studies [7, 8] and lumbar spine support [9], making this a logical choice for division and separation as part of an abdominal wall reconstruction.

This chapter will focus on separation of the external oblique muscle with detachment of its medial insertion just lateral to the rectus muscle, combined with posterior rectus sheath mobilization. This is currently the most widely practiced method for component separation utilized for the purpose of a midline abdominal wall reconstruction. For the remaining part of this chapter, the term component separation (CS) will refer to release of the external oblique and posterior rectus sheath as described above. Additionally, prosthetic-related issues such as type and placement are beyond the scope of this chapter and are discussed elsewhere in this book.

Indications and Relative Contraindications

It is important to note that a component separation technique is only one technical part of an abdominal wall reconstruction. Other technical components of an abdominal wall reconstruction include suturing technique, prosthetic use and placement, management of the excess skin and subcutaneous tissue, and management of concomitant procedures such as gastrointestinal and gynecological procedures to name a few. In general, the indications for utilizing a component separation technique should be based on the aligned goals of the patient and surgeon, anatomic details of the

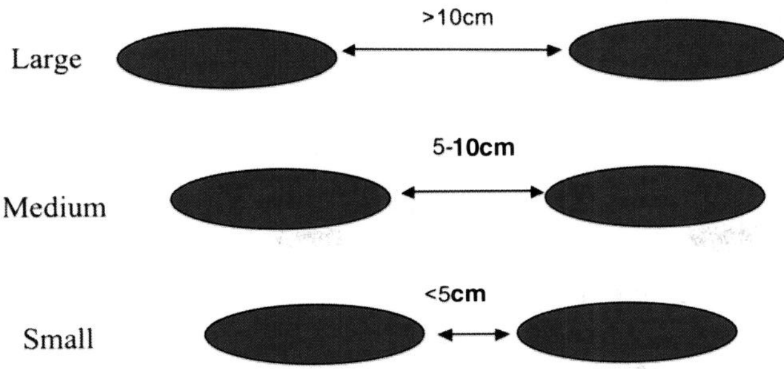

Fig. 27.1. Sizing the hernia defect. Midline hernia defects are measured as the gap between the medial borders of the rectus muscles as one defect, regardless of the size and number of hernia sacs seen on the physical examination. This may be accomplished with physical examination alone or with CT scanning depending on the clinical scenario. Small (<5 cm), medium (5–10 cm), and large (>10 cm) defects are based on the width between the rectus muscles, not the length of the defect. Component separation should usually be done for medium-sized defects where deformity is a significant problem, or avoidance of a permanent synthetic prosthesis is desired for infectious related concerns. Most large defects should be repaired with the assistance of a component separation technique, unless limited by obesity or active smoking.

hernia (size, shape, and location), and the clinical scenario (medical history, urgency of operation). While there are exceptions to every rule, this technique should be utilized when there is a significant deformity of the abdominal, and correction of that deformity is important to the patient. In general, it is appropriate to consider CS as part of an abdominal wall reconstruction when there is a medium to large size defect (Fig. 27.1), reduction of the viscera is feasible (not limited by obesity or loss of domain), and the patient is not actively smoking. A list of factors associated with the decision making about abdominal wall reconstruction utilizing CS is listed in Table 27.1.

Clinical examples of when you may not want to perform CS as part of the operation include morbid obesity with a large defect and no major deformity. This is particularly true if the fat distribution has a significant visceral component, making reduction of the viscera with complete closure of the midline tenuous or not possible. Currently, there is no way to determine this other than looking at the patient and/or a CT scan of the abdomen and estimating whether or not the viscera will fit inside a closed abdominal wall. Component separation generally requires the tissues to heal together, and active smoking is known to increase wound complications and reduce healing and would be considered a relative contraindication in a completely elective setting [6].

Table 27.1. Indications and relative contraindications for utilizing component separation techniques.

	Indications	Relative contraindications (precautions)
Defect size medium to large	X	
Deformity significant	X	
Patient desires correction of deformity	X	
Obesity—limiting reduction of viscera		X
Active smoking		X
Active infection		X

In general, most of the indications should be present, and as many as possible relative contraindications should be absent. Combined excision of excess skin and subcutaneous tissue may also be employed, and nicotine testing can confirm smoking cessation. Control of infection preoperatively is best when possible

Technique

The concept is straightforward, but there are clearly some technical pitfalls and pearls that are important to a successful outcome. The steps of this procedure are (in no particular order):

1. Division of the medial attachment of the external oblique muscle only (lateral to the rectus abdominis muscle).
2. Separation of the internal and external oblique muscles.
3. Mobilization of the posterior rectus sheath.
4. Midline closure (commonly performed with closure of the posterior rectus sheath, followed by closure of the linea alba/anterior rectus sheath to approximate the rectus muscles).

The order of the procedures will depend on the operative plan, which in turn depends somewhat on the goals of the operation. For example, if there is significant excess skin and subcutaneous tissue from a large hernia sac and/or significant weight loss, this is often excised as part of the operation to avoid problems with postoperative seroma, excessive tension on the closure due to the weight of the excess tissue, and persistent abdominal wall deformity. If this portion of the operation is being done first, then the incision for this will dictate exposure for the external oblique release. In the case where the incision for this will allow fairly easy access to the full length of the medial attachment of the external oblique, this portion of the CS can be performed through the existing incision. In the case where the incision is not enough to allow proper exposure, large skin flaps from the midline incision or laterally based vertical flaps or "tunnels" can be utilized for proper exposure. If excess skin excision is not being performed, then large skin flaps from a midline incision or transverse laterally based incisions will be required for exposure of the external oblique medially. It is important to note that the blood supply to the skin of the abdominal wall comes from the laterally based intercostal, subcostal, and lumbar arteries, and medially based deep inferior and superior epigastric arteries, along with direct branches of cutaneous vessels from the circumflex iliac and superficial epigastric networks [10]. These perforator sparing have been utilized to reduce wound complication rates, primarily related to tissue ischemia and infection.

Open Exposure of the External Oblique

When gaining exposure to the anterior abdominal wall for the external oblique release, preservation of as much of the blood supply as possible is important to avoid wound complications. Raising large flaps of skin from a midline incision was originally described and has been associated with significant wound morbidity. Sparing the periumbilical perforators (based on the deep epigastric network) is advantageous to reducing ischemia of the wound edges, which in turn reduces wound complications. This can be accomplished with transverse incisions in the lateral abdomen, through which laterally based vertical flaps (lateral to the periumbilical perforators) are raised to expose the medial border of the external oblique along its length. Lighted retractors or a laparoscope can be used to assist in lighting and retraction. Alternatively, if there is the need for a long, inferior transverse incision to excise excess skin, subcutaneous tissue, and hernia sac, laterally based vertical flaps can be made from below, also using lighted retractors or a laparoscope as needed for lighting and retraction. These techniques are collectively referred to as "perforator-sparing" CS techniques.

External Oblique Division and Separation

There are two steps in the external oblique release—(1) division of the medial attachment and (2) separation of the external and internal oblique muscles. With all open techniques, the first step is to divide the medial attachment of the external oblique.

Full division will extend from above the costal margin to near the inguinal ligament. For defects that are confined to the lower or upper abdomen, the division may be confined to the relevant portion only, particularly if the defect is not too large. Partial division of the medial attachment of the external oblique however may not yield the best benefit in terms of postoperative tension caused by lateral muscle contracture during a variety of Valsalva maneuvers. One of the major pitfalls of this is dividing the common attachment to the entire lateral muscle complex. To avoid this, it is usually easiest to start over the external oblique muscle fibers, rather than over the aponeurosis. This is best accomplished by scoring the overlying fascia with a monopolar instrument where you can visualize the muscle belly. Once the muscle fibers are exposed, separate the external oblique muscle fibers with a blunt-tipped clamp, spreading the fibers in a plane parallel to the direction they are positioned anatomically. Once the whitish color of the internal oblique fascia is identified, you do not want to continue any deeper. The clamp can then be placed in between the oblique muscles, parallel to the insertion of the external oblique, and the monopolar electrosurgical device utilized to divide the muscle longitudinally along its length. The laterally cut edge still can then be grasped with Allis clamps to lift the external oblique to allow the separation of the oblique muscles to occur.

Separating the oblique muscles is very straightforward, as they are only held together by a network of flimsy fibro-areolar connective tissue. Each strand of connective tissue is not strong, but collectively they act as resisters in series and are very strong. This separation is more important for medial mobilization and closure and does not contribute to the concept of postoperative tension during Valsalva maneuvers. With Allis clamps lifting the cut edge of the laterally attached external oblique, simple blunt dissection is then utilized to accomplish the separation of the two oblique muscles. At the lateral aspect of the separation will be neurovascular bundles, and identification of these should serve as the terminus of the separation. Knowledge of these, along with the expected position of the origins of the oblique muscles, should minimize the risk of injuring these neurovascular structures.

Posterior Rectus Sheath

It is important to identify the medial border of the rectus muscle prior to beginning. This can best be accomplished by lifting the edge of the laparotomy incision near the abdominal wall with Kocher clamps. Grasp the hernia sac to avoid damaging the portion of the rectus sheath you will eventually be sewing together. Then, by visual inspection and manual palpation, you should be able to identify the medial border of the rectus muscle. Use the monopolar cautery to longitudinally make an incision at the medial border of the rectus, or slightly anteriorly. Once you identify the muscle fibers, enlarge the opening until you can insert an index finger which can be used to sweep the posterior rectus sheath away from the muscle and as a marker for where to continue the division of the posterior rectus sheath. This should be accomplished along the length of the incision, making sure to go both above and below the borders of the hernia defect. For a long midline incision, this typically extends from the xiphoid process to the pubic symphysis. Below the arcuate line, the mobilization consists of the bladder and extraperitoneal fat in the space of Retzius. Pitfalls of this include dividing the posterior rectus sheath too far posteriorly, as this will increase the difficulty in closing this layer if that technique is being utilized. Existing or previous ostomies placed through the rectus muscle can make this mobilization difficult at the location of the current or former ostomy. If the posterior sheath is to be closed, then this site can be closed transversely once the midline is closed. When closing the posterior rectus sheath, take care not to put sudden tension on the sutures while pulling them taut after placement. Also, pulling at a low angle (laterally) rather than a 90° angle (straight up) can avoid tearing the posterior sheath. It is also important to utilize the short suture technique described by Isrealsson and colleagues to distribute the tension over a wider surface area [11].

Despite an initial tension on the closure, once the posterior sheath is completely closed, the tension often seems negligible. The closure should generally be accomplished vertically until the arcuate line is reached, at which point the peritoneum overlying the bladder mobilization can be brought up and closed to the arcuate line transversely. Long-acting absorbable suture is probably the best, and the use of barbed suture material may distribute the tension over an even greater surface area and reduce the chance of dehiscence and make this often difficult closure more easily accomplished by the surgeon.

The Anterior Rectus Sheath and Linea Alba

Once the posterior rectus sheath has been mobilized (and closed in many cases), the rectus muscles are then reapproximated by suturing together the anterior sheath, scar tissue, and remains of the linea alba. It is important to note that the sutures should again be placed with the short suture technique, taking care to avoid incorporating muscle tissue and/or attenuated scar/anterior sheath. This will minimize tissue ischemia and allow the rectus muscles to be reapproximated [12]. While the short suture technique was proven to reduce hernia formation and infection rates for closure of primary and midline laparotomies, its use in abdominal wall reconstruction is logical, as the technique is based on the physics of broadening the surface area over which the tension will be distributed and reducing the amount of tissue within the suture line, thus reducing tissue ischemia within the suture line. These facts are no different for hernia repair than for primary laparotomy closure.

Outcomes

Recurrence rates of primary closure of incisional hernia vary widely but are generally considered to be high and are reported to be 63% in a long-term follow-up study of primary vs. prosthetic repair [13].

Primary closure with the addition of a component separation (without the use of mesh and without the short suture technique) reduces recurrence rates to between 0 and 20% [5]. When utilizing large skin flaps from a midline incision to expose the external oblique muscles, wound complication rates related to ischemia (20%), infection (40%), and dehiscence (43%) are often serious and require reoperation in as much as 20% of the cases [10]. Utilizing a perforator-sparing or endoscopic technique, the rate of serious wound complications decreases dramatically [14–17].

It is important to note, however, that the suturing technique is also likely to influence the recurrence rates. As mentioned above, the principles of the short suture technique should be no different for hernia repair than for primary laparotomy closure. Furthermore, if a suture fails after utilizing the short suture technique, the resulting gap in the tissue is small and more likely to be filled in with scar tissue rather than develop into another hernia defect [12]. It is therefore logical that application of the short suture technique for midline closure of hernia defect after a component separation would serve to further reduce the recurrence rates. Use of a prosthesis is also a factor that will undoubtedly affect recurrence rates but is beyond the scope of this chapter. It is also worth mentioning that a recurrence is not the sole metric of success or failure. For example, consider a patient with a 15-cm-wide midline defect and overlying skin graft that is completely disabled from the abdominal wall defect. Repair of this hernia utilizing a component separation technique without a permanent prosthesis might result in a small recurrence at the superior aspect of the midline closure. Despite the fact that there is a recurrent hernia, the patient is typically still fully functional without symptoms and has many options for repair, or observation. From the typical patient's perspective, despite the existence of a recurrent hernia, the operation was a complete success.

Conclusion

In summary, open component separation can be described by a variety of techniques. The most commonly utilized technique involves detaching the insertion of the external oblique along its length lateral to the rectus abdominis muscles and separating the external oblique muscle from the internal oblique. This may be accomplished with or without the mobilization of the posterior rectus sheath and with or without the use of a prosthetic. Primary closure of the midline (posterior and anterior rectus sheaths) should be performed using a short suture technique in which 5–8-mm bites of tissue are taken with each bite in terms of both depth and travel, taking care to avoid incorporating muscle and attenuated fascia within the suture line. This technique should be used selectively for patients with medium to large defects as described in Table 27.1. The benefits of component separation performed in this manner are twofold: (1) medial mobilization of the rectus muscles and (2) reduced postoperative tension on the midline closure. Recurrence rates in the 5–20% range should be expected, and recurrences are typically smaller and easier to deal with compared to the hernia at the time of reconstruction with CS. A perforator-sparing technique is best when possible and should yield wound complication rates that should be less than 10% and generally minor in severity.

References

1. Larson GM, Harrower HW. Plastic mesh repair of incisional hernias. Am J Surg. 1978;135(4):559–63.
2. Mahorner H. Umbilical and ventral herniae. Ann Surg. 1940;111(6):979–91.

3. Gibson C. Operation for the cure of large ventral hernia. Ann Surg. 1920; 72(2):214–7.
4. Ramirez OM, Ruas E, Dellon AL. "Components separation" method for closure of abdominal-wall defects: an anatomic and clinical study. Plast Reconstr Surg. 1990;86(3):519–26.
5. Shell DH, de la Torre J, Andrades P, Vasconez LO. Open repair of ventral incisional hernias. Surg Clin North Am. 2008;88:61–83.
6. Blatnik JA, Krpata DM, Novitsky YW, Rosen MJ. Does a history of wound infection predict postoperative surgical site infection after ventral hernia repair? Am J Surg. 2012;203(3):370–4. discussion 374.
7. Abe T, Kusuhara N, Yoshimura N, et al. Differential respiratory activity of four abdominal muscles in humans. J Appl Physiol. 1996;80(4):1379–89.
8. de Troyer A, Estenne M, Ninane V, Van Gansbeke D, Gorini M. Transversus abdominis muscle function in humans. J Appl Physiol. 1990;68(3):1010–6.
9. Gracovetsky S, Farfan H, Helleur C. The abdominal mechanism. Spine. 1985;10(4): 317–24.
10. Lowe JB, et al. Risks associated with "component separation" for closure of complex abdominal wall defects. Plast Reconstr Surg. 2003;111(3):1276–83.
11. Cengiz Y, Blomquist P, Israelsson LA. Small tissue bites and wound strength: an experimental study. Arch Surg. 2001;136(3):272–5.
12. Millbourn D, Cengiz Y, Israelsson LA. Effect of stitch length on wound complications after closure of midline incisions: a randomized controlled trial. Arch Surg. 2009;144(11):1056–9.
13. Burger JW, Luijendijk RW, Hop WC, Halm JA, Verdaasdonk EG, Jeekel J. Long-term follow-up of a randomized controlled trial of suture versus mesh repair of incisional hernia. Ann Surg. 2004;240:578–85.
14. Lowe JB, Garza JR, Bowman JL, Rohrich RJ, Strodel WE. Endoscopically assisted "components separation" for closure of abdominal wall defects. Plast Reconstr Surg. 2000;105:720.
15. Saulis AS, Dumanian GA. Periumbilical rectus abdominis perforator preservation significantly reduces superficial wound complications in separation of parts hernia repair. Plast Reconstr Surg. 2002;109(7):2275–80. discussion: 2281–2.
16. Giurgius M, Bendure L, Davenport DL, Roth JS. The endoscopic component separation technique for hernia repair results in reduced morbidity compared to the open component separation technique. Hernia. 2012;16(1):47–51. Epub 2011 Aug 11.
17. Harth KC, Rose J, Delaney CP, Blatnik JA, Halaweish I, Rosen MJ. Open versus endoscopic component separation: a cost comparison. Surg Endosc. 2011;25(9): 2865–70. Epub 2011 Jun 3.

28. Endoscopic Component Separation

Michael J. Rosen

Indications and Contraindications

Abdominal wall reconstruction is a major surgical procedure requiring careful preoperative clearance. Smoking cessation and weight loss are strongly encouraged (I believe smoking cessation is mandatory), nutritional status is optimized, and cardiac status is stratified. Indications for an endoscopic component separation include those defects that the surgeon feels will not be reapproximated without myofascial advancement flaps. There is no absolute minimal or maximal defect that precludes this procedure although some general recommendations can be made. Defects less than 8–10 cm wide often do not require additional release. Defects over 20 cm wide are often too large to bring together with a standard endoscopic component separation. Defects close to the xiphoid process or suprapubic area will not obtain similar advancement as those around the umbilicus. Another major consideration that is difficult to measure preoperatively is the innate compliance of the abdominal wall. Multiply recurrent hernias often have stiff noncompliant abdominal walls, and this procedure will not result in substantial myofascial advancement.

This procedure can be performed at the time of open abdominal wall reconstruction or as an entirely minimally invasive reconstruction using laparoscopic techniques to repair the hernia defect. Both will be described below. In general, if the surgeon is performing an open reconstruction and the placement of the mesh requires large skin undermining, an open component separation should be performed. Likewise, if excess skin is being resected or a panniculectomy is planned, an open approach is warranted. If the procedure is being performed entirely laparoscopically, defects smaller than 6 cm in width usually do not require an endoscopic component separation and can often be closed with standard techniques.

B.P. Jacob and B. Ramshaw (eds.), *The SAGES Manual of Hernia Repair*,
DOI 10.1007/978-1-4614-4824-2_28,

The endoscopic component separation provides approximately up to 85 % of the release as a standard open procedure. Therefore, if the surgeon deems a component separation is necessary, the endoscopic approach is usually warranted. However, in patients with prior transverse incisions extending into the lateral abdominal wall, or have undergone a prior open component separation, the endoscopic approach is relatively contraindicated. In these cases, the balloon dissectors will often tear the abdominal wall if excessive scar tissue is present and the planes are fixed.

Patient Preparation and Room Setup

Equipment needs include a 10-mm, 30° laparoscope; preperitoneal inguinal hernia balloon dissector (Covidien, Norwalk, CT); 30-mL balloon-tipped trocar (Covidien, Norwalk, CT); laparoscopic trocar, an ultrasonic dissector or LigaSure™ device (Covidien, Norwalk, CT); and/or laparoscopic scissors with cautery. Patients receive appropriate preoperative antibiotics and invasive monitoring as needed. Epidural catheters may be placed for postoperative pain control (routine in my practice).

Patient Positioning

Patients are placed in the supine position with both arms abducted. Access to the posterior axillary line is important to place the lateral abdominal trocar during the endoscopic component separation and can be limited if the arm is tucked at the sides.

Trocar Position of Endoscopic Component Separation

Three trocars per side are placed. The initial port is placed off the tip of the 11th rib and provides access for the balloon dissector. Another port is placed in the posterior axillary line just inferior to the initial port. A third port is placed through the released external oblique, in line with the cephalad transection point.

The Technique of Endoscopic Component Separation

A cutdown incision is performed off the tip of the eleventh rib. It is critical that this incision is made lateral to the linea semilunaris to avoid placing the balloon in the rectus sheath. This port should be placed lateral enough to allow space between the linea semilunaris and the trocar, enabling complete cephalad dissection. In my opinion, this is the most important step in the operation, and the anatomy must be clearly identified. Therefore, in obese patients, I extend this incision to the appropriate size to permit clear identification of the fibers of the external oblique. The subcutaneous tissue and Scarpa fascia are bluntly separated, and the external oblique is grasped with Kocher clamps.

If a midline open incision has been performed, the lateral edge of the rectus muscle may be palpated through the incision and may help to better determine the location for the initial 10-mm endoscopic incision.

Depending on how far lateral you have performed your cutdown, the external oblique can be only fascia or fascia and muscle. It is important to confirm this anatomy, to avoid cutting too deep into the internal oblique. The external oblique fibers are split and bluntly separated. An S retractor gently creates the plane underneath the external oblique and above the internal oblique heading in a caudal direction.

A standard preperitoneal inguinal hernia balloon dissector is placed underneath the external oblique and passed inferiorly toward the pubic tubercle. This balloon should be guided laterally to avoid injuring the linea semilunaris. If prior transverse incisions are encountered, the balloon might not be able to traverse the scar tissue and should be aborted and the intermuscular space created under direct vision.

The balloon is insufflated under direct vision, and the orientation of the external oblique fibers ("hands in pockets"), internal oblique fibers ("hands on the hips"), and the linea semilunaris are identified.

The shape of the standard preperitoneal inguinal hernia balloon dissector usually does not permit cephalad dissection of the external oblique off the costal margin. Therefore, the balloon is removed, and a finger is placed in the intermuscular space, and the dissection is bluntly carried out over the costal margin using a sweeping motion. If this space is not created at this point, the dissection planes can be confusing laparoscopically and may result in a technical error. Remember the external oblique inserts 5–7 cm above the costal margin and should be cleared off the costal margin to permit the muscles to slide medially.

A balloon-tipped trocar is secured in the space to prevent air leakage. One should avoid the use of a triangular-shaped structural balloon at this point because it can result in obliteration of the dissection space. Insufflation pressures of 10–12 mmHg are used.

The inferior space can be bluntly created with a 30°, 10-mm laparoscope to complete the dissection of the intermuscular space to the posterior axillary line and inguinal ligament.

The second port is placed in the posterior axillary line. This port is placed as far laterally as possible to provide the appropriate angle to release the external oblique, 2 cm lateral to the linea semilunaris.

Using scissors with cautery, in the posterior axillary port, and the camera in the cutdown port, the external oblique is incised from the cephalad as much as possible to the inguinal ligament/pubic tubercle. Great care should be taken to complete the release lateral to the linea semilunaris.

Extra release can be achieved by continuing the dissection superficially through Scarpa fascia. The majority of the blood supply runs superficial to this layer and will not be disturbed.

The third port is placed through the released external oblique in the lower abdomen. This port is placed medial to the original cutdown port in the line that the external oblique will be transected when going over the costal margin. This orientation is important because the cephalad portion of the dissection can be challenging as it is performed in a reverse camera orientation.

The camera is then placed in the lower abdominal trocar, and the scissors are placed in the lateral port, and the cephalad dissection is completed separating the external oblique off the costal margin. The external oblique is carefully separated off the costal margin to provide a clear plane and trajectory when transecting the external oblique. This avoids releasing the linea semilunaris or dissecting underneath the costal margin.

Once the dissection of the external oblique is completed, the camera is positioned in the lateral port, and the LigaSure™ ultrasonic dissector is placed in the inferior port. Since the external oblique is fairly muscular at the cephalad portion, I prefer to use LigaSure™, as simple cautery can result in troublesome bleeding.

The external oblique is transected several centimeters above the costal margin. The exact cephalad extent of the transection of the external oblique is variable, but it should be at least 5 cm above the superior extent of the hernia defect and, likely, at least 3–4 cm above the costal margin.

A bilateral component separation is preferred in most patients to provide symmetric distribution of tension on the closure.

The next steps depend on whether the endoscopic component separation is being performed in conjunction with an open mesh placement or as an entirely minimally invasive repair.

Open Mesh Placement

Midline laparotomy is performed (if not performed before the endoscopic component separation), and bowel work is completed as necessary.

Retrorectus Placement

My preferred space for mesh placement is in the posterior rectus space. By using this technique, skin flaps are not necessary for wide mesh overlap. Drains are routinely placed above the mesh and below the rectus muscle. Although some authors describe continuing the dissection through the linea semilunaris into the lateral abdominal plane during a retrorectus repair, this should be avoided if a component separation has been performed. If the external oblique is released and then the transversus abdominis is intentionally or unintentionally released, the lateral abdominal wall is only supported by the internal oblique, which likely will result in at least a bulge if not a hernia.

Minimally Invasive Abdominal Wall Reconstruction

In patients with defects less than 10–12 cm, without a complex scar requiring revision, and in who a standard laparoscopic ventral hernia repair with mesh is not deemed sufficient an entirely minimally invasive reconstruction can be performed. In this repair, the endoscopic component separation is preformed first to avoid leaking from the ports. After completing the bilateral components separation, the ports for the intraperitoneal hernia repair are then placed into the abdominal cavity. The posterior surface of the entire anterior abdominal wall is freed of adhesions. The hernia defect is measured internally using spinal needles in conjunction with a 15-cm ruler in a rostrocaudal and medial-lateral orientation.

Next, the fascial defect is reapproximated. We do not typically excise the hernia sac or remove the peritoneum from the fascia, but this is an option. A small stab wound in the skin is made just above the hernia, and a suture passer is placed with a #1 polypropylene suture through the skin and through the fascial edge of the hernia defect. This is retrieved with a laparoscopic grasper, the suture passer is then removed and passed through the same skin incision to the contralateral side of the hernia defect, and the suture is retrieved. A series of these interrupted sutures are placed throughout the length of the hernia defect to allow a secure musculofascial approximation. The insufflation pressure is decreased, and the sutures are tied with the knots below the skin on the fascia. Given the fact that these sutures are typically placed under a fair amount of tension, the repair may become disrupted. Therefore, we feel it is important to size the mesh based on the original measurements of the defect with at least 4 cm of overlap. An appropriately sized piece of prosthesis is placed intraperitoneally and secured with transfascial sutures. A laparoscopic tacker is then used to secure the mesh to the abdominal wall. Placing additional transfascial sutures can off-weight the forces on the midline closure to the lateral abdominal wall with the mesh.

Complications

The absence of skin flaps significantly reduces wound morbidity. We have experienced one case of a postoperative hematoma at the external oblique muscular release above the costal margin. At that location, the external oblique is quite muscular and should be controlled with the LigaSure to prevent this complication.

Similar to open component separation, it is important to avoid transecting the linea semilunaris. If one divides this structure, there is a full thickness defect in the lateral abdominal wall that will result in a hernia that may be difficult to repair. Maintaining the transection line at least 2 cm lateral to the linea semilunaris can avoid this problem. Patients with massive hernias (>20 cm) or loss of domain should typically be approached with other reconstructive measures, as an endoscopic component separation often is not adequate.

Suggested Readings

Harth KC, Rosen MJ. Endoscopic versus open component separation in complex abdominal wall reconstruction. Am J Surg. 2010;199(3):342–6. discussion 346–7.

Rosen MJ, Fatima J, Sarr MG. Repair of abdominal wall hernias with restoration of abdominal wall function. J Gastrointest Surg. 2010a;14(1):175–85.

Rosen MJ, Jin J, McGee M, Marks J, Ponsky J. Laparoscopic component separation in the single stage treatment of infected abdominal wall prosthetic removal. Hernia. 2007a;11(5):435–40.

Rosen MJ, Reynolds HL, Champagne B, Delaney CP. A novel approach for the simultaneous repair of large midline incisional and parastomal hernias with biological mesh and retrorectus reconstruction. Am J Surg. 2010b;199(3):416–20. discussion 420–1.

Rosen MJ, Williams C, Jin J, McGee M, Marks J, Ponsky J. Laparoscopic versus open component separation: a comparative analysis in a porcine model. Am J Surg. 2007b;194(3):385–9.

29. Technique: Laparoscopic Ventral/Incisional Hernia Repair

Archana Ramaswamy

Ventral hernias may be primary or incisional. Primary central hernias may be classified as umbilical, paraumbilical, lumbar, epigastric, and spigelian. Incisional hernias have incidence rates greater than 15% and are likely related to incision size, as well as closure technique [1], postoperative complications such as infection and patient factors including diabetes, smoking, and immunosuppressant use. Patients seek repair most commonly for discomfort, decreased abdominal wall function, and less commonly for bowel obstruction or bowel ischemia. It is estimated that 300,000 ventral hernias are repaired in Europe and 400,000 in the USA each year [2].

History of Laparoscopic Ventral Hernia Repair

Open suture ventral hernia repair was the standard of care for many years. The long-term outcomes of this technique were questioned when recurrence rates of 18–63% were published [3]. Open repair with mesh was then demonstrated to have lower recurrence rates in a randomized study of moderate size hernias (<6 cm) where recurrence rates were statistically lower in the mesh group (43% vs. 23%) at 3 years [4]. As mesh utilization for open ventral hernia repair was being adopted, various locations were being utilized for mesh placement including inlay, onlay, and underlay (retrorectus, extra- and intraperitoneal). The lowest recurrence rates were noted with underlay placement [5]. In parallel with these studies was the publication of the first technical description of laparoscopic ventral hernia repair [6]. The technique described in 1993 utilized PTFE mesh with fixation with staples to the anterior abdominal

B.P. Jacob and B. Ramshaw (eds.), *The SAGES Manual of Hernia Repair*,
DOI 10.1007/978-1-4614-4824-2_29,

wall. There have been various mesh and fixation options introduced since then, but the basic technique has remained unchanged.

Patient Selection

As there is still limited penetration of laparoscopic ventral hernia repair among general surgeons, complex cases should be reserved to those past their learning curve. Though there is no defined learning curve for this procedure, the most severe complications are related to laparoscopic adhesiolysis and bowel injury [7]. Operative time (including abdominal access, adhesiolysis, and mesh placement) is increased when associated with patient variables comprising the following: greater BMI, higher ASA classification, prior ventral hernia repairs, suprapubic location, bowel adhesion to the abdominal wall or hernia sac, larger hernia defect, incarcerated hernia contents, and decreased postgraduate year of the surgical assistant [8]. Though some of these are variables only identifiable intraoperatively, others can be assessed preoperatively to select operative candidates. Appropriate case selection for the novice includes primary hernias or first-time incisional hernias of small to moderate size in normal-weight healthy patients. Once a comfort level is reached with straightforward cases, then, atypical locations, recurrent hernias, large defects, and components separation may be added to the surgeon's armamentarium. Operative planning can be aided by CT scans to define hernia size and potential issues with loss of domain. Patient comorbidities, such as diabetes, immunosuppression, obesity, and smoking, may be related to increased complications, complexity of surgery, and recurrence [9–12]. These factors should be addressed preoperatively when possible.

Operative Setup

The patient is placed supine, with alterations in positioning for atypical locations. The arms are generally both tucked if the patient's girth allows it, to allow the surgeon enough mobility to perform adhesiolysis and fixation in the lower quadrants. A Foley catheter may be placed if a lengthy procedure is envisioned, or if the hernia extends well below the umbilicus. A monitor on each side of the table is necessary as the surgeon/assistant will frequently need to work from both sides of the patient for adhesiolysis and for mesh fixation (Fig. 29.1).

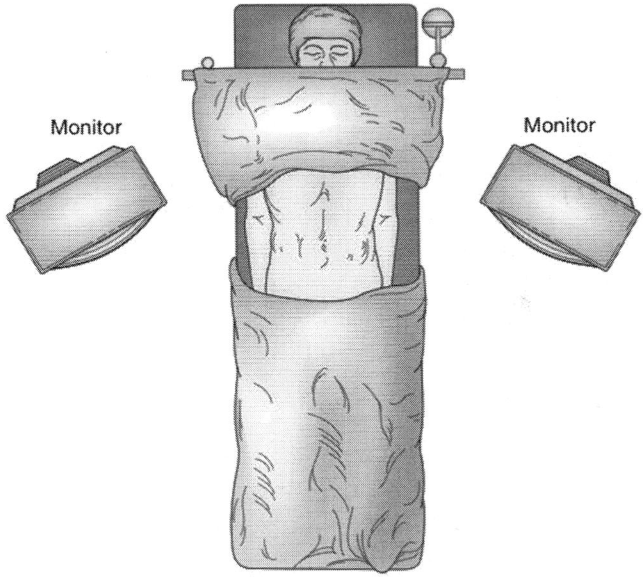

Fig. 29.1. Patient and monitor positioning.

Abdominal Access

Access methods have been described via closed techniques (Veress needle and optical trocar) as well as open techniques. The basic concept is to gain access away from the hernia defect, in an area which should presumably have a paucity of adhesions (Fig. 29.2).

Adhesiolysis and Hernia Reduction

Adhesiolysis and hernia reduction may be straightforward or may take up the majority of the operative time. Hernia size and number of previous repairs may help predict an increased time for adhesiolysis and aid operative planning [8]. Adhesiolysis is generally safer using blunt and sharp dissection with avoidance of energy sources. Energy sources may cause an injury which is not visible at the time of surgery but may have a lateral thermal spread, which can result in a delayed leak. A missed bowel injury is also possible when dissecting without the use

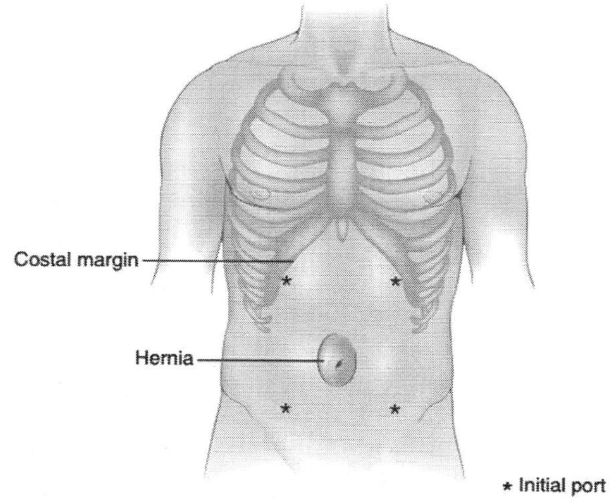

Fig. 29.2. Recommended locations for port insertion.

of energy sources. The bowel should be examined after completion of adhesiolysis. Though most serosal injuries are unlikely to be significant, their closure is recommended to avoid the uncommon instances where it may progress to a full-thickness injury. Management of bowel injury is discussed elsewhere. Bleeding may occur during adhesiolysis and can usually be managed by application of clips, or focal use of energy.

Complete adhesiolysis of the abdominal wall is generally performed since hernias other than the palpable one are not infrequently identified. At the least, 5 cm of abdominal wall needs to be cleared on either side of the fascial defect to allow adequate overlap of mesh with healthy fascia. Inferiorly, this may require mobilization of the bladder and identification of Cooper's ligament and superiorly, transection of the falciform ligament. With umbilical hernias, it is important to remember that it is often preperitoneal fat which is herniated, and an adequate laparoscopic hernia repair cannot be completed without preperitoneal dissection and reduction of these contents.

Reduction of chronically incarcerated contents may be challenging. A hand-over-hand technique and use of external pressure may be helpful. If no progress is being made, consideration should be given to making a small incision over the hernia defect and performing adhesiolysis within the sac to allow reduction, or to converting to a completely open approach (Figs. 29.3 and 29.4).

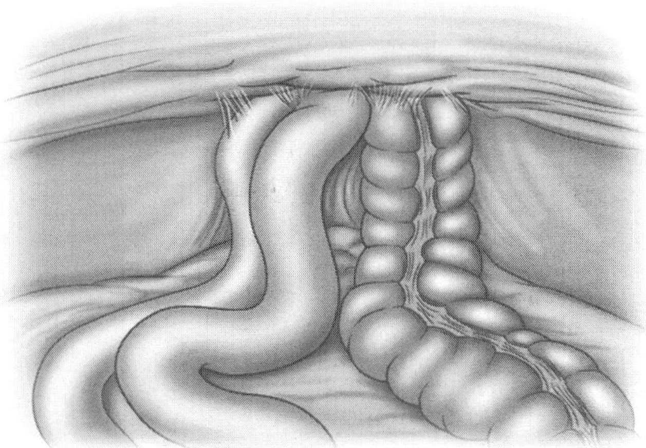

Fig. 29.3. Initial view of unreduced hernia.

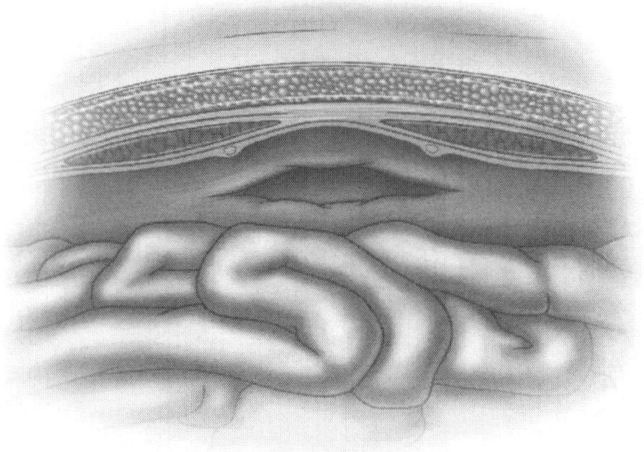

Fig. 29.4. Hernia defect following hernia reduction.

Hernia Sizing and Mesh Selection

The hernia defect may be measured intracorporeally using a suture held between two graspers. Alternatively, the defect can be measured externally using small-gauge or spinal needles. The defect edges are marked on the abdominal wall, and a ruler used to measure the defect size. The measurements may be more accurate with the abdomen desufflated. This external method can be used in most patients with small- to medium-sized hernias who are not obese. In obese individuals and/or those with complex hernias, the discrepancy between intra-abdominal and extra-abdominal measurements may be significant and leads to oversizing of the mesh. Mesh should be selected to provide ~5-cm overlap onto healthy tissue. A Swiss cheese defect may require less, and a large single defect may require a larger piece of mesh. The mesh should be marked, generally in one location (e.g., top). This will help orient the mesh internally both in the craniocaudal plane and with regard to the side which will lie toward the abdominal wall. There are different methods of mesh fixation which guide any further preparation of the mesh prior to insertion. Most experts do feel that transfascial sutures are necessary and will place four cardinal sutures through the mesh with the tails being left long to grasp and bring out. Permanent suture is generally recommended in this situation, and Gore-Tex® suture is used by many. The mesh should then be centered on the hernia defect, and the abdominal wall marked for location of suture retrieval. Recently, there have been advocates of midline closure in laparoscopic ventral hernia repair. This will be discussed elsewhere in detail, but closure can be accomplished with transfascial sutures. The width of the mesh when the midline has been closed may not have to based on the original preclosure hernia defect, though this is not clear, since some of these sutures placed under tension can be occasionally be heard breaking when the patient is extubated and coughs forcefully.

Mesh Insertion and Fixation

The mesh can be rolled tightly and inserted through the 10-mm port or the incision with the port removed. A laparoscopic grasper inserted through a trocar on the contralateral side and brought out through the 10-mm port incision can facilitate this task. The mesh can then be unrolled using two graspers. The cardinal transfascial sutures can then be retrieved (Fig. 29.5). The mesh should be stretched out, after retrieval of the first two sutures, to confirm the position of planned retrieval of the remaining sutures (Fig. 29.6). These can then be tied down, and point fixation undertaken around the circumference of the mesh at 1–2-cm

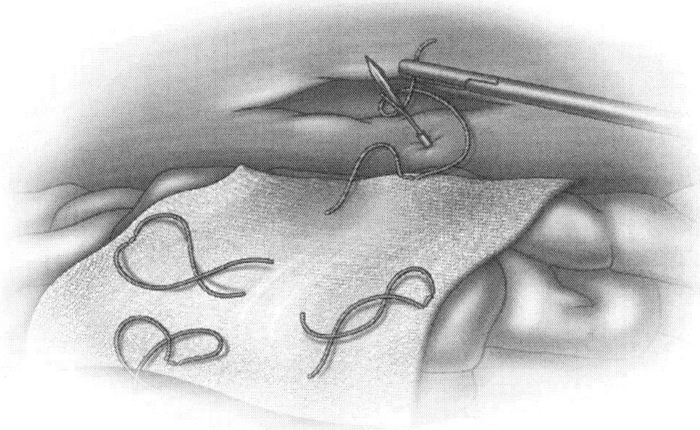

Fig. 29.5. Retrieval of first transfascial suture.

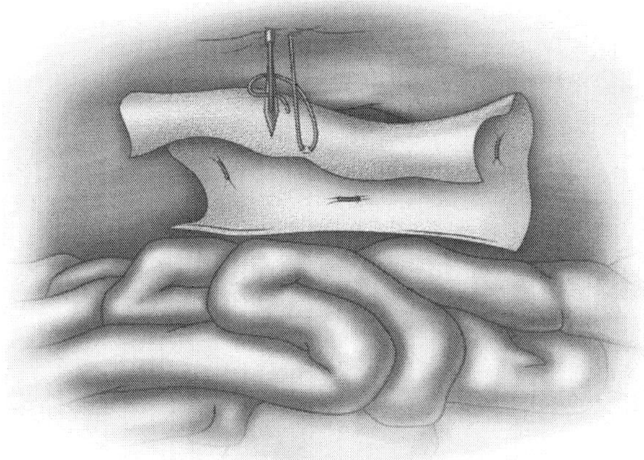

Fig. 29.6. Retrieval of final cardinal transfascial suture.

intervals (Fig. 29.7). Additional transfascial sutures may be placed at 3–5-cm intervals. This basic technique has been described with outcomes published on a case series of 850 patients with a recurrence rate of 4.7% and a mesh infection rate of 0.7% [13]. Others have questioned the need for transfascial sutures and have described the double-crown technique, which utilizes two rows of point fixation without transfascial suture fixation. Results have been published demonstrating low recurrence rates

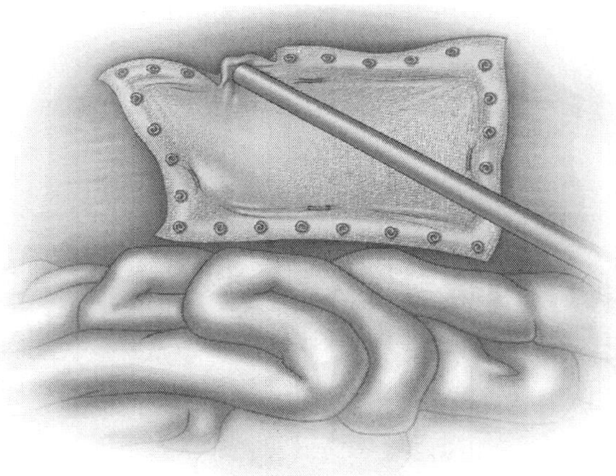

Fig. 29.7 Circumferential tacking.

[14, 15], though the purported benefit of decreased pain due to lack of transfascial fixation has not borne out in a randomized trial [16].

Outcomes

Specific complications and their management are discussed elsewhere. Generally speaking, laparoscopic ventral hernia repair has been increasing in practice without the benefit of impressive randomized trial data. Most of the randomized studies have been small, so summary measures have been examined. A meta-analysis of eight randomized trials demonstrated hospital stay and infection rates (not requiring mesh removal) which favored laparoscopy but no differences in bowel injury, seroma, and hernia recurrence [17]. A systematic review of 11 randomized trials and comparative studies concluded that there was no evidence that the laparoscopic approach is better or worse than open, though the data suggested that the laparoscopic approach is associated with a lower recurrence rate, shorter hospital stay, and fewer complications [18]. A recent Cochrane review identified 11 randomized trials and concluded that there appeared to be a lower wound infection rate in the laparoscopic group, with a shorter hospital stay in the majority of studies, but no differences were identified in recurrence rates [2]. A summary of the randomized trials is presented in Table 29.1.

Table 29.1. Comparison of outcomes of randomized trials of laparoscopic versus open ventral hernia repair.

Author	**Year**	**No. of patients**	**Recurrence**		**Any complication**		**Enterotomy**		**Seroma/ hematoma**		**Surgical site infection**	
			Lap	**Open**	**Lap**	**Open**	**Lap**	**Open**	**Lap**	**Open**	**Lap**	**Open**
Itani [19]	2010	146	12.3%	8.2%	31.5%	47.9%	4.1%	0	11.0%	27.4%	5.5%	24.7%
Asencio [20]	2009	84	9.7%	7.9%	33.3%	5.1%	2.2%	0	31.1%	5.1%	0	0
Pring [21]	2008	54	3.3%	4.2%	36.7%	54.2%	0	0	16.7%	33.3%	3.3%	16.7%
Olmi [22]	2007	170	2.3%	1.1%	16.4%	29.4%	0	0	7.1%	4.7%	1.2%	8.2%
Navarra [23]	2007	24	0	0	16.7%	8.3%	0	0	16.7	0	0	8.3%
Misra [24]	2006	62	6.3%	3.3%	21.2%	42.4%	0	0	12.1%	3.0%	6.1%	33.3%
Moreno-Egea [25]	2002	22	0	0	0	36.3%	0	0	0	36.3%	0	0
Carbajo [26]	1999	60	0	6.7%	6.7%	66.7%	0	6.7%	3.3%	36.7%	0	10%

Conclusion

Laparoscopic ventral hernia repair is a procedure which is gaining popularity. It has an unknown but probably short learning curve for simple cases; however, atypical locations and complex cases should be reserved for when expertise has been gained. Level 1 studies have provided limited evidence of clear superiority over open repair, but many have been plagued with short follow-up (<2 years).

References

1. Cengiz Y, Mansson P, Israelsson LA. Conventional running suture and continuous double loop closure: an experimental study of wound strength. Eur J Surg. 2000;166(8):647–9.
2. Sauerland S, Walgenbach M, Habermalz B, Seiler CM, Miserez M. Laparoscopic versus open surgical techniques for ventral or incisional hernia repair. Cochrane Database Syst Rev. 2011, (3).
3. Shell D, de la Torre J, Andrades P, Vasconez L. Open repair of ventral incisional hernias. Surg Clin North Am. 2008;88(1):61–83.
4. Luijendijk RW, Hopp WC, van den Tol MP, et al. A comparison of suture repair with mesh repair for incisional hernia. N Engl J Med. 2000;343(6):392–8.
5. Rudmik LR, Schieman C, Dixon E, Debru E. Laparoscopic incisional hernia repair: a review of the literature. Hernia. 2006;10(2):110–9.
6. LeBlanc KA, Booth WV. Laparoscopic repair of incisional abdominal hernias using expanded polytetrafluoroethylene: preliminary findings. Surg Laparosc Endosc. 1993;3(1):39–41.
7. LeBlanc KA, Elieson MJ, Corder 3rd JM. Enterotomy and mortality rates of laparoscopic incisional and ventral hernia repair: a review of the literature. JSLS. 2007;11(4):408–14.
8. Jenkins E, Yom V, Melman L, et al. Clinical predictors of operative complexity in laparoscopic ventral hernia repair: a prospective study. Surg Endosc. 2010;24:1872–7.
9. Chang EI, Galvez MG, Padilla BE, Freise CE, Foster RD, Hoffman WY. Ten-year retrospective analysis of incisional herniorrhaphy following renal transplantation. Arch Surg. 2011;146(1):21–5.
10. Bege T, Berdah SV, Moutardier V, Brunet C. Risks related to tobacco use in general and intestinal surgery. J Chir. 2009;146(6):532–6.
11. Finan KR, Vick CC, Kiefe CI, Neumayer L, Hawn MT. Predictors of wound infection in ventral hernia repair. Am J Surg. 2005;190(5):676–81.
12. Tsereteli Z, Pryor A, Heniford BT, Park A, Voeller G, Ramshaw BJ. Laparoscopic ventral hernia repair (LVHR) in morbidly obese patients. Hernia. 2008;12:233–8.
13. Heniford BT, Park A, Ramshaw BJ, Voeller G. Laparoscopic repair of ventral hernias nine years' experience with 850 consecutive hernias. Ann Surg. 2003;238(3):391–9.

14. Morales-Conde S, Cadet H, Cano A, Bustos M, Morales-Mendez S. Laparoscopic ventral hernia repair without sutures–double crown technique: our experience after 140 cases with a mean follow-up of 40 months. Int Surg. 2005;90(3 Suppl):S56–62.
15. Baccari P, Nifosi J, Ghirardelli L, Staudacher C. Laparoscopic incisional and ventral hernia repair without sutures: a single-center experience with 200 cases. J Laparoendosc Adv Surg Tech A. 2009;19(2):175–9.
16. Wassenaar E, Schoenmaeckers E, Raymakers J, van der Palen J, Rakic S. Mesh-fixation method and pain and quality of life after laparoscopic ventral or incisional hernia repair: a randomized trial of three fixation techniques. Surg Endosc. 2010;24(6):1296–302.
17. Forbes SS, Eskicioglu C, McLeod RS, Okrainec A. Meta-analysis of randomized controlled trials comparing open and laparoscopic ventral and incisional hernia repair with mesh. Br J Surg. 2009;96:851–8.
18. Clarabelle T, Pham C, Perera D, Watkin S, Maddern GJ. Laparoscopic ventral hernia repair: a systematic review. Surg Endosc. 2009;23:4–15.
19. Itani KM, Hur K, Kim LT, Anthony T, Berger DH, Reda D, Neumayer L, Veterans Affairs Ventral Incisional Hernia Investigators. Comparison of laparoscopic and open repair with mesh for the treatment of ventral incisional hernia: a randomized trial. Arch Surg. 2010;145(4):322–8.
20. Asencio F, Aguilo J, Peiro S, Carbo J, Ferri R, Caro F, Ahmad M. Open randomized clinical trial of laparoscopic versus open incisional hernia repair. Surg Endosc. 2009;23:1441–8.
21. Pring CM, Tran V, O'Rourke N, Martin IJ. Laparoscopic versus open ventral hernia repair: a randomized controlled trial. Aust N Z J Surg. 2008;78(10):903–6.
22. Olmi S, Scaini A, Cesana GC, Scaini L, Erba E. Laparoscopic versus open incisional hernia repair: an open randomized controlled study. Surg Endosc. 2007;21:555–9.
23. Navarra G, Musolino C, De Marco ML, Bartolotta M, Barbera A, Centorrino T. Retromuscular sutured incisional hernia repair: a randomized controlled trial to compare open and laparoscopic approach. Surg Laparosc Endosc. 2007;17(2):86–90.
24. Misra MC, Bansal VK, Kulkarni MP, Pawar DK. Comparison of laparoscopic and open repair of incisional and primary ventral hernia: results of a prospective randomized study. Surg Endosc. 2006;20(12):1839–45.
25. Moreno-Egea A, Carrasco L, Girela E, Martín JG, Aguayo JL, Canteras M. Open vs. laparoscopic repair of spigelian hernia: a prospective randomized trial. Arch Surg. 2002;137(11):1266–8.
26. Carbajo MA, del Olmo JC M, Blanco JI, de la Cuesta C, Toledano M, Martín F, Vaquero C, Inglada L. Laparoscopic treatment vs. open surgery in the solution of major incisional and abdominal wall hernias with mesh. Surg Endosc. 1999;13(3):250–2.

30. Loss of Abdominal Domain

Victor B. Tsirline, Igor Belyansky, David A. Klima, and B. Todd Heniford

Over two million laparotomies are performed every year in the United States. 5% to 20% of these cases lead to incisional hernia formation [1], some leading to large abdominal wall defects with loss of domain. Approximately 160,000 ventral hernia repairs are performed annually, with a recurrence rate of 5–20% in uncomplicated hernias and low-risk individuals. The success of the hernia operations diminishes with larger hernia defects, obesity, and multiple reoperations [2]. In patients with complex abdominal hernias and loss of domain, recurrence rates of up to 67% have been reported [3]. Such cases require particular expertise in evaluation, counseling, and multimodality treatment in order to achieve long-term success. This chapter will address some of the theoretical principles and practical considerations in the management of patients with loss of abdominal domain.

Definitions

In 1943, Dr. Ivan Goni Moreno published a paper on the treatment of chronic abdominal hernias where the visceral contents have lost their "derecho de domicilio" (right of domain). The literature most commonly defines loss of abdominal domain as the inability of the abdominal cavity to accommodate the viscera, without prohibitively high intraabdominal pressures (>15 mmHg) [2]. Chevrel in 1987 described abdominal ventral hernias whose contents were held in place by adhesions and not reducible, thus losing their right of domain [4], as applied to large abdominal defects >10–15 cm [5] or areas >100–225 cm^2 [6, 7]. Others have defined loss of domain as extrusion of 15–20% or more of abdominal volume

B.P. Jacob and B. Ramshaw (eds.), *The SAGES Manual of Hernia Repair*,
DOI 10.1007/978-1-4614-4824-2_30,

[8], as reducing such or greater volume of tissue into the abdominal cavity is likely to require significant physiologic adaptation. Most experts agree that evisceration of more than 50% of abdominal contents into the hernia requires specialized strategies for successful repair [9].

Pathophysiology and Biomechanics

Loss of abdominal domain implies the absence of mechanical strength in the anterior abdominal wall, with unopposed protrusion of the abdominal viscera, leading to loss of structural integrity of the torso. The pathophysiology and biomechanics differ from those of ordinary ventral hernias, where tissue herniates through a well-defined fascial defect due to increased intraabdominal pressure and may result in incarceration and strangulation. Patients may experience discomfort due to intermittent herniation/reduction, acute obstruction, or chronic mental strangulation in the ventral defect. In contrast, with loss of abdominal domain, there is lack of confinement of the intraabdominal contents, resulting in low intraabdominal pressure and chronic, gravity-induced stretch of the viscera. Voluntary straining and postural reflex contraction of the residual abdominal muscles lead to progressive retraction laterally because the muscles on each side of the hernia are not mechanically coupled.

Causes and Challenges

Ventral hernias of all sizes tend to enlarge over time. As the abdominal circumference increases, the tension in the abdominal wall and at the edge of the growing defect increases according to LaPlace's law. Eventually, this leads to loss of domain with musculofascial tissues retracting laterally. The challenge in repairing such defects, rather than bridging a gap and preventing recurrence, is the restoration of a physiologic, mechanical, and functional covering around the eviscerated abdominal structures, if possible.

Patient history is important, as loss of domain often results from an abdominal catastrophe requiring either extensive abdominal debridement, such as traumatic injuries or infection, or a prolonged open abdomen, due to peritonitis and intestinal edema [10–12]. In the latter case, the abdominal wall recedes laterally due to the unopposed lateral forces on the oblique muscles. During the acute hospitalization, the abdominal wall coverage may be temporized by using an absorbable mesh or a biologic graft, which usually stretches over time. Epidermal coverage in the acute setting is often accomplished using split-thickness skin grafts, which are aesthetically unappealing and lack thermal, mechanical, and regenerative properties of natural cutaneous and subcutaneous tissues.

Morbidity of Loss of Domain

Loss of abdominal domain is often morbid, and patients usually describe poor overall quality of life. This comes from a combination of postural musculoskeletal dysfunction, chronic gastrointestinal pathology, and psychosocial issues. Lack of abdominal functional musculature causes significant activity limitation and leads to chronic progressive strain on the lumbar spine, often resulting in chronic back pain. Obesity is commonplace among patients with loss of domain, as a result of restricted mobility. Gastrointestinal dysfunction with pain and chronic intestinal incarceration is common. Abdominal wall dysfunction often produces significant thoracic impairment. Spinal kyphosis resulting from loss of anterior torsal integrity can lead to reduced thoracic volume and decreases the inspiratory capacity. Lack of abdominal muscular function can also reduce inspired volumes.

Finally, the cosmetic considerations add to the overall morbidity. The disfigured abdomen, distorted by scars, obesity, and inability to exercise maintain a normal physical appearance, carries a large psychological burden. Many patients with loss of abdominal domain are significantly distressed and unable to change the progressive course of their condition without surgical intervention.

Evaluation

General Preoperative Considerations

Taking into account preoperative considerations, patients with loss of abdominal domain may be classified into discrete categories based on the following [13]:

- Presence of contamination
- Size of the fascial defect
- Volume of the hernia sac relative to peritoneum

Patients with loss of domain not only present with difficult to repair abdominal wall defects but they often have dramatically thin or excess skin, chronic nonhealing abdominal wounds, fistulas, and stomas. These issues significantly complicate the general problems of returning the bowel to the peritoneal cavity and closing the abdomen. The issues above require planning, preparation, and technical factors that exponentially add to the difficulty of the abdominal reconstruction. Management of the chronic wounds, fistulas, stomas, etc., requires significantly greater time commitment, tools, and frequently a team approach. Each complicating factor may change the approach, mesh choice, position of the mesh, and closure techniques.

Volume Measurement

Preoperative physical examination is important; however, it is somewhat unreliable in estimating the hernia sac volume for multiple reasons. External circumference of the hernia sac has been shown to have poor correlation to the hernia sac volume [14]. Therefore, preoperative imaging is often helpful. CT of the abdomen may suggest whether abdominal wall reconstruction will be feasible. There has been considerable interest in CT volumetric analysis of patients with loss of domain undergoing abdominal reconstruction [15–17]. Both the peritoneal cavity and the hernia sac can be approximated as ellipse, with craniocaudal (D_{CC}), anteroposterior (D_{AP}), and horizontal (D_H) diameter measurements from the CT slices [17]. In this model, the volume of each compartment can be estimated as

$$\text{Volume} = \frac{\pi}{6} \times D_{CC} \times D_{AP} \times D_{H}.$$

Advanced geometric models can be employed in computer-aided CT volumetrics to yield more accurate results. Incisional hernia volume of less than 20% of peritoneal volume was found to be highly predictive of being able to reduce the hernia contents and close the abdomen without causing a compartment syndrome. Patients whose hernia sac volume was more than 20% of the peritoneal volume could require bridging devices or visceral resection and risked excessive abdominal pressures postoperatively [15].

While the latter group had slightly higher BMI (39 kg/m^2 vs. 37 kg/m^2), this was not an independent predictor of postoperative compartment syndrome. The surface area of the hernia was not useful in predicting the feasibility of the operation.

Preoperative Preparation

Preoperative preparation is an important part of repairing large hernias. Patients' quality of life should be taken into account in setting realistic postoperative expectations with regard to the rehabilitation process, goal activity level, and aesthetics. Patients must be warned of the very high likelihood of wound complications, which will require additional time and effort on their part throughout the recovery period. Serious systemic complications and even mortality are more than just theoretical risks in major abdominal wall reconstructions.

Preoperative weight loss can dramatically aid the success of the operation and lower the incidence of postoperative complications. Reduction in the intraabdominal fat content will effectively result in lower intraabdominal pressures after return of hernia sac contents into the peritoneal cavity and can reduce the need for component separation. Cardiovascular, pulmonary, and endocrine benefits of weight loss reduce the risk of anesthesia-related complications, and improved baseline mobility hastens postoperative rehabilitation and lowers the incidence of deep vein thrombosis. Weight loss reduces intraabdominal pressure [18], which correlates with a significant incidence of recurrence [1]. There are also studies that have demonstrated a correlation with an increased infection rate in patients with a higher body mass index. Preoperative weight loss should be attempted, whether through lifestyle modification or surgically—unfortunately, the latter option is often not feasible.

Smoking cessation is a must. Given the ultimate increase in intraabdominal pressure when a large hernia is repaired, maximizing a patient's pulmonary function is appropriate. Cigarette smoking effect on tissue perfusion is an extremely important concern. Wound infection rates are significantly higher in smokers. However, if a patient quits smoking for as little as 3 weeks prior to a major operation, he can reduce the possibility of infection as much as 50% [19]. In our specialized hernia center, we conduct preoperative urine cotinine testing (positive for approximately 2 weeks after smoke exposure) prior to proceeding with a restoration of abdominal domain. If it is positive, the operation may be canceled.

In addition to the standard preoperative antibiotic and thromboembolic prophylaxis, many surgeons prescribe a bowel prep the day before surgery in order to minimize contamination in case bowel resection has to be performed, although the incidence of central volume-related problems at the time of surgery carries its own set of risks. Some advocate low-fiber diet the week prior to surgery [16]. Routine use of prophylactic inferior vena cava filters has been described, particularly with the use of preoperative progressive pneumoperitoneum (PPP) [9].

Preoperative Progressive Pneumoperitoneum

Pioneered by an Argentinian surgeon Ivan Goni Moreno in 1940s, this technique is based on the principle of progressive stretching of the abdominal wall in order to lengthen the musculofascial tissues that are used for subsequent abdominal reconstruction. Three weeks prior to surgery, a tunneled, intraperitoneal catheter is inserted with a subcutaneous port or penetrating the skin. Every other day, the abdomen is insufflated with sterile air, with the gas acting as a tissue expander. There is no consensus on the type of gas, the optimal amount of insufflation, or duration of therapy.

McAdory et al. described using medical grade air insufflated to the degree tolerated by patient, every 1–2 days for 7 days, followed by repeat CT scan; based on whether the abdominal viscera returned into the abdomen or not, the therapy was continued, or surgery was undertaken [9]. Dumont et al. in France used every other day insufflation of air for 2 weeks, as long as the patients remained asymptomatic of shoulder pain, shortness of breath, or subcutaneous emphysema [14]. Mayagoitia and colleagues in Mexico used Seldinger technique to place a percutaneous catheter, with daily insufflation of atmospheric air at 1,000–2,000 cc, not to exceed the abdominal pressure of 15 mmHg, continued for 9–15 days for ventral abdominal defects [20]. Toniato et al. from Italy performed progressive pneumoperitoneum on an outpatient basis using a percutaneous catheter inserted in the left iliac region to insufflate nitrous oxide every other day for 8–16 days, each session using 1,000–1,500 cc more than the previous, for a total of up to 38 L [16]. A similar approach was reported by Caldironi et al. 10 years prior [21]. Willis et al. from Aachen, Germany used daily injections of air via percutaneous catheter placed in the left upper quadrant, ranging from 1,000 to 4,000 cc based on patient symptoms of shoulder pain or maximum intraabdominal pressure of 15 mmHg [22].

Effects of Progressive Pneumoperitoneum

Despite over two dozen reports in the literature describing the utility of progressive preoperative pneumoperitoneum in the treatment of patients with loss of abdominal domain, little quantitative data has been collected. A recent CT-based analysis of 61 patients undergoing preoperative pneumoperitoneum for 2 weeks showed an increase of rectus abdominis muscle width from approximately 10–11 cm on each side and the length of anterolateral muscles from an average of 20–24 cm, despite insufflation of a total of 13 L of air on average [14]. Such small geometric yield could hardly facilitate bridging of giant ventral defects measuring on average 10 cm across in this study. Therefore, it has been suggested that progressive preoperative pneumoperitoneum works primarily by forcing preoperative physiologic adaptation to higher intraabdominal pressures, allowing the patients to tolerate greater aponeurotic tension postoperatively. We find it most effective in patients with loss of domain through small defects. A venous thromboembolic event is a possibility during progressive pneumoperitoneum. Inability to tolerate progressive pneumoperitoneum may be a marker of postoperative inability to tolerate increased intraabdominal pressures and may be a contraindication for proceeding with the operation [16].

Surgical Techniques

Surgeons performing complex abdominal wall reconstructions should have in their arsenal a number of techniques specifically developed for such extreme ventral hernias. The goals are similar to any hernia repair: restoration of the abdominal wall continuity with native tissues and/or permanent prosthesis with ample mesh-fascial overlap and without excessive tension or intraabdominal pressure. The challenges in patients with loss of domain stem from (1) excessive extra-abdominal visceral content, (2) lack of lateral musculofascial tissue for adequate mesh fixation, (3) altered abdominal wall mechanics and three-dimensional nature of the defect, and (4) the presence of contamination either from wound infections or exposure to intestinal contents via fistula, stomas, or concomitant bowel resection [8].

Many techniques have been developed to address the above challenges. Native tissue coverage for loss of domain restoration is important but not always attainable. It provides not only a durable, adaptive, and fairly infection resistant barrier but, importantly, an innervated musculofascial anterior mechanical support. To accomplish this task, surgeons have used fascial tissue expanders to stretch receded fascia, progressive pneumoperitoneum, and serial prosthesis placements such as with a repair of a congenital gastroschisis. Many authors recommend separation of component whenever possible to achieve midline fascial reapproximation. Pedicle flaps have been utilized but do not maintain true muscle contraction and will stretch or protrude with time.

Prosthetic Mesh Reinforcement

The use of mesh in repair of incisional and ventral hernias has been shown to reduce recurrence by 50% or more compared to primary repair [23]. In the case of giant ventral hernias and loss of abdominal domain, some form of reinforcement is mandatory in order to provide supporting framework for the newly reconstructed abdominal wall [24]. Still prosthetic reinforcement is not a simple and complete answer in these patients. Inlay fascial reinforcement has been shown to have inferior durability compared to fascial sublay or onlay mesh placement [25] and has a limited role in the reconstruction of the abdominal domain. While the onlay mesh technique has the advantage of ease of placement for small ventral hernias, its use in complex abdominal reconstructions is more difficult to justify due to the higher risk of postoperative wound complications [7].

Alternatively, a two-layer reinforcement of the abdominal wall has been described [26]. This technique involves intraperitoneal placement of a coated synthetic sublay and a second synthetic fascial onlay. The advantages of this approach are wide mesh-tissue overlap and more even distribution of tension forces between tissue planes. The use of a lightweight, large pore polypropylene may lead to a reduced foreign body sensation and a reduced risk of infection [27]. Advocates of this approach argue that it obviates the need for native tissue reinforcement vis-a-vis component separation; however, no comparative data are available.

Preperitoneal Reinforcement

In most patients with loss of abdominal domain, despite often far lateral recession of the musculofascial tissues, the peritoneum is present and typically readily identifiable throughout the visceral coverage. Once identified, the preperitoneal plane can be developed laterally to the psoas muscles, inferiorly below the pubis, and onto the diaphragm superiorly. The peritoneum can then be closed over the intestine with a running absorbable suture [28]. Such wide preperitoneal dissection and closure of the peritoneum yields several advantages. Closing the peritoneum makes it so no bowel retraction is needed while the components' separation is performed or, more importantly, the mesh is placed. Additionally, dissection and closure of the peritoneum allows the surgeon to separate the mesh from the intestine and, therefore, select a mesh without the costly barriers that are designed to prevent intestinal ingrowth. As well, mesh can be placed to cover the entire abdomen and beyond—the flank and diaphragm. It allows a surgeon to cover or reinforce an aggressive components separation with mesh, extending it beyond the cut edges of the external oblique. An attempt is made to close the fascia in the midline, in order to restore functional abdominal wall and provide a native tissue barrier between the underlying mesh and the superficial tissues, as the risk of wound complication is high in these patients. Panniculectomy is performed as necessary, and talc is applied subcutaneously as a rule to reduce seroma formation and lower the risk of subsequent wound infections and breakdown [29].

Mesh Fixation

Loss of domain repairs is often hindered by the need for sufficient and strong tissue on which to anchor the mesh. The use of metal supports to secure mesh to bone has been suggested [30]; however, long-term discomfort, technical complexity, and complications inherent to the use of prosthetic materials have limited the widespread use of this method [2]. The standard for fixation in large hernias, whether performed open or laparoscopically, is full thickness, permanent sutures. Their holding strength is 2.5-fold greater than tacks [31], they can be easily applied at the pubis, edge of the ribs, or iliac crest, and they are truly cost effective.

Biologic Mesh for Loss of Domain

The role of biologic mesh for abdominal wall reconstruction is fairly specialized, and its use should be judicious [32]. Biologic prostheses can stretch over time when used as a bridge, and most will eventually lose structural strength and event rate. Data for cases where it is used as a buttress for fascial reinforcement appear more promising. The patients should be counseled about the goals and expectations of mesh selection, especially in light of very high costs of bioprosthetics.

Separation of Components

Various authors advocate the use of temporary, biologic, or composite materials [33], but most agree that native tissue coverage should be maximized during abdominal wall reconstruction for loss of domain [8]. The value of primary fascial closure in large ventral defects with loss of abdominal domain has been documented in multiple studies [34, 35]. In patients with loss of abdominal domain, lack of native, innervated tissue leads to diminished mobility and can result in increased mesh sensation and impaired dynamics of the trunk. Component separation, first described in the US literature by Ramirez in 1990, is the first-line strategy to extend the musculofascial coverage of the abdomen [36]. Component separation may be performed in several ways: by dividing the anterior or posterior rectus sheath, the external or internal oblique fascia, or transversus abdominis or certain combinations of Fig. 30.1. Patients with loss of abdominal domain must be carefully assessed intraoperatively for the presence and integrity of the rectus abdominis and oblique muscle bilaterally, and the feasibility of component separation in the light severe lateral recession and the choice of procedure must be made accordingly [37]. The risk of lateral recurrence must not be ignored; in patients with loss of domain, this is especially pertinent and is yet another reason for wide prosthetic reinforcement. The major limitation of this technique in the face of domain loss is lack of sufficient native tissue to afford a durable abdominal closure [33]. Patient satisfaction and quality of life improvement are high [38].

Tissue Grafts and Abdominoplasty

The inability to accomplish native skin and subcutaneous closure has been correlated with an up to 30% recurrence rate [39, 40], although the causal relationship has not been proven. When the residual abdominal tissue is insufficient to provide coverage, autologous tissue grafts may be an appropriate alternative, but they are infrequently used. These may be musculofascial or musculocutaneous flaps and are usually supplied by one major artery. Tensor fascia lata flap was the earliest, described in 1946,

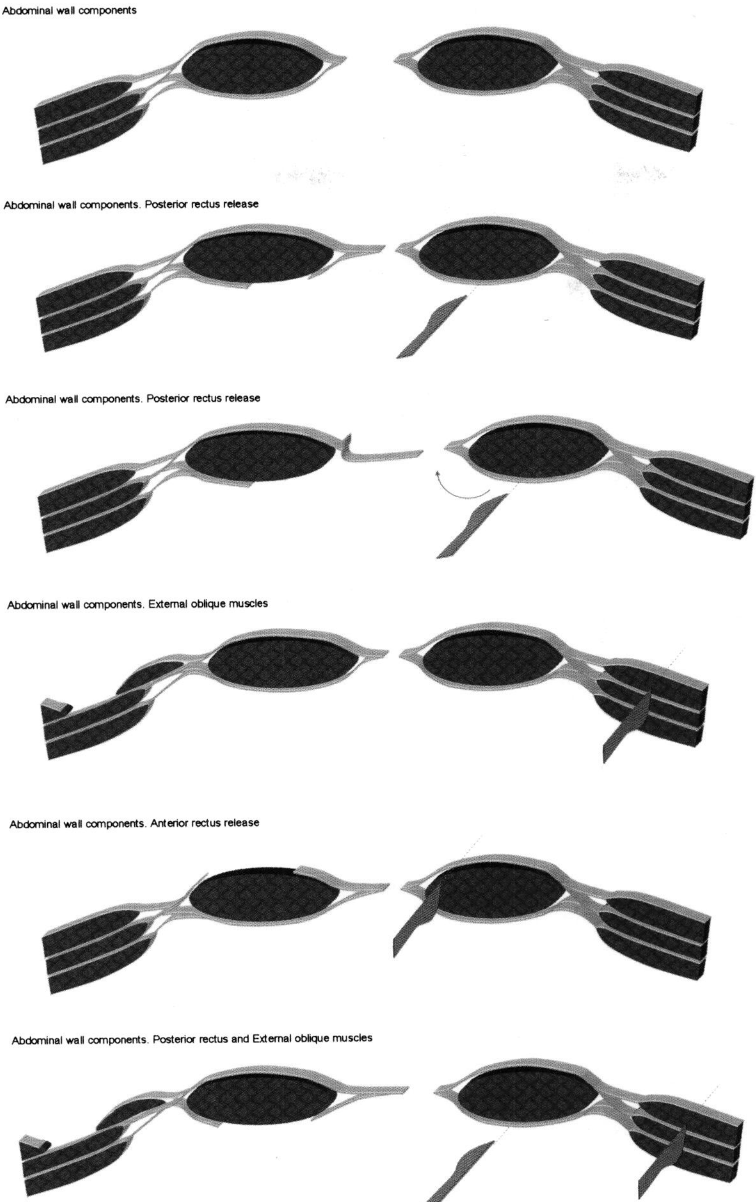

Fig. 30.1. Anatomic diagram of abdominal components separation techniques.

and may be suitable for lower abdominal wall defects [41]. It may be performed as a simple, rotational, or free flap; however, they are extremely painful. Other options include latissimus dorsi and rectus femoris flaps; however, up to 50% shrinkage of the denervated muscular component results in high recurrence rate [42]. Recently, the use of anterolateral thigh free flap has been reported with promising results [43, 44]. Overall, the results of the tissue transfer flaps have been discouraging because of the insufficient tensile strength, risk of flap necrosis, donor site complications, and lack of muscle innervation, which results in eventration.

In addition to preoperative pneumoperitoneum described earlier, tissue expanders have been used with moderate success. These can be placed subcutaneously, between internal and external oblique or transversus abdominis muscles [42]. There are case reports of autologous tissue expansion by virtue of pregnancy leading to successful primary repair with fair outcomes. The role of endogenous hormones in facilitating tissue expansion and long-term effects remains unclear. In general, tissue expansion is more effective for subcutaneous tissues compared to musculofascial components.

Reconstruction in a Contaminated Field

Abdominal wall reconstruction should be performed acute in the presence of a contaminated field or bowel edema. In such cases, various strategies have been used, all providing the temporary coverage while the bowel edema subsides and the infection resolves. The simplest acute method is the use of negative pressure closure, where the omentum or artificial protective covering is placed over the bowel and the abdominal wall is bridged with a sponge or towel and gentle continuous suction is applied over the top, such as with the use of the wound VAC [45]. Vicryl mesh may be used as temporary coverage, with a later skin graft, when gross infection or contamination is present. Because the material dissolves in 2–4 weeks, 100% hernia recurrence rate is to be expected. Despite its temporary nature, Vicryl stimulates a significant inflammatory reaction, and bowel fistulization has been reported [46]. Biologic mesh provides another coverage option in a contaminated field, leading to at least 80% hernia recurrence without subsequent definitive reconstruction. Traditionally, the use of heavyweight polypropylene mesh in contaminated field was contraindicated due to high infection rates, mesh extrusion, and fistulization rates of up to 50% in the acute management [47]. The newer lightweight polypropylene prostheses are less inflammatory and more amenable to bacterial eradication.

Staged Repair with Serial Excisions

Aside from the added time, resources, and expenses, the use of serial mesh excisions provides a robust method for loss of domain reconstruction [10, 33]. This approach takes advantage of the adaptive elasticity of the muscle and fascia of the abdominal wall, in a sense, reversing the process of loss of abdominal domain. The first operation proceeds similarly to other techniques. Once the eviscerated contents are reduced into the abdomen, the dimensions of the ventral defect are measured, and exactly shaped Gore-Tex prosthesis is sutured in the inlay position under moderate tension to produce gradual medialization of the edges of the defect. The superficial wound is closed in the usual fashion. Patients are taken back to the operating room repeatedly every 2–4 days. At surgery, the tension on the mesh is qualitatively ascertained, and several centimeters of mesh are excised from the middle, and the mesh is sutured together to maintain medial tension on the edges of the defect. In the final stage, the mesh is completely excised, and the fascia is closed primarily in the midline, with optional sublay mesh reinforcement. Component separation may be added to facilitate midline closure [33].

Laparoscopic Repair

Patients with loss of abdominal domain are often not considered minimally invasive candidates, and most surgeons use open repairs for these hernias. Nonetheless, the feasibility of a laparoscopic repair of giant ventral hernias has been demonstrated in multiple studies [2, 48]. Laparoscopic approaches carry low wound complication rate, which can benefit patients who otherwise suffer 30–50% complication rates. The laparoscopic technique is an intraperitoneal sublay—similar to conventional ventral hernia repairs. Please refer to the Laparoscopic Repair chapter in this text. The laparoscopic approach for loss of domain requires an alteration of this technique including trocar placement above the mesh.

Outcomes and Complications

Postoperative Management

Patients with loss of abdominal domain who undergo extensive abdominal wall reconstructions are particularly prone to wound-related complications. The use of JP drains, subcutaneous and over the mesh, are commonplace. Abdominal binders are used for patient comfort only and have not been shown to impact rates of seroma formation. The use of subcutaneous talc after fascial closure has proven to reduce the postoperative seroma formation, decrease drain duration, and lower subsequent wound complications [29]. Previously, wound complication rates of 30–50% were not uncommon. Fortunately, most wound problems are limited in nature and respond to local wound care and antibiotics. Early mobilization, respiratory therapy, and rehabilitation are important in this population. Pain control can be an issue, and epidural anesthesia is often employed.

Long-Term Outcomes

Although wound complications are common in the short term, the majority of patients are fully recovered by 6 months after the operation. Satisfaction levels are high among patients, even those who suffer wound complications, because of the dramatically improved quality of life. The literature suggests good results long term after staged abdominal reconstructions using a combination of prosthetic reinforcement and separation of components. DiCocco et al. reported at a mean follow-up of 5 years, recurrence rate of 14%, with approximately half occurring within 18 months and the rest within 48 months after the abdominal reconstruction. They showed no association of recurrence with comorbidities, defect size, or time to reconstruction; however, female gender and BMI were associated with higher recurrence rates [49]. Long-term quality of life is similar among patients undergoing conventional open ventral hernia repairs and those with components separation [38].

References

1. Heniford BT, et al. Laparoscopic repair of ventral hernias: nine years' experience with 850 consecutive hernias. Ann Surg. 2003;238(3):391–9. discussion 399–400.
2. Baghai M, et al. Technique of laparoscopic ventral hernia repair can be modified to successfully repair large defects in patients with loss of domain. Surg Innov. 2009;16(1):38–45.
3. Park A, Birch DW, Lovrics P. Laparoscopic and open incisional hernia repair: a comparison study. Surgery. 1998;124(4):816–21. discussion 821–2.
4. Chevrel JP, Caix M. Surgery of the abdominal wall. Berlin: Springer; 1987.

5. Korenkov M, et al. Classification and surgical treatment of incisional hernia. Results of an experts' meeting. Langenbecks Arch Surg. 2001;386(1):65–73.
6. Parker 3rd HH, et al. Laparoscopic repair of large incisional hernias. Am Surg. 2002;68(6):530–3. discussion 533–4.
7. Bernard C, et al. Repair of giant incisional abdominal wall hernias using open intraperitoneal mesh. Hernia. 2007;11(4):315–20.
8. Kingsnorth AN, et al. Open mesh repair of incisional hernias with significant loss of domain. Ann R Coll Surg Engl. 2004;86(5):363–6.
9. McAdory RS, Cobb WS, Carbonell AM. Progressive preoperative pneumoperitoneum for hernias with loss of domain. Am Surg. 2009;75(6):504–8. discussion 508–9.
10. Vertrees A, et al. Early definitive abdominal closure using serial closure technique on injured soldiers returning from Afghanistan and Iraq. J Am Coll Surg. 2006;202(5):762–72.
11. Xiao SC, et al. Repair of complex abdominal wall defects from high-voltage electric injury with two layers of acellular dermal matrix: a case report. J Burn Care Res. 2009;30(2):352–4.
12. Tang R, et al. Immediate repair of major abdominal wall defect after extensive tumor excision in patients with abdominal wall neoplasm: a prospective review of 27 cases. Ann Surg Oncol. 2009;16(10):2895–907.
13. Rosen M. Loss of domain - definition and management. SAGES 12th world congress of endoscopic surgery. Washington, DC. April 15, 2010.
14. Dumont F, et al. Progressive pneumoperitoneum increases the length of abdominal muscles. Hernia. 2009;13(2):183–7.
15. Sabbagh C, et al. Peritoneal volume is predictive of tension-free fascia closure of large incisional hernias with loss of domain: a prospective study. Hernia. 2011;15(5):559–65.
16. Toniato A, et al. Incisional hernia treatment with progressive pneumoperitoneum and retromuscular prosthetic hernioplasty. Langenbecks Arch Surg. 2002;387(5–6):246–8.
17. Tanaka EY, et al. A computerized tomography scan method for calculating the hernia sac and abdominal cavity volume in complex large incisional hernia with loss of domain. Hernia. 2010;14(1):63–9.
18. Cobb WS, et al. Normal intraabdominal pressure in healthy adults. J Surg Res. 2005;129(2):231–5.
19. Lindstrom D, et al. Effects of a perioperative smoking cessation intervention on postoperative complications: a randomized trial. Ann Surg. 2008;248(5):739–45.
20. Mayagoitia JC, et al. Preoperative progressive pneumoperitoneum in patients with abdominal-wall hernias. Hernia. 2006;10(3):213–7.
21. Caldironi MW, et al. Progressive pneumoperitoneum in the management of giant incisional hernias: a study of 41 patients. Br J Surg. 1990;77(3):306–7.
22. Willis S, Schumpelick V. Use of progressive pneumoperitoneum in the repair of giant hernias. Hernia. 2000;4(2):105–11.
23. Luijendijk RW, et al. A comparison of suture repair with mesh repair for incisional hernia. N Engl J Med. 2000;343(6):392–8.
24. Joels CS, et al. Abdominal wall reconstruction after temporary abdominal closure: a ten-year review. Surg Innov. 2006;13(4):223–30.

25. de Vries Reilingh TS, et al. Repair of large midline incisional hernias with polypropylene mesh: comparison of three operative techniques. Hernia. 2004;8(1):56–9.
26. Moreno-Egea A, et al. Repair of complex incisional hernias using double prosthetic repair: single-surgeon experience with 50 cases. Surgery. 2010;148(1):140–4.
27. Cobb WS, Kercher KW, Heniford BT. The argument for lightweight polypropylene mesh in hernia repair. Surg Innov. 2005;12(1):63–9.
28. Novitsky YW, et al. Open preperitoneal retrofascial mesh repair for multiply recurrent ventral incisional hernias. J Am Coll Surg. 2006;203(3):283–9.
29. Klima DA, et al. Application of subcutaneous talc in hernia repair and wide subcutaneous dissection dramatically reduces seroma formation and post-operative wound complications. Am Surg. 2011;77(7):888–94.
30. Yee JA, et al. Bone anchor mesh fixation for complex laparoscopic ventral hernia repair. Surg Innov. 2008;15(4):292–6.
31. Joels CS, et al. Evaluation of adhesion formation, mesh fixation strength, and hydroxyproline content after intraabdominal placement of polytetrafluoroethylene mesh secured using titanium spiral tacks, nitinol anchors, and polypropylene suture or polyglactin 910 suture. Surg Endosc. 2005;19(6):780–5.
32. Pomahac B, Aflaki P. Use of a non-cross-linked porcine dermal scaffold in abdominal wall reconstruction. Am J Surg. 2010;199(1):22–7.
33. Lipman J, Medalie D, Rosen MJ. Staged repair of massive incisional hernias with loss of abdominal domain: a novel approach. Am J Surg. 2008;195(1):84–8.
34. Lowe 3rd JB, et al. Risks associated with "components separation" for closure of complex abdominal wall defects. Plast Reconstr Surg. 2003;111(3):1276–83. quiz 1284–5; discussion 1286–8.
35. Rios A, et al. Factors that affect recurrence after incisional herniorrhaphy with prosthetic material. Eur J Surg. 2001;167(11):855–9.
36. Ramirez OM, Ruas E, Dellon AL. "Components separation" method for closure of abdominal-wall defects: an anatomic and clinical study. Plast Reconstr Surg. 1990;86(3):519–26.
37. Levine JP, Karp NS. Restoration of abdominal wall integrity as a salvage procedure in difficult recurrent abdominal wall hernias using a method of wide myofascial release. Plast Reconstr Surg. 2001;107(3):707–16. discussion 717–8.
38. Klima DA, et al. Prospective comparison of component separation versus conventional open ventral hernia repair in patients with large ventral hernias. San Francisco: American Hernia Society; 2011.
39. Girotto JA, et al. Recalcitrant abdominal wall hernias: long-term superiority of autologous tissue repair. Plast Reconstr Surg. 2003;112(1):106–14.
40. Lowe JB, et al. Endoscopically assisted "components separation" for closure of abdominal wall defects. Plast Reconstr Surg. 2000;105(2):720–9. quiz 730.
41. Wangensteen OH. Repair of large abdominal defects by pedicled fascial flaps. Surg Gynecol Obstet. 1946;82:144–50.
42. Van Geffen HJ, Simmermacher RK. Incisional hernia repair: abdominoplasty, tissue expansion, and methods of augmentation. World J Surg. 2005;29(8):1080–5.

43. Kuo YR, et al. One-stage reconstruction of large midline abdominal wall defects using a composite free anterolateral thigh flap with vascularized fascia lata. Ann Surg. 2004;239(3):352–8.
44. Berrevoet F, et al. The anterolateral thigh flap for complicated abdominal wall reconstruction after giant incisional hernia repair. Acta Chir Belg. 2010;110(3):376–82.
45. Miller PR, et al. Prospective evaluation of vacuum-assisted fascial closure after open abdomen: planned ventral hernia rate is substantially reduced. Ann Surg. 2004;239(5):608–14. discussion 614–6.
46. Fabian TC, et al. Planned ventral hernia. Staged management for acute abdominal wall defects. Ann Surg. 1994;219(6):643–50. discussion 651–3.
47. Jernigan TW, et al. Staged management of giant abdominal wall defects: acute and long-term results. Ann Surg. 2003;238(3):349–55. discussion 355–7.
48. Ferrari GC, et al. Laparoscopic management of incisional hernias ≥15 cm in diameter. Hernia. 2008;12(6):571–6.
49. DiCocco JM, et al. Long-term follow-up of abdominal wall reconstruction after planned ventral hernia: a 15-year experience. J Am Coll Surg. 2010;210(5):686–95. 695–8.

31. Drains, Pain Pumps, and Abdominal Binders

Chris Edwards

Some aspects of surgery rely heavily on science to tell the surgeon how to perform a certain procedure or determine which adjunctive modality should be used at a certain time. Some aspects of surgery rely on surgical science to develop algorithms of patient care and to standardize best practices. Some aspects of surgery rely more heavily on tradition than on hard scientific fact usually in areas where surgical science is hard to produce or inconsistent. Some areas are a true blend of the science of surgery and the art of surgery. This is certainly true when discussing current strategies regarding drains, pain pumps, and abdominal binders for the laparoscopic treatment of hernia.

This is certainly one area where surgical science is lacking. There simply is a paucity of true surgical research in this area of hernia repair. Many surgeons rely on the advice of others and the traditions that have been passed down from their mentors as to when these adjuncts to hernia repair are used. This chapter is an attempt to consolidate what little research is available and to provide the author's current practice regarding the use of drains, pain pumps, and abdominal binders for laparoscopic hernia repair.

Drains

There are many types of drains available for surgical practice today. Open or closed drainage of hernia repair has been described. The scope of this writing is not to describe the types of drains available but to describe the use during laparoscopic hernia repair.

B.P. Jacob and B. Ramshaw (eds.), *The SAGES Manual of Hernia Repair*,
DOI 10.1007/978-1-4614-4824-2_31,

The primary purpose of the use of any drain is to be able to evacuate blood, pus, or fluid from a surgical site. The benefits of this in hernia repair may be to decrease seroma formation, to remove infected material from a surgical site, or to allow more rapid healing of wounds by the use of negative pressure. Drains used for open treatment of hernia are often used to evacuate the accumulation of seroma fluid.

The use of drains during laparoscopic hernia repair is often controversial. There truly is minimal data published on this topic. The use of drains for laparoscopic hernia repair should be balanced by the possibility of introducing an outside contaminant with the benefit of removing seroma fluid. Closed suction drains placed over a permanent prosthetic material should be avoided as the author feels this can lead to a portal of infection to the mesh often used for laparoscopic hernia repair. One of the key benefits of laparoscopic hernia repair is the decreased risk of wound infection and mesh infection [1, 2]. It simply does not make sense to leave a tract for the possible contamination of a mesh material by the use of a drain.

However, the data on the use of drains during laparoscopic mesh hernia repair is minimal. In fact, Kaafarani et al. list the placement of a surgical drain as an independent risk factor for the development of surgical site infection after laparoscopic ventral hernia repair [3]. Other studies have found inconclusive evidence on whether the use of a drain over mesh hernia repairs yields an increase in surgical site infections or not during incisional hernia repair [4].

One recent study is worth looking into that advocates the use of closed suction drainage during laparoscopic total extraperitoneal (TEP) inguinal hernia repair. This study by Ismail et al. reviewed 929 patients (1,753) hernias where laparoscopic TEP hernia repair was performed. Eight hundred forty-nine (1,607) patients had drains placed where 80 (146) patients did not. Seroma formation was significantly less in the drain group (0.75 %) compared to the open group (15.1 %). No infections were identified in either group supporting the use of drains in this procedure [5]. Still, the data suggesting routine drainage for mesh hernia repair is sparse, and the author does not recommend the use of drains in this setting. Furthermore, the author feels that the risk of even one mesh infection during laparoscopic repair outweighs the benefits of decreased seroma formation that typically clears spontaneously without complication.

However, one example where drains should be used liberally is in abdominal wall reconstruction. Drains should be used during component's release incisional hernia repair in the submuscular spaces that are created during this particular type of procedure. Drains used in this fashion will help reduce seroma formation and allow the negative pressure to help "seal" these spaces and improve healing. Furthermore, the evacuation of this fluid can certainly help limit the accumulation of old hematoma and seroma that can predispose to abscess formation in the often medically complex patients where this procedure is performed. The technique should attempt to separate any prosthetic with drains to limit contamination of the mesh. These drains left in the submuscular spaces should be left longer than most other procedures where mesh is used typically. Most surgeons remove drains when the volume of fluid being drained reaches a certain minimal amount. However, with components release where large sub- or intramuscular flaps are created, the author feels it is useful to leave these drains in for 2–3 weeks sometimes for the negative pressure to help close these spaces and speed healing.

Overall, minimal data supports the use of drains during laparoscopic mesh hernia repair. Several studies emphasize the use of drains to increase the incidence of surgical site and mesh infections when used in this matter. Some studies may demonstrate the use of drains to decrease seroma rates, but the author feels that the prevention of this relatively benign complication not to be worth the risk of mesh infection that the drain may cause. If the surgeon can separate the mesh from the site needed for drainage however as in certain abdominal wall reconstruction techniques, then drains may prove useful. More data needs to be evaluated.

Binders

Many surgeons feel that the use of abdominal binders after laparoscopic ventral hernia repair may have many advantages. The possible advantages include less pain, possibility of lower recurrence, and the possibility of fewer seromas. Like the use of drains after laparoscopic hernia repair, there is a paucity of data for this.

The most common binders used in the United States are relatively inexpensive elasticized products with Velcro fixation. The benefits of these binders are that they are cheap and easy to place. They are also readily available at any medical supply store. These are usually placed immediately after the procedure. Many surgeons claim that these binders add support to the repair; however, there is no clear evidence in the literature to support this for laparoscopic repair.

One of the most common findings after laparoscopic incisional hernia repair is postoperative seroma. These are all usually benign but can be disconcerting to the patient and confused with early recurrence to the inexperienced clinician. Dr. LeBlanc feels that the use of binders may decrease the incidence of this common finding after surgery [6]. However, this author could not find any comparative analysis in the literature to support this.

There does seem to be some support in the literature for the use of binders to benefit postoperative pain after laparoscopic hernia repair. Cheifetz et al. found a significant reduction in pain 1, 3, and 5 days after surgery with the use of binders. They also found improvement in the ability to ambulate afterward in a randomized control trial [7]. Larson et al. also demonstrated an improvement in pain scores of about half that without binders in a prospective randomized control study of 54 patients [8].

A criticism of binders is that there may be a decrease in the patient's ability to breathe. This may lead to poor respiratory function and the associated problems of atelectasis, postoperative fever, and pneumonia following an especially painful procedure. Larson and Cheifitz groups both looked at this as well and found no reduction in pulmonary function as measured by pulmonary function testing with the use of abdominal binders after major abdominal surgery [7, 8].

The author feels that binders can help with pain if the patient feels that this will be the case. The authors do not routinely use binders after laparoscopic ventral hernia repair unless asked by the patient. There is no clear evidence that binders reduce the incidence of seroma formation or reduce the recurrence rate. However, pain control does seem to be improved. The drawback however is that many patients feel that the binder is "prescribed" for them and they often wear it to excess, including in the shower. The author has seen some very foul binders come back in to the office raising the question of hygiene for these patients. Overall, binders may have a utility for pain control but have not shown a clear cut benefit in other postoperative improvements in laparoscopic incisional hernia repair.

Pain Pumps

Pain control after laparoscopic surgery is a huge topic and best suited for its own chapter. The general feeling that the laparoscopic approach is a less painful approach should not mean to say that laparoscopic treatment of hernia is a painless procedure. In fact, the author believes that the laparoscopic approach provides access to perform a much more thorough dissection than an open approach. The laparoscopic approach also allows for more broad mesh placement which can irritate a very sensitive peritoneum and provide significant postoperative pain. The use of postoperative pain pumps can be one way to minimize this pain after surgery.

Pain control after laparoscopic surgery can consist of a variety of modalities. Intravenous and oral narcotics, anti-inflammatory, epidural catheter infusions, regional anesthetic blocks, and placement of pain pumps are a few of these modalities. This discussion will center on what the literature supports for the placement of pain pumps after laparoscopic hernia repair.

Epidural catheter pumps have been demonstrated to be a successful pain control strategy for a number of open procedures. However, the routine use of epidural catheters for laparoscopic hernia repair is not universally accepted or understood. There is minimal data supporting this. This author feels however that a laparoscopic repair of a large ventral hernia is a very painful procedure. This author also routinely uses epidural catheter and patient-controlled pumps for its administration after their repair. The data is not published yet, but this author has seen a reduction in length of stay by 2 days as well as a faster recovery of gastrointestinal function after the use of epidural catheters for laparoscopic repair of ventral hernias over 30 cm^2. In fact, an ad hoc analysis of the authors' data supported early closure of the trial due to favorable results. These findings are to be presented later this year.

There are problems associated with epidural catheters however. Weakness and numbness are some common side effects. Urinary retention is also common. A lot of these factors are technique driven and depend on the anesthetists' skill at placing the catheter. In summary, it is reasonable to consider an epidural catheter for pain control after any large laparoscopic ventral hernia repair.

The uses of regional anesthetic pumps are commonplace as well. The most common is a Silastic-type catheter attached to a continuously infusing reservoir of local anesthetic designed to administer a set amount of local anesthesia to the surgery site. The use for open inguinal hernia repair is present with Stewart et al. and Sanchez et al. presenting their data in 2004 demonstrating lower mean pain scores and less rescue aesthesia with the use of these pumps in open inguinal hernia repair. This difference persisted even after removal of the pump [9, 10]. However, Rosen et al. did not see a difference in pain scores with the use of these pumps after laparoscopic ventral hernia repairs in 73 patients [11].

An interesting corollary of this is the use of regional block anesthesia with or without the use of pumps. There has been interest in the administration of local anesthetic to the preperitoneal space for the use of both open and laparoscopic procedures. This is commonly called transversus abdominis plane (TAP) block. Heil et al. reported a benefit in pain scores when used for outpatient open inguinal hernia repair [12], while Ahmed et al. reported a benefit with laparoscopic incisional hernia repair [13]. Data on this technique is sparse but carries the benefit of no additional short-term catheter.

Conclusion

The use of drains, binders, and pain pumps is largely driven by anecdotal evidence only. Few studies really support or disprove these techniques in regard to laparoscopic hernia repair. However, these techniques may prove beneficial in the long run and require further study.

References

1. Sains PS, et al. Outcomes following laparoscopic versus open repair of incisional hernia. World J Surg. 2006;30(11):2056–64.
2. Sauerland S, et al. Laparoscopic versus open surgical techniques for ventral or incisional hernia repair. Cochrane Database Syst Rev. 2011;3:CD007781.
3. Kaafarani HMA, et al. Predictors of surgical site infection in laparoscopic and open ventral incisional herniorrhaphy. J Surg Res. 2010;163(2):229–34.
4. Gurusamy KS (2007) Wound drains after incisional hernia repair. Cochrane Database Syst Rev. 2007; (1):CD005570.
5. Ismail M, et al. Impact of closed-suction drain in preperitoneal space on the incidence of seroma formation after laparoscopic total extraperitoneal inguinal hernia repair. Surg Laparosc Endosc Percutan Tech. 2009;19(3):263–6.
6. LeBlanc KA. Laparoscopic incisional and ventral hernia repair: complications—how to avoid and handle. Hernia. 2004;8(4):323–31.
7. Cheifetz O, et al. The effect of abdominal support on functional outcomes inpatients following major abdominal surgery: a randomized controlled trial. Physiother Can. 2010;62(3):242–53.
8. Larson CM, et al. The effect of abdominal binders on postoperative pulmonary function. Am Surg. 2009;75(2):169–71.

9. Stewart A, et al. Randomized trial of a pain control infusion pump following inguinal hernia repair. ANZ J Surg. 2004;4(10):873–6.
10. Sanchez B, et al. Local anesthetic infusion pumps improve postoperative pain after inguinal hernia repair: a randomized trial. Am Surg. 2004;70(11):1002–6.
11. Rosen MJ, et al. Prospective randomized double-blind placebo-controlled trial of postoperative elastomeric pain pump devices used after laparoscopic ventral hernia repair. Surg Endosc. 2009;23(12):2637–43.
12. Heil JW, et al. Ultrasound-guided transversus abdominis plane catheters and ambulatory perineural infusions for outpatient hernia repair. Reg Anesth Pain Med. 2010;35(6):556–8.
13. Ahmed M, et al. A simple technique of regional anesthesia to reduce opioid requirements postoperatively in laparoscopic incisional hernia repairs. Surg Laparosc Endosc Percutan Tech. 2011;21(2):e70–1.

Part VII
Outcomes and Complications Following Ventral and Incisional Hernia Repair

32. Skin Necrosis After Open Component Separation: Prevention and Management

Jignesh V. Unadkat and Dinakar Golla

Component separation as popularized by Ramirez et al. [1] has been the mainstay of autologous abdominal wall reconstruction for complex defects especially with loss of domain. This method allows closure of significant midline defects up to 12, 20, and 10 cm in the upper, middle, and lower abdomen, respectively [2]. Using this technique, hernia recurrence rates have been significantly reduced compared to primary repair [3]. One obvious drawback of the procedure is the extensive dissection of the skin and subcutaneous tissue to access the external oblique muscle for subsequent release. Significantly higher wound complication rates have been reported with skin necrosis occurring in up to 40 % of the patients [4]. In the presence of preexisting infection, this rate is even higher [5].

Anatomy

The abdominal wall has a robust blood supply [6]. Huger divided the anterior abdominal wall into three zones. Zones I and II, the mid-abdomen and lower abdomen, respectively, are supplied by the vascular arcade of the superior and inferior deep epigastric arteries supplemented by branches from the superficial inferior epigastric and superficial circumflex iliac arteries to the lower abdominal wall. Zone III is supplied by the intercostal, subcostal, and lumbar arteries that course toward the midline. The neurovascular bundle exists between the internal oblique and transversalis muscles. As such, there is a relatively avascular and nerve-sparing plane between the external and internal oblique muscles,

B.P. Jacob and B. Ramshaw (eds.), *The SAGES Manual of Hernia Repair*,
DOI 10.1007/978-1-4614-4824-2_32,

providing the anatomic basis for separating the component parts of the abdominal wall musculature. Blood supply to the skin is provided by superficial and deep vascular systems. In the lower abdomen, direct superficial cutaneous supply comes from superficial circumflex and superficial inferior epigastric arteries and in the upper abdomen from the branches off of the subcostal and intercostal arteries. These branches originate lateral and course toward the midline. In the midline, the abdomen is supplied predominantly by the indirect blood supply coming via the musculocutaneous perforators off the deep epigastric arcade. These perforators are predominantly grouped around the umbilicus.

Pathophysiology

Midline incision to access the hernia sac divides any crossing blood vessels. As such, the midline skin relies on the blood supply from lateral sources and deep sources, that is, the periumbilical perforators. In a wide abdomen, wherein the midline skin is distant from the lateral limits of the abdomen, direct lateral superficial blood supply is limited. Furthermore, wide undermining of the subcutaneous flaps to access the external oblique muscle divides the musculocutaneous perforators, thereby rendering the abdominal midline skin and subcutaneous areas avascular. This consequently leads to skin infection and necrosis [7] and fat necrosis leading to tissue loss, leaving the midline facial closure exposed and prone to infections [8].

Prevention

Clearly, gentle skin and soft tissue handling is a prerequisite in preventing most wound complications. One must be cognizant of potential wound healing complications in patients with several comorbidities including but not limited to obesity, diabetes, smoking, and immunosuppressed status. Following component separation, the key to preventing skin necrosis lies in prevention of severance of blood supply to the abdominal skin:

1. Careful planning of incision and assessment of any previous abdominal scars will allow preservation of blood supply to the midline skin. Presence of right subcostal scar would preclude undermining of the right adipocutaneous flap superiorly.

Similarly, transverse scar for renal transplantation would preclude undermining of lower adipocutaneous flaps.

2. Preventing widespread undermining of the adipocutaneous flaps would prevent disruption of blood supply to the medial skin edges. A number of methods have been undertaken to access the external oblique musculature without significant undermining of the adipocutaneous flaps. Maas et al. [9] used a separate longitudinal incision 15 cm laterally from the medial skin edge to access the external oblique aponeurosis. In their small series of four patients, none had hernia recurrence or skin necrosis. Lowe et al. [10] used balloon dissection of a subcutaneous pocket via two small lateral incisions on either side of the abdomen to access the external oblique. Following this, the external oblique muscle was released endoscopically. In their series of 37 patients, none of the endoscopic group patients had any infection, ischemia, or dehiscence compared to the open approach groups of patients.
3. Preserving the periumbilical musculocutaneous perforators would maintain blood supply to the medial skin edges. Dumanian et al. [8] carefully dissected the adipocutaneous flaps off the external oblique muscle taking care to preserve the periumbilical perforators. They performed lateral dissection from the defect edges to expose the linea semilunaris both superior and inferior to the umbilicus and connecting the two areas via a tunnel lateral to the perforators. Using this technique, in a series of 41 patients, they obtained significantly lower incidence of superficial skin complications even in the presence of contamination/enterocutaneous fistulae. A modification described later [3] involved the use of 6–8-cm transverse subcostal incisions bilaterally to access the linea semilunaris rather than any subcutaneous dissections.
4. A simple key to prevent skin necrosis would be to predict its occurrence. This idealistic approach, albeit with extreme uncertainty, can be adapted in a patient such as one who is an overweight individual with diabetes, who has had multiple previous abdominal surgeries, and presents with gross contamination. Excising the excess medial tissue, enough to allow primary closure, much like a vertical panniculectomy, would remove the potentially threatened skin and subcutaneous tissue that may have gone onto ischemic necrosis. In addition, infraumbilical hernias maybe approached via a standard panniculectomy

approach with excision of threatened tissue at closure. Some authors [3] have implemented short-term subatmospheric pressure dressings as an immediate dressing. This has led to decreased soft tissue loss and consequent infections.

Management

Management of skin necrosis following component separation presents a potential challenge. Firstly, the patient usually has had multiple abdominal surgeries, often through the same incision. Repeated attempts at hernia repair induce significant scar formation within the potential dead space created by elevation of adipocutaneous flaps. This scar is avascular which potentiates wound complications. In addition, many patients have had prior infections or infected mesh repairs. Several patients have numerous comorbidities further impairing the ability for wound healing.

Once skin and soft tissue necrosis has occurred, complete debridement of the necrotic tissues is mandated. All attempts to maintain integrity of the underlying fascial closure should be made. Soft tissue debridement can be undertaken using chemical, mechanical, or surgical methods. Chemical methods involve usage of enzymatic agents. Mechanical debridements involve regular dressing changes using wet-to-dry dressings or moist dressings as warranted. Above methods help in situations where in there is limited or superficial tissue necrosis. Full-thickness adipocutaneous necrosis warrants excision of the affected area either by the bedside or in the office or in the operative room depending on the extent of involvement.

Once all necrotic tissue is excised, the next step would be reconstructing the defect. Depending on the amount of abdominal soft tissue excess, it may be possible to advance the remaining abdominal wall to approximate in the midline. Sometimes, depending on the status of the wound and the condition of the patient, it may be necessary to temporize the wound before implementing final reconstruction. Application of subatmospheric pressure dressing, especially in abdominal contaminated fields, has been shown to enable the growth of healthy granulation tissue [11]. Subsequently, these areas can be reconstructed by advancing surrounding healthy tissue as described above or application of a split-thickness skin graft.

Conclusion

Hernia repair using the component separation method is safe, effective, and reliable. Using the standard open technique, undermining of the adipocutaneous tissue to access and release the external oblique musculature is fraught with increased incidence of skin and subcutaneous tissue necrosis. Good planning and several modifications to the standard technique have demonstrated effectiveness in reduction in the rate of wound complications.

References

1. Ramirez OM, Ruas E, Dellon AL. "Components separation" method for closure of abdominal-wall defects: an anatomic and clinical study. Plast Reconstr Surg. 1990;86(3):519–26.
2. Shestak KC, Edington HJ, Johnson RR. The separation of anatomic components technique for the reconstruction of massive midline abdominal wall defects: anatomy, surgical technique, applications, and limitations revisited. Plast Reconstr Surg. 2000;105(2):731–8. quiz 9.
3. Ko JH, Wang EC, Salvay DM, Paul BC, Dumanian GA. Abdominal wall reconstruction: lessons learned from 200 "components separation" procedures. Arch Surg. 2009;144(11):1047–55.
4. Nguyen V, Shestak KC. Separation of anatomic components method of abdominal wall reconstruction—clinical outcome analysis and an update of surgical modifications using the technique. Clin Plast Surg. 2006;33(2):247–57.
5. Rosen MJ, Jin J, McGee MF, Williams C, Marks J, Ponsky JL. Laparoscopic component separation in the single-stage treatment of infected abdominal wall prosthetic removal. Hernia. 2007;11(5):435–40.
6. Huger Jr WE. The anatomic rationale for abdominal lipectomy. Am Surg. 1979;45(9):612–7.
7. Feng LJ, Price DC, Mathes SJ, Hohn D. Dynamic properties of blood flow and leukocyte mobilization in infected flaps. World J Surg. 1990;14(6):796–803.
8. Sukkar SM, Dumanian GA, Szczerba SM, Tellez MG. Challenging abdominal wall defects. Am J Surg. 2001;181(2):115–21.
9. Maas SM, van Engeland M, Leeksma NG, Bleichrodt RP. A modification of the "components separation" technique for closure of abdominal wall defects in the presence of an enterostomy. J Am Coll Surg. 1999;189(1):138–40.
10. Lowe JB, Garza JR, Bowman JL, Rohrich RJ, Strodel WE. Endoscopically assisted "components separation" for closure of abdominal wall defects. Plast Reconstr Surg. 2000;105(2):720–9. quiz 30.
11. Baharestani MM, Gabriel A. Use of negative pressure wound therapy in the management of infected abdominal wounds containing mesh: an analysis of outcomes. Int Wound J. 2011;8(2):118–25.

33. Recurrent Incisional Hernia Repair

John G. Linn and Dean J. Mikami

Repairing recurrent incisional hernias comprises thousands of operations performed nationwide each year. Patients suffering from these abdominal wall defects constitute a true challenge to general, minimally invasive, and plastic surgeons across the country. Traditional approaches to repairing these hernias, including open suture and mesh repair, have been plagued by repeated recurrences in both the short and long term. Other options, such as abdominal wall myofascial advancement flaps and laparoscopic approaches to incisional hernias have been proposed as superior alternatives with the potential for lower recurrence rates. Dozens of different mesh prostheses are available for recurrent hernia repairs, yet none offers a panacea immune to recurrence or other complications. Knowledge of all these options is required to provide the best possible care for patients with these difficult problems.

Scope of the Problem

In 1997, Luijendijk published a series of primary midline incisional hernias repaired using an interrupted mattress suture, vertical Mayo repair. They demonstrated a recurrence rate of nearly 50% at 5-year follow-up [1]. Later, the same group published the results of a multicenter trial which randomized patients to either mesh or primary suture repair of incisional hernias. Recurrence rates of 43% with primary suture repair and 24% with mesh repair were seen at 3-year follow-up [2]. While this second paper is often used to demonstrate the superiority of mesh repair compared to suture repair, the fact remains that despite good surgical technique using prosthetic, up to 1/4 of patients will suffer from a hernia recurrence in only 3 years. For those repaired primarily, the risk of recurrence is even higher, creating a huge group of patients with recurrent

B.P. Jacob and B. Ramshaw (eds.), *The SAGES Manual of Hernia Repair*,
DOI 10.1007/978-1-4614-4824-2_33,

hernias that seek further surgical treatment. In 1993, Hesselink examined a series of over 300 patients who underwent primary incisional hernia repair and concluded that better techniques in hernia surgery were badly needed [3]. A population-based study of incisional hernia repairs in Washington state in 2003 demonstrated that despite significant increase in the use of mesh over a 12-year period, the cumulative reoperation rate, used as a surrogate for recurrence, was over 20% [4].

Etiology and Pathophysiology of Recurrence

While the problem is significant, the underlying etiology of recurrence after a previous hernia repair is still poorly understood. Traditional surgical teaching links hernia recurrence to tension either created or not relieved during the repair operation. The use of "tension-free mesh repair" in inguinal hernias has certainly offered an improvement in recurrence rate from tissue repair alone. However, surgeons tend to believe that most of their own incisional hernia repairs are done without tension, and most published series describe a tension-free technique. Still, incisional hernia repairs recur at an extremely high rate. Therefore, the pathophysiology of recurrence likely has more to it than simply tension alone.

Patient-related factors, such as obesity, diabetes, tobacco use, and medications that impair wound healing such as steroids, have often been cited as risk factors for incisional hernia recurrence [5, 6]. Many of these factors, however, are difficult to cure or alter when patients present with symptomatic hernias. Patients with these comorbid conditions will continue to present with recurrent incisional hernias, and surgeons should focus on aspects of repair that can be controlled.

Local wound problems such as wound infection, hematoma, or mesh infection requiring removal seem to predispose patients to recurrence as well [7]. Providing adequate tissue coverage of mesh prostheses, judicious use of subcutaneous drains that may serve as routes of bacterial infection, and careful hemostatic technique may minimize the potential for these complications that have long-term consequences.

Mesh prostheses, which should probably be utilized for almost all recurrent incisional hernias, have different degrees of tensile strength, cross-linking, elasticity, durability, and contraction/shrinkage after implantation. Animal data suggests that using polypropylene mesh probably alters the elastic properties of the abdominal wall [8], which may help decrease recurrence. Elasticity will likely vary with different types of mesh, and poor understanding of this factor may predispose some patients to recurrence.

While surgical factors are important to consider, molecular alterations in collagen composition may prove to be underlying causes of hernia recurrence. A decrease in the ratio of type I to type III collagen has been implicated in the pathogenesis of inguinal hernia recurrence [9]. While matrix metalloproteinases (MMPs) have been implicated in the pathogenesis of both abdominal aortic aneurysm formation and inguinal hernia recurrence [10], their role in incisional hernia recurrence has been more difficult to elucidate and remains controversial [10, 11]. Some data suggests that fibroblast expression of MMPs may vary with the type of prosthetic material [11].

The last factor that surgeons can control is the technical aspects of mesh placement and fixation. Awad and colleagues performed an exhaustive review of technical factors that led to recurrence in published series of ventral hernia repair with mesh over the last 40 years. Types of mesh placement described included the following: (1) sandwich, in which prostheses are placed both anterior and posterior to the fascia; (2) onlay, in which mesh prostheses are secured to the anterior surface of the fascia, which is closed primarily; (3) inlay, in which the mesh is used as a bridge between two sides of fascia; (4) retrorectus or Rives-Stoppa repair, in which the mesh is placed deep to the rectus muscles between the anterior and posterior fascia layers, which are both closed primarily; and (5) intraperitoneal, as performed with a laparoscopic incisional hernia repair. Recurrence rates were highest among patients undergoing inlay and onlay mesh placement, which is supported by other reviews [12, 13]. Specific etiologies of hernia recurrence that seemed most common were inadequate mesh fixation, lateral mesh detachment, and mesh infection. Based on these findings, they proposed a specific classification system for mechanism of recurrence. Technical factors include mesh infection, mesh lateral distraction secondary to either inadequate fixation or inadequate overlap, and "missed" hernia [12]. Wassenaar reported a series of recurrences after 505 laparoscopic hernia repairs with polytetrafluoroethylene (PTFE). Interestingly, patients undergoing non-midline hernia repair, such as subcostal incisional hernia, had a much higher recurrence rate. While the groups were not equal due to a much smaller number of subcostal hernias, it does suggest that laparoscopic repair of subcostal incisional hernias is more difficult than midline hernias and that technical failure may increase recurrence rates. Most midline incisional hernia recurrences were immediately adjacent to the edge of the mesh, suggesting either a missed hernia or an overall weakness of the previously closed fascia [14].

Specific Challenges

Recurrent incisional hernias may present specific challenges during repair which are usually irrelevant to primary incisional hernia. Several unanswered questions remain regarding these challenges. For those hernias previously repaired with mesh, should it be removed at a second operation? Should colostomies be resited during the repair of recurrent incisional and parastomal hernias? Should the presence of these factors dictate which type of prosthetic is selected? Patients with prior colostomy or ileostomy incisions have additional levels of complexity that may make further recurrence even more difficult to prevent. Abdominal wall vascular supply may be interrupted so that standard repair techniques cannot be applied.

Finally, the repair of recurrent incisional hernias lends itself well to the old adage that "the first repair has the best chance to be the last repair." These patients have already failed an attempt at repair, and the likelihood of success probably decreases with each subsequent recurrence [3]. While surgeons cannot realistically expect to have recurrence-free complex hernia practices, proper patient selection, timing of surgery, and choice of surgical approach are paramount in the battle to minimize recurrence in this challenging patient population.

Open and Laparoscopic Approaches to Recurrent Incisional Hernias

Modified Rives-Stoppa Repair

Careful consideration of mesh placement relative to the anterior rectus sheath fascia should be included in the discussion of open recurrent incisional hernia repair. As suggested by the review from Awad previously cited, inlay and onlay open mesh repairs tend toward higher recurrence rates compared to sublay or underlay techniques.

The most commonly described technique for open mesh underlay is a modification of the Rives-Stoppa repair [15]. For the purposes of this discussion, this includes techniques described as "preperitoneal," "extraperitoneal," or "retromuscular" as well. Specifically, this technique involves several steps: (1) complete dissection and reduction of the hernia sac and its contents into the abdominal cavity, which may include lysis of adhesions and removal of other prosthetic material; (2) creation of a wide retrorectus plane, in which the posterior rectus sheath and peritoneum are dissected off the posterior surface of the rectus abdominis muscle and potentially further extended to the most lateral aspects of the abdominal wall; (3) primary closure of the posterior rectus sheath and/or peritoneum, to create a natural tissue barrier to avoid prosthetic contact with the viscera; (4) placement of a widely overlapped, permanent mesh prosthesis into the retrorectus space and securing it circumferentially; and (5) closure of the anterior rectus sheath [16].

This technique offers several advantages that help counteract some of the factors that may lead to recurrence. It is done in a relative tension-free fashion and excludes the mesh prosthesis from the viscera, reducing the potential for mesh infection and fistula formation. The retrorectus space is well vascularized, and the size of the space allows for a huge surface area for tissue ingrowth into the mesh. Finally, it theoretically allows the mesh to augment the strength of the abdominal wall when intra-abdominal pressure increases since the mesh lies deep to the anterior fascia [17].

Data supporting the use of this approach for recurrent incisional hernias are included in larger series of open Stoppa repairs for all incisional hernias. The Mayo Clinic series of 254 patients with complex incisional hernias repaired using this technique included 76 patients with recurrent hernias, some multiply recurrent. The majority of these hernias were midline incisional hernias, and most were repaired using polypropylene mesh. Overall hernia recurrence with mean follow-up of 70 months was 5%, though this was for the entire cohort, not just recurrent hernias. Interestingly, recurrence was much more common in patients who had wound infections [17]. Novitsky et al. published a series of 32 patients who underwent repair of *multiply* recurrent incisional hernias with open preperitoneal technique. Over half the patients were morbidly obese, and comorbidities such as diabetes, pulmonary disease, and smoking were common. Again, polypropylene mesh was used with very large surface area for ingrowth (mean 937 cm [2]). Mean follow-up of 28 months yielded only a single recurrence, occurring in a patient who required partial mesh removal due to infection. In their discussion, the authors stress the advantage of wide mesh overlap, which in some cases measured 8–10 cm [18]. Another series with mean follow-up of 34 months included 15 recurrent hernias repaired with modified Rives-Stoppa technique; only 1 recurrence occurred in a patient requiring mesh removal for infection [19].

There are drawbacks to this approach, however. The retromuscular dissection can be bloody, and it creates a large space which can be a source of hemorrhage in the early postoperative period. Additionally, the neurovascular innervation to the muscles of the abdominal wall lies just lateral to the rectus muscle, and significant long-term morbidity can result if this is injured. An earlier series reported high long-term postoperative pain scores in a significant proportion of patients, occurring in up to 27%. The use of slowly absorbing sutures may help minimize this potential complication.

Laparoscopic Recurrent Incisional Hernia Repair

Laparoscopic incisional hernia repair was introduced in the 1990s with the potential advantages of smaller incisions, less postoperative narcotic use, shorter hospital stay, and faster return to normal activity compared to open repair [20, 21]. The laparoscopic repair is performed with 3–5 ports placed on the lateral aspect of the abdominal wall. Once adhesiolysis and hernia reduction are completed, the mesh is inserted through a port and affixed to the abdominal wall. This can be achieved in a number of ways, with transfascial sutures, tacking devices, and adhesive sealants. This offers the same theoretical advantage as the Stoppa repair, with the mesh placed posterior to the abdominal wall as an augmentation. It also allows the surgeon to visualize the entire abdominal wall, preventing the potential for missed hernias described by Wassenaar [14]. It allows a potentially more accurate estimation of mesh overlap at the edges of the defect, which may help prevent the "edge of the mesh" recurrences described by Awad.

Several series of laparoscopic repair of recurrent incisional hernia have shown durability of the repairs at intermediate follow-up. Verbo and colleagues published a series of 41 recurrent hernias repaired using PTFE mesh. Patients underwent clinical exam and ultrasound examination at 6 and 12 months postoperatively, and only 1 recurrence was identified at mean follow-up of 38 months [22]. A prospective study by Uranues showed only three recurrences in 85 patients undergoing laparoscopic repair of multiply recurrent hernias with mean follow-up of 41 months. Interestingly, patients were followed with health-related quality of life scoring 2 years after surgery, and scores were significantly improved [23]. Both series included patients with larger hernias, and many had prior mesh repairs.

The question of superiority between laparoscopic and open recurrent incisional hernia repairs has not been borne out in the literature. Bingener compared two cohorts of patients undergoing laparoscopic incisional hernia repair to a group of patients undergoing open mesh *onlay*, which showed equivalent recurrence at long-term follow-up. Patients undergoing open repair had twice the rate of major morbidity as patients in the laparoscopic cohort [24]. A meta-analysis of randomized controlled trials comparing laparoscopic and open repair of any incisional hernia, not only recurrent hernias, showed no significant difference in recurrence rate between the two approaches. Laparoscopic hernia repair had a relative risk = 0.22 of wound infection compared to open repair. There was also a trend toward decreased mesh infection and bleeding complications with the laparoscopic approach [25]. An earlier series from the Cleveland Clinic showed similar recurrence rates for laparoscopic and open hernia repairs; however, patients who required conversion to open repair from a laparoscopic attempt had significantly higher recurrence. It is important to note the follow-up period in this study was 5 years, and the 25–30% overall recurrence rate after mesh repair may be a more accurate estimation of long-term recurrence with either technique [26].

Refinements to the technique of laparoscopic hernia repair may help reduce recurrence rates in these complex hernias. A major difference between the laparoscopic and open repairs is that open repair usually involves closure of the fascia anterior to the mesh underlay, which increases the surface area for potential mesh ingrowth and adds another barrier to mesh infection. Traditionally, laparoscopic hernia repair has not included primary closure of the fascial defect with mesh underlay. Some data suggests that this may reduce recurrence rate compared to standard techniques; this also creates a greater surface area for laparoscopic mesh fixation to the fascia, preventing mesh migration [27, 28]. Laparoscopic approaches to recurrent incisional hernias will likely continue to increase in utilization, and other technical considerations may help prevent recurrence.

Component Separation

While laparoscopic and open Stoppa repairs of recurrent incisional hernias rely heavily on prosthetic augmentation of the abdominal wall, autologous tissue closure of large, midline incisional hernia defects can be accomplished with abdominal wall component separation. This repair can be extremely valuable in patients with obvious contraindication to synthetic mesh placement, such as in contaminated fields. Synonymous techniques include "separation of parts," "bilateral myofascial release," and "sliding myofascial flap." Described by Ramirez in 1990, this technique allows a surgeon to increase the volume of the abdominal cavity by transposing the muscle layers of the abdominal wall while preserving neurovascular supply.

For recurrent incisional hernia repair that likely involves visceral adhesions, this technique requires several steps: (1) the abdomen is entered through a midline incision and a complete lysis of adhesions is performed; (2) the lateral most aspect of the rectus abdominis muscle is palpated; (3) the skin and subcutaneous fat are elevated from the anterior fascia, taking care to preserve the perforating branches of the epigastric and circumflex iliac vessels; (4) the external oblique aponeurosis is incised 2 cm lateral to the rectus muscle border and carried cranially to the costal margin, then caudally to the iliac crest; (5) the external and internal oblique muscles are bluntly separated from one another, allowing a release of the external layer so the rectus muscle may be advanced, tension-free, to the midline; (6) the same steps are repeated on the opposite side. This allows for advancement of the rectus muscle 3–5 cm in the upper abdomen, 7–10 cm in the mid abdomen, and 1–3 cm in the lower abdomen. If additional release is required, the posterior sheath can be separated from the rectus muscle, though this increases the risk of lateral abdominal wall defects postoperatively [29]. This allows closure of defects up to 15–20 cm in the midline with the standard approach, though other authors would dispute that such a large degree of mobilization is routinely achieved [30].

Results of component separation for recurrent incisional hernia should be considered in light of the types of hernias for which the technique is usually applied: very large, multiply recurrent hernias in challenging patients that may involve removal of other mesh prostheses or skin-graft removal. DiBello published a series of 35 patients with large (>10 cm), recurrent incisional hernias repaired with component separation and selective mesh underlay. Mean follow-up of 22 months yielded a recurrence rate of 9% [31]. Another retrospective cohort study of 284 patients with recurrent hernias demonstrated a recurrence rate of 22% in hernias repaired with component separation [32].

While these results are very good for large, recurrent incisional hernias, the operation carries significant risk of wound complications due to the large subcutaneous space created by the superficial dissection, which may predispose patients to infection. A series from the Netherlands demonstrated a 32% wound complication rate in 43 patients undergoing component separation for large incisional hernias [33]. A modification of the midline-subcutaneous dissection technique, popularized by Dumanian and others, avoids the creation of these large subcutaneous flaps. Instead, 6–8-cm transverse incisions are created at the anterior axillary line just below the costal margin. With the assistance of long, narrow retractors, the external oblique muscle is divided adjacent to the semilunar line, and this is carried from the costal margin to the iliac crest [34]. This allows preservation of the perforator blood supply to the skin and subcutaneous fat, which is particularly important in patients who have undergone prior stoma creation, which interrupts abdominal wall blood supply [29]. Others have used a combined endoscopic-open approach to component separation. This uses two or three trocars placed on either lateral abdominal wall. Using a technique similar to totally extraperitoneal laparoscopic inguinal hernia repair, the external oblique is incised, and the space between the external and internal oblique layers is balloon dissected. The external oblique fascia is divided vertically as with open component separation, and the dissection is repeated on the contralateral side [30, 35]. This may offer some benefit to standard open fascial release, but probably does not offer significant advantage over the technique that uses bilateral transverse incisions.

The use of mesh underlay for augmentation may provide additional value in combination with component separation. Some authors advocate the use of a dual-sided mesh such as PTFE or a coated polyester mesh placed intra-abdominally [31]. Others will place soft polypropylene intra-abdominally with omental coverage of the viscera [34]. One series showed zero recurrences with soft polypropylene mesh underlay in 18 patients at 1-year follow-up [34].

Special Techniques

Repair of recurrent incisional hernias in challenging patient populations, such as the morbidly obese, deserves special attention. These patients are more likely to develop primary incisional hernias, and recurrence rates after incisional hernia repair in the obese are higher than in lean patients [5, 36]. While the lofty goal of significant weight loss prior to elective hernia repair is admirable, the success and compliance with this plan is probably suboptimal. Wound complications after infraumbilical hernia repair are difficult to prevent, and removal of the redundant skin and subcutaneous fat over the infraumbilical abdomen during recurrent hernia repair may improve wound complication rates.

Given the association between wound complications, mesh infection, and hernia recurrence, consideration of this technique should be given to obese patients with lower midline incisional hernias. A series of 24 component separation hernia repairs combined with panniculectomy in obese patients showed four recurrences at 1 year [37]. In another study, a retromuscular mesh repair combined with a panniculectomy in 47 patients for repair of recurrent incisional hernias produced a recurrence rate of 8% [38]. However, others have demonstrated a significantly higher rate of wound complications *with* panniculectomy [39]. We would suggest that this combined approach to recurrent hernia repair with pannus removal should be carefully applied in select patients who will derive the greatest benefit from it.

Summary

Recurrent incisional hernias continue to be a challenging problem for both patients and surgeons. While the use of prosthetic material for nearly all recurrent hernias and advances in the knowledge of pathophysiology of hernia recurrence have helped reduce both recurrence rates and operative morbidity, a significant number of patients will unfortunately suffer yet another recurrent hernia. Basic investigation into the molecular mechanisms behind hernia recurrence will continue. Careful attention to the factors that lead to these recurrences may help in the planning of future operations. Refinements in surgical technique will continue to evolve. We remain optimistic that these advances will help our understanding of the appropriate treatments for recurrent hernias, reducing both the morbidity and the rate of recurrence.

References

1. Luijendijk RW, Lemmen MH, Hop WC, Wereldsma JC. Incisional hernia recurrence following “vest-over-pants” or vertical Mayo repair of primary hernias of the midline. World J Surg. 1997;21:62–5. discussion 6.
2. Luijendijk RW, Hop WC, van den Tol MP, et al. A comparison of suture repair with mesh repair for incisional hernia. N Engl J Med. 2000;343:392–8.
3. Hesselink VJ, Luijendijk RW, de Wilt JH, Heide R, Jeekel J. An evaluation of risk factors in incisional hernia recurrence. Surg Gynecol Obstet. 1993;176:228–34.

4. Flum DR, Horvath K, Koepsell T. Have outcomes of incisional hernia repair improved with time? A population-based analysis. Ann Surg. 2003;237:129–35.
5. Sugerman HJ, Kellum Jr JM, Reines HD, DeMaria EJ, Newsome HH, Lowry JW. Greater risk of incisional hernia with morbidly obese than steroid-dependent patients and low recurrence with prefascial polypropylene mesh. Am J Surg. 1996;171:80–4.
6. Anthony T, Bergen PC, Kim LT, et al. Factors affecting recurrence following incisional herniorrhaphy. World J Surg. 2000;24:95–100. discussion 1.
7. Rios A, Rodriguez JM, Munitiz V, Alcaraz P, Perez D, Parrilla P. Factors that affect recurrence after incisional herniorrhaphy with prosthetic material. Eur J Surg. 2001;167:855–9.
8. DuBay DA, Wang X, Adamson B, Kuzon Jr WM, Dennis RG, Franz MG. Mesh incisional herniorrhaphy increases abdominal wall elastic properties: a mechanism for decreased hernia recurrences in comparison with suture repair. Surgery. 2006;140:14–24.
9. Zheng H, Si Z, Kasperk R, et al. Recurrent inguinal hernia: disease of the collagen matrix? World J Surg. 2002;26:401–8.
10. Antoniou SA, Antoniou GA, Granderath FA, Simopoulos C. The role of matrix metalloproteinases in the pathogenesis of abdominal wall hernias. Eur J Clin Invest. 2009;39:953–9.
11. Rosch R, Lynen-Jansen P, Junge K, et al. Biomaterial-dependent MMP-2 expression in fibroblasts from patients with recurrent incisional hernias. Hernia. 2006;10:125–30.
12. Awad ZT, Puri V, LeBlanc K, et al. Mechanisms of ventral hernia recurrence after mesh repair and a new proposed classification. J Am Coll Surg. 2005;201:132–40.
13. Klinge U, Conze J, Krones CJ, Schumpelick V. Incisional hernia: open techniques. World J Surg. 2005;29:1066–72.
14. Wassenaar EB, Schoenmaeckers EJ, Raymakers JT, Rakic S. Recurrences after laparoscopic repair of ventral and incisional hernia: lessons learned from 505 repairs. Surg Endosc. 2009;23:825–32.
15. Stoppa RE. The treatment of complicated groin and incisional hernias. World J Surg. 1989;13:545–54.
16. Temudom T, Siadati M, Sarr MG. Repair of complex giant or recurrent ventral hernias by using tension-free intraparietal prosthetic mesh (Stoppa technique): lessons learned from our initial experience (fifty patients). Surgery. 1996;120:738–43. discussion 43–4.
17. Iqbal CW, Pham TH, Joseph A, Mai J, Thompson GB, Sarr MG. Long-term outcome of 254 complex incisional hernia repairs using the modified Rives-Stoppa technique. World J Surg. 2007;31:2398–404.
18. Novitsky YW, Porter JR, Rucho ZC, et al. Open preperitoneal retrofascial mesh repair for multiply recurrent ventral incisional hernias. J Am Coll Surg. 2006;203:283–9.
19. Bauer JJ, Harris MT, Gorfine SR, Kreel I. Rives-Stoppa procedure for repair of large incisional hernias: experience with 57 patients. Hernia. 2002;6:120–3.
20. Ramshaw BJ, Esartia P, Schwab J, et al. Comparison of laparoscopic and open ventral herniorrhaphy. Am Surg. 1999;65:827–31. discussion 31–2.
21. Park A, Birch DW, Lovrics P. Laparoscopic and open incisional hernia repair: a comparison study. Surgery. 1998;124:816–21. discussion 21–2.
22. Verbo A, Petito L, Manno A, et al. Laparoscopic approach to recurrent incisional hernia repair: a 3-year experience. J Laparoendosc Adv Surg Tech A. 2007;17:591–5.

23. Uranues S, Salehi B, Bergamaschi R. Adverse events, quality of life, and recurrence rates after laparoscopic adhesiolysis and recurrent incisional hernia mesh repair in patients with previous failed repairs. J Am Coll Surg. 2008;207:663–9.
24. Bingener J, Buck L, Richards M, Michalek J, Schwesinger W, Sirinek K. Long-term outcomes in laparoscopic vs. open ventral hernia repair. Arch Surg. 2007;142:562–7.
25. Forbes SS, Eskicioglu C, McLeod RS, Okrainec A. Meta-analysis of randomized controlled trials comparing open and laparoscopic ventral and incisional hernia repair with mesh. Br J Surg. 2009;96:851–8.
26. Ballem N, Parikh R, Berber E, Siperstein A. Laparoscopic versus open ventral hernia repairs: 5 year recurrence rates. Surg Endosc. 2008;22:1935–40.
27. Banerjee A, Beck C, Narula VK, Linn JG, Noria S, Zagol BR, Mikami DJ. Laparoscopic ventral hernia repair—does primary repair in addition to placement of mesh decrease recurrence? Surg Endosc. 2012;26(5):1264–8.
28. Franklin Jr ME, Gonzalez Jr JJ, Glass JL, Manjarrez A. Laparoscopic ventral and incisional hernia repair: an 11-year experience. Hernia. 2004;8:23–7.
29. Bleichrodt RP, de Vries Reilingh TS, Malyar A, et al. Component separation technique to repair large midline hernias. Operat Tech Gen Surg. 2004;6(3):179–88.
30. Rosen MJ, Fatima J, Sarr MG. Repair of abdominal wall hernias with restoration of abdominal wall function. J Gastrointest Surg. 2010;14:175–85.
31. DiBello Jr JN, Moore Jr JH. Sliding myofascial flap of the rectus abdominus muscles for the closure of recurrent ventral hernias. Plast Reconstr Surg. 1996;98:464–9.
32. Girotto JA, Chiaramonte M, Menon NG, et al. Recalcitrant abdominal wall hernias: long-term superiority of autologous tissue repair. Plast Reconstr Surg. 2003;112:106–14.
33. de Vries Reilingh TS, van Goor H, Rosman C, et al. "Components separation technique" for the repair of large abdominal wall hernias. J Am Coll Surg. 2003;196:32–7.
34. Ko JH, Wang EC, Salvay DM, Paul BC, Dumanian GA. Abdominal wall reconstruction: lessons learned from 200 "components separation" procedures. Arch Surg. 2009;144:1047–55.
35. Rosen MJ, Jin J, McGee MF, Williams C, Marks J, Ponsky JL. Laparoscopic component separation in the single-stage treatment of infected abdominal wall prosthetic removal. Hernia. 2007;11:435–40.
36. Heniford BT, Park A, Ramshaw BJ, Voeller G. Laparoscopic repair of ventral hernias: nine years' experience with 850 consecutive hernias. Ann Surg. 2003;238:391–9. discussion 399–400.
37. Reid RR, Dumanian GA. Panniculectomy and the separation-of-parts hernia repair: a solution for the large infraumbilical hernia in the obese patient. Plast Reconstr Surg. 2005;116:1006–12.
38. Berry MF, Paisley S, Low DW, Rosato EF. Repair of large complex recurrent incisional hernias with retromuscular mesh and panniculectomy. Am J Surg. 2007;194:199–204.
39. Harth KC, Blatnik JA, Rosen MJ. Optimum repair for massive ventral hernias in the morbidly obese patient-is panniculectomy helpful? Am J Surg. 2011;201:396–400. discussion.

34. Chronic Mesh Infections

Andrei Churyla and Andrew B. Lederman

The use of synthetic mesh has become the standard for repair of many types of hernias since mesh repairs have significantly lower rates of hernia recurrence [1–3]. However, with the use of synthetic meshes comes the risk of infection. While the majority of mesh infections are acute infections, presenting either early in the postoperative period or as delayed infections, chronic mesh infections may also develop.

Chronic mesh infections can result from various clinical scenarios. Often chronic infections result from untreated or incompletely treated acute infections or from attempts at mesh salvage when acutely infected. While mesh explantation is the primary treatment for acute mesh infection, attempts at mesh salvage via antibiotics and percutaneous drainage, dressing changes, or negative pressure wound therapy may result in chronic infection.

Presentation

Synthetic mesh can harbor bacteria and may present as an indolent infection several years after implantation [4, 5]. Chronic mesh infections may present without an acute phase, as a chronic non-healing wound, sinus tract, or a wound with cycles of spontaneous closure followed by wound dehiscence and drainage. Sinus tracts or associated enterocutaneous fistulae tend to be very low output and may even appear to heal only to spontaneously drain in the future.

Diagnosis is usually based on a history of mesh implantation and the presence of an associated chronic wound. A history of postoperative wound infection, previous mesh infections, or sepsis should raise a suspicion of mesh infection. Systemic signs of infection are variable. Fever, leukocytosis, elevated erythrocyte sedimentation rate or other

B.P. Jacob and B. Ramshaw (eds.), *The SAGES Manual of Hernia Repair*, DOI 10.1007/978-1-4614-4824-2_34,

markers of inflammation are unreliable indicators of chronic mesh infection. Imaging with CT scan, white blood cell nuclear medicine scan, or sinogram may be useful to demonstrate inflammation or fluid around mesh, but the diagnostic yield is variable. The best diagnostic test is usually to probe an open wound with a cotton swab or finger, often making the diagnosis by palpating the rough edge of exposed mesh. Percutaneous drainage of suspected infections or fluid collections might prove infection, but also introduce the risk of infecting a potentially sterile mesh; drainage is more useful as a therapeutic maneuver for known infections rather than a diagnostic test.

Biomaterials

The type of mesh may influence the risk of developing chronic infections. The ability of bacteria to adhere to mesh is affected by the surface area of the mesh, the hydrophilic or hydrophobic nature of the material, and the pore size of the mesh. Additionally, mesh coatings and composite meshes made of more than one type of material also influence the potential for infections.

Multifilament meshes, typically made from polypropylene, have a significantly greater surface area for bacterial adherence and may be more prone to infection. This results in a higher rate of fistula formation and persistence of bacteria when attempts are made to salvage mesh [6, 7]. Monofilament mesh limits the adherence of bacteria and may be less prone to chronic infection.

Microporous mesh, such as PTFE or ePTFE with a pore <10 μm, will allow adherence of bacteria, but the pores are too small to admit leukocytes. This small pore size limits the propensity to form adhesions but increases the risk of infection. When mesh gets infected, microporous mesh generally cannot be salvaged since infection cannot be cleared through immune response. In contrast, macroporous prostheses, typically polypropylene or polyester, allow for ingrowth of fibroblasts, macrophages, and collagen fibers. While this ingrowth may limit the risk of infection, it increases mesh contraction with scar formation. Although macroporous mesh may have a lower risk of infection, the higher risk of adhesion formation, erosion, and fistula formation make it a poor choice inside the peritoneum.

Composite mesh such as combination ePTFE and polypropylene presents a different problem. The different components stimulate a different immune response, causing fibroblast ingrowth, fibrin deposition, and mesh contraction at different rates depending on the layer. As the two layers of mesh contract at different rates, the layers tend to delaminate despite sutures securing them together. The mesh delamination creates a dead space between the mesh layers that may be prone to infection. Furthermore, the delamination may expose adhesiogenic polypropylene mesh to the bowel, that could lead to fistula formation.

Mesh coatings such as carboxymethylcellulose-sodium hyaluronate are highly hydrophilic and have been demonstrated in vitro to separate from the less hydrophilic polypropylene mesh. This leads to an increase in bacterial adherence compared to uncoated mesh [8].

Microbiology

Infection of a bioprosthesis by bacteria is dependent upon the ability of bacteria to adhere to mesh. While surface characteristics of the prosthetic play a role, adhesion is partly a function of the hydrophobicity and hydrophilicity of the microorganism itself [8]. For example, a hydrophobic organism such as Staphylococci binds with difficulty to a hydrophilic surface [9]. Gram-negative bacteria such as *Escherichia coli* and *Pseudomonas aeruginosa* bind with difficulty to hydrophobic mesh such as PTFE [10].

The source of the bacterial inoculation is frequently skin flora, either from contamination during the time of mesh placement or from postoperative wound complications. Staphylococcus species, including methicillin-sensitive *Staphylococcus aureus* (MSSA), methicillin-resistant *Staphylococcus aureus* (MRSA), *Staphylococcus epidermidis*, and *Streptococcus* species including group B organisms are common isolates. Skin flora that produce biofilms on the prosthetics, such as *S. epidermidis*, are particularly difficult to eradicate, and are often the reason for the chronic nature of the mesh infection. Antibiotic therapy with a first-generation cephalosporin or vancomycin may be useful in conjunction with surgical drainage or mesh explantation.

Gram-negative bacteria, including *Enterobacteriaceae* and anaerobic bacteria are less common isolates. Potential sources of contamination include direct contamination from wound infections, intra-abdominal infections or fistulae, or rarely hematogenous seeding. Rarely, fungal or atypical organisms can cause chronic mesh infections.

Management

Chronic mesh infections have an indolent presentation without signs of systemic infection. This allows for careful planning to control infection, remove unsalvageable mesh, resect gastrointestinal fistulae, and repair any resulting hernia. The standard for chronic mesh infection is mesh explantation and reconstruction. Prior to surgery, any cellulitis or acute abscess is controlled with antibiotics and drainage as necessary. Suspected fistulae may be studied with CT or sinogram to demonstrate the anatomy. The operative approach generally involves resection of sinus tracts, removing the infected mesh, and reconstructing the abdominal wall. Chronic gastrointestinal fistulae are resected, and an anastomosis can usually be safely created as long as the patient has fully recovered from previous abdominal surgery and has a good nutrition status. Reconstruction of the abdominal wall is often the most difficult task and may be accomplished with primary closure or component separation techniques. Biologic mesh may be useful as an adjunct to reinforce the tissue repair. Implantation of a prosthetic is not recommended due to the high risk of recurrent infection. Delayed closure after mesh explantation is also reported, utilizing negative pressure wound therapy (NPWT) or other wound care techniques as an interim.

Mesh salvage has also been reported but has limited success. This approach uses long-term antibiotic therapy, minimal debridement of visibly infected tissue or mesh, and often NPWT. Mesh salvage is only possible when infection is limited and the majority of mesh is incorporated into the abdominal wall. Although there are case reports of successful mesh salvage of PTFE, since PTFE is microporous and tends to have limited incorporation, it is much less likely to be successfully treated nonoperatively when compared to macroporous mesh.

Percutaneous drainage, open drainage, or serial debridements are usually necessary in order to achieve success with mesh salvage. These patients can usually be managed as an outpatient and rarely require inpatient care or procedures. There are several reports that describe good outcomes with long-term antibiotic irrigation of infected sinus tracts or cavities with mesh involvement [11]. The local or topical application of high-concentration antibiotics may help with mesh salvage.

The salvage of chronically infected mesh is only possible in certain circumstances [12]. The infection needs to be isolated to a small portion of the mesh, not involving the entire mesh. Macroporous mesh that allows for greater encapsulation with scar has a higher rate of mesh salvage than microporous mesh. While there are case reports of PTFE salvage, the lack of incorporation of PTFE into tissue generally precludes mesh salvage.

References

1. Grant AM. Open mesh versus non-mesh repair of groin hernia: meta-analysis of randomized trials based on individual patient data [corrected]. Hernia. 2002;6:130–6.
2. Birolini C, Utiyama EM, Rodrigues Jr AJ, Birolini D. Elective colonic operation and prosthetic repair of incisional hernia: does contamination contraindicate abdominal wall prosthesis use? J Am Coll Surg. 2000;191:366–72.
3. Leber GE, Garb JL, Alexander AI, Reed WP. Long-term complications associated with prosthetic repair of incisional hernias. Arch Surg. 1998;133:378–82.
4. Mann DV, Prout J, Havranek E, et al. Late-onset deep prosthetic infection following mesh repair of inguinal hernia. Am J Surg. 1998;176:12–4.
5. Taylor SG, O'Dwyer PJ. Chronic groin sepsis following tension-free inguinal hernioplasty. Br J Surg. 1999;86:562–5.
6. Amid PK, Shulman AG, Lichtenstein IL, et al. Biomaterials for abdominal wall hernia surgery and principles of their applications. Langenbecks Arch Surg. 1994;379:168–71.
7. Demiter S, Gecim IE, Aydinuraz K, et al. Affinity of Staphylococcus epidermidis to various prosthetic graft materials. J Surg Res. 2001;99:70–4.
8. Aydinuraz K, Agalar C, Agalar F, et al. In vitro S. epidermidis and S. aureus adherence to composite and lightweight polypropylene grafts. J Surg Res. 2009;157:e79–86.
9. Reifsteck F, Wee S, Wilkinson BJ. Hydrophobicity—hydrophilicity of staphylococci. J Med Microbiol. 1987;24:65–73.
10. Engelsman AF, Gooitzen MD, van der Mei HC, et al. In vivo evaluation of bacterial infection involving morphologically different surgical meshes. Ann Surg. 2010;251(1):133–7.
11. Trunzo JA, Ponsky JL, et al. A novel approach for salvaging infected prosthetic mesh after ventral hernia repair. Hernia. 2009;13:545–9.
12. http://sageswiki.org/index.php?title=Use_of_synthetic_mesh_in_the_infected_field. Accessed 5 July 2011.

35. Adhesions After Lap Ventral: Do They Matter?

Dennis L. Fowler

The Incidence and Consequences of Intra-abdominal Adhesions

Intra-abdominal adhesions are the cause of significant morbidity and mortality. Beyond the technical challenge posed by adhesions, they cause enormous human suffering and cost to society. In 1994, a comprehensive report based on the National Hospital Discharge Survey indicated that 303,836 patients underwent adhesiolysis [1]. These procedures were associated with 846,415 inpatient days and incurred $1.3 billion in hospital and surgeon costs. Ten years later, those numbers had increased slightly. In 2004, more than 342,000 patients underwent adhesiolysis [2]. Many other patients who did not require adhesiolysis were admitted to the hospital with either a bowel obstruction or complaints of pain caused by adhesions. Many other patients are afflicted with infertility caused by adhesions [3–5].

In addition to the human and financial cost of treating conditions that are caused by adhesions, they are commonly the cause of adverse consequences during surgery for conditions unrelated to the adhesions themselves. The presence of adhesions increases the chance of converting a laparoscopic operation to an open operation, increases the time required to enter the abdomen, and is the primary cause of bowel injury at the time of trocar insertion during laparoscopic surgery [6]. In short, adhesions are frequently the cause of a significant technical complication during an operation.

Although any condition inciting an inflammatory response may cause intra-abdominal adhesions, by far, the most common cause of adhesions is previous surgery. Until the late twentieth century, surgeons performed essentially all abdominal surgery with an open laparotomy, and up to 95% of patients who undergo a laparotomy develop adhesions [7, 8]. Depending

B.P. Jacob and B. Ramshaw (eds.), *The SAGES Manual of Hernia Repair*,
DOI 10.1007/978-1-4614-4824-2_35,

on the underlying disease and the nature of the procedure at the time of the primary surgical procedure, up to 30% of patients will develop a bowel obstruction secondary to adhesions after a laparotomy. [9] After any colon resection, patients have a 5–10% chance of an adhesion-related admission within 5 years, and the incidence of adhesion-related admission within 5 years after proctocolectomy is 15.4% [10, 11].

The size and orientation of the laparotomy incision may be factors in the development of adhesions, but there is no reliable method to prevent adhesions during surgery [12]. Anecdotal experience and some initial observational studies suggested that laparoscopic surgery resulted in fewer and less severe adhesions than those caused by laparotomy [13]; however, other studies regarding adhesions after colorectal surgery suggest that the incidence of adhesions is not significantly different between open and laparoscopic colectomy [14].

Some of the important factors that increase the likelihood of extensive adhesion formation include ischemia, surgical trauma, inflammation, hemorrhage, thermal injury, and reactions to foreign bodies [15]. Although foreign bodies such as gloves, powders, sutures, sponges, and irrigating solutions all incite a response that can lead to adhesion formation, the foreign body of most concern in this discussion is hernia mesh.

Prosthetic Mesh as a Cause of Adhesions

Most surgeons have seen extensive, dense adhesions between polypropylene mesh and viscera at the time of re-exploration in patients with previously placed intraperitoneal mesh. Because these findings often led to difficult operations and sometimes caused complications, surgeons became reluctant to place mesh intraperitoneally. The occasional occurrence of these extremely difficult situations has led to attempts to develop mesh that would incite fewer adhesions. The main concern on reoperation after previous intra-abdominal mesh placement is the ingrowth that can occur between the viscera and a macroporous mesh. Adherence (adhesions) without ingrowth results in minimal to moderate effort to lyse the adhesions. But, with ingrowth, the mesh may need to be cut off of the abdominal wall, or a bowel resection may need to be performed to complete an operation. In rare cases, ingrowth may also lead to fistula or abscess formation.

There is no widely accepted method for determining the extent and density of adhesions in the peritoneal cavity short of abdominal exploration. Because it is unethical to subject patients to repeat laparotomy or laparoscopy simply to explore for the presence of adhesions, investigators cannot conclusively determine the extent and density of adhesions formed after mesh placement. We really only know the extent of adhesion formation in the small, but significant, percent of patients who require a repeat operation after mesh placement. For this reason, to evaluate meshes that were designed to prevent adhesions, investigators have documented for several types of new meshes the extent and density of adhesion formation at either laparoscopy or necropsy in several animal studies [16–27].

These studies typically compare the extent and severity of adhesion formation after placement of a composite mesh (two layers) or coated mesh (single layer) with the extent and severity of adhesion formation after placement of a single-layer uncoated mesh, usually polypropylene. The composite mesh is designed to enable excellent tissue ingrowth into one layer while preventing adhesion formation and/or ingrowth into the other layer. The layer designed to lie against the abdominal wall is called the parietal layer, and the layer designed to lie against the omentum or viscera is called the visceral layer.

The parietal layer is usually a porous synthetic mesh with interstices into which the body can grow. The porous layer should enable firm incorporation of the mesh into the parietes. The visceral layer is microporous, usually either expanded polytetrafluoroethylene (ePTFE) or an anti-adhesive material such as a hydrophilic anti-adhesive collagen layer, a hyaluronate/carboxymethylcellulose combination, or polyvinylidene fluoride although other materials have also been tested. A coated mesh is a single-layer mesh that is coated with a material to prevent adhesions, such as a hydrogel.

Most studies in the animals documented tissue ingrowth into the parietal layer of the composite or coated mesh that was equivalent to ingrowth into plain polypropylene but with fewer and less dense adhesions to the visceral layer than to plain polypropylene. Based on the results of animal studies, surgeons often choose a composite mesh hoping that fewer serious adhesions will form. However, there are no human studies confirming this. Despite the belief that the composite meshes cause fewer intraperitoneal adhesions, there continues to be occasional anecdotal reports of serious adhesions caused by composite meshes [28] (Fig. 35.1).

Some investigators have reported successful identification and documentation of the location and density of intraperitoneal adhesions with the use of abdominal ultrasound [29]; however, not all investigators have found the use of ultrasound to accurately identify adhesions.

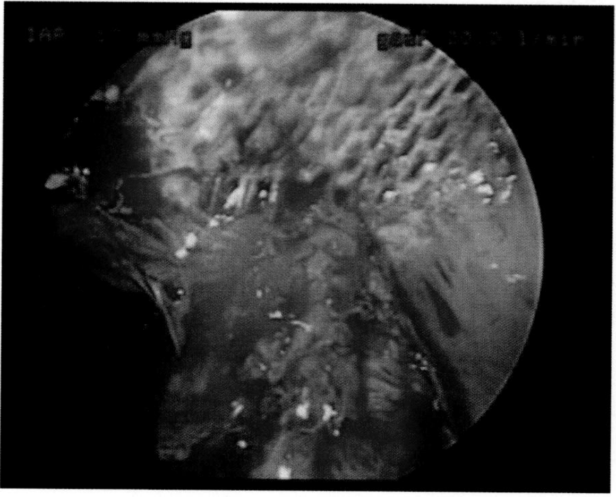

Fig. 35.1. Intraoperative photograph showing dense adhesions between a composite mesh and the small intestine.

Conclusions

There is no experimental evidence from human studies that one mesh is better than another, despite evidence in animal studies that some meshes incite fewer and less dense adhesions. However, the severity of the adhesion problem is clear, and the role of mesh in the formation of adhesions is clear. Based on the evidence from animal studies and solid theoretical reasons, the use of a composite mesh with an anti-adhesive layer seems appropriate when hernia repair requires intraperitoneal mesh [30].

Summary

Adhesions are a serious and very significant cause of morbidity and mortality in the USA. Many synthetic mesh products incite extensive and dense adhesion formation in the abdominal cavity if placed intraperitoneally. Because it is necessary to use mesh in many patients who require hernia repair, it is theoretically and experimentally desirable to use a mesh designed to reduce adhesion formation if intraperitoneal placement of mesh is necessary.

References

1. Ray NF, Denton WG, Thamer M, et al. Abdominal adhesiolysis: inpatient care and experience in the Unites States in 1994. JACS. 1998;186:1–9.
2. DeFrances CJ, Podgornik MN. 2004 National hospital discharge survey. Advance data from vital and healthc statistics; no 371. Hyattwsville, MD: National Center for Health Statistics. 2006.
3. Latenser B. Commentary (A novel hydrogel-coated polyester mesh prevents post-surgical adhesions in a rat model). J Surg Res. 2011;166:73–4.
4. Judge TW, Parker DM, Dinsmore RC. Abdominal wall hernia repair: a comparison of Sepramesh and Parietex composite mesh in a rabbit hernia model. J Am Coll Surg. 2007;204:76.
5. Emans PJ, Schreinemacher MH, Gijbels MJ, et al. Polypropylene meshes to prevent abdominal herniation. Can stable coatings prevent adhesions in the long term? Ann Biomed Eng. 2009;37:410.
6. van Goor H. Consequences and complications of peritoneal adhesions. Colorectal Dis. 2007;2:25–34.
7. Lower AM, Hawthorn RJ, Ellis H, O'Brien F, Buchan S, Crowe AM. The impact of adhesions on hospital readmissions over ten years after 8849 open gynaecological operations: an assessment from the Surgical and Clinical Adhesions Research Study. BJOG. 2000;107(7):855–62.
8. Fukuhira Y, Ito M, Kakenko H, et al. Prevention of postoperative adhesions by a novel honeycomb-patterned poly(lactide) film in a rat experimental model. J Biomed Mater Res B Appl Biomater. 2008;86B:353.
9. Ellis H, Moran BJ, Thompson JN, et al. Adhesion-related hospital readmissions after abdominal and pelvic surgery: a retrospective cohort study. Lancet. 1999;353(9163): 1476–80.
10. Parker MC, Wilson MS, Menzies D, et al. The SCAR-3 study: 5-year adhesion-related readmission risk following lower abdominal surgical procedures. Colorectal Dis. 2005;7(6):551–8.
11. Parikh JA, Ko CY, Magard MA, et al. What is the rate of small bowel obstruction after colectomy? Am Surg. 2008;74:1001–5.
12. van der Wal JBC, Lordens GIT, Vrijland WW, et al. Adhesion prevention during laparotomy. Ann Surg. 2011;253(6):1118–21.
13. Barmparas G, Branco BC, Schnuriger B, et al. The incidence and risk factors of post-laparotomy adhesive small bowel obstruction. J Gastrointest Surg. 2010;14:1619–28.
14. Khury E, Schwenk W, Gaupset R, et al. Long-term outcome of laparoscopic surgery for colorectal cancer: a Cochrane systematic review of randomized controlled trials. Cancer Treat Rev. 2008;34:498–504.
15. Liakakos T, Thomakos N, Fine P, et al. Peritoneal adhesions: etiology, pathophysiology, and clinical significance. Dig Surg. 2001;18:260–73.
16. Goldberg JM, Toledo AA, Mitchell DE. An evaluation of the Gore-Tex surgical membrane for the prevention of postoperative peritoneal adhesions. Obstet Gynecol. 1987;70(6):846–8.

17. Duffy AJ, Hogle NJ, LaPerle KM, et al. Comparison of two composite meshes using two fixation devices in a porcine laparoscopic ventral hernia repair model. Hernia. 2004;8:358–64.
18. McGinty JJ, Hogle NJ, McCarthy H, et al. A comparative study of adhesion formation and abdominal wall ingrowth after laparoscopic ventral hernia repair in a porcine model using multiple types of mesh. Surg Endosc. 2005;19(6):786–90.
19. Gonzalez R, Rodeheaver GT, Moody DL, et al. Resistance to adhesion formation: a comparative study of treated and untreated mesh products placed in the abdominal cavity. Hernia. 2004;8:213–9.
20. Harrell AG, Novitsky YW, Peindl RD, et al. Prospective evaluation of adhesion formation and shrinkage of intra-abdominal prosthetics in a rabbit model. Am Surg. 2006;72(9):808–13.
21. Novitsky YW, Harrell AG, Cristiano JA, et al. Comparative evaluation of adhesion formation, strength of ingrowth, and textile properties of prosthetic meshes after long-term intra-abdominal implantation in a rabbit. J Surg Res. 2007;140(1):6–11.
22. Jacob B, Hogle NJ, Durak E, et al. Tissue ingrowth and bowel adhesion formation in an animal comparative study: polypropylene vs. Proceed® vs. Parietex Composite®. Surg Endosc. 2007;21(4):629–33.
23. Novitsky YW, Harrell AG, Hope WW, et al. Meshes in hernia repair. Surg Technol Int. 2007;16:123–7.
24. Gruber-Blum S, Petter-Puchner AH, Brand J, et al. Comparison of three separate antiadhesive barriers for intraperitoneal onlay mesh hernia repair in an experimental model. Br J Surg. 2010;98:442–9.
25. Fortelny RH, Petter-Puchner AH, Glaser KS, et al. Adverse effects of polyvinylidene fluoride-coated polypropylene mesh used for laparoscopic intraperitoneal onlay repair of Incisional hernia. Br J Surg. 2010;97:1140–5.
26. Letter 1 and Letter 2 re: Fortelny, et al. in BJS;97:1140–5. Br J Surg. 2011;98:156–60.
27. Bringman S, Conze J, Cuccurulla D, et al. Hernia repair: the search for ideal meshes. Hernia. 2010;14:81–7.
28. Jenkins ED, Yom V, Melman L, et al. Prospective evaluation of adhesion characteristics to intraperitoneal mesh and adhesiolysis-related complications during laparoscopic re-exploration after prior ventral hernia repair. Surg Endosc. 2010;24:3002–7.
29. Arnaud JP, Hennekinee-Mucci S, Pessaux P, et al. Ultrasound detection of visceral adhesion after intraperitoneal ventral hernia treatment: a comparative study of protected versus unprotected meshes. Hernia. 2003;7:85–8.
30. Eriksen JR, Gogenur I, Rosenberg J. Choice of mesh for laparoscopic ventral hernia repair. Hernia. 2007;11:481–92.

36. Chronic Pain After Ventral Hernia Repair

Victor B. Tsirline, David A. Klima, Igor Belyansky, and Kent W. Kercher

Prior to the widespread use of synthetic mesh for ventral hernia repair (VHR), recurrence after primary fascial repair was an accepted yet disappointing complication in up to 67% of repairs [1]. Mesh reinforcement has now helped to drastically reduce recurrence rates to <10% in a majority of studies [1–6] with only the most complicated repairs having higher recurrence rates of up to 29% [7–10]. With an ever increasing number of VHR performed in the United States (now reaching an estimated 250,000 annually) [11] and advancements in hernia repair techniques and materials, attention has become increasingly focused on functional outcomes, quality-of-life measures, and aesthetics. Chronic pain, specifically, has dominated the literature with regard to inguinal hernia repair for years and more recently has become a major focus in VHR [12, 13]. While the incidence of chronic pain after VHR is variable, surgeons may choose not to operate on an asymptomatic patient for fear of the chronic consequences patients may face. In the subsequent text, we seek to define chronic pain and help identify the etiologies, treatments, and plausible efforts to avoid pain in this relatively common procedure.

Definitions

The International Association for the Study of Pain (IASP) defines chronic pain as pain lasting more than 3 months after insult. In defining post-herniorrhaphy pain, it is important to distinguish between surgical and neuropathic pain. Surgical pain is inevitable, generally uniform, and resolves over time. It arises from a combination of sharp skin incision,

B.P. Jacob and B. Ramshaw (eds.), *The SAGES Manual of Hernia Repair*,
DOI 10.1007/978-1-4614-4824-2_36,

tension at the fixation points, and postoperative inflammation due to tissue dissection and mesh implantation. The healing and scarring is 90% complete at 6 weeks and most patients have no signs of surgical pain by 6 months. In contrast, neuropathic pain is typically caused by direct injury to a sensory nerve. This trauma can subsequently result in spontaneous firing of the injured or impinged neuronal fibers and aberrant repair of the nerve fibers leading to chronic pain sensation. Neuropathic pain may present as chronic pain sensation, hyperesthesia, sensitivity to temperature or light touch, altered sensation, or even phantom pain (rarely in the case of hernia repair). While neuropathic pain may be confined to the specific area of injury, it can frequently be referred to specific anatomic areas innervated by the injured nerve, which may be remote from the site of herniorrhaphy, thus making identification of the offending source difficult.

Incidence

While most surgeons utilize 3 months as a defining time point for chronic pain, definitions are mixed throughout the literature with differences in severity and duration as the predominate causes for discrepancy. Because of this variability, the reported rate of chronic pain can be as high as 43% [14]. However, review of the literature using the above guidelines suggests that the rate of significant chronic postoperative pain after VHR is 1–6% [12, 13, 15]. As with inguinal herniorrhaphy, it has been noted that younger patients have a greater tendency to report persistent pain than older patients [16]. Whether recurrent or first-time hernia repairs are associated with a greater likelihood of chronic pain is not clear, with mixed results reported in the literature. Several recent studies found no effect of hernia location or mesh size on subacute postoperative pain scores [16, 17].

Causes of Chronic Pain

The causes of chronic pain after ventral hernia repair are unfortunately poorly understood. Despite this, surgeon experience and literature have focused on one of three major etiologies, which include transfascial fixation, mesh selection, and surgical technique. Other less likely etiologies of chronic pain include adhesions and microabrasion of the parietal peritoneum. Nonetheless, recent studies have established that preoperative pain is likely the best predictor of postoperative pain and should be controlled for in all studies evaluating chronic pain. In fact, a recent review of 226 VHR in patients who were asymptomatic or minimally symptomatic preoperatively yielded no patients with chronic postoperative pain [18].

Sutures, Tacks, and Glue

The placement of mesh, while beneficial for limiting hernia recurrence, is not without consequences. Fixation of mesh to the abdominal wall is an important step in minimizing recurrences. Transfascial sutures have become the most commonly utilized fixation technique in both laparoscopic and open repairs. Patients who experience prolonged postoperative pain after ventral or incisional hernia repair often complain of focal pain at the site of transfascial suture fixation. This is usually described as a pulling sensation exacerbated by abdominal stretch, leading many surgeons to believe that chronic pain arises predominantly from the transfascial fixation. The finding that local anesthetic injection at suture sites sometimes resolves this chronic problem further supports this notion [19]. The mechanism of transfascial suture site pain is poorly understood; possible explanations include intercostal nerve entrapment, local muscle ischemia, and mesh contraction leading to persistent nerve irritation. Opponents argue that patients report persistent pain in 7.4% of cases without transabdominal suture fixation [20] and 2.5% of cases where only fibrin glue is used for fixation [21, 22]. Other authors have reported statistically higher pain scores with suture fixation during the first month postoperatively with no differences at 6 months and thereafter [23].

Tacks, fascial staples, and other mechanical anchoring devices also embed themselves in the fascia and are used primarily in laparoscopic repair. They, however, do not traverse the entire abdominal wall and thus are theorized to cause less pain and nerve impingement. In a randomized trial of metallic tacks versus absorbable or nonabsorbable suture fixation, Wassenaar showed no difference in pain between groups at 6 weeks or 3 months postoperatively or any difference in change from preoperative to postoperative pain levels [24]. Similar findings were reported in case–control studies comparing multiple (20 or more) transfascial sutures with tacks, limited transfascial sutures (typically four) with tacks, and tacks alone [25, 26]. In a recent series of 1,242 laparoscopic VHR, transfascial suture fixation plus tacks was associated with slightly higher incidence of chronic pain (16.4%) compared to tacks alone (13.3%) but did not reach statistical significance ($p<0.078$) [27]. While fibrin glue holds promise in reducing the incidence of chronic pain, randomized prospective trials comparing glue against tacks and transabdominal sutures are needed to establish its efficacy and confirm its utility with regard to durability, safety, recurrence rates, and complications related to mesh displacement.

Laparoscopic Versus Open Repair

Multiple studies over the past decade have documented improved patient satisfaction with laparoscopic compared to open repairs [16, 17, 28]. However, in long-term follow-up, postoperative chronic pain occurred in 10–19% of patients after abdominal wall hernia repair, with no significant difference in the median visual analog scale (VAS) score between open and laparoscopic groups [29]. While surgical pain, hospital length of stay, and recovery time are usually less after laparoscopic repair, it is important to distinguish these from chronic postoperative pain. The former is likely secondary to smaller incisions and less surgical pain, while the latter is more likely a combination of the prosthesis, fixation, technique, and patient-related factors than the surgical approach.

Effects of Mesh

While the routine use of mesh in hernia repair has overwhelmingly reduced recurrence rates, it has brought about new challenges such as altered abdominal wall compliance, adhesion formation, and foreign-body reaction—all of which could contribute to chronic postoperative pain [25, 30]. The inflammatory reaction associated with mesh enhances scar formation and potentially strengthens the repair but is inevitably associated with some degree of added discomfort. The inflammatory-mediated process of scar formation and remodeling is almost complete by 90 days and is thus likely not the cause of chronic pain. The mesh material itself tends to undergo contraction, with traditional heavyweight polypropylene, contracting up to 12% despite proper fixation [23]. At the extremes, in patients with mesh-related pain, mesh shrinkage of up to

63% has been documented [25]. Mesh shrinkage may continue for 6 months or longer, resulting in pain from tissue abrasion, tension on the transfascial sutures, and foreign-body sensation. The role of mesh contraction is supported by findings of reduced postoperative pain with lightweight mesh compared to heavyweight mesh, the latter being more prone to contraction and fibrosis. In a study comparing Marlex (Bard, heavyweight), Atrium (medium weight), and Vypro (Ethicon, lightweight) meshes, after 4 months postoperatively, paraesthesias were noted in 58%, 16%, and 4% of patients, respectively. Patients complained of symptoms during activity in 17%, 16%, and 7%, and at rest in 9%, 3%, and 0% of cases, respectively [31].

Other Theories

While surgical technique, mesh type, and mechanical fixation are major factors in postoperative pain after VHR, there are other considerations that may be important. Adhesions have been suggested by Carbajo et al. as 7.4% of patients in their series reported prolonged postoperative pain despite the absence of transfascial mesh fixation [20]. Others have demonstrated the role of polyester-based materials in adhesion formation leading to visceral pain [17]. These authors and others have argued that adhesion formation could be a significant source of postoperative pain and emphasized the value of complete adhesiolysis during incisional hernia repair [32, 33]. Adhesiolysis does come with its own risk, and we do not necessarily adhere to this model, especially if the adhesions do not interfere with the placement of the mesh or the adequacy of hernia repair. Microabrasion of the highly sensitive parietal peritoneum may also be a cause of chronic pain, especially with the implant of mesh, which may be continuously irritated by wrinkles or contraction of the prosthetic. This may perhaps lead to more generalized chronic pain which cannot be well localized.

Time Course of Chronic Pain

Most patients undergoing ventral or incisional hernia repair, whether open or laparoscopic, experience a significant amount of surgical pain, requiring intravenous or enteral narcotic medications. Acute postoperative pain typically begins to resolve within 1–2 weeks after surgery. The hernia literature commonly documents mild to moderate pain at 6-week follow-up, with significant reduction by 6 months after surgery [29]. In most studies comparing different mesh types, implantation techniques, and fixation modalities, no differences in pain are seen between groups at 6 months postoperatively [17, 34]. Therefore, it may be prudent to postpone surgical revisions due to persistent pain until 6 months after surgery or later. Nerve irritation will often resolve spontaneously as the inflammatory response subsides and the scar tissue reorganizes. We have found in our experience consistent trends of slightly increased pain by 1 month postoperatively compared to preoperative levels, with significant decline in pain by 6 months after surgery, with similar levels at 1-year and 2-year follow-up [18].

Patient Satisfaction

Patient satisfaction after VHR is >85% in most studies, despite 20–38% of patients experiencing occasional pain, 43% altered abdominal wall mobility, 31% foreign-body sensation, and 13% using medications for pain relief [35, 36]. On the other hand, functional outcome and recurrence appears to play a major role in patient satisfaction. Snyder et al. showed that patients who had a recurrence were four times more likely to report unsatisfactory outcomes [16]. In addition, patients with active recurrence were more likely to have moderate to severe sensory and affective pain, higher levels of pain at rest, and more movement limitation secondary to pain. The type of repair alone did not appear to have an effect on patient satisfaction. Multiple studies document overall improved quality of life (physical and mental component summary scores on the Short Form SF-36 questionnaire) in patients after surgery compared to before surgery, for both open and laparoscopic procedures [24, 37], despite the real incidence of chronic pain in some of these patients.

Pain Assessment

Patient quality of life and satisfaction with surgery should be differentiated from pain and discomfort related to abdominal defect repair and mesh implantation. SF-36 is a well-established quality-of-life instrument, which takes into account the patient's psychological perception, emotions, attitudes, and physical capabilities. While SF-36 provides a global quality-of-life picture, pain assessment is most commonly performed and reported in the literature on a subjective visual analog scale (0–10 or 0–100, the upper limit being the worst possible pain). Lack of specific definition of the VAS scale as well as variation in the meaning of "worst pain ever" between individuals or throughout the course of treatment serves as a major source of type I error in identifying statistically significant differences in pain between groups. Furthermore, there is no uniform agreement on what constitutes a clinically significant score or change on the VAS scale.

More robust and extensively validated instruments for postoperative pain and functional assessment are available such as the Carolinas Comfort Scale™ (CCS) and McGill Pain Scale [38]. The CCS is a 23-item questionnaire through which patients report not only pain but also severity of mesh sensation and degree of movement limitation on a 6-point Likert scale for a predefined set of activities such as sitting, walking, coughing, and exercise. The Carolinas Comfort Scale has been shown to be more sensitive and specific for hernia repair outcomes than generic health questionnaires [39] and should be strongly considered for measuring hernia surgery quality-of-life outcomes.

Treatment

The most common treatment of acute postoperative pain is systemic or oral opioid analgesia, despite the recognized side effects of nausea, constipation, pruritus, and sedation. The use of local anesthesia has been advocated based, and several randomized trials have been conducted for inguinal herniorrhaphy analgesia [40, 41]. Patients who received bupivacaine infusion pumps had significantly lower narcotic requirements during the first five postoperative days; many (up to 24%) required no narcotic medications. Some authors suggest that, unlike systemic narcotics, the use of local anesthesia to prevent the sensation of pain may be associated with less catecholamine release, less vasoconstriction, better tissue perfusion, and ultimately improved wound healing. Additionally, local anesthetic infusion provides faster therapeutic levels than systemic opioids, with significantly better pain control on postoperative day 1 [41]. The use of elastomeric pumps has shown promise in reducing narcotic requirements and hospital stay after donor nephrectomy and colon resection. However, a recent randomized double-blind trial showed no differences in pain levels, narcotic requirements

(40.8–44.5 mg/day vs. 32.1–52.2 mg/day for the first three postoperative days), return of bowel function (2.7 days vs. 2.6 days), or hospital stay (3.7 days vs. 3.6 days) [42].

Chronic pain after hernia repair has many potential causes and is likely multifactorial. The importance of perioperative pain control cannot be understated, because incisional pain, if inadequately controlled, may sensitize the patient to subsequent discomfort related to tissue healing and remodeling. At 6 weeks postoperative, most patients have only mild to moderate pain which continues to improve over time. Therefore, reassurance and supplementation with oral nonsteroidal anti-inflammatory medications is a prudent initial strategy. An exception to this strategy may be the rare patient with severe, focal, neuropathic pain immediately after surgery, indicating mechanical nerve entrapment, which demands prompt surgical revision. Analgesics such as gabapentin and pregabalin have been extensively investigated for the treatment and prevention of postoperative pain after many operations including inguinal hernia repairs [43, 44]. When oral analgesic therapy fails and persistent pain is well localized, as may be the case in 1–3% of the patients [12, 19, 45], injection of local anesthetic should be performed. The transabdominal suture site is injected circumferentially with 25–30 mL of 0.25% bupivacaine with 1:200,000 epinephrine and 1% lidocaine at the level of the abdominal musculature, using a blunted 22-G needle. The needle is blunted so that the surgeon can feel the tip of the needle penetrate the anterior fascia. The majority of patients (92%) have complete relief of their symptoms and require only a single injection [19]. The theory is that the temporary blockade of the afferent pain signal allows the hypersensitivity to subside, resulting in a "resetting" of the sensory nerves with subsequent long-term pain relief.

Techniques for Prevention

Despite many controversies in the literature regarding various operative approaches, mesh choices, and repair techniques, the following principles should be considered in an attempt to reduce the risk of chronic postoperative pain. Patients with evidence of extensive adhesions may benefit from an open, extraperitoneal approach to eliminate intraperitoneal sources of pain. Laparoscopy minimizes the skin and subcutaneous soft tissue dissection with resultant inflammatory response at the risk of transabdominal suture pain and peritoneal irritation by the prosthetic.

In either case, liberal use of local anesthesia around sutures sites should be employed at the time of surgery to minimize the risk of pain sensitization. Lightweight mesh materials are less prone to shrinkage, postoperative scarring, and adhesion formation and are generally favored; however, they should not be used at the expense of the durability of the repair. Given the surgeon's individual experience, skill set, and judgment, a mesh should be chosen that will provide the most durable repair, since recurrence is a strong predictor of chronic pain, whether physiologic or psychological in nature. Likewise, a fixation method should be chosen based on its durability; a combination of four transfascial sutures and non-excessive use of tacks spaced evenly at 5–7 mm along the entire mesh perimeter is a reasonable starting point. Excessive traction on the transfascial fixation sutures or stretching of the mesh should be avoided as this can lead to persistent pain, possibly on the basis of tissue ischemia. For this reason, the insufflation should be reduced during laparoscopic mesh fixation in order to bring the abdominal wall to its resting configuration prior to tying down the transfascial fixation sutures.

Selective strategies for suture fixation in laparoscopic ventral hernia repair may be an appropriate response to the recognition that suture fixation of mesh contributes to acute and chronic postoperative pain. Despite this reality, more aggressive mesh fixation is probably warranted in patients at high risk for hernia recurrence. This approach includes the use of multiple transfascial fixation sutures, additional tacks, and generous (5 cm or more) mesh-fascial overlap on all sides of the defect. High-risk patients may be identified preoperatively based on the presence of morbid obesity (up to fivefold higher recurrence risk), multiple previous recurrences, and comorbidities that may impair wound healing, as well as large (>10 cm), central defects as opposed to "Swiss cheese" defects [46]. While aggressive fixation strategies in high-risk patients may increase postoperative discomfort or mesh sensation, the benefit of avoiding recurrence is unequivocal in select patient groups. In contrast, fewer sutures are probably required in nonobese patients with small fascial defects in whom wide mesh overlap can be achieved.

Summary

Chronic pain after ventral hernia repair is complex in nature and is likely multifactorial in etiology. While no strategy has been shown to completely eliminate pain after VHR, we advocate the use of light- to mid-weight mesh with a limited number of transabdominal sutures and/or tacks. Laparoscopy may limit immediate postoperative surgical pain but does not appear to have an effect on the incidence of chronic postoperative pain. Any changes in mesh choice or surgical technique should not come at the expense of a durable repair as hernia recurrence in and of itself can result in significant postoperative pain and discomfort along with the need for reoperation. Postoperative pain control, nonsteroidal anti-inflammatory therapy, and reassurance for up to 6 weeks are effective in treating postoperative pain in the majority of patients. When severe, focal, neuropathic pain is present immediately after surgery, local injection or surgical release may be necessary. Chronic pain after VHR is a more challenging problem. Effective management in these patients often requires a combination of local injection, formal sensory nerve blocks, and the use of systemic neuropathic pain modulators.

References

1. Burger JW, Luijendijk RW, Hop WC, Halm JA, Verdaasdonk EG, Jeekel J. Long-term follow-up of a randomized controlled trial of suture versus mesh repair of incisional hernia. Ann Surg. 2004;240(4):578–83. discussion 583–5.
2. Berger D, Bientzle M, Muller A. Postoperative complications after laparoscopic incisional hernia repair. Incidence and treatment. Surg Endosc. 2002;16(12):1720–3.
3. Luijendijk RW, Hop WC, van den Tol MP, et al. A comparison of suture repair with mesh repair for incisional hernia. N Engl J Med. 2000;343(6):392–8.
4. Bencini L, Sanchez LJ, Bernini M, et al. Predictors of recurrence after laparoscopic ventral hernia repair. Surg Laparosc Endosc Percutan Tech. 2009;19(2):128–32.
5. Koehler RH, Voeller G. Recurrences in laparoscopic incisional hernia repairs: a personal series and review of the literature. JSLS. 1999;3(4):293–304.
6. Rosen M, Brody F, Ponsky J, et al. Recurrence after laparoscopic ventral hernia repair. Surg Endosc. 2003;17(1):123–8.
7. Clarke JM. Incisional hernia repair by fascial component separation: results in 128 cases and evolution of technique. Am J Surg. 2010;200(1):2–8.
8. Anthony T, Bergen PC, Kim LT, et al. Factors affecting recurrence following incisional herniorrhaphy. World J Surg. 2000;24(1):95–100. discussion 101.
9. de Vries Reilingh TS, Bodegom ME, van Goor H, Hartman EH, van der Wilt GJ, Bleichrodt RP. Autologous tissue repair of large abdominal wall defects. Br J Surg. 2007;94(7):791–803.
10. Sailes FC, Walls J, Guelig D, et al. Synthetic and biological mesh in component separation: a 10-year single institution review. Ann Plast Surg. 2010;64(5):696–8.
11. Breuing K, Butler CE, Ferzoco S, et al. Incisional ventral hernias: review of the literature and recommendations regarding the grading and technique of repair. Surgery. 2010;148(3):544–58.

12. LeBlanc KA, Whitaker JM, Bellanger DE, Rhynes VK. Laparoscopic incisional and ventral hernioplasty: lessons learned from 200 patients. Hernia. 2003;7(3):118–24.
13. Heniford BT, Park A, Ramshaw BJ, Voeller G. Laparoscopic repair of ventral hernias: nine years' experience with 850 consecutive hernias. Ann Surg. 2003;238(3):391–9. discussion 399–400.
14. Alfieri S, Amid PK, Campanelli G, et al. International guidelines for prevention and management of post-operative chronic pain following inguinal hernia surgery. Hernia. 2011;15:239–49.
15. Kehlet H. Chronic pain after groin hernia repair. Br J Surg. 2008;95(2):135–6.
16. Snyder CW, Graham LA, Vick CC, Gray SH, Finan KR, Hawn MT. Patient satisfaction, chronic pain, and quality of life after elective incisional hernia repair: effects of recurrence and repair technique. Hernia. 2010;15:123–9.
17. Eriksen JR, Poornoroozy P, Jorgensen LN, Jacobsen B, Friis-Andersen HU, Rosenberg J. Pain, quality of life and recovery after laparoscopic ventral hernia repair. Hernia. 2009;13(1):13–21.
18. Klima DA, Tsirline VB, Belyansky I, et al. Minimally symptomatic patients undergoing ventral hernia repair have improved quality of life: a prospective multinational review. Paper presented at American Hernia Society, San Francisco, CA, 19 Mar 2011.
19. Carbonell AM, Harold KL, Mahmutovic AJ, et al. Local injection for the treatment of suture site pain after laparoscopic ventral hernia repair. Am Surg. 2003;69(8):688–91. discussion 691–2.
20. Carbajo MA, Martp del Olmo JC, Carbajo JI, Blanco MA, et al. Laparoscopic approach to incisional hernia. Surg Endosc. 2003;17(1):118–22.
21. Canziani M, Frattini F, Cavalli M, Agrusti S, Somalvico F, Campanelli G. Sutureless mesh fibrin glue incisional hernia repair. Hernia. 2009;13(6):625–9.
22. Olmi S, Scaini A, Erba L, Croce E. Use of fibrin glue (Tissucol) in laparoscopic repair of abdominal wall defects: preliminary experience. Surg Endosc. 2007;21(3):409–13.
23. Beldi G, Wagner M, Bruegger LE, Kurmann A, Candinas D. Mesh shrinkage and pain in laparoscopic ventral hernia repair: a randomized clinical trial comparing suture versus tack mesh fixation. Surg Endosc. 2010;25:749–55.
24. Wassenaar E, Schoenmaeckers E, Raymakers J, van der Palen J, Rakic S. Mesh-fixation method and pain and quality of life after laparoscopic ventral or incisional hernia repair: a randomized trial of three fixation techniques. Surg Endosc. 2010;24(6):1296–302.
25. LeBlanc KA, Whitaker JM. Management of chronic postoperative pain following incisional hernia repair with Composix mesh: a report of two cases. Hernia. 2002;6(4):194–7.
26. Nguyen SQ, Divino CM, Buch KE, et al. Postoperative pain after laparoscopic ventral hernia repair: a prospective comparison of sutures versus tacks. JSLS. 2008;12(2):113–6.
27. Sharma A, Mehrotra M, Khullar R, Soni V, Baijal M, Chowbey PK. Laparoscopic ventral/incisional hernia repair: a single centre experience of 1,242 patients over a period of 13 years. Hernia. 2010;15:131–9.
28. Hope WW, Lincourt AE, Newcomb WL, Schmelzer TM, Kercher KW, Heniford BT. Comparing quality-of-life outcomes in symptomatic patients undergoing laparoscopic or open ventral hernia repair. J Laparoendosc Adv Surg Tech A. 2008;18(4):567–71.

29. Kurmann A, Visth E, Candinas D, Beldi G. Long-term follow-up of open and laparoscopic repair of large incisional hernias. World J Surg. 2011;35(2):297–301.
30. Müller M, Klinge U, Conze J, Schumpelick V. Abdominal wall compliance after Marlex® mesh implantation for incisional hernia repair. Hernia. 1998;2(3):113–7.
31. Welty G, Klinge U, Klosterhalfen B, Kasperk R, Schumpelick V. Functional impairment and complaints following incisional hernia repair with different polypropylene meshes. Hernia. 2001;5(3):142–7.
32. Carbajo Caballero MA, Martin del Olmo JC, Blanco JI, Martin F, Cuesta MT. Therapeutic value of laparoscopic adhesiolysis. Surg Endosc. 2001;15(1):102–3.
33. Malik E, Berg C, Meyhofer-Malik A, Haider S, Rossmanith WG. Subjective evaluation of the therapeutic value of laparoscopic adhesiolysis: a retrospective analysis. Surg Endosc. 2000;14(1):79–81.
34. Beldi G, Ipaktchi R, Wagner M, Gloor B, Candinas D. Laparoscopic ventral hernia repair is safe and cost effective. Surg Endosc. 2006;20(1):92–5.
35. Langer C, Schaper A, Liersch T, et al. Prognosis factors in incisional hernia surgery: 25 years of experience. Hernia. 2005;9(1):16–21.
36. Paajanen H, Hermunen H. Long-term pain and recurrence after repair of ventral incisional hernias by open mesh: clinical and MRI study. Langenbecks Arch Surg. 2004;389(5):366–70.
37. Mussack T, Ladurner R, Vogel T, Lienemann A, Eder-Willwohl A, Hallfeldt KK. Health-related quality-of-life changes after laparoscopic and open incisional hernia repair: a matched pair analysis. Surg Endosc. 2006;20(3):410–3.
38. Melzack R. The short-form McGill pain questionnaire. Pain. 1987;30(2):191–7.
39. Heniford BT, Walters AL, Lincourt AE, Novitsky YW, Hope WW, Kercher KW. Comparison of generic versus specific quality-of-life scales for mesh hernia repairs. J Am Coll Surg. 2008;206(4):638–44.
40. LeBlanc KA. Incisional hernia repair: laparoscopic techniques. World J Surg. 2005;29(8):1073–9.
41. Schurr MJ, Gordon DB, Pellino TA, Scanlon TA. Continuous local anesthetic infusion for pain management after outpatient inguinal herniorrhaphy. Surgery. 2004;136(4):761–9.
42. Rosen MJ, Duperier T, Marks J, et al. Prospective randomized double-blind placebo-controlled trial of postoperative elastomeric pain pump devices used after laparoscopic ventral hernia repair. Surg Endosc. 2009;23:2637–43.
43. Ho KY, Gan TJ, Habib AS. Gabapentin and postoperative pain—a systematic review of randomized controlled trials. Pain. 2006;126(1–3):91–101.
44. Sen H, Sizlan A, Yanarates O, et al. A comparison of gabapentin and ketamine in acute and chronic pain after hysterectomy. Anesth Analg. 2009;109(5):1645–50.
45. Bower CE, Reade CC, Kirby LW, Roth JS. Complications of laparoscopic incisional-ventral hernia repair: the experience of a single institution. Surg Endosc. 2004;18(4):672–5.
46. Novitsky YW, Cobb WS, Kercher KW, Matthews BD, Sing RF, Heniford BT. Laparoscopic ventral hernia repair in obese patients: a new standard of care. Arch Surg. 2006;141(1):57–61.

37. Enterotomy During Hernia Repair

Ross F. Goldberg and C. Daniel Smith

An obvious enterotomy or bowel injury that can lead to an enterotomy can occur during abdominal access, lysis of adhesions, or hernia reduction during any hernia repair [1].

Incidence

In a recent review of the literature, the enterotomy rate during ventral hernia repair (of over 3,900 patients) was determined to be 1.78% [2]. Eighty-two percent of these enterotomies are noticed at the time of the operation (total of 1.5% of all patients), while the remainder go unrecognized [2]. The overall incidence of occult enterotomies was 0.33%, resulting in the death of 2.8% of patients [2]. It was also found that these enterotomies could occur in either a laparoscopic or open hernia repair, and some are missed even during an open repair [2].

Diagnosis

Recognized enterotomies are, by namesake, apparent during the operation. Spillage of the intestinal contents is sometimes evident, indicating that there is a perforation of the bowel wall. However, sometimes an enterotomy can be made without spillage, and therefore high index of suspicion is paramount. Whether operating with the laparoscope or open techniques, if there is a chance an enterotomy was made, the surgeon should do everything to ensure it was treated.

Occult enterotomies are more difficult to diagnose. As the name would suggest, these injuries are not recognized during the operation and

B.P. Jacob and B. Ramshaw (eds.), *The SAGES Manual of Hernia Repair*,
DOI 10.1007/978-1-4614-4824-2_37,

are found postoperatively. If a patient develops fever, tachycardia, pain, or abdominal distention in the immediate postoperative setting, bowel injury with possible intestinal spillage needs to be seriously considered. This concern increases if the patient has a concurrent leukocytosis. If a patient develops these symptoms, especially within the first few days after the hernia repair, radiographic imaging, such as CT scans, usually does not provide definitive diagnosis of bowel injury. If there is a concern for a bowel injury, the best approach for diagnosis is early reoperation, either through a laparoscopic or open approach. A CT scan failing to demonstrate extravasation of contrast does not rule out a bowel enterotomy, and this fact cannot be overstated enough. If there is a chance that a patient is decompensating because of an enterotomy, and there is no other feasible explanation for the current symptoms, then the patient should be explored.

Management

There are a variety of approaches to repairing an enterotomy, which is dependent on several situational factors including whether the injury is found at the time of the primary operation or in the postoperative period. Factors that help decide the appropriate course of action include the patient's medical condition, the type of bowel injured (the majority being small bowel), the presence and amount of gross spillage, the extent of the lysis of adhesions, and the size of the hernia defect [1]. The approach to the repair is also dependent on the surgeon's comfort level and experience, requiring the surgeon to use their best judgment in any given situation.

Enterotomy/Bowel Injury at the Time of Primary Operation

In the case of a bowel injury recognized at the time of the primary surgery, one option to consider is immediate conversion from a laparoscopic to an open operation, allowing for either a primary repair of the injured bowel or a bowel resection with primary anastomosis. This would then allow for completion of the adhesiolysis. Depending on the nature and severity of the injury, along with the surgeon's experience, the injury can also be repaired laparoscopically. Regardless of the approach to repairing the bowel, it is imperative that the rest of the bowel be examined to rule out other potential injuries.

The hernia itself could then be repaired from a few approaches. First, there is the primary repair, using suture material only with no mesh implantation. If this approach is feasible, it removes the possibility of foreign material becoming infected due to possible contamination from the bowel. But this approach still leaves the patient at risk for recurrence, especially if the hernia defect is large in size and under tension when repaired. The patient can also be followed for several months, and once they are healed from their enterotomy repair, they could be offered another operation at which the permanent mesh can be placed.

Another approach would be to use a temporary mesh, either a biologic or a mesh made of an absorbable material. This approach allows for a hernia repair while reducing the risk of a mesh infection. Even the timeline to insert such a mesh in the face of an enterotomy is up for debate in the literature. One approach is to place the mesh in the same operative setting, immediately after the enterotomy is repaired. Another approach is to repair the enterotomy, temporarily close the incision by just suturing skin closed and place the patient on antibiotics anywhere from 3 days to 1 week, then returning the patient to the operating room to place a permanent mesh prior to the formation of any dense intestinal adhesions. The purpose of this delayed approach is to further reduce the risk of infection in the setting of the hernia repair. While the risk is less, there is still a chance for mesh infection, requiring further interventions including possible mesh removal and wound debridement.

Another suggested approach is that if the injury is recognized early, with limited spillage, then the injury can be repaired primarily and the prosthetic repair completed at that time. While there is some data on this approach, the number of patients treated this way is very small. The obvious concern is that with a prosthetic mesh and potential for infection, further operative interventions if the mesh becomes infected may be necessary.

A recent review of the literature by LeBlanc et al. helps reflect the different approaches used for recognition and repair of enterotomies and subsequent hernia repairs, shown here in Table 37.1 [2].

Regardless of the approach taken, it is paramount that these issues be discussed with the patient preoperatively. It is imperative that the patient be made aware of the possible issues that could occur and different avenues of repair of an injury if it were to occur.

Table 37.1. Method of recognized enterotomy repair and hernia repair [2].

		Method of enterotomy repair		Method of hernia repair	
Reference	**Conversion**	**Open**	**Lap**	**Open**	**Lap**
Kyzer [3]	2/2	2	0	2	0
Roth [4]	1/2	1	1	1	1[a]
Birgisson [5]	0/2	0	2	0	1, 1[a]
Parker [6]	1/2	1	1	0	2[a]
Bageacu [7]	3/3	3	0	3	0
Ben-Haim [8]	4/4	4	0	4	0
Berger [9]	2/3	2	1	0	2, 1[a]
Gillian [10]	0/3	0	3	0	3
Eid [11]	1/1	1	0	1	0
Carbajo [12]	1/9	1	8	1	8
LeBlanc [13]	2/2	2	0	2	0
Heniford [14]	2/12	2	10	1	7, 4[a]
Franklin [15]	0/5	0	5	0	5
Holzman [16]	1/1	1	0	1	0
Ramshaw [17]	0/1	0	1	0	1
Robbins [18]	1/1	1	0	1	0
Wright [19]	3/3	3	0	3	0
Total (%)	24/56 (43)	24/56 (43)	32/56 (57)	20/56 (36)	27/56 (48) 9/56 (16)[a]

From Ref. [2] with permission

[a]Delayed laparoscopic repair

Concern for Enterotomy/Bowel Injury at Time of Primary Operation

If there is a concern for an injury while performing the primary operation, the bowel should be run in its entirety once more. If there is an area of concern, or an area of serosal injury, suturing can be done to attempt to prevent an eventual enterotomy; this can be done laparoscopically. If there is high suspicion, and laparoscopic exploration fails to reveal the location, then conversion to open should occur and the bowel should be run extracorporeally. If there is no gross spillage, according to the literature review, the surgeon may choose to proceed with synthetic mesh implantation, but the patient needs to be closely monitored postoperatively for any signs of sepsis, including fever, tachycardia, leukocytosis, and abdominal pain that is out of proportion. Should that occur, then the patient must be returned to the operating room to have the mesh removed.

The only sure way to prevent a mesh infection in the setting of an intraoperative enterotomy is to avoid any implantation of synthetic nonabsorbable mesh. An enterotomy and the surgeon's plan, should one occur, should be discussed with the patient ahead of time and included in the informed consent.

Occult Enterotomy/Bowel Injury

If there is a missed or delayed thermal injury that results in enterotomy, the patient will present with signs and symptoms of sepsis. If there is concern for or evidence of a bowel injury, then an emergent operation is warranted; typically this should be done via an open approach. With the presence of gross spillage, the mesh has to be removed regardless of any other intervention. This is then followed by a thorough examination of the abdominal cavity, with either direct repair of the injured bowel or, more likely, resection of the injured segment of bowel. Depending on the amount of intestinal spillage, a decision can be made either to anastomose in that setting or to bring out an ostomy and plan for a delayed repair. In the setting of gross sepsis, the hernia defect can be closed primarily or with an absorbable product, with the plan on returning to the operating room at a later date for a more definitive repair.

Avoidance

While a bowel injury can always occur during these operations, care must be taken to decrease the risk of an injury as much as possible. When gaining abdominal access, it is recommended to always enter the abdomen under direct vision, especially in a patient with previous abdominal operations. This can be done either via an open Hassan technique, or using an optical trocar. These approaches help to reduce the incidence of trocar injury to the underlying bowel.

When performing adhesiolysis, it is recommended to only use cold instruments, such as laparoscopic shears. An energy source should never be attached to the instrument performing the dissection, thereby removing the risk of thermal injury to underlying tissue/bowel.

Finally, if there is a concern for bowel injury, or there is an area of bowel that could be problematic in the future, the area can be buttressed with simple serosal sutures. All of this can be performed laparoscopically.

At the end of every hernia repair, the involved or manipulated bowel should be visualized to look for any signs of injury, and this final assessment and absence of bowel injury are documented in the operative note. This becomes important in cases of occult injury to document nothing at the time of surgery.

Conclusion

There is no standard approach to enterotomy management in the setting of a hernia repair. The factors affecting the treatment path include the severity and nature of the injured bowel, presence of gross spillage, and surgeon's expertise and comfort level, which results in options for both laparoscopic and open repairs. As demonstrated in the literature, multiple options exist, and all are reasonable choices, as long as they are done safely, minimizing the risk to the patient.

References

1. Ramshaw B. Laparoscopic ventral hernia repair—managing and preventing complications. Int Surg. 2005;90:S48–55.
2. LeBlanc KA, Elieson MJ, Corder 3rd JM. Enterotomy and mortality rates of laparoscopic incisional and ventral hernia repair: a review of the literature. JSLS. 2007;11:408–14.
3. Kyzer S, Alis M, Aloni Y, Charuzi I. Laparoscopic repair of postoperation ventral hernia. Early postoperation results. Surg Endosc. 1999;13:928–31.
4. Roth JS, Park AE, Witzke D, Mastrangelo MJ. Laparoscopic incisional/ventral herniorraphy: a five year experience. Hernia. 1999;3:209–14.
5. Birgisson G, Park AE, Mastrangelo Jr MJ, Witzke DB, Chu UB. Obesity and laparoscopic repair of ventral hernias. Surg Endosc. 2001;15:1419–22.
6. Parker 3rd HH, Nottingham JM, Bynoe RP, Yost MJ. Laparoscopic repair of large incisional hernias. Am Surg. 2002;68:530–3. discussion 533–4.
7. Bageacu S, Blanc P, Breton C, et al. Laparoscopic repair of incisional hernia: a retrospective study of 159 patients. Surg Endosc. 2002;16:345–8.
8. Ben-Haim M, Kuriansky J, Tal R, et al. Pitfalls and complications with laparoscopic intraperitoneal expanded polytetrafluoroethylene patch repair of postoperative ventral hernia. Surg Endosc. 2002;16:785–8.
9. Berger D, Bientzle M, Muller A. Postoperative complications after laparoscopic incisional hernia repair. Incidence and treatment. Surg Endosc. 2002;16:1720–3.

10. Gillian GK, Geis WP, Grover G. Laparoscopic incisional and ventral hernia repair (LIVH): an evolving outpatient technique. JSLS. 2002;6:315–22.
11. Eid GM, Prince JM, Mattar SG, Hamad G, Ikrammudin S, Schauer PR. Medium-term follow-up confirms the safety and durability of laparoscopic ventral hernia repair with PTFE. Surgery. 2003;134:599–603. discussion 603–4.
12. Carbajo MA, del Olmo Martp JC, Blanco JI, et al. Laparoscopic approach to incisional hernia. Surg Endosc. 2003;17:118–22.
13. LeBlanc KA, Whitaker JM, Bellanger DE, Rhynes VK. Laparoscopic incisional and ventral hernioplasty: lessons learned from 200 patients. Hernia. 2003;7:118–24.
14. Heniford BT, Park A, Ramshaw BJ, Voeller G. Laparoscopic repair of ventral hernias: nine years' experience with 850 consecutive hernias. Ann Surg. 2003;238:391–9. discussion 399–400.
15. Franklin Jr ME, Gonzalez Jr JJ, Glass JL, Manjarrez A. Laparoscopic ventral and incisional hernia repair: an 11-year experience. Hernia. 2004;8:23–7.
16. Holzman MD, Purut CM, Reintgen K, Eubanks S, Pappas TN. Laparoscopic ventral and incisional hernioplasty. Surg Endosc. 1997;11:32–5.
17. Ramshaw BJ, Esartia P, Schwab J, et al. Comparison of laparoscopic and open ventral herniorrhaphy. Am Surg. 1999;65:827–31. discussion 831–2.
18. Robbins SB, Pofahl WE, Gonzalez RP. Laparoscopic ventral hernia repair reduces wound complications. Am Surg. 2001;67:896–900.
19. Wright BE, Niskanen BD, Peterson DJ, et al. Laparoscopic ventral hernia repair: are there comparative advantages over traditional methods of repair? Am Surg. 2002;68:291–5. discussion 295–6.

38. Chronic Seroma

Morris Franklin Jr., Richard Alexander, Gerardo Lozano, and Karla Russek

Definition

A seroma is a collection of liquefied fat, serum, and lymphatic fluid in a closed space. The fluid is usually clear, yellow, and somewhat viscous and is found in the subcutaneous layer of the skin. Seromas represent the most benign complications after an operative procedure and are particularly likely to occur when large skin flaps are developed in the course of the operation, as is often seen with mastectomy, axillary dissection, groin dissection, and large ventral hernias [1].

There has been no consistent definition of chronic seroma in the literature, although it has been documented most frequently when it is symptomatic, bothersome to the patient, palpable, fluctuant, tense, and requires at least one needle aspiration [2–4]. In contrast, in a published study [5], seroma was documented only when multiple aspirations were required, or if insertion of a new drain was necessary in persistent cases. Similarly, other studies used the term seroma if a verified volume of more than 5–20 ml of fluid was obtained by puncture and aspiration [6], whereas some studies have used ultrasonography to verify seroma [7].

Seroma formation is one of the most commonly reported complications after laparoscopic and open hernia surgery. It occurs early after operation in virtually all patients, to some extent. Virtually all seromas resolve spontaneously over a period of weeks to months, with fewer than 5% persisting for more than 8 weeks. Because of this, seromas are rarely clinically significant [8].

B.P. Jacob and B. Ramshaw (eds.), *The SAGES Manual of Hernia Repair*,
DOI 10.1007/978-1-4614-4824-2_38,

Physiology

Postoperative fluid collections represent sequelae of events that ultimately contribute to negative soft tissue healing events [9]. It has been demonstrated that seroma is not merely an accumulation of serum, but exudate resulting from an acute inflammatory reaction, and concluded that seroma formation reflects an increased intensity and prolongation of the first phase of wound repair. Mc Caul et al. [10] have also demonstrated that drainage fluid has a composition different from that of lymph but similar to that of inflammatory exudate.

Seroma formation can be seen as a consequence of the inflammatory foreign body reaction with monocytes and macrophages involved at the interface of connective tissue and implant. These cells produce a variety of cytokines, which regulate the local immune response, wound healing, and scar formation [11].

On the other hand, Wu et al. [12] have reported an increase of vascular endothelial growth factor (VEGF) and a decrease of endostatin in drainage fluid immediately after surgery. VEGF is a known mediator of angiogenesis, vascular proliferation, and permeability, and endostatin is a potent inhibitor of angiogenesis [13, 14]. Therefore, these changes may not only reflect induction of angiogenesis as a physiologic response to operative trauma but also enhanced accumulation of fluid.

Heidemann et al. showed that stabilizing the pH value in the environment of implants for several weeks improves the biocompatibility by reducing adverse tissue reactions [15]. Though the risk of seroma formation increases when mesh is used for repair, little is known about the genesis of seroma formation. Alloplastic mesh prosthesis leads to a multitude of tissue reactions, including the postoperative release of cytokines and the formation of seroma sometimes persistent for months [16].

Presentation

A seroma is usually manifested as a localized and well-circumscribed swelling, pressure or discomfort, and occasional drainage of clear liquid from the immature surgical wound. A study by Bernatchez et al. [11] showed that the total drainage output within the first few postoperative days was significantly elevated in patients with subsequent seroma formation.

Prevention

Prevention of seroma formation may be achieved by placing suction drains under the skin or in any potential dead space created. Premature removal of drains frequently results in large seromas that require aspiration under sterile conditions, followed by placement of a pressure dressing. Abdominal binders worn by patients for up to 6 weeks after the hernia repair have been advocated by surgeons as they believe the extra pressure applied across the abdominal wall may increase fluid movement and decrease the incidence of seroma formation [17].

The effects of electrocautery on tissues are an acknowledged risk factor for seroma formation. Two prospective clinical trials were conducted where randomized breast cancer patients underwent surgery with electrocautery and scalpel, respectively; they confirmed a lower incidence of seroma formation with the latter technique. However, few surgeons are willing to relinquish the convenience and improved hemostasis associated with electrocautery dissection [4].

In cases of hernia surgery, it has been suggested that cauterization of the hernia sac together with a central full-thickness suture to reduce dead space seems to prevent seroma formation [18].

There have been attempts to prevent or decrease seroma formation as the application of tetracycline and/or bovine thrombin as sclerosing agents, but they have not worked well. Fibrin glues, patches, and sealants appear promising, but they too have proven to not be useful for the prevention of seromas. Additional strategies promoted especially for open-component separation techniques include quilting sutures to fix the skin flaps to the abdominal wall and minimize dead space and the use of aerosolized talc to induce tissue adherence of skin flaps to the abdominal wall musculofascial in the early postoperative period.

Treatment

A seroma that reaccumulates after several aspirations can be evacuated by opening the incision and packing the wound with saline-moistened gauze to allow healing by secondary intention. In the presence of synthetic mesh, the best option may be open drainage in the operating room with the incision closed to avoid exposure and infection of the mesh; closed suction drains are generally placed. An infected seroma is also treated by open drainage, typically without skin closure. However, the presence of synthetic mesh in these cases may prevent the wound from healing. Management of the mesh depends on the severity and extent of infection. In the absence of severe sepsis, spreading cellulitis, or the presence of localized infection, the mesh can be left in situ and removed at a later date when the acute infectious process has resolved. Granulation tissue may grow into and over the mesh. This is especially true for the less dense, wider pore types of mesh and least likely for PTFE mesh. If the mesh does not integrate well into the tissue and signs of infection are not resolving, the mesh will most likely need to be removed and the wound managed with open wound care [1].

References

1. Surgical complications. In: Townsend CM (eds) Sabiston textbook of surgery, 18th ed. Saunders. 2008; (15).
2. Kuroi K, Shimozuma K, Taguchi T, Imai H, Yamashiro H, Ohsumi S, Saito S. Pathophysiology of seroma in breast cancer. Breast Cancer. 2005;12(2):288–93.
3. Bryant M, Baum M. Postoperative seroma following mastectomy and axillary dissection. Br J Surg. 1987;74:1187.
4. Porter KA, O'Connor S, Rimm E, Lopez M. Electrocautery as a factor in seroma formation following mastectomy. Am J Surg. 1998;176:8–11.
5. Burak WE, Goodman PS, Young SC, Farrar WB. Seroma formation following axillary dissection for breast cancer: risk factors and lack of influence of bovine thrombin. J Surg Oncol. 1997;64:27–31.
6. Tejler G, Aspegren K. Complications and hospital stay after surgery for breast cancer: a prospective study of 385 patients. Br J Surg. 1985;72:542–4.
7. Puttawibul P, Sangthong B, Maipang T, Sampao S, Uttamakul P, Apakupaul N. Mastectomy without drain at pectoral area: a randomized controlled trial. J Med Assoc Thai. 2003;86:325–31.
8. Souba WW. Laparoscopic hernia repair. In: ACS surgery principles practice. WebMD Professional Publishing, Inc.
9. Bullocks J, Basu B, Hsu P, Singer R. Prevention of hematomas and seromas. Semin Plast Surg. 2006;20(4):233–40.
10. Mc Caul JA, Aslaam A, Spooner RJ, Louden I, Cavanagh T, Purushotham AD. Aetiology of seroma formation in patients undergoing surgery for breast cancer. Breast. 2000;9:144–8.
11. Bernatchez SF, Parks PJ, Gibbons DF. Interaction of macrophages with fibrous materials in vitro. Biomaterials. 1996;17:2077–86.
12. Wu FP, Hoekman K, Meijer S, Cuesta MA. VEGF and endostatin levels in wound fluid and plasma after breast surgery. Angiogenesis. 2003;6:255–7.

13. Toi M, Matsumoto T, Bando H. Vascular endothelial growth factor: its prognostic, predictive, and therapeutic implications. Lancet Oncol. 2001;2:667–73.
14. Folkman J. Endogenous angiogenesis inhibitors. APMIS. 2004;112:496–507.
15. Heidemann W, Jeschkeit-Schubbert S, Ruffieux K, Fischer JH, Jung H, Krueger G, Wintermantel E, Gerlach KL. pH stabilization of predegraded PDLLA by an admixture of water soluble sodium hydrogen phosphate—results of an in vitro- and in vivo-study. Biomaterials. 2002;23:3567–74.
16. Klink CD, Binnebosel M, Lucas AH, Schachtrupp A, Klinge U, Shumpelick V, Junge K. Do drainage liquid characteristics serve as predictors for seroma formation after incisional hernia repair? Hernia. 2010;14:175–9.
17. Jin J, Schomisch S, Rosen M. In vitro evaluation of the permeability of prosthetic meshes as the possible cause of postoperative seroma formation. Surg Innov. 2009;16(2):129–33.
18. Tsimoyiannis EC, Tsimogiannis KE, Pappas-Gogos G. Seroma and recurrence in laparoscopic ventral hernioplasty. JSLS. 2008;12(1):51–7.

Part VIII
Current Debates in Ventral and Incisional Hernia Repair

39. Bridging Versus Closing the Defect During Laparoscopic Ventral Hernia Repair

Yuri W. Novitsky

Benefits of Laparoscopy in Ventral Hernia Repair

Hernia repair continues to be one of the most common procedures performed by general surgeons. With the advent of laparoscopy, minimally invasive techniques have been employed in abdominal wall reconstructions in an effort to reduce postoperative morbidity and wound complications. In fact, over the last decade, laparoscopic repair has been utilized for repairs of many ventral hernia defects due to its efficacy and safety [1–3]. Compared to open repairs, laparoscopic ventral hernia repair (LVHR) has been shown to result in reduced wound complications, quicker recovery of bowel function, shorter hospital stay, and improved cosmesis [4–6]. In addition, appropriately performed laparoscopic repair has also been associated with low recurrence rates [1, 5, 7]. Not surprisingly, LVHR has been proposed as the gold standard for many ventral hernia repairs [7, 8].

Drawbacks of Traditional LVHR

Despite a multitude of perioperative advantages, there are several drawbacks to the use of laparoscopic techniques. Postoperative seroma is a common complication of a traditional LVHR [9]. Reduction of the viscera followed by mesh "patching" of the hernia defect results in a potential space that is filled with serous fluid postoperatively. Such seromas are common and typically do not require intervention; however, they may be a source of postoperative discomfort and wound-related

B.P. Jacob and B. Ramshaw (eds.), *The SAGES Manual of Hernia Repair*,
DOI 10.1007/978-1-4614-4824-2_39,

morbidity. Furthermore, traditional laparoscopic repairs have been associated with bulging at the site of the hernia repair. While laparoscopic underlay mesh repair is a true "tension-free" technique, it leaves behind adynamic, "bridged" areas of the abdominal wall. Lack of anatomic reconstruction and medialization of rectus muscles, in turn, often leads to various degrees of visceral bulging at the site of a hernia defect. Although this fact has received little attention in the majority of LVHR literature, practicing surgeons have long been frustrated by this shortcoming of a traditional laparoscopic technique.

Goals of Repair

As with any other surgical procedure, there are several goals that should be achieved during a given ventral hernia repair. First, the operation needs to be conducted safely with minimal risks to the patient. This is achieved via proper patient selection, careful abdominal access, and meticulous adhesiolysis, among other are key safety principles. Next, a surgeon should strive to minimize postoperative infectious complications and limit other long-term adverse side effects of a herniorrhaphy. Appropriate mesh selection is paramount, especially during laparoscopic ventral hernia repair. Finally, an operation should be aimed at providing a durable and lasting repair with minimal chance of recurrence. Important principles in this regard have been reported to be complete adhesiolysis, appropriate mesh sizing with sufficient overlap, as well as permanent transabdominal fixation. In addition to these principles, reconstruction of an abdominal wall that resembles native anatomy has recently emerged as another key component of a ventral hernia repair.

Defect Closure

When addressing ventral hernia repair, abdominal wall mechanics/physics is an important topic that necessitates some discussion. Pascal's principle states that pressure applied to a confined fluid is transmitted throughout the fluid and container walls by the same amount [10]. Additionally, a hernia defect is akin to a vascular aneurysm, with respect to a focal weakness or thinning of its wall. According to an extension of the law of Laplace [11], as the abdominal wall radius increases and thickness decreases, wall tension across the hernia defect is greatly increased. Because a hernia defect provides an outlet for abdominal pressure, the force applied across the defect is increased substantially. As discussed by Agarwal et al. [8], mesh covering the defect in a traditional "bridged" fashion bears this multiplied intra-abdominal pressure point, possibly leading to mesh instability, excessive suture tension, and bulging [8]. Thus, it can be hypothesized that by closure of the defect, abdominal wall integrity is restored, leading to equalized pressure and tension across the abdominal wall and intra-abdominally placed mesh.

Overall, it appears that the impetus for the modern trend of "anatomic" repairs stems from surgeons' three major frustrations associated with traditional repairs: seromas, persistence of palpable defect, and bulging at the site of a "bridged" defect. By closing the defect, the rectus abdominis muscles are re-approximated, and the major insertion point of abdominal musculature, the linea alba, is restored. Closure of the defect results in a near total decrease of the "dead" space and thus minimizes the risks of postoperative seromas. Although objective data are lacking, hernia repair with defect closure also likely contributes to restoration of a functional and dynamic abdominal wall. We recently reported our early experience with routine defect closure during laparoscopic hernia repair [12]. Our laparoscopic "shoelace" repair combined techniques of both primary defect closure and mesh prosthesis placement for reinforcement. Although we were not able to evaluate "functionality" of the abdominal wall, routine defect closure resulted in subjective elimination of adynamic areas of the abdominal wall and postoperative bulging at the site of the hernia defects.

Technical Considerations and Outcomes

Several techniques for defect closure have recently been described. Palanivelu et al. have utilized continuous intracorporeal sutures for defect closure with subsequent intraperitoneal onlay mesh repair [13]. However, in addition to technical challenges of this approach, running closure may not be applicable to wider defects. Agarwal et al. presented a series of patients undergoing laparoscopic ventral hernia repair with rather cumbersome transabdominal "double-breasted" defect closure. They achieved fascial closure with interrupted sutures followed by mesh reinforcement [14]. They reported no infectious complications, no visible bulging, and no recurrences at mean follow-up of 34 months. Cheala et al. published a series of nearly 400 patients with defect closure. They utilized a laparoscopic "transparietal U reverse suturing technique." In short, the stitch is placed transabdominally along one side of the defect, and a horizontal mattress stitch is formed intracorporeally through the contralateral side. The tail of the stitch is then retrieved through the original skin incision utilizing a suture passer. At a mean follow-up of 28 months, they reported 2% rate of seromas, 1.8% rate of chronic pain, and only a 1.5% recurrence rate. Importantly, they found a 1.3% incidence of postoperative bulging at the site of the hernia defect. The authors emphasized the importance of complete "reconstructive" defect closure to minimize complications and recurrences [15]. As mentioned above, we recently reported our series of 47 consecutive patients undergoing LVHR with defect closure [12]. Our technique has several unique elements. Briefly, we achieve pneumoperitoneum using an optical trocar in the subcostal area. The hernia sac is usually left in situ. Using a laparoscopic suture passer, the hernia defect is closed with multiple figure-of-eight stitches using a permanent monofilament suture. Each stitch is placed through a stab incision in the skin (traversing the hernia sac) and incorporates 1–2 cm of fascia on each side. Once all the stitches are placed, the pneumoperitoneum is released, and the knots are tied in the subcutaneous tissue. To facilitate closure, the knots are tied sequentially, starting at the superior and inferior aspects of the defect first and moving toward the center. The mesh is then tailored to achieve at least a 5-cm overlap above and below the defect. Importantly, the width of the mesh is not calculated according to the original width of the defect. Instead, we use 14–16 cm wide mesh which allows for about 7–8 cm of overlap in each lateral direction from the newly re-created linea alba/midline. The use of narrower meshes facilitates mesh positioning and allows us to avoid "bisecting" the abdominal cavity with large, wide meshes. Furthermore, smaller meshes should result in a reduction in the overall foreign body response and fibrotic reactions to the mesh. With diminished lateral scar tissue to the mesh, patients should experience improved mobility and decreased long-term postoperative discomfort. Such reduction in the width of the mesh implant is one of the major benefits of our laparoscopic "shoelacing" technique. The mesh is then secured with transabdominal sutures and tacks. Finally, full-thickness, nonabsorbable U-stitches are placed every 3–4 cm on each side of the midline closure. These stitches are a key component to our technique as they transfer any tension at the midline closure throughout the large portion of the mesh. We strongly believe that these "buttress" stitches not only allow for "downsizing" of the mesh width but also relieve tension in the newly re-created linea alba and assist with creation of physiologic tension throughout the entire abdominal wall. Not surprising, we found no instances of postoperative seromas or bulging at the hernia site. In addition, we detected no recurrences at a mean 10-month follow-up [12].

Defect Closure: Who Needs It?

A major goal of any ventral hernia repair should be the reconstructions of a functional, dynamic abdominal wall. Traditional LVHR relies on intraperitoneal "patching" of defects as an underlay. However, such bridging technique fails to close the actual defect and may result in adynamic areas of abdominal wall. Clinically, this may lead to bulging at the site of hernia repair, especially in the long term. Moreover, significant seroma accumulation may occur in the created dead space above the mesh patch. By closing the hernia defect, medialization of the rectus muscles occurs, clearly allowing for a better functional and cosmetic reconstruction. Two major reasons exist against routine application of defect closure during LVHR. First, this step adds time to the operation as well as an additional technical challenge. Secondly, transabdominal closure of large defects seems to cause significant additional incisional discomfort with unclear long-term implications on chronic pain. As a result, the pros and cons of defect closures have to be compared on an individual patient-to-patient basis. In my view, most defects in younger, active patients should be closed routinely. In addition, thinner patients are more likely to notice persistent defects and bulging and would also benefit from defect closure during LVHR. Older patients, on the other hand, are unlikely to derive any benefits from a "dynamic" reconstructed abdominal wall and are likely best served by a traditional LVHR. Similarly, morbidly obese patients are less likely to enjoy the benefits of defect closure. As defect closure gains wider implementation, the benefits and disadvantages of this approach should become clearer. A recently initiated prospective randomized trial at out institution should add to the knowledge base of LVHR with defect closure. This type of evidence may help to determine the subgroup of patients who stand to benefit from this modification of a traditional LVHR technique.

References

1. Heniford BT, Park A, Ramshaw BJ, Voeller G. Laparoscopic repair of ventral hernias: nine years' experience with 850 consecutive hernias. Ann Surg. 2003;238:391–9.
2. Carbajo MA, Martin del Olmo JC, Blanco JI, de la Cuesta C, Toledano M, Martin F, Vaquero C, Inglada L. Laparoscopic treatment vs. open surgery in the solution of major incisional and abdominal wall hernias with mesh. Surg Endosc. 1999;13:250–2.
3. Sajid MS, Bokhari SA, Mallick AS, Cheek E, Baig MK. Laparoscopic versus open repair of incisional/ventral hernia: a meta-analysis. Am J Surg. 2009;197:64–72.

4. Lomanto D, Iyer SG, Shabbir A, Cheah WK. Laparoscopic versus open ventral hernia mesh repair: a prospective study. Surg Endosc. 2006;20:1030–5.
5. Ramshaw BJ, Esartia P, Schwab J, Mason EM, Wilson RA, Duncan TD, Miller J, Lucas GW, Promes J. Comparison of laparoscopic and open ventral herniorrhaphy. Am Surg. 1999;65:827–31. discussion 831–822.
6. Bencini L, Sanchez LJ, Boffi B, Farsi M, Scatizzi M, Moretti R. Incisional hernia: repair retrospective comparison of laparoscopic and open techniques. Surg Endosc. 2003;17:1546–51.
7. Novitsky YW, Cobb WS, Kercher KW, Matthews BD, Sing RF, Heniford BT. Laparoscopic ventral hernia repair in obese patients: a new standard of care. Arch Surg. 2006;141:57–61.
8. Agarwal BB, Agarwal S, Mahajan KC. Laparoscopic ventral hernia repair: innovative anatomical closure, mesh insertion without 10-mm transmyofascial port, and atraumatic mesh fixation: a preliminary experience of a new technique. Surg Endosc. 2009;23:900–5.
9. White TJ, Santos MC, Thompson JS. Factors affecting wound complications in repair of ventral hernias. Am Surg. 1998;64:276–80.
10. Giancoli DC. Physics: principles with applications. 4th ed. Englewood Cliffs, NJ: Prentice Hall; 1995.
11. Sabiston DC, Townsend CM. Sabiston textbook of surgery: the biological basis of modern surgical practice. 18th ed. Philadelphia, PA: Saunders/Elsevier; 2008.
12. Orenstein SB, Dumeer JL, Monteagudo J, Poi MJ, Novitsky YW. Outcomes of laparoscopic ventral hernia repair with routine defect closure using "Shoelace" technique. Surg Endosc. 2011;25:1452–7.
13. Palanivelu C, Jani KV, Senthilnathan P, Parthasarathi R, Madhankumar MV, Malladi VK. Laparoscopic sutured closure with mesh reinforcement of incisional hernias. Hernia. 2007;11:223–8.
14. Agarwal BB, Agarwal S, Gupta MK, Mishra A, Mahajan KC. Laparoscopic ventral hernia meshplasty with "double-breasted" fascial closure of hernial defect: a new technique. J Laparoendosc Adv Surg Tech A. 2008;18:222–9.
15. Cheala E, Thoma M, Tatete B, Lemye AC, Dessily M, Alle JL. The suturing concept for laparoscopic mesh fixation in ventral and incisional hernia repair: mid-term analysis of 400 cases. Surg Endosc. 2007;21:391–5.

40. Bridging versus Closing the Defect During Laparoscopic Ventral Hernia Repair: It Is OK to Bridge

Stephen M. Kavic and Adrian Park

Our surgical approach to the repair of incisional and ventral hernias has evolved dramatically only over the last two decades. Reports that surgeons yearly repair nearly 200,000 incisional hernias in the United States [1] contribute to making the lowly hernia a most important topic of discussion. This chapter reviews the rationale for laparoscopic ventral hernia repair and discusses the advantages offered by using a permanent prosthetic for bridging the hernia defect. In considering the optimal management and repair of hernias, we take into account conceptual arguments, technical considerations, practical advantages, and experience.

Bridging Versus Closing: Hernia Consequences and Repair

The pathophysiology of hernia formation is well described in detail in this volume's earlier chapters and elsewhere [2]. Failure of a defect once established to heal is due to the pressure that remains and exceeds the native resistance of the abdominal wall [3]. As such, any repair of an incisional or ventral hernia must address the pressures that exist on the anterior abdominal wall in order to optimize the repair and to minimize the likelihood of recurrence.

It is commonly stated that the forces that create a hernia will actually reinforce the strength of a laparoscopic repair [4]. Pascal's principle—modified to the irregular contour of the abdominal wall—suggests that the intra-abdominal pressure will maintain the prosthetic against the inner aspects of the abdominal wall [2].

B.P. Jacob and B. Ramshaw (eds.), *The SAGES Manual of Hernia Repair*,
DOI 10.1007/978-1-4614-4824-2_40,

In the abdominal midline, hernias most commonly develop in the postoperative setting. This represents the simplest scenario of acquired hernia development, where the surgically altered tissues no longer have structural integrity.

Pain is widely recognized as the predominant symptom of ventral or incisional hernias. Activity limitation and aesthetic distress may also present as reasons to repair. In addressing the symptoms, the surgeon, mindful of incarceration risk, avoids the life-threatening complication of strangulation, estimated to occur in approximately 5 % of patients with a ventral hernia [5, 6].

Traditionally, hernia repairs have been accomplished with an open incision, reduction of hernia contents, excision of the sac, and primary repair of the native fascia. The hernia recurrence rate, however, was found to be unacceptably high. As recognized with inguinal hernias many decades ago, the enemy of a primary repair is tension. As ventral hernias enlarge, it becomes increasingly difficult to reapproximate the tissues without undue tension.

Primary repair was compared with mesh use in a multicenter trial conducted by Luijendijk et al. Its convincingly decisive conclusion demonstrated reduction in the recurrence rate of midline abdominal herniation with the use of mesh [7]. Systematic reviews, since undertaken, have strongly promoted the employment of mesh, relating its use to an at least 50 % decrease in the rate of hernia recurrence [8, 9]. Little debate remains regarding the use of mesh, now considered the gold standard of abdominal wall hernia repair.

Components separation also has been advocated as a means of minimizing the tension on a midline closure [10, 11]. Several disadvantages are, however, associated with this technique. It is a substantial operative procedure. Although occasionally performed with laparoscopic assistance, the greatest tension decrease is achieved when done in an open fashion, and this is accompanied with increased wound complication risks ranging from overt infection to skin necrosis. When the ultimate measure of an operation—its success rate at treating the underlying condition—is applied to separation of components for hernia repair, the recurrence rates that have been produced are variable at best and often disappointing [12, 13]. Better operative results are achieved with this technique when it is augmented with use of resorbable mesh, an addition that may considerably increase the expense of the procedure [14].

Bridging a hernia defect satisfies the conceptual requirements of a successful hernia repair. Specifically, it addresses the pressures that perpetuate a hernia, avoids the consequence of strangulation of entrapped viscera, and provides for a tension-free environment to maintain durability of repair.

Technical Considerations

Laparoscopic ventral hernia repair is a well-established technique. The procedure may be complicated but has the advantage of conceptual simplicity. After adhesiolysis through a lateral approach, a bridging mesh may be introduced and secured intracorporeally, deep to the fascia and the peritoneum. Care is taken to ensure adequate overlap—generally considered to be 5 cm or greater—of the hernia defect.

Importantly, use of a bridging mesh largely preserves the abdominal domain. Although the physical space for the viscera is necessarily smaller than that of the extended hernia sac, the volume of the abdominal compartment is retained. In reapproximating the midline, too significant a decrease in the abdominal cylinder could occur, resulting at the extreme in compressed viscera and development of the abdominal compartment syndrome. More commonly, the patient suffers some degree of diaphragmatic restriction and pulmonary compromise.

Practical Advantages

Use of mesh in laparoscopic ventral hernia repair to bridge a hernia defect is safe, rapid, and efficacious as research has demonstrated. Even in the face of such data, some may claim that it remains a fundamentally better operation to align and approximate the edges of the hernia defect. The arguments for this go beyond the desire to add a novel approach to hernia repair. Specifically, the detractors of the established technique may challenge the modifications of the fundamental technique, the functional result of the repair, and the cosmetic outcome.

No substitute exists, however, for actual data. In the case of bridging the laparoscopic hernia defect, many large-scale series—summarized in Table 40.1—demonstrate excellent long-term outcomes. In fact, laparoscopic ventral hernia repair may be considered the standard of care [34].

Table 40.1. Large series (>100 cases) of laparoscopic incisional hernia repair using mesh.

Author	Year	*n*	BMI	Defect (cm^2)	Patch (cm^2)	Prior repair (%)	Conversion (%)	Patch material	Trans-fascial sutures	Complications		Recurrence		
										Total (%)	Seroma (%)	LOS (d)	(%)	F/U (m)
Alkhoury [15]	2011	141	31	144	257	NS	0	PP	N	8	1	1.1	6	40
Bageacu [16]	2002	159	NS	NS	NS	23	14	PTFE	Y	44	16	3.5	16	49
Ben-Haim [17]	2002	100	NS	NS	NS	25	4	PTFE	N	24	11	5	2	14
Berger [18]	2002	150	29	94	350	13	2	PTFE	Y	97	93	9.1	3	15
Bower [19]	2004	100	34	124	280	32	1	PTFE	Y	15	1	NS	2	6.5
Carbajo [20]	2003	270	NS	145	300	27	1	PTFE	N	15	12	1.5	4	44
Chowbey [21]	2000	202	NS	NS	NS	NS	1	PP	N	30	25	1.8	1	35
Franklin [22]	2004	384	NS	NS	NS	NS	4	PP, PTFE	N	10	3	2.9	3	47
Frantzides [23]	2004	208	NS	173	NS	NS	0	PTFE	N	3	NS	1.4	1	24
Gillian [24]	2002	100	NS	NS	NS	NS	0	Composix	N	7	3	NS	1	NS
Heniford [25]	2003	850	32	118	344	34	4	PTFE	Y	13	3	2.3	5	20
Kirshtein [26]	2002	103	34	175	324	41	3	PTFE	N	6	0	3.1	4	26
LeBlanc [27]	2003	200	NS	111	258	21	4	PTFE	Y	18	NS	1.3	7	36
Olmi [28]	2006	178	30	144	NS	NS	0	Polyester	Y	7	4.4	2.1	2.5	12
Perrone [29]	2005	121	35	109	256	29	10	PTFE, PP	Y	27	9	1.7	9	22
Rosen [30]	2003	100	31	96	354	38	12	PTFE, PP	Y/N	14	4	1.8	17	30
Sharma [31]	2011	1,242	32	26	NS	NS	1.5	PTFE, PP	Y/N	67	31	NS	4.4	65
Toy [32]	1998	144	NS	98	216	26	0	PTFE	Y	26	16	2.3	4	8
Ujiki [33]	2004	100	33	97	259	24	3	PTFE	Y	23	13	2	6	3

NS not specified

Modifications

Type of mesh used and the means of mesh fixation constitute the most common modifications in the laparoscopic ventral hernia repair. Although initially the types of mesh were fairly limited, a large variety of available implants now exists [35]. With these mesh materials, it is entirely probable that some will prove to be superior in the long term, and some may even prove unacceptable. Regarding biologic mesh, the argument has been advanced that its use in bridging a defect does not result in a durable hernia repair [13]. Derisively, its use has been labeled as resulting in the "world's most expensive hernia sac" [14]. The contention is easily avoided through use of a permanent prosthetic.

Mesh Fixation

The standard of mesh fixation remains permanent trans-fascial sutures accompanied by edge fixation [36]. The degree of overlap of the hernia defect has been recommended to be 5 cm by most authorities, and many place tacking points approximately 1 cm apart along the circumference. However, there is substantial variation in this model, and it is this variation that may account for differences in result.

Functional Repair Results

A criticism of the bridging technique centers on the fact that it does not recreate physiology, only static anatomy. The abdominal wall continues to move and flex, which may lead to distortion of properly placed mesh [37]. Additionally, even if the mesh itself is flexible, the scar tissue surrounding the operative site may not be, leading to poor functional outcomes. Although mesh repairs resolve the majority of hernia complications, they are imperfect substitutes for the patient's actual abdominal wall.

The abdominal wall is indeed a complex arrangement of overlapping layers of muscle and connective tissue. Yet, it is precisely this complexity that should dissuade us from oversimplified attempts to re-create the dynamic interplay of its individual layers. It is possible to bridge the defect and achieve a functional result. It may not be possible to reapproximate the midline in mass fashion and achieve a complete restoration of normal function.

It has been recently suggested that primary closure of the defect may be accomplished laparoscopically with improved physiologic results [38]. Little data exists, however, to support this claim. There have been no studies documenting significant impairment of abdominal wall function using bridging techniques nor demonstrations of superior function with midline closure. At present, what constitutes the most optimal functional outcome of abdominal wall remains speculative only.

Cosmetic Repair Results

Few would argue against the cosmetic benefits of laparoscopic surgery in comparison with open surgery. Some advantages, however, exist in regard to open excisional techniques that may be potentially contributory to a cosmetically superior result.

The skin and hernia sac is left in situ above a bridging hernia repair. In most instances, this does not result in any significant complication or cosmetic deformity. It is true that a widened scar from initial incision is better addressed by excision. Circumstances where the skin does not have an acceptable appearance following laparoscopic repair may be addressed at any point in a secondary operation. In addition, some centers have suggested that the positive impact of laparoscopic surgery is more pronounced in patients with larger hernias, and laparoscopy is more strongly indicated in patients with large defects [39].

Although the development of a seroma may be a consequence of a laparoscopic ventral hernia repair, it is seldom of true clinical significance. The use of a postoperative abdominal binder has been advocated to minimize seroma formation, with at least some anecdotal success [40]. Reports regarding the high rate of seroma resolution without intervention as well as the excellent cosmetic results of the laparoscopic technique are common [41].

Conclusion

The laparoscopic ventral hernia repair is the standard of care for the repair of incisional and ventral hernias. As described, it involves bridging the fascial defect, which produces good results that have been reproduced in multiple centers. Although select patients may be considered for open repairs or alternative approaches, bridging the defect remains the quality option and should remain the standard approach for laparoscopic repair.

References

1. Franz MG, Kuhn MA, Nguyen K, et al. Transforming growth factor beta-2 lowers the incidence of incisional hernias. J Surg Res. 2001;97(2):109–16.
2. Park AE, Roth JS, Kavic SM. Abdominal wall hernias. Curr Prob Surg. 2006;43(5):321–75.
3. Turner PL, Park AE. Laparoscopic repair of ventral incisional hernias: pros and cons. Surg Clin North Am. 2008;88(1):85–100.
4. Louis D, Stoppa R, Henry X, Verhaeghe P. Postoperative eventration. Apropos of 247 surgically treated cases. J Chir (Paris). 1985;122(10):523–7.
5. Courtney CA, Lee AC, Wilson C, O'Dwyer PJ. Ventral hernia repair: a study of current practice. Hernia. 2003;7(1):44–6.
6. Kulah B, Duzgun AP, Moran M, Kulacoglu IH, Ozmen MM, Coskun F. Emergency hernia repairs in elderly patients. Am J Surg. 2001;182(5):455–9.
7. Luijendijk RW, Hop WC, van den Tol MP, et al. A comparison of suture repair with mesh repair of incisional hernia. N Eng J Med. 2000;343(6):392–8.
8. Rudmik LR, Schieman C, Dixon E, Debru E. Laparoscopic hernia repair: a review of the literature. Hernia. 2006;10(2):110–9.
9. Scott NW, McCormack K, Graham P, Go PM, Ross SJ, Grant AM. Open mesh versus non-mesh for repair of femoral and inguinal hernia. Cochrane Database Syst Rev. 2002;(4):CD002197.
10. Ramirez OM, Ruas E, Dellon AL. "Components separation" method for closure of abdominal-wall defects: an anatomic and clinical study. Plast Reconstr Surg. 1990;86(3):519–26.
11. van Geffen HJ, Simmermacher RK, van Vroonhoven TJ, van der Werken C. Surgical treatment of large contaminated abdominal wall defects. J Am Coll Surg. 2005;201(2):206–12.
12. Hultman CS, Tong WM, Kittinger BJ, Cairns B, Overby DW, Rich PB. Management of recurrent hernia after components separation: 10-year experience with abdominal wall reconstruction at an academic medical center. Ann Plast Surg. 2011;66(5):504–7.
13. Ko JH, Wang EC, Salvay DM, Paul BC, Dumanian GA. Abdominal wall reconstruction: lessons learned from 200 "components separation" procedures. Arch Surg. 2009;144(11):1047–55.
14. Blatnik J, Jin J, Rosen M. Abdominal hernia repair with bridging acellular dermal matrix—an expensive hernia sac. Am J Surg. 2008;196(1):47–50.
15. Alkhoury F, Helton S, Ippolito RJ. Cost and clinical outcomes of laparoscopic ventral hernia repair using intraperitoneal mesh. Surg Laparosc Endosc Percutan Tech. 2011;21(2):82–5.

16. Bageacu S, Blanc P, Breton C, et al. Laparoscopic repair of incisional hernia: a retrospective study of 159 patients. Surg Endosc. 2002;16(2):345–8.
17. Ben-Haim M, Kuriansky J, Tal R, et al. Pitfalls and complications with laparoscopic intraperitoneal expanded polytetrafluoroethylene patch repair of postoperative ventral hernia: lessons from the first 100 consecutive cases. Surg Endosc. 2002;16(5):785–8.
18. Berger D, Bientzle M, Müller A. Postoperative complications after laparoscopic incisional hernia repair. Incidence and treatment. Surg Endosc. 2002;16(12):1720–3.
19. Bower CE, Reade CC, Kirby LW, Roth JS. Complications of laparoscopic incisional-ventral hernia repair: the experience of a single institution. Surg Endosc. 2004;18(4):672–5.
20. Carbajo MA, Martp del Olmo JC, Blanco JI, et al. Laparoscopic approach to incisional hernia. Lessons learned from 270 patients over 8 years. Surg Endosc. 2003;17:118–22.
21. Chowbey PK, Sharma A, Khullar R, Mann V, Baijal M, Vashistha A. Laparoscopic ventral hernia repair. J Laparoendosc Adv Surg Tech. 2000;10(2):79–84.
22. Franklin Jr ME, Gonzalez Jr JJ, Glass JL, Manjarrez A. Laparoscopic ventral and incisional hernia repair: an 11-year experience. Hernia. 2004;8(1):23–7.
23. Frantzides CT, Carlson MA, Zografakis JG, Madan AK, Moore RE. Minimally invasive incisional herniorrhaphy: a review of 208 cases. Surg Endosc. 2004;18(10):1488–91.
24. Gillian GK, Weis WP, Grover G. Laparoscopic incisional and ventral hernia repair (VH): an evolving outpatient technique. JSLS. 2002;6(4):315–22.
25. Heniford BT, Park A, Ramshaw BJ, Voeller G. Laparoscopic repair of ventral hernias: nine years' experience with 850 consecutive hernias. Ann Surg. 2003;238(3):391–9.
26. Kirshtein B, Lantsberg L, Avinoach E, Bayne M, Mizrahi S. Laparoscopic repair of large incisional hernias. Surg Endosc. 2002;16(12):1717–9.
27. LeBlanc KA, Whitaker JM, Bellanger DE, Rhynes VK. Laparoscopic incisional and ventral hernioplasty: lessons learned from 200 patients. Hernia. 2003;7(3):118–24.
28. Olmi S, Erba L, Magnone S, Bertolini A, Croce E. Prospective clinical study of laparoscopic treatment of incisional and ventral hernia using a composite mesh: indications, complications and results. Hernia. 2006;10(3):243–7.
29. Perrone JM, Soper NJ, Eagon JC, et al. Perioperative outcomes and complications of laparoscopic ventral hernia repair. Surgery. 2005;138(4):708–15.
30. Rosen M, Brody F, Ponsky J, et al. Recurrence after laparoscopic ventral hernia repair. A five-year experience. Surg Endosc. 2003;17(1):123–8.
31. Sharma A, Mehrotra M, Khullar R, Soni V, Baijal M, Chowbey PK. Laparoscopic ventral/incisional hernia repair: a single centre experience of 1,242 patients over a period of 13 years. Hernia. 2011;15(2):131–9.
32. Toy FK, Bailey RW, Carey S, et al. Prospective, multicenter study of laparoscopic ventral hernioplasty. Preliminary results. Surg Endosc. 1998;12(7):955–9.
33. Ujiki MB, Weinberger J, Varghese TK, Murayama KM, Joehl RJ. One hundred consecutive laparoscopic ventral hernia repairs. Am J Surg. 2004;188(5):593–7.
34. Sauerland S, Walgenbach M, Habermalz B, Seiler CM, Miserez M. Laparoscopic versus open surgical techniques for ventral or incisional hernia repair. Cochrane Database Syst Rev. 2011;16(3):CD007781.

35. Shankaran V, Weber DJ, Reed 2nd RL, Luchette FA. A review of available prosthetics for ventral hernia repair. Ann Surg. 2011;253(1):16–26.
36. Cobb WS, Kercher KW, Heniford BT. Laparoscopic repair of incisional hernia. Surg Clin North Am. 2005;85(1):91–103.
37. Schumpelick V, Klinge U. Prosthetic implants for hernia repair. Br J Surg. 2003;90(12):1457–8.
38. Orenstein SB, Dumeer JL, Monteagudo J, Poi MJ, Novitsky YW. Outcomes of laparoscopic ventral hernia repair with routine defect closure using "shoelacing" technique. Surg Endosc. 2011;25(5):1452–7.
39. Arteaga-Gonzalez I, Martin-Malagon A, Fernandez EM, Carrillo-Pallares A. Which patients benefit most from laparoscopic ventral hernia repair? A comparative study. Surg Laparosc Endosc Percutan Tech. 2010;20(6):391–4.
40. LeBlanc KA. Laparoscopic incisional and ventral hernia repair: complications—how to avoid and handle. Hernia. 2004;8(4):323–31.
41. Misra MC, Bansal VK, Kulkarni MP, Pawar DK. Comparison of laparoscopic and open repair of incisional and primary ventral hernia: results of a prospective randomized study. Surg Endosc. 2006;20(12):1839–45.

41. The Bariatric Patient with a Complex Ventral Hernia

Jenny J. Choi and Alfons Pomp

The overall incidence and complexity of ventral and incisional hernias have increased. Patients live longer, accumulating comorbidities, and undergo more surgeries. Moreover, obesity is now a worldwide epidemic. Wound infections and incisional hernia formation more frequently complicate laparotomies on obese patients with a large abdominal girth. The management of hernias continues to evolve as we learn more about genetic predisposition and the pathophysiology of the disease. There are now multiple options for hernia repair. What historically began as the primary repair of simple ventral hernias has evolved to mesh repair of larger hernias and now encompasses complex procedures such as multiple layers of component separation complemented with synthetic and biologic mesh. With increasing numbers of bariatric procedures performed, hernias in these patients have now emerged as an important topic that needs to be addressed both preoperatively and postoperatively.

Morbidly obese patients are at an increased risk for primary as well as incisional hernias. Studies have shown that obese patients have increased intra-abdominal pressures (IAP) when compared to normal weight control patients [1, 2]. When comparing obese patients (mean BMI 55 ± 2 kg/m^2) to controls, the mean IAP for the morbidly obese group was 12 ± 0.8 cm H_2O, significantly increased when compared to controls with IAP$=0 \pm 2$ cm H_2O. Obese patients consistently had elevated intra-abdominal pressures when compared to normal-weighed controls during the activities of daily living such as walking, climbing stairs, coughing, and lifting. Increased IAP puts added stress on the abdominal wall and tensile strength of the mesh. Obese patients are also more likely to be afflicted with weight-related comorbidities, which also predispose the development of hernias. A study looking at 62 patients with a mean BMI of 49 revealed that systemic hypertension,

B.P. Jacob and B. Ramshaw (eds.), *The SAGES Manual of Hernia Repair*,
DOI 10.1007/978-1-4614-4824-2_41,

the American Society of Anesthesiologists (ASA) physical status score, and body mass index (BMI) were predictors of elevated IAP [3]. Risk factors for developing abdominal wall hernias include smoking, advanced age, wound infection, multiple surgeries, and chronic medical conditions such as chronic obstructive pulmonary disease, diabetes, and immunosuppression. Given these findings, it is not surprising that potential bariatric patients are more predisposed to primary ventral hernias as well as developing postoperative hernias. Open bariatric surgery is associated with an incidence of incisional hernias of ~20% [4–6]. With laparoscopy now more customary, the number of large incisional hernias has decreased, but port-site hernias can still occur. The specific incidence of port hernias in the bariatric surgery population is not known, but in general, these hernias typically occur within 3–4 years after surgery at rates of 0.8–2.8% [7, 8].

The recurrence rates of incisional hernias have also been shown to be higher in the obese population. Many studies have shown a statistically significant higher incidence of incisional hernia in patients with BMI > 35 [9–12]. However, a retrospective study of 168 patients, specifically comparing morbidly obese to normal body weight patients, showed no difference in the complication or recurrence rates at 19-month follow-up after laparoscopic hernia repair [13]. Regardless, the morbidly obese patients tend to have larger fascial defects, and recurrence may occur up to 10 years postoperatively [14]. Thus, the timing of most durable ventral hernia repair may well be after significant weight loss which is usually accompanied by at least a partial resolution of medical comorbidities.

Management

The management of concomitant ventral hernia at the time of primary bariatric surgery remains controversial. Datta et al. have shown that the incidence of ventral hernia at the time of gastric bypass was quite common. Of the 325 patients operated in their series, 26 had a ventral hernia, an incidence of 8% [15]. This rate is even higher when combined with those patients who also have known and symptomatic incisional or ventral hernias. The ultimate goal is to perform the primary bariatric surgery safely and avoid postoperative complications. However, there may be an increased risk of complications if these hernias are not addressed at the time of primary bariatric surgery.

Currently, there is no consensus regarding the best option for bariatric surgery patients with ventral hernias. There are essentially three surgical options when an unsuspected hernia is encountered during the performance of a gastric bypass, which is defined as a clean-contaminated case. The most straightforward option is to simply note the presence of the hernia in the operative report and "leave it alone." This approach offers certain advantages including expediting the operative time and avoiding hernia repair complications. The downside is painful incarceration and/or bowel obstructions that are the well-documented possible sequelae of untreated hernias, and immediate postoperative gastric bypass patients have even greater risks. Incarceration and potential proximal bowel obstruction can stress fresh anastomoses, and disruption can cause leaks. Given that these patients are already considerably medically compromised due to their morbid obesity, this can be a potentially life-threatening complication.

Another option is primary closure, especially in smaller (<3–4 cm) hernias, a strategy which sidesteps the potential of mesh placement in a clean-contaminated field. This approach may not be appropriate as an oft-cited study suggests that more than one-third of patients who had deferred treatment of their hernias during laparoscopic Roux-en-Y gastric bypass experienced subsequent development of small bowel obstruction. 85 patients who had ventral hernias at the time of gastric bypass had either no treatment, primary repair, or repair with small intestinal submucosa (SIS). There was a 22% recurrence in the primary repair group, and 36% developed bowel obstruction due to incarceration in no treatment group [16].

Another smaller study examined 27 preoperative bariatric patients with complex recurrent ventral hernias. Seven patients underwent ventral hernia repair simultaneously (primary and biologic mesh), and all others were deferred. All seven of the repaired hernias recurred, and one patient in the deferred group needed an urgent operation for incarceration [17]. Clearly, there is a relatively high risk of complications if complex hernias are not treated at the time of gastric bypass.

For simple small defects that measure <3–4 cm and already have viable omentum in the hernia sac and are out of the operative field, the risk of incarceration still appears minimal, and these may be left in situ. The omentum in the sac may actually act like a "plug" and prevent bowel incarceration and obstruction. Then there are small hernias that are symptomatic or do not contain anything within the hernia sac. While all symptomatic hernias must be addressed at the time of bariatric surgery since clinical symptoms are likely secondary to intermittent bowel incarceration and obstruction, these small-necked hernias may be more likely to cause incarceration (or a partial Richter's type hernia). Postoperative ileus and bowel distension is common after bariatric surgery, which may increase the risk of incarceration. Small defects <3–4 cm may be closed primarily with a suture passer at the time of bariatric surgery. Although, as mentioned, the recurrence may be as high as 25%, this may bridge the patients during the early, crucial postoperative period [16].

For larger symptomatic hernias and complex hernias, studies have shown that the rate of hernia recurrence is largely based on initial size of the defect, and these hernias cannot be closed primarily [13]. The best option may be repair with biologic or synthetic mesh. Recurrent hernias with multiple small defects or those with mesh from previous surgeries are also difficult to deal with. Since the likelihood of recurrence and bowel obstruction is high, these hernias must also be addressed, likely with mesh.

Surgeons are justifiably concerned with mesh infection and recurrence of hernia when performing primary clean-contaminated bariatric surgery concomitantly with complex hernia repair. The previously cited study by Eid et al. showed no recurrence of hernia when mesh repair with SIS was performed. However, there were significant perioperative complications as wound infection occurred in 25% and seroma in 33% of these patients [16]. Biologic mesh is not an ideal solution. It is expensive, and significant rates of early and midterm recurrences, especially when this type of mesh is used to bridge fascial defects, have been reported [18]. Another, more recent, retrospective study of 325 gastric patients, 26 of whom had ventral hernia, underwent primary and prosthetic mesh repair. Surprisingly, 2 of the 8 patients who had primary repair had postoperative small bowel obstruction, while those with mesh repair had none [15]. This same study also showed no mesh infection when gastric bypass was performed simultaneously with synthetic mesh ventral hernia repair. Thus, it appears that complex hernias may be repaired with either synthetic or biologic mesh, depending on the surgeon's comfort level.

Now that sleeve gastrectomy is an accepted part of the bariatric armamentarium [19], this may be the bariatric procedure of choice if a patient has a complex hernia. Sleeve gastrectomy allows for minimal manipulation of the bowel and does not dislocate the bowel that then may potentially incarcerate. The peritoneum is never appreciably exposed to enteric contents, and there is minimal risk of mesh infection. These patients are less likely to develop ileus or bowel distension since there are no anastomoses. For those with a large complex hernia or those with chronically incarcerated but nonobstructed bowel, sleeve gastrectomy may be a very safe option.

Occasionally, there are large, complex hernias that may preclude the surgeon from performing any intra-abdominal procedure prior to repairing the hernia. These hernias need to be repaired as a separate procedure prior to any elective bariatric surgery. Those patients with very large, chronic incisional hernias (>25–30 cm) will pose a problem for the surgeon in many aspects. Given the lack of fascia and chronically distended bowel, access into the peritoneum for insufflation to perform laparoscopy or adequate exposure for open surgery may be nearly impossible. The loss of domain with pneumoperitoneum will also be prohibitive for this type of patient, and ventilation, venous return, and tissue oxygenation will be compromised. This can lead to multiple complications including prolonged intubation, cardiac depression, and poor wound healing [20, 21]. Thus, the hernia must be dealt with first. In this scenario, the patient may need component separation and a staged ventral hernia repair prior to an elective bariatric surgery [22].

Another subset of patients with chronic fistulas or infected mesh from previous hernia repair will also require definitive hernia repair prior to bariatric surgery. The presence of an ongoing infection and further exposure of mesh will put the patient at risk for multiple postoperative complications. An attempt to remove the infected mesh in order to completely resolve the infection should be done before proceeding with (elective) bariatric surgery.

Conclusion

Whether an incisional hernia is simple or large and complex, the repair must be tailored to each individual bariatric patient. Clearly the lowest recurrence and complication rates will be realized if hernia repair is deferred until maximal weight loss is accomplished, with the added benefit that concurrent abdominoplasty can be performed. For some, small, incidentally discovered hernias, deferred management may be appropriate, but close follow-up is necessary. There appears to be good data at present however to make a case that primary repair is usually not sufficient as definitive therapy even for small, but clinically significant, defects, but it still may be applicable as a bridge repair during the immediate postoperative period. While infection rates are not common when prosthetics are used concomitantly with gastric bypass, mesh use in clean-contaminated cases remains debatable. If biologic mesh is used, substantial recurrence rates (and expense!) are important considerations. Despite some encouraging safety data that synthetic mesh should be considered in the repertoire of techniques to repair incisional hernia during gastric bypass, the use of this type of prosthetic material remains controversial.

References

1. Lambert DM, Marceau S, Forse RA. Intra-abdominal pressure in the morbidly obese. Obes Surg. 2005;15(9):1225–32.
2. Cobb WS, Burns JM, Kercher KW, Matthews BD, Norton JH, Heniford BT. Normal intraabdominal pressure in healthy adults. J Surg Res. 2005;129(2):231–5.
3. Varela JE, Hinojosa M, Nguyen N. Correlations between intra-abdominal pressure and obesity-related co-morbidities. Surg Obes Relat Dis. 2009;5(5):524–8.
4. Sugarman HJ, Kellum JM, Reines HD, DeMaria EJ, Newsome HH, Lowry JW. Greater risk of incisional hernia with morbidly obese than steroid dependent patients and low recurrence with prefascial polypropylene mesh. Am J Surg. 2006;171:80–4.
5. Alper D, Ramadan D, Vishne T, et al. Silastic ring vertical gastroplasty—long-term results and complications. Obes Surg. 2000;10:250–4.
6. Paran H, Shargian L, Schwarz I, Gutman M. Long-term follow-up on the effect of Silastic ring vertical gastroplasty on weight and co-morbidities. Obes Surg. 2007;17:737–41.
7. Tonouchi H, Ohmori Y, Kobayashi M, Kusunoki M. Trochar site hernia. Arch Surg. 2004;139:1248–56.
8. Hussain A, Mahmood H, Singhal T, et al. Long-term study of port-site incisional hernias after laparoscopic procedure. JSLS. 2009;13:346–9.
9. Bageacu S, Blanc P, Breton C, Gonzalez M, Porcheron J, Chabert M, Balique JG. Laparoscopic repair of incisional hernia: a retrospective study of 159 patients. Surg Endosc. 2002;16:345–8.
10. Raftopoulos I, Vanuno D, Khorsand J, Ninos J, Kouraklis G, Lasky P. Outcome of laparoscopic ventral hernia repair in correlation with obesity, type of hernia, and hernia size. J Laparoendosc Adv Surg Tech. 2002;12:425–9.
11. Rosen M, Brody F, Ponsky J, Walsh RM, Rosenblatt S, Duperier F, Fanning A, Siperstein A. Recurrence after laparoscopic ventral hernia repair. Surg Endosc. 2003;17:123–8.
12. Novitsky YW, Cobb WS, Kercher KW, Matthews BD, Sing RF, Heniford BT. Laparoscopic ventral hernia repair in obese patients: a new standard of care. Arch Surg. 2006;141:57–61.
13. Ching SS, Sarela AI, Dexter SP, Hayden JD, McMahon MJ. Comparison of early outcomes for laparoscopic ventral hernia repair between nonobese and morbidly obese

patient populations. Surg Endosc. 2008;22(10):2244–50.

14. Heniford BT, Park A, Ramshaw BJ, Voeller G. Laparoscopic repair of ventral hernias: nine years' experience with 850 consecutive hernias. Ann Surg. 2003;238:391–4.
15. Datta T, Eid G, Nahmias N, Dallal RM. Management of ventral hernias during laparoscopic gastric bypass. Surg Obes Relat Dis. 2008;4(6):754–7.
16. Eid GM, Mattar SG, Hamad G, Cottam DR, Lord JL, Watson A, Dallal RM, Schauer PR. Repair of ventral hernias in morbidly obese patients undergoing laparoscopic gastric bypass should not be deferred. Surg Endosc. 2004;18:207–10.
17. Newcomb WL, Polhill JL, Chen AY, Kuwada TS, Gersin KS, Getz SB, Kercher KW, Heniford BT. Staged hernia repair preceded by gastric bypass for the treatment of morbidly obese patients with complex ventral hernias. Hernia. 2008;12(5):465–9.
18. Jin J, Rosen MJ, Blatnik J, et al. Use of acellular dermal matrix for complicated ventral hernia repair: does technique affect outcomes? J Am Coll Surg. 2007;205(5):654–60.
19. Brethauer SA, Hammel JP, Schauer PR. Systematic review of sleeve gastrectomy as staging and primary bariatric procedure. Surg Obes Relat Dis. 2009;5(4):469–75.
20. Paajanen H, Laine H. Operative treatment of massive ventral hernia using polypropylene mesh: a challenge for surgeon and anaesthesiologist. Hernia. 2005;9:62–7.
21. Molloy RG, Moran KT, Waldron RP, Brady MP, Kirwan WO. Massive incisional hernia: abdominal wall replacement with Marlex mesh. Br J Surg. 1991;78(2):242–4.
22. Rao RS, Gentileschi P, Kini SU. Management of ventral hernias in bariatric surgery. Surg Obes Relat Dis. 2011;7(1):110–6.

42. Open Versus Endoscopic Component Separation: How to Choose One or the Other

Eduardo Parra-Davila, Juan J. Diaz-Hernandez, and Carlos M. Ortiz-Ortiz

The repair of massive ventral hernias has remained a challenging problem for surgeons. Primary repair is rarely successful and has associated recurrence rates of 18–62% depending on the defect size [1–4]. The addition of synthetic mesh decreases recurrence rates significantly from 2 to 32% [1, 3–6]. The use of large sheets of synthetic material for hernia repair often results in a rigid, noncompliant, adynamic abdominal wall and in most cases is contraindicated in the setting of contamination. The principles of ventral hernia repair are well established: wound closure should be free of excessive tension, sutures should be placed in healthy tissue, and strong suture material should be used to support the wound through the critical period of healing [7].

To allow a patient who presents with a ventral hernia to regain dynamic support of the abdominal wall, the fascial edges need to be reapproximated. This may not be an appropriate repair for all patients, but techniques that ease tension on the midline and have less potential complications will probably increase in popularity.

Open separation of components, as championed by Ramirez [8], has enable rectus muscle medialization in patients with midline defect up to 20 cm in size. Several series have reported recurrence rates from 5 to 30% [9–11]. More recently, the component separation technique (CST) has been performed with several modifications including reinforcement with biological or synthetic mesh to improve results. Additionally, the endoscopic approach has been described by Rosen [12].

B.P. Jacob and B. Ramshaw (eds.), *The SAGES Manual of Hernia Repair*, DOI 10.1007/978-1-4614-4824-2_42,

Description of Component Separation Technique and Modifications

Open Component Separation Technique

The incision at the skin is done longitudinally or horizontally (suprapubic) in most cases. The skin and subcutaneous fat are dissected free from the anterior rectus sheath and the aponeurosis of the external oblique muscle. The aponeurosis of the external oblique muscle is transected longitudinally about 3 cm lateral from the rectus sheath, including the muscular part that inserts on the thoracic wall, which extends at least 5–7 cm cranially of the costal margin. The external oblique muscle is separated from the internal oblique muscle as far lateral as possible. The posterior rectal sheath is separated from the rectus abdominis muscle if tension-free closure is not possible. The fascia is closed in the midline with a running #1 PDS (polydioxanone) suture of at least four times the length of the incision. The skin is closed over at least two suction drains.

Open Component Separation Technique with Reinforcement of Mesh

Same technique as described above but with the following reinforcement with mesh:

(a) Onlay synthetic large pore or biological mesh.
(b) Underlay intraperitoneal (with adhesion barrier) or biological mesh.
(c) Retromuscular mesh placement (large pore synthetic or biologic).
(d) Preperitoneal mesh placement (allows a macroporous mesh to be placed with wider coverage than the lateral border or the rectus muscle).
(e) Bridging an already component separation that does not reach for complete closure of the midline. Mesh reinforcement is usually underlain (biologic or synthetic).

Endoscopic Component Separation Technique

The operation can begin with a 1-cm incision made just below the costal margin or at the lower quadrants of the abdomen, depending on surgeon's preference. Alternatively, a midline open incision with lysis of adhesions can be performed first. The endoscopic incision is made lateral to the rectus abdominis muscle. If an open midline incision is already made, it can help to identify the lateral border of the rectus muscle by palpating it through the midline incision. The subcutaneous tissue is dissected to expose the external oblique fascia. The aponeurosis is separated, and further dissection follows the direction of the muscle fibers encountering the space between the external and the internal oblique muscle. The hernia balloon dissector is introduced, and the space is created usually with several insufflations with the balloon pump. Then a balloon port is inserted to maintain insufflation of 10–12 mmHg. The 5-mm 30° laparoscope is used to place a second 5-mm trocar laterally at the posterior axillary line approximately at the level of the umbilicus. With a grasper and/or scissors, the space is completed to expose the external oblique aponeurosis from the costal margin to the inguinal ligament. Then the external oblique is released under direct visualization using coagulating scissors.

Endoscopic CST with Laparoscopic Ventral Hernia Repair

The endoscopic CST is performed as described as above, without a midline open incision. After this, the trocars are placed intraperitoneally for the dissection and reduction of the hernia contents. The hernia defect is closed with sutures to approximate the fascia to the midline. This technique can also be followed by intraperitoneal reinforcement with synthetic (with adhesion barrier) or biological mesh.

There have been reports of accomplishing an average of 86% of the myofascial advancement using the endoscopic CST approach without the elevation of the skin flaps. Any additional release can be achieved with incision of the posterior rectus sheath if necessary [12] (Figs. 42.1 and 42.2).

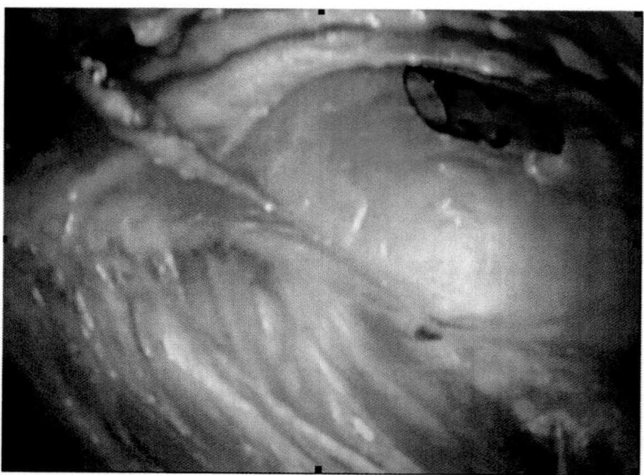

Fig. 42.1. Endoscopic separation of external oblique fascia.

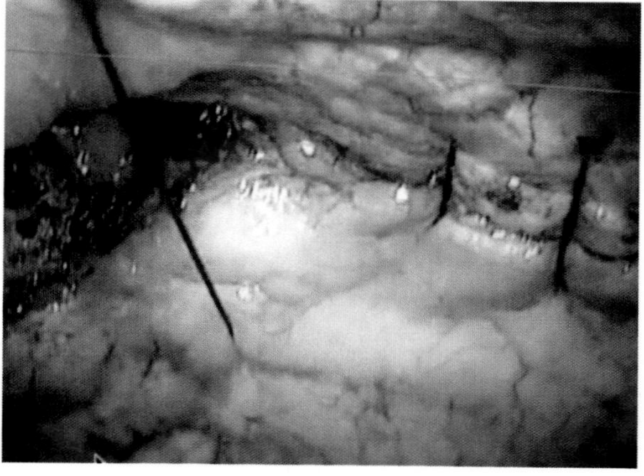

Fig. 42.2. Laparoscopic closure of hernia defect.

Open Ventral Hernia Repair with Endoscopic Component Separation

This technique includes the usual dissection for the open ventral hernia repair combined with the endoscopic approach for the component separation technique to avoid the open dissection of the abdominal wall flaps. The reinforcement of the repair is performed usually intraperitoneally with synthetic (with adhesion barrier) or biological mesh. The fascia is approximated at the midline with a running #1 PDS (polydioxanone) suture.

Indications for CST

(a) Limited contaminated or clean contaminated fields.
(b) History of recurrence after several previous repairs.
(c) Large hernia defects including loss of domain.
(d) When restoration of physiology of abdominal wall is imperative (patient with hernia and neo-bladder).
(e) Cosmetic restoration.
(f) Hernia with tension when attempting closure of fascia.

There are a number of surgeon-, hernia type, and patient-dependent factors that will eventually contribute to the surgical techniques chosen to complete any given hernia operation. Some of the intraoperative decisions regarding choosing a component release may be influenced by the following hernia and patient characteristics:

Extension of Hernia Sac Laterally to the Semilunaris Line and Complex Surgery that Involves the Lateral Abdominal Wall

The fibrosis and/or scar tissue from previous surgery makes the endoscopic CST approach more difficult. The CST in these patients is usually performed by open technique (Fig. 42.3).

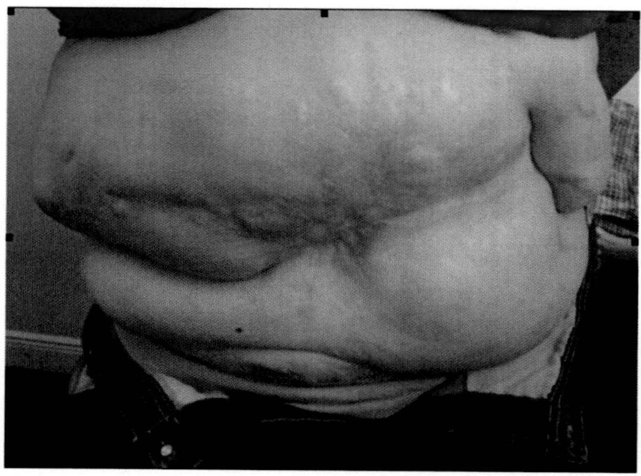

Fig. 42.3. Multiple and extensive abdominal wall surgeries.

Need for Wound Revision

If the dissection requires a vast removal of soft tissue, the endoscopic approach may not provide an advantage. This dissection will expose most of the area needed to perform an open CST.

Need for Mesh Explantation

To be able to remove an onlay mesh, a vast subcutaneous flap dissection is required, making an open CST a better choice (Fig. 42.4). If the mesh was placed as an underlay, the CST can be performed endoscopically or open depending on the surgeon's preference since the subcutaneous space has not been violated.

Presence of Ostomy

Most surgeons do not perform a bilateral CST in the presence of an ostomy (Fig. 42.5). The unilateral approach for the CST can be performed open or endoscopically, including mesh reinforcement.

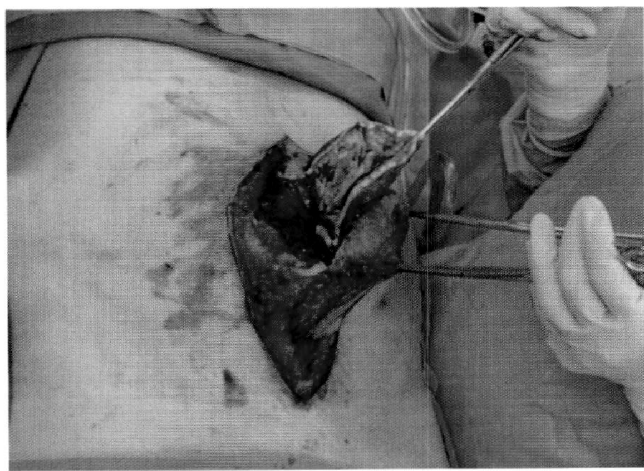

Fig. 42.4. Removal of infected onlay mesh.

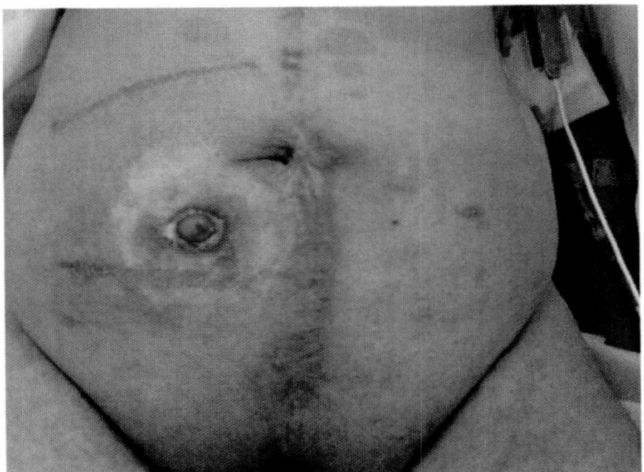

Fig. 42.5. Multiple parastomal hernia repairs.

Need for Panniculectomy

This technique requires bilateral abdominal wall flaps that will expose the aponeurosis of the external oblique for open CST (Fig. 42.6).

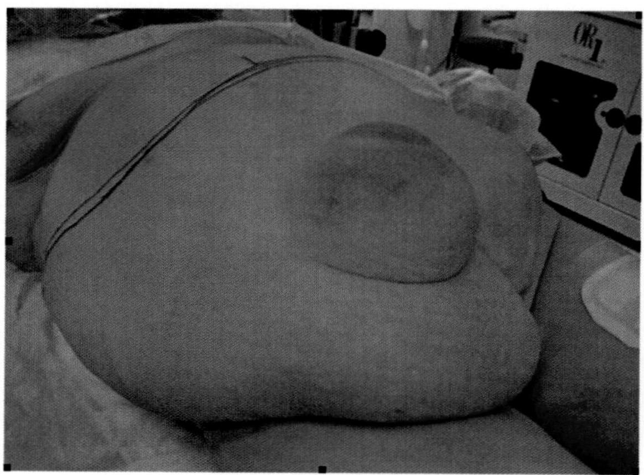

Fig. 42.6. Medically necessary panniculectomy.

Presence of Abdominal Contamination

In the setting of limited and controlled contamination, the endoscopic approach provides the release of the fascia in a clean space not in continuity with the midline incision. This potentially decreases the incidence of postoperative wound infections.

Intraoperative Assessment of Tension

During the operation, if an open midline incision is made first, an assessment of tension and abdominal wall compliance can be done by placing clamps on rectus muscle medial fascia and pulling them to the midline. Although this is a very imprecise measure, this may help determine the best approach for component separation: open or endoscopic.

In summary, the Achilles tendon of the open CST is the wound infection, hematoma, seroma, and abdominal wall flap necrosis that are reported in 12–67% of cases [8–11, 13–19]. Other reports in the literature show an overall complication rates that were similar for endoscopic CST (32%) and open CST (35%). Comparison between endoscopic CST and open CST showed comparable hernia recurrence rates (endoscopic CST 17% and open CST 21%) [20].

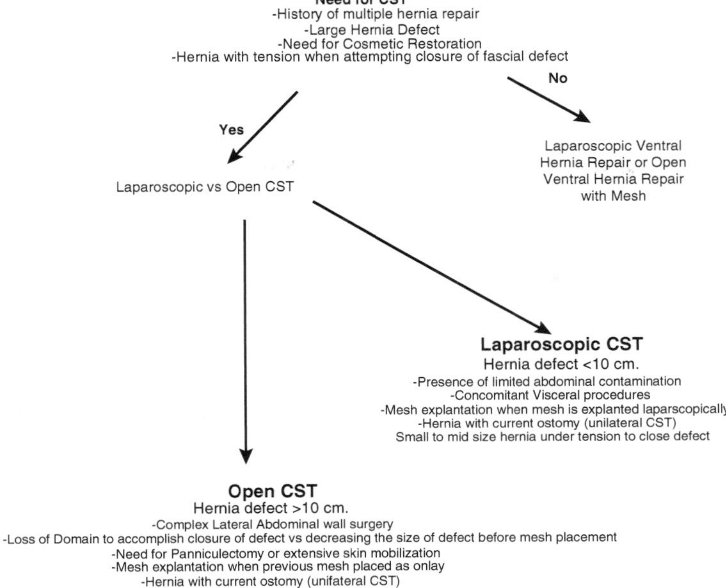

Fig. 42.7. A decision-making flowchart for the need for CST.

We believe that medialization of the rectus muscle is imperative for improving abdominal wall function. The CST with muscle advancement increases the abdominal wall circumference to enlarge the intraperitoneal space for those patients afflicted with large ventral hernias and loss of domain. The placement of mesh for reinforcement of the repair decreases the recurrence rate of the CST, and the rectus medialization decreases the risk of mesh eventration. This technique is not indicated for the small "average" ventral hernia when the fascia can be easily approximated or in patients with multiple small (<2 cm) "Swiss cheese" hernias. In our experience with open CST, we have accomplished more advancement of the abdominal wall when compared to the endoscopic CST. For this reason, we use the endoscopic CST for selected cases of midsize (<10 cm), usually midline primary or first recurrent hernias. Please refer to Fig. 42.7 for a decision-making flowchart.

References

1. Burger JW, Luijendijk RW, Hop WC, et al. Long-term follow-up of a randomized controlled trial of suture versus mesh repair of incisional hernia. Ann Surg. 2004; 240:578–85.
2. Millikan KW. Incisional hernia repair. Surg Clin North Am. 2003;83:1223–34.
3. Sauerland S, Schmedt CG, Lein S, et al. Primary incisional hernia repair with or without polypropylene mesh: a report on 384 patients with 5-year follow-up. Langenbecks Arch Surg. 2005;390:408–12.
4. Luijendijk RW, Hop WC, van den Tol MP, et al. A comparison of suture repair with mesh repair for incisional hernia. N Engl J Med. 2000;343:392–8.
5. Lomanto D, Iyer SG, Shabbir A, et al. Laparoscopic versus open ventral hernia mesh repair: a prospective study. Surg Endosc. 2006;20:1030–5.
6. Novitsky YW, Porter JR, Rucho ZC, et al. Open preperitoneal retrofascial mesh repair for multiply recurrent ventral incisional hernias. J Am Coll Surg. 2006;203:283–9.
7. Larson GM. Ventral hernia repair by the laparoscopic approach. Surg Clin North Am. 2000;80:1329–40.
8. Ramirez OM, Ruas E, Dellon AL. "Components separation" method for closure of abdominal-wall defects: an anatomic and clinical study. Plast Reconstr Surg. 1990; 86:519–26.
9. de Vries Reilingh TS, van Goor H, Rosman C, et al. "Components separation technique" for the repair of large abdominal wall hernias. J Am Coll Surg. 2003; 196:32–7.
10. Shestak KC, Edington HJ, Johnson RR. The separation of anatomic components technique for the reconstruction of massive midline abdominal wall defects: anatomy, surgical technique, applications, and limitations revisited. Plast Reconstr Surg. 2000;105:731–9.
11. DiBello Jr JN, Moore Jr JH. Sliding myofascial flap of the rectus abdominus muscles for the closure of recurrent ventral hernias. Plast Reconstr Surg. 1996;98:464–9.
12. Rosen MJ, Williams C, Jin J, McGee MF, Schomisch S, Marks J, Ponsky J. Laparoscopic versus open-component separation: a comparative analysis in a porcine model. Am J Surg. 2007;194:385–9.
13. Girotto JA, Mascus K, Redett R, et al. Closure of chronic abdominal wall defects: a long-term evaluation of the components separation method. Ann Plast Surg. 1999;42:385–94.
14. Cohen M, Morales Jr R, Fildes J, et al. Staged reconstruction after gunshot wounds to the abdomen. Plast Reconstr Surg. 2001;108:83–92.
15. Jernigan TW, Fabian TC, Croce MA, et al. Staged management of giant abdominal wall defects: acute and long-term results. Ann Surg. 2003;238:349–55.
16. Kuzbari R, Worseg AP, Tairych G, et al. Sliding door technique for the repair of midline incisional hernias. Plast Reconstr Surg. 1998;101:1235–42.
17. Lowe III JB, Lowe JB, Baty JD, et al. Risks associated with "components separation" for closure of complex abdominal wall defects. Plast Reconstr Surg. 2003;111:1276–83.

18. Sukkar SM, Dumanian GA, Szczerba SM, et al. Challenging abdominal wall defects. Am J Surg. 2001;181:115–21.
19. Ennis LS, Young JS, Gampper TJ, et al. The "open-book" variation of component separation for repair of massive midline abdominal wall hernia. Am Surg. 2003; 69:733–42.
20. Tong WMY, Hope W, Overby DW, Hultman CS. Comparison of outcome after mesh-only repair, laparoscopic component separation, and open component separation. Ann Plast Surg. 2011;66:551–6.

43. Absorbable Fixation Materials: A Critical Appraisal

Kevin El-Hayek and Matthew Kroh

Hernia repair is one of the most common procedures performed around the world, with an estimated 1,000,000 such repairs being performed per year in the United States alone [1–4]. The most common types include repairs of inguinal, ventral or incisional, and hiatal hernias. Standard herniorrhaphy prior to the 1950s primarily involved direct tissue re-approximation; however, this technique was associated with reported recurrence rates of 25–54% [5–9]. Subsequent development of prosthetic mesh implantation decreased recurrence rates significantly; however, a trade-off of more mesh-related complications has ensued. These complications include infection, visceral adhesions, fistulae, and obstructions among others [10, 11]. In response to these complications, more sophisticated mesh products have been designed to provide a durable repair with adequate tissue ingrowth while maintaining a less inflammatory barrier against the intra-abdominal viscera.

In conjunction with increased technology of mesh products, fixation devices have evolved as well. Historically, the only options for mesh fixation were sutures of varying degrees of absorbability and permanence. The influx of laparoscopy in general surgery has ushered in new options for fixation, including tacking devices and sealants. Laparoscopic ventral hernia repair is associated with lower recurrence rates, lower mesh infection rates, fewer postoperative complications, and shorter hospital stays [12–14]. Though the majority of operative repairs, including laparoscopy, are performed using permanent sutures or tacks, there is currently an opportunity to limit the amount of foreign material by using absorbable fixation devices. The goal of this chapter is to review the materials and methods involved in the use of absorbable fixation for inguinal and ventral hernias.

B.P. Jacob and B. Ramshaw (eds.), *The SAGES Manual of Hernia Repair*,
DOI 10.1007/978-1-4614-4824-2_43,

Principles of Mesh Fixation

The physical and physiologic changes that exist at the time of hernia repair and subsequent to implantation ultimately dictate long-term efficacy. Discussion of fixation devices is therefore dependent on a brief review of their interactions with various mesh types. Mesh material is a critical consideration when preparing to repair a hernia. Characteristics of mesh to consider prior to implantation include material, pore size, and density [15, 16]. Mesh material will dictate the degree of inflammatory response and the ultimate scar plate that is deposited. This interaction will in large part determine the strength of a repair. Pro-inflammatory materials such as polypropylene and polyester generate excellent tissue ingrowth but are also prone to adhesion formation when exposed to viscera [10]. The structure of mesh will also guide tissue ingrowth and ultimately stability. The porosity of the mesh weave will to varying degrees allow for native tissue infiltration. Microporous mesh (<10–75 μm) such as ePTFE has the advantage of causing less visceral adhesions; however, tissue ingrowth is also decreased. Macroporous (>75 μm) mesh provides much better tissue ingrowth; however, this mesh can lead to more dense adhesions [15, 16]. Consideration of porosity is important when selecting fixation devices as mesh that is less porous will require greater fixation than mesh that allows for better tissue ingrowth. Finally, mesh density may dictate fixation material penetration, which in turn determines adequate security.

Once the mesh is chosen, how to secure the mesh becomes relevant. The fixation technique must provide adequate stability to ensure that the mesh does not migrate. Migration and mesh shrinkage are two common causes of hernia recurrence. During ventral hernia repair, data has shown that greater fascial overlap, typically at least 3–5 cm, will decrease recurrence rates [17]. If the fixation material and method do not provide adequate strength to maintain proper orientation, the mesh can pull away due to normal body movements. The time and strength required of such a fixation device is variable based on anatomic location of mesh repair, for example, inguinal versus abdominal wall, and the specific to the type of mesh used, based on material and porosity.

In addition to adequate strength, fixation materials must provide durability. Additionally, mesh fixation involves limiting postoperative complications such as foreign body reaction, infection, and pain. There are many absorbable materials in use today which purport to have many of these positive properties while limiting the negative properties of mesh fixation.

Composition and Properties of Absorbable Fixation Materials

Currently, permanent fixation is commonly used for hernia repair. Specifically for abdominal wall repair with synthetic mesh, permanent transfascial suture fixation has shown excellent strength [18, 19]. Transfascial fixation with permanent suture remains the gold standard in laparoscopic ventral hernia repair, but these are not without complication [20]. When used to secure mesh laparoscopically, transfascial fixation sutures traverse all layers of the abdominal wall in a mass closure technique. From a strength standpoint, this is ideal. In a porcine model of mean tensile strength, transfascial sutures were found to be 2.5 times stronger than tack placement in securing polypropylene mesh [19]. However, this technique can also result in significant patient pain. Studies have shown that placement of sutures using this technique for mesh fixation during ventral hernia repair can result in chronic and often difficult to manage pain [21, 22]. Even after surgical suture removal, pain may not be mitigated in these patients. Though still considered the most durable long-term option for mesh fixation, these unique complications from permanent suture fixation have prompted investigation into other materials.

Absorbable Suture

Sutures are foreign bodies and as such, illicit reaction from adjacent tissue. The development of absorbable suture was designed to limit this reaction as most tissues, once approximated, will adhere to one another without permanent fixation. There are numerous types of absorbable sutures. The main variants include material, braidedness, and absorption profile. These sutures range from beef or sheep submucosa to synthetic material such as polyglactin and poliglecaprone. Their absorption profiles vary from 40 to >200 days. The main mechanism for absorption is via hydrolization and enzymatic degradation when the body recognizes this foreign material [23]. Transfascial suture fixation is currently the most common form of mesh fixation during open and laparoscopic ventral hernia repair, and typically this is performed with permanent suture.

Absorbable Fasteners

Though transfascial suture fixation is the most common method to secure mesh, there is a trend toward fastening devices such as tacks. These devices are more common in laparoscopic repair but are also used during open repair. The technology has evolved and includes medical skin staples, helical fasteners, and other specialty tacking devices [24, 25]. Tack fixation of mesh during laparoscopic hernia repair has the advantage of being relatively easy to dispense and to secure the mesh, but the depth of penetration into the soft tissue is limited by the design of the tack, the thickness of mesh being used, and the adequacy with which the tack is seated into the abdominal wall. These concerns have prompted many surgeons to use tacks in conjunction with transfascial suture fixation, with the idea that the tacks will help position the mesh for ultimate transfascial suture placement. Tacks also keep the periphery of the mesh annealed to the abdominal wall until re-peritonealization takes place, a process that typically takes 7–10 days [6]. The suture is then designed to stabilize the mesh for robust tissue ingrowth and durable mesh fixation. With mesh products that allow for fast and significant tissue ingrowth, some authors have proposed not using transfascial suture fixation, though studies have shown increased rates of hernia recurrence when PTFE mesh is used without suture fixation [12]. However, composite materials may allow better tissue ingrowth resulting in accelerated healing times and stronger repairs [26]. Other authors have shown that use of tacks as an adjunct or replacement for sutures reduces time and possibly even postoperative pain [22].

Permanent metallic fixation devices work well in securing the mesh long enough for reperitonealization and stabilization. However, concerns exist about leaving these permanent materials in place. Complications such as adhesions to metallic tack heads and tack migration from the abdominal wall into the viscera have been shown to result in small bowel obstruction and even perforation [27–30]. Such complications have led to the development of absorbable fixation devices. There are currently three companies with absorbable fixation systems on the market: Covidien (AbsorbaTack™), Bard Davol (SorbaFix™, PermaSorb™), and Ethicon (Securestrap™).

Covidien: AbsorbaTack™

The Covidien AbsorbaTack™ was released in 2008. There are both long and short 5-mm versions of the delivery system for use in laparoscopic and open repair. These devices have 15 or 30 tacks for the long delivery system and 20 tacks for the short delivery system. There is no pilot tip in this design for engaging soft tissue. The fasteners are composed of poly(glycolide-co-L-lactide) (PGLA) and have a tapered screwlike tip. There is a 1.0-mm head with a total length of 5.1 mm. A significant absorption period occurs at 3–5 months via hydrolysis into glycolic and lactic acid, which are then metabolized completely by 12 months. When in vitro shear strength was tested by Covidien, AbsorbaTack™ screws had 39 lbf initially, which ultimately degraded to 19 lbf at 8 weeks [31].

Bard Davol: SorbaFix™ and PermaSorb™

The Bard Davol SorbaFix™ was released in 2009. A 5-mm delivery system is used with either 15 or 30 fasteners. Fasteners are composed of poly(D,L)-lactide (PDLLA) and are shaped with a blunt screwlike tip. The head length is 0.8 mm with a 6.7-mm total length. There is a sharp pilot tip on the delivery system that is needed for engaging tissue. Material degradation involves a process of hydrolysis and enzymatic metabolism. Sixty days postimplantation, the fastener maintains 100% of original strength, while degradation is nearly complete at 1 year. Preclinical, company-based studies revealed that burst strength remained seven times higher than the intra-abdominal pressure requirement at 56 days [32].

The Bard Davol PermaSorb™ is another option for hernia fixation and differs mainly in design when compared to SorbaFix™. The PermaSorb fasteners are also made of PDLLA but are configured with two staggered hooklike projections off a central shaft to allow for a mesh and tissue fixation. Because the fasteners are composed of the same material as SorbaFix™, the absorption profiles are similar.

Ethicon: Securestrap™

The Securestrap was released by Ethicon in 2011. A 5-mm delivery system is used with 25 total fasteners. These fasteners are designed in a strap-like configuration with fixation points on both sides. When fully deployed, there is a low-profile area exposed which is designed to limit foreign body reaction. Ethicon sponsored studies revealed that the Securestrap™ maintained significant shear strength in relation to angle of deployment. Absorption occurs via a hydrolysis and metabolism mechanism [33].

Fibrin Sealants

Interest in adhesive products for hernia fixation stemmed from a desire to limit the foreign body reaction following placement of mesh and permanent suture in hernia repair. The first materials used were synthetic cyanoacrylate-based glues, and while they showed promise for hernia fixation, they were also associated with cytotoxicity, carcinogenicity, and severe tissue inflammation [34–37]. Due to these unwanted side effects, the use of nonsynthetic fibrin sealant products has been recommended in lieu of synthetic-based glues. Baxter Healthcare offers two such options for fibrin sealant products: Tisseel™ and Artiss™.

Baxter Healthcare: Tisseel™ and Artiss™

Tisseel™ and Artiss™ are adhesive agents procured from human fibrinogen and thrombin. An initial formulation of Tisseel™ received FDA approval in 1998, while an upgraded formulation received approval in 2006. Artiss™ was approved for use in 2008. The concentration of human thrombin is 500 IU/ml in Tisseel™ and 4 IU/ml in Artiss™. When mixed with human fibrinogen, these preparations mimic the final stage of blood coagulation pathway. Tisseel™ is indicated as an adjunct to hemostasis in several operations including those involving cardio-pulmonary bypass as well as treatment of splenic injury following trauma. It is also indicated for use as an adjunct to prevent anastomotic leakage in colonic anastomoses. Indication for use of Artiss™ is limited to prepared wound beds for patients undergoing autologous skin grafting. There is no indication for hemostasis. Fibrin sealant use in hernia repair is considered "off-label"; however, investigators have studied it in both animal and human trials [38, 39]. It is important to note that while these sealants are considered absorbable, there is a small risk of human disease transmission as they are procured from human plasma.

Clinical Use of Absorbable Fixation Materials

Inguinal Hernia Repair

The typical method of mesh fixation in open repair of inguinal hernia is that of direct suture. In a large cohort study, Novik et al. studied the use of permanent suture, long-term absorbable suture (i.e., PDS), and short-term absorbable suture (i.e., Vicryl) fixation of mesh in over 80,000

Lichtenstein herniorrhaphies [40]. This group found that there was no advantage in using permanent versus long-term absorbable suture in terms of hernia recurrence. However, the use of short-term absorbable suture was associated with a twofold increased risk of hernia recurrence versus long-term absorbable or permanent suture, discouraging use of short-term absorbable sutures for open hernia repair.

For laparoscopic inguinal herniorrhaphy, the discussion regarding mesh fixation is more controversial, with multiple questions regarding type and extent of fixation [41]. Lau performed a randomized trial comparing mechanical stapling versus fibrin sealant in patients undergoing bilateral endoscopic totally extraperitoneal inguinal hernioplasty (TEP). In this study, he found a significant reduction in postoperative analgesics in the fibrin sealant group; however, there was a higher incidence of postoperative seroma in this group when compared to the mechanical staple group (17.4% vs. 5.3%) [42]. Because of such findings, investigators began to study nonfixation in laparoscopic inguinal hernia repair, hoping to find equivalent outcomes with less pain and seroma. A multicenter, blinded, randomized trial by Taylor et al. sought to evaluate this postulate. In this study, investigators learned that following unilateral repair, the nonfixated group had significantly less groin pain. Likewise, following bilateral repair when each side was randomized to fixation or nonfixation, the nonfixated side was more comfortable than the fixated side (47% vs. 9%; $P=0.006$). When more than six tacks were used, there was also greater pain than when six or fewer tacks were used (40% vs. 22%; $P=0.008$) [43].

Incisional/Ventral Hernia Repair

Data regarding absorbable fixation methods during open ventral hernia repair is relatively sparse, being limited to animal studies and small case series. A comparative study by Grommes et al. in a porcine ventral hernia model tested nonabsorbable suture, absorbable suture, fibrin glue, and nonfixation of retrorectus mesh implantation. In this study, there was no mesh dislocation or migration, and tensile strength of mesh integration was similar in all four groups. The technique of this repair did require fascial re-approximation in front of the mesh [44].

Similar to laparoscopic inguinal hernia repair, a significant controversy exists in relation to mesh fixation during laparoscopic ventral hernia repair. There are several key differences that make mesh fixation a more complex discussion in laparoscopy. While hernia sac excision and abdominal wall dissection is common in open repair, often the hernia sac and abdominal wall tissue are not disturbed during laparoscopic repair. Such differences allow for different variety of mesh choice for open repair, as intraperitoneal exposure of the mesh can be avoided. During laparoscopy, the mesh is typically placed in an intraperitoneal position, with at least one aspect exposed to viscera. For this reason, mesh selection becomes paramount. First, in order to limit intraperitoneal complications such as adhesions or fistulae, anti-adhesive barriers should be employed on the visceral side of the mesh [6]. Also, significant overlap of 3–5 cm around the defect is important to allow for adequate ingrowth and to compensate for possible mesh shrinkage, as the area covering the defect will not be in contact with any tissue in many cases [17].

In a porcine model of hernia repair comparing absorbable tacks to metal tacks, Duffey et al. showed equivalent mesh incorporation with both permanent and absorbable fasteners. In this model, transfascial fixation was not used [45]. Hollinsky et al. studied mesh fixation via transfascial fixation, a permanent fastener (Covidien ProTack™), and two absorbable fasteners (Covidien AbsorbaTack™, and I-Clip™) in rats. Retention strength was significantly higher (8.7 N/cm [2]) in the transfascial fixation group than that of ProTack™ (5.6 N/cm [2]) or AbsorbaTack™ (5.7 N/cm [2]). The authors also found that the I-Clip™ had poor retention strength, while the ProTack™ was associated with significantly more adhesions [46].

In humans, significant debate regarding increased postoperative pain with use of transfascial fixation led several investigators to compare this approach with alternative fixation materials. Beldi et al. found that pain at 6 weeks was significantly higher when transfascial fixation sutures were used compared with tacks in a series of laparoscopic hernia repairs. While recurrence rates were similar at 6 months, this group did note that mesh shrinkage was also greater with metal tack fixation [47]. Morales-Conde proposed a "double-crown" technique using permanent fasteners and reported a 2.14% recurrence rate after 140 repairs [48]. Wassenaar et al. also compared three groups of patients who underwent laparoscopic ventral hernia repair: those with absorbable sutures and tack fixation, those with double-crown tack fixation and no sutures, and those with nonabsorbable suture with tack fixation. These investigators found no difference in postoperative pain or quality of life scores at 2 weeks, 6 weeks, and 3 months postoperatively [49]. Likewise, Nguyen et al. showed equivalent narcotic usage, hospital stay, and return to work in patients who underwent either primarily transfascial fixation versus primarily tack fixation [50].

Conclusion

Based on a critical review of the literature, there are still many unanswered questions regarding the use of absorbable fixation materials. Two inseparable factors for successful hernia repair are mesh selection and mesh fixation, and inappropriate choice of either can lead to operative failure. Currently, absorbable fixation methods appear to show promise, but further study needs to more clearly evaluate the device efficacy against proposed benefits of less foreign material. Future studies should be aimed at areas such as cost analysis, nonfixation methods, and long-term outcomes.

References

1. Cassar K, Munro A. Surgical treatment of incisional hernia. Br J Surg. 2002;89(5): 534–45.
2. Luijendijk RW, Hop WC, van den Tol MP, et al. A comparison of suture repair with mesh repair for incisional hernia. N Engl J Med. 2000;343(6):392–8.
3. Oelschlager BK, Pellegrini CA, Hunter J, et al. Biologic prosthesis reduces recurrence after laparoscopic paraesophageal hernia repair: a multicenter, prospective, randomized trial. Ann Surg. 2006;244(4):481–90.
4. Rutkow IM. Demographic and socioeconomic aspects of hernia repair in the United States in 2003. Surg Clin North Am. 2003;83(5):1045–51. v–vi.
5. Turner PL, Park AE. Laparoscopic repair of ventral incisional hernias: pros and cons. Surg Clin North Am. 2008;88(1):85–100. viii.
6. Matthews BD. Absorbable and nonabsorbable barriers on prosthetic biomaterials for adhesion prevention after intraperitoneal placement of mesh. Int Surg. 2005;90 (3 Suppl):S30–4.
7. Read RC, Yoder G. Recent trends in the management of incisional herniation. Arch Surg. 1989;124(4):485–8.
8. Luijendijk RW, Lemmen MH, Hop WC, Wereldsma JC. Incisional hernia recurrence following "vest-over-pants" or vertical Mayo repair of primary hernias of the midline. World J Surg. 1997;21(1):62–5. discussion 66.
9. Hesselink VJ, Luijendijk RW, de Wilt JH, Heide R, Jeekel J. An evaluation of risk factors in incisional hernia recurrence. Surg Gynecol Obstet. 1993;176(3):228–34.
10. Bachman S, Ramshaw B. Prosthetic material in ventral hernia repair: how do I choose? Surg Clin North Am. 2008;88(1):101–12.
11. Forbes SS, Eskicioglu C, McLeod RS, Okrainec A. Meta-analysis of randomized controlled trials comparing open and laparoscopic ventral and incisional hernia repair with mesh. Br J Surg. 2009;96(8):851–8.

12. Heniford BT, Park A, Ramshaw BJ, Voeller G. Laparoscopic repair of ventral hernias: nine years' experience with 850 consecutive hernias. Ann Surg. 2003;238(3):391–9. discussion 399–400.
13. McGreevy JM, Goodney PP, Birkmeyer CM, Finlayson SR, Laycock WS, Birkmeyer JD. A prospective study comparing the complication rates between laparoscopic and open ventral hernia repairs. Surg Endosc. 2003;17(11):1778–80.
14. Topart P, Ferrand L, Vandenbroucke F, Lozac'h P. Laparoscopic ventral hernia repair with the Goretex Dualmesh: long-term results and review of the literature. Hernia. 2005;9(4):348–52.
15. Phillips JD, Nagle AP. Minimally invasive approaches to incisional hernia repairs. J Long Term Eff Med Implants. 2010;20(2):117–28.
16. Greca FH, de Paula JB, Biondo-Simoes ML, et al. The influence of differing pore sizes on the biocompatibility of two polypropylene meshes in the repair of abdominal defects. Experimental study in dogs. Hernia. 2001;5(2):59–64.
17. Doctor HG. Evaluation of various prosthetic materials and newer meshes for hernia repairs. J Minim Access Surg. 2006;2(3):110–6.
18. Joels CS, Matthews BD, Kercher KW, et al. Evaluation of adhesion formation, mesh fixation strength, and hydroxyproline content after intraabdominal placement of polytetrafluoroethylene mesh secured using titanium spiral tacks, nitinol anchors, and polypropylene suture or polyglactin 910 suture. Surg Endosc. 2005;19(6):780–5.
19. van't Riet M, de Vos van Steenwijk PJ, Kleinrensink GJ, Steyerberg EW, Bonjer HJ. Tensile strength of mesh fixation methods in laparoscopic incisional hernia repair. Surg Endosc. 2002;16(12):1713–6.
20. LeBlanc KA. Laparoscopic incisional hernia repair: are transfascial sutures necessary? A review of the literature. Surg Endosc. 2007;21(4):508–13.
21. Bellows CF, Berger DH. Infiltration of suture sites with local anesthesia for management of pain following laparoscopic ventral hernia repairs: a prospective randomized trial. JSLS. 2006;10(3):345–50.
22. Carbonell AM, Harold KL, Mahmutovic AJ, et al. Local injection for the treatment of suture site pain after laparoscopic ventral hernia repair. Am Surg. 2003;69(8):688–91. discussion 691–682.
23. Ethicon (homepage on the Internet) (2011) http://www.ecatalog.ethicon.com/sutures-absorbable. Accessed 29 May 2011.
24. Dion YM, Laplante R, Charara J, Marois M. The influence of the number of endoclips and of mesh incorporation on the strength of an experimental hernia patch repair. Surg Endosc. 1994;8(11):1324–8.
25. Hollinsky C, Gobl S. Bursting strength evaluation after different types of mesh fixation in laparoscopic herniorrhaphy. Surg Endosc. 1999;13(10):958–61.
26. Greenstein AJ, Nguyen SQ, Buch KE, Chin EH, Weber KJ, Divino CM. Recurrence after laparoscopic ventral hernia repair: a prospective pilot study of suture versus tack fixation. Am Surg. 2008;74(3):227–31.
27. Ladurner R, Mussack T. Small bowel perforation due to protruding spiral tackers: a rare complication in laparoscopic incisional hernia repair. Surg Endosc. 2004;18(6): 1001.

28. Peach G, Tan LC. Small bowel obstruction and perforation due to a displaced spiral tacker: a rare complication of laparoscopic inguinal hernia repair. Hernia. 2008;12(3):303–5.
29. Karahasanoglu T, Onur E, Baca B, et al. Spiral tacks may contribute to intra-abdominal adhesion formation. Surg Today. 2004;34(10):860–4.
30. Byrd JF, Agee N, Swan RZ et al. Evaluation of absorbable and permanent mesh fixation devices: adhesion formation and mechanical strength. Hernia. 2011;15(5): 553–8. Epub 2011 May 19.
31. Covidien AbsorbaTack (2011) http://www.covidien.com/hernia/us/fixation/absorbatack. Accessed 30 May 2011.
32. Bard Davol SorbaFix (2011) http://www.davol.com/products/soft-tissue-reconstruction/fixation/sorbafix-absorbable-fixation-system/. Accessed 31 May 2011.
33. Ethicon Securestrap (2011) http://www.ethicon360.com/products/ethicon-securestrap. Accessed 31 May 2011.
34. Jourdan IC, Bailey ME. Initial experience with the use of N-butyl 2-cyanoacrylate glue for the fixation of polypropylene mesh in laparoscopic hernia repair. Surg Laparosc Endosc. 1998;8(4):291–3.
35. Leggat PA, Kedjarune U, Smith DR. Toxicity of cyanoacrylate adhesives and their occupational impacts for dental staff. Ind Health. 2004;42(2):207–11.
36. Samson D, Marshall D. Carcinogenic potential of isobutyl-2-cyanoacrylate. J Neurosurg. 1986;65(4):571–2.
37. Fortelny RH, Petter-Puchner AH, Walder N, et al. Cyanoacrylate tissue sealant impairs tissue integration of macroporous mesh in experimental hernia repair. Surg Endosc. 2007;21(10):1781–5.
38. Baxter Healthcare Tisseel (2011) http://www.baxter.com/healthcare_professionals/products/tisseel.html. Accessed 31 May 2011.
39. Baxter Healthcare Artiss (2011) http://www.baxter.com/downloads/healthcare_professionals/products/ARTISS_PI.pdf. Accessed 31 May 2011.
40. Novik B, Nordin P, Skullman S, Dalenback J, Enochsson L. More recurrences after hernia mesh fixation with short-term absorbable sutures: a registry study of 82 015 Lichtenstein repairs. Arch Surg. 2011;146(1):12–7.
41. Leung D, Ujiki MB. Minimally invasive approaches to inguinal hernia repair. J Long Term Eff Med Implants. 2010;20(2):105–16.
42. Lau H. Fibrin sealant versus mechanical stapling for mesh fixation during endoscopic extraperitoneal inguinal hernioplasty: a randomized prospective trial. Ann Surg. 2005;242(5):670–5.
43. Taylor C, Layani L, Liew V, Ghusn M, Crampton N, White S. Laparoscopic inguinal hernia repair without mesh fixation, early results of a large randomised clinical trial. Surg Endosc. 2008;22(3):757–62.
44. Grommes J, Binnebosel M, Klink CD, von Trotha KT, Junge K, Conze J. Different methods of mesh fixation in open retromuscular incisional hernia repair: a comparative study in pigs. Hernia. 2010;14(6):623–7.
45. Duffy AJ, Hogle NJ, LaPerle KM, Fowler DL. Comparison of two composite meshes using two fixation devices in a porcine laparoscopic ventral hernia repair model. Hernia. 2004;8(4):358–64.

46. Hollinsky C, Kolbe T, Walter I, et al. Tensile strength and adhesion formation of mesh fixation systems used in laparoscopic incisional hernia repair. Surg Endosc. 2010;24(6): 1318–24.
47. Beldi G, Wagner M, Bruegger LE, Kurmann A, Candinas D. Mesh shrinkage and pain in laparoscopic ventral hernia repair: a randomized clinical trial comparing suture versus tack mesh fixation. Surg Endosc. 2011;25(3):749–55.
48. Morales-Conde S, Cadet H, Cano A, Bustos M, Martin J, Morales-Mendez S. Laparoscopic ventral hernia repair without sutures—double crown technique: our experience after 140 cases with a mean follow-up of 40 months. Int Surg. 2005;90(3 Suppl):S56–62.
49. Wassenaar E, Schoenmaeckers E, Raymakers J, van der Palen J, Rakic S. Mesh-fixation method and pain and quality of life after laparoscopic ventral or incisional hernia repair: a randomized trial of three fixation techniques. Surg Endosc. 2010;24(6):1296–302.
50. Nguyen SQ, Divino CM, Buch KE, et al. Postoperative pain after laparoscopic ventral hernia repair: a prospective comparison of sutures versus tacks. JSLS. 2008;12(2): 113–6.

44. Biologic Mesh: When and Why—A Critical Appraisal

Jaime A. Cavallo, Corey R. Deeken, and Brent D. Matthews

Ventral Hernia Repair Reinforcement

The US Markets for Soft Tissue Repair Report prepared by the Millennium Research Group estimates that 305,900 ventral hernia repair were performed in the United States in 2006 [1], reaffirming ventral hernia repair as one of the most common procedures in general surgery. The 10-year cumulative rate of recurrence for suture repair of ventral hernias is as high as 63%, which contributes to the high incidence of repair [2]. Significant risk factors for recurrence include surgical technique, history of previous failed hernia repairs, large hernia size, obesity, smoking habits, and patient comorbidities that contribute to diminished soft tissue integrity. To reduce recurrence to a 10-year cumulative rate <32%, level A and B evidence supports reinforcement with synthetic or biologic materials for all incisional ventral hernia repairs [2, 3]. Likely attributable to these evidence-based recommendations for material reinforcement, it is estimated that synthetic or biologic reinforcement materials were used in nearly 95% of the ventral hernias performed in the United States in 2006 [1]. Market analysts predict a 7% annual growth rate in the $1 billion United States soft tissue repair device industry, largely impelled by costly biologic scaffold materials for ventral hernia repair. The aging patient population, the prevalence of comorbidities contributing to diminished soft tissue integrity, the high incidence of obesity, and the rising demand for bariatric procedures with high potential for sequelae of incisional ventral hernias are major factors driving the anticipated market expansion for ventral hernia reinforcement materials. In particular, demand for biologic scaffold materials is expected

B.P. Jacob and B. Ramshaw (eds.), *The SAGES Manual of Hernia Repair*,
DOI 10.1007/978-1-4614-4824-2_44,

to expand based on preclinical evidence that biologic materials enable revascularization of soft tissue repair sites and improved pathogen clearance in contaminated and infected surgical sites [4, 5], clinical evidence that biologic materials do not necessarily require removal when exposed or infected [6–8].

Biologic Scaffolds for Abdominal Wall Reconstruction

As the strength layer of the abdominal wall, fascial layers are composed predominantly of fibroblasts and the extracellular matrix components that these cells secrete: collagen, elastin, proteoglycans, and fibronectin. A high collagen and elastin content is responsible for the great tensile strength and elasticity of fascia. The consistency of fascia is determined by the total proteoglycan surface area, which is responsible for binding cations and attracting water molecules. Fibronectins aid in the attachment of cells to the extracellular matrix and therefore play an important role in wound healing.

Biologic scaffolds composed of mammalian extracellular matrices possess favorable characteristics for cell attachment, proliferation, and differentiation and therefore serve as archetypal substrates for soft tissue repair. The ideal biologic scaffold for abdominal wall reconstruction closely resembles the native extracellular matrix of the host tissue, possesses biomechanical properties that approximate the dynamics of the abdominal wall, gradually degrades to allow for neovascularization and high-integrity host tissue regeneration, avoids a biologic footprint that could elicit a chronic inflammatory immune response and fibrosis from the host, resists new infection and optimizes pathogen clearance from contaminated and infected surgical sites, and provides an effective and durable soft tissue repair. Biologic grafts used in abdominal wall soft tissue repair are mostly porous acellular extracellular matrix constructs from dermal, fascial, pericardial, or intestinal submucosal tissue of cadaveric human, porcine, or bovine origin (Table 44.1). The characteristics of the native species, donor, and tissue type of the scaffold determine the remnant three-dimensional protein infrastructure following proprietary manufacturing processes to decellularize, enhance, and sterilize the material for clinical use. Some remaining source growth factors remain in the scaffold and serve as chemotactic signals for host fibroblasts and endothelial cells after implantation. The gradual degradation of the

Table 44.1. Biologic scaffolds for abdominal wall reconstruction.

Product	Manufacturer	Source	Cross-linking process	Sterilization process	Storage/ shelf-life	Cost/cm^2
Xenografts						
Biodesign™ Surgisis® and Biodesign™ Surgisis® FM Hernia Grafts	Cook® Medical (Bloomington, IN)	Porcine small intestine submucosa; FM = fenestrated matrix		Ethylene oxide	Room temperature/ 18 months	\$10–20
CollaMend™ and CollaMend™ FM Implants	Davol, Inc./C. R. Bard (Warwick, RI)	Porcine dermis; FM = fenestrated matrix	1-Ethyl-(3-dimethylaminopropyl)-carbodiimide hydrochloride (EDC)	Ethylene oxide	Room temperature	\$10–20
Peri-Guard® Repair Patch	Synovis® Surgical Innovations (St. Paul, MN)	Bovine pericardium	Glutaraldehyde	Ethanol, propylene oxide, sodium hydroxide	Room temperature	<\$10
Permacol™ Surgical Implant	Covidien Surgical (Norwalk, CT)	Porcine dermis	Hexamethylene diisocyanate (HDMI)	Gamma irradiation	Room temperature	\$20–30
Strattice™ Reconstructive Tissue Matrix	LifeCell Corporation (Branchburg, NJ)	Porcine dermis		Electron beam irradiation	Room temperature	\$20–30
SurgiMend® Collagen Matrix	TEI Biosciences, Inc. (Boston, MA)	Fetal bovine dermis		Ethylene oxide	Room temperature/3 years	\$20–30

(continued)

Table 44.1. (continued)

Product	Manufacturer	Source	Cross-linking process	Sterilization process	Storage/ shelf-life	Cost/cm²
Veritas® Collagen Matrix	Synovis® Surgical Innovations (St. Paul, MN)	Bovine pericardium		Sodium hydroxide, electron beam irradiation	Controlled room temperature	\$20–30
XenMatrix™ Surgical Graft	Davol, Inc./C. R. Bard (Warwick, RI)	Porcine dermis		Electron beam irradiation	Room temperature	\$20–30
Allografts						
AlloDerm® Regenerative Tissue Matrix	LifeCell Corporation (Branchburg, NJ)	Human dermis		Aseptically processed	Freeze-dried, refrigerated/ 2 years	≥\$30
AlloMax™ Surgical Graft	Davol, Inc./C. R. Bard (Warwick, RI)	Human dermis		Tutoplast® process, low-dose gamma irradiation	Room temperature	≥\$30
FlexHD® Acellular Dermis	Musculoskeletal Transplant Foundation/ Ethicon, Inc. (Somerville, NJ)	Human dermis		Aseptically processed; passes U.S. Pharmacopeia Standard 71 for sterility	Room temperature	≥\$30

Data compiled from the manufacturer-provided instructions for product use, the International Consensus expert working group on acellular matrices for soft tissue repair [9], and Deeken et al. [26]

biologic scaffold by host macrophages and matrix metalloproteinases (MMPs) allows for simultaneous tissue remodeling through infiltration of host cells, neovascularization, and regeneration of the dynamic extracellular matrix. A semiquantitative histologic scoring system for biologic scaffold tissue remodeling has been described on the basis of six characteristics: cellular infiltration, cellular types present, host extracellular matrix deposition, scaffold degradation, fibrous encapsulation, and neovascularization (Table 44.2). Biologic scaffolds possess varying degrees of biocompatibility and biodegradability based on their resulting molecular composition and can therefore have substantial impact on the host tissue response, the constructive remodeling of the substrate tissue, and the integrity of the tissue repair.

Modifications During Manufacture

During manufacture into biologic scaffolds, mammalian extracellular matrices undergo a variety of chemical and mechanical processes to render the scaffold free of immunogenic agents and safe for therapeutic application: decellularization, sterilization, and preservation for storage. Ideally, manufacturing processes should achieve these objectives while minimizing disruption to the native scaffold structure. The molecular structures of the extracellular matrix components are conserved across animal species and demonstrate immunologic tolerance as allografts and xenografts [9]. Manufacturing processes that alter the molecules of the native scaffold may lead to more rapid in vivo degradation of the scaffold, inflammatory cell response, and fibrotic encapsulation preventing cellular infiltration and neovascularization, thus ultimately favoring scar formation rather than constructive tissue remodeling in the host [10].

Detergents used to extract cells and antigenic agents from the scaffold have the ability to deform collagen and negatively impact the mechanical properties of the scaffold [11]. For Food and Drug Administration (FDA) clearance of all xenographic scaffolds, the products must be sterilized to reduce the risk of infectious disease transmission. Chemical sterilization with glutaraldehyde or ethylene oxide may leave residual by-products that elicit an inflammatory response and alter the mechanical properties of the scaffold, whereas radiation sterilization may disrupt the native scaffold architecture, cause unintended molecular bonding, and alter the mechanical properties of the scaffold [9, 11, 12]. Materials that remain hydrated during storage tend to evacuate soluble growth factors, while scaffolds that are preserved in dehydrated form can develop ultrastructural

Table 44.2. Semiquantitative histologic scoring system of tissue remodeling characteristics for explants of biologic scaffolds.

Score	**0**	**1**	**2**	**3**
Cellular infiltration	Zero cells in contact with scaffold	Cells contact periphery, no penetration into scaffold	Cells infiltrate scaffold, but none reach center	Cells penetrate into center of scaffold
Cell types ("inflammatory cells" include neutrophils, macrophages, and foreign body giant cells)	Inflammatory cells present, no fibroblasts	Primarily inflammatory cells, few fibroblasts	Primarily fibroblasts, few inflammatory cells	Fibroblasts only, no inflammatory cells
Host extracellular matrix deposition	No host ECM deposition	Host ECM deposited at periphery of scaffold	Host ECM deposited inside scaffold, but not at the center	Host ECM deposited inside scaffold, including the center
Scaffold degradation	Original scaffold intact, borders clearly demarcated	Scaffold partially degraded, layers separated by cells, blood vessels, host tissue, etc.	Scaffold extremely degraded, difficult to distinguish scaffold from host tissue	Scaffold completely degraded, no evidence of original scaffold
Fibrous encapsulation	Extensive encapsulation (50–100% of periphery)	Moderate encapsulation (25–50% of periphery)	Mild encapsulation (<25% of periphery)	No fibrous encapsulation
Neovascularization	Zero blood vessels present	Vessels present at scaffold periphery, no penetration into scaffold	Vessels infiltrate scaffold but none reach center of scaffold	Vessels penetrate into center of scaffold

Histologic scoring system of six characteristics of biologic scaffold tissue remodeling: cellular infiltration, cell type, extracellular matrix (ECM) deposition, scaffold degradation, fibrous encapsulation, and neovascularization. Note that higher scores indicate more favorable remodeling characteristics of the biologic scaffold

(From ref. [24], with permission)

collapse, unintended molecular bonding, and restricted cellular infiltration [8, 13]. Manufacturing processes have also been shown to greatly affect the macrophage profile of the host response and the pathway to constructive remodeling versus chronic inflammation and scar formation [14]. Manufacturing processes, therefore, have the potential to produce direct effects on the durability of the tissue repair and the clinical treatment outcomes. Many of these processes remain proprietary, deterring further scientific investigation of their potential impact on clinical outcomes.

Collagen Cross-linking

Collagen cross-linking processes create bonds between collagen triple helices intending to stabilize the scaffold and reduce enzymatic degradation by MMPs. Often, these processes do not confer control over the degree of collagen cross-linking, create short and inflexible bonds that restrict early cellular infiltration, or leave residual chemical by-products that elicit an inflammatory response [10, 11, 15, 16]. Various degrees of collagen cross-linking may also occur as an unintended consequence of other proprietary manufacturing processes. The clinical benefit of cross-linked collagen scaffolds remains to be proven. Preclinical studies by Deeken et al. have demonstrated no significant difference in the tensile strength [17] of the surgical repair site (Fig. 44.1) and earlier cellular infiltration, extracellular matrix deposition, and neovascularization in non-cross-linked materials compared to cross-linked materials explanted from a porcine model of ventral hernia repair. However, by 12 months postimplantation, cross-linked and non-cross-linked explants demonstrated no significant differences in cell types, cellular infiltration, scaffold degradation, extracellular matrix deposition, fibrotic encapsulation, or neovascularization [18, 19] (Fig. 44.2). Further investigation of the comparative clinical effectiveness of cross-linked and non-cross-linked materials is warranted.

Scaffold Fenestration

A host inflammatory cell response to a biologic scaffold may elicit fibrotic encapsulation of the graft leading to a reduction in both infiltration of host cells and neovascularization. The resulting dead space at the graft-tissue interface may lead to increased clinical incidence of seromas, wound complications, and infections [20–23]. Fenestrated grafts that

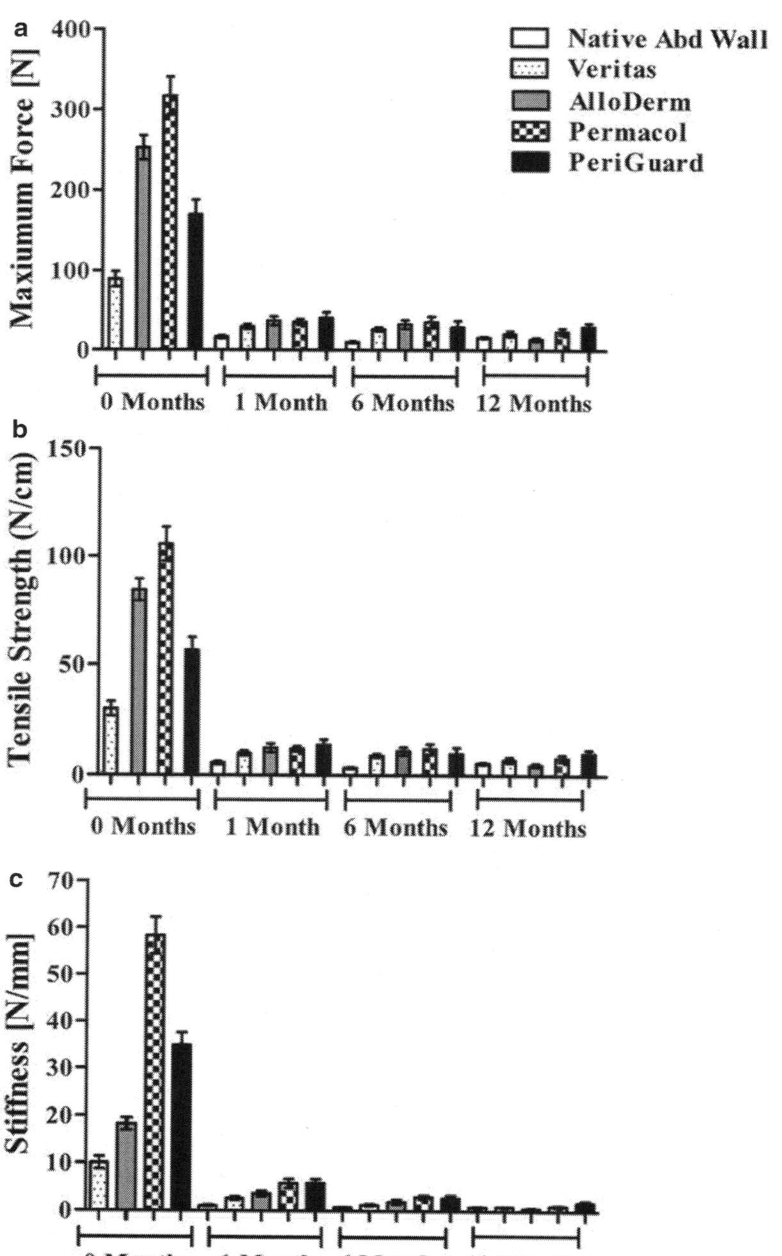
a
Maxiumum Force [N]
400
300
200
100
0
Native Abd Wall
Veritas
AlloDerm
Permacol
PeriGuard
0 Months
1 Month
6 Months
12 Months
b
Tensile Strength (N/cm)
150
100
50
0
0 Months
1 Month
6 Months
12 Months
c
Stiffness [N/mm]
70
60
50
40
30
20
10
0
0 Months
1 Month
6 Months
12 Months

allow the passage of fluid and the deposition of host tissue through pores have been proposed as one potential solution. Preclinical studies by Matthews et al. have demonstrated increased tissue incorporation at fenestrated sites compared with nonfenestrated grafts up to 6 months postimplantation in a porcine model of ventral hernia repair [24, 25] (Fig. 44.3). Conclusive long-term clinical studies comparing the clinical effectiveness of commercially available fenestrated and nonfenestrated scaffolds are lacking.

De Novo Scaffold Properties

The de novo biomechanical, thermal, and degradation properties of 12 biologic scaffolds FDA-approved for abdominal wall reconstruction applications were recently evaluated [26]. Thermal analysis using modulated differential scanning calorimetry demonstrated significantly higher melting temperatures for cross-linked bovine pericardium and porcine dermis compared to their non-cross-linked counterparts. Degradation by collagenase digestion assay revealed significantly longer resistance to enzymatic digestion by cross-linked bovine pericardium compared to non-cross-linked bovine pericardium. The suture retention strengths for all 12 scaffolds exceeded the threshold value of 20 N suggested for hernia repair applications [27, 28] (range 23.75–127.20 N), with cross-linked materials generally exhibiting lower suture retention strengths than non-cross-linked materials. The tear resistance for only 6 of the 12 scaffolds exceeded the threshold value of

Fig. 44.1. Biomechanical properties of cross-linked and non-cross-linked biologic scaffolds explanted from a porcine model of ventral hernia repair. Biomechanical characteristics of mesh-repaired sites over time compared with de novo strength and native porcine abdominal wall: (**a**) maximum load (Newtons [N]), (**b**) tensile strength (N/cm), and (**c**) stiffness (N/mm). All four meshes were significantly stronger and stiffer at time 0 compared with their corresponding repair sites (mesh-abdominal wall tissue composites) after 1, 6, or 12 months ($p<0.01$ for all comparisons). Although significant differences were observed between the strength and stiffness for each of the four meshes at time 0, no significant differences in strength or stiffness were observed between mesh-repair sites at 1, 6, or 12 months due to the type of mesh used to repair the defect ($p>0.05$ in all cases). In addition, no significant differences in strength or stiffness of the repair sites were detected over time for any of the meshes studied ($p>0.05$ in all cases). Abd = abdominal (From ref. [19], with permission).

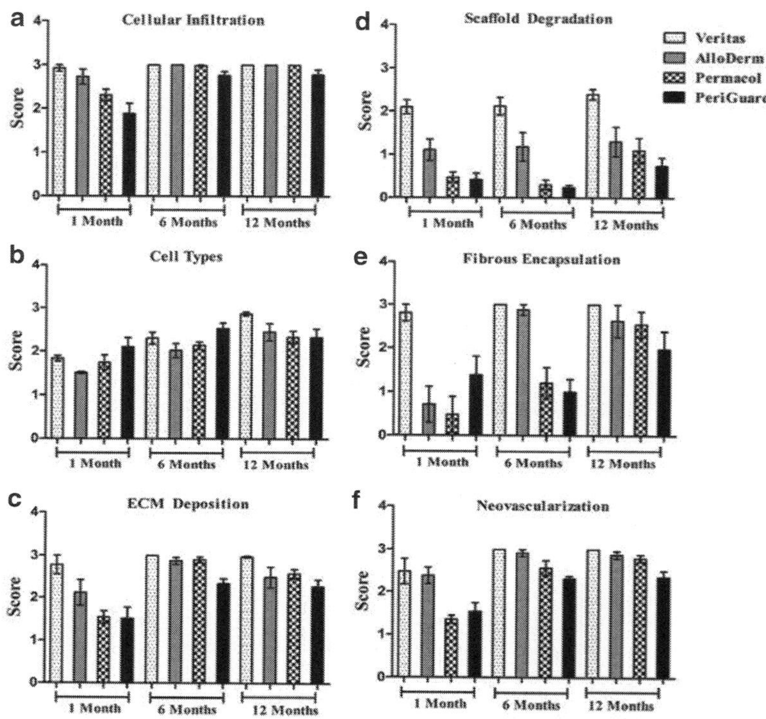

Fig. 44.2. Tissue remodeling characteristics of cross-linked and non-cross-linked biologic scaffolds explanted from a porcine model of ventral hernia repair. Histologic scores, separated by mesh type and length of time in vivo: (**a**) cellular infiltration scores, (**b**) cell type scores, (**c**) extracellular matrix (ECM) deposition scores, (**d**) scaffold degradation scores, (**e**) fibrous encapsulation scores, and (**f**) neovascularization scores (From ref. [19], with permission).

20 N suggested for hernia repair applications [27, 28] (range 10.10–84.73 N), with cross-linked materials exhibiting significantly lower tear resistance strengths than non-cross-linked materials. The uniaxial tensile strength was significantly greater for cross-linked compared to non-cross-linked bovine pericardium. The ball burst strength of all 12 scaffolds exceeded the 50 N/cm threshold suggested for hernia repair applications [27, 28] (range 66.2–1028.0 N/cm), and 9 of the 12 scaffolds exhibited ball burst strain within the physiologic range of 10–30% suggested for hernia repair applications [27, 28] (range 5.85–26.22%). Cross-linked materials generally exhibited significantly lower ball burst strengths compared to non-cross-linked materials. No clear trends were

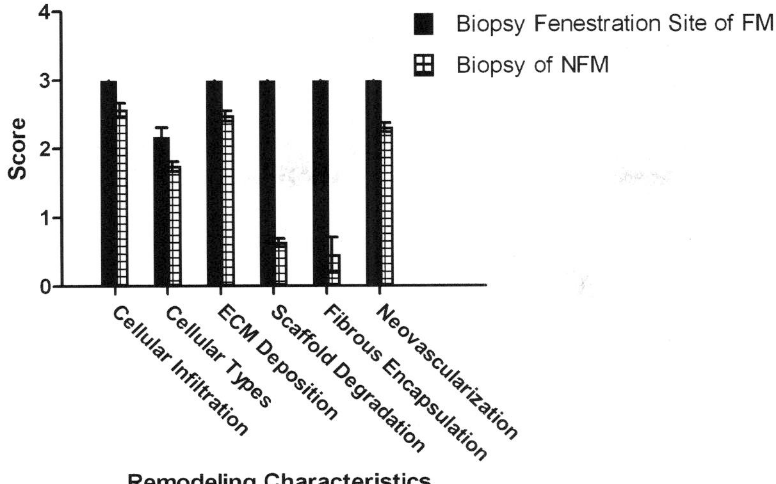

Fig. 44.3. Tissue remodeling characteristics of fenestrated and nonfenestrated biologic scaffolds explanted from a porcine model of ventral hernia repair. Histologic scores of biopsies at the fenestration sites of a fenestrated cross-linked porcine dermal matrix (FM) compared to biopsies of a nonfenestrated cross-linked porcine dermal matrix (NFM) explanted after 6 months from a porcine model of ventral hernia repair: cellular infiltration scores, cellular type scores, extracellular matrix (ECM) deposition scores, scaffold degradation scores, fibrous encapsulation scores, and neovascularization scores [25].

otherwise noted between cross-linked and non-cross-linked materials, suggesting the potential role of source factors and other proprietary manufacturing processes.

Appropriate and Inappropriate Indications for Use

Graded Risk for Postoperative Surgical Site Occurrence

As an instrument to assist surgeons in stratifying the risk of a postoperative surgical site occurrence (SSO) after abdominal wall reconstruction, the Ventral Hernia Working Group (VHWG) developed a novel grading system based on characteristics of both the patient and the hernia defect [29]. Grade 1 (low-risk) ventral hernias are clean, uncontaminated surgical sites of patients without a history of comorbidities or wound infection. The VHWG recommends that patient factors and the clinical judgment of the surgeon should be weighed in the choice of appropriate repair materials for grade 1 ventral hernias. Grade 2 (comorbid) ventral hernias are clean, uncontaminated surgical sites of patients with comorbidities that increase the risk for surgical-site infection. The VHWG notes that the relative contribution of different patient comorbidities (i.e., diabetes mellitus, obesity) to the risk of a surgical site occurrence is a matter of consideration and debate. Therefore, the VHWG advises that surgeons must continue to rely on their clinical judgment for the identification and appropriate treatment of grade 2 ventral hernias until comparative data is available. The VHWG suggests that patients with comorbidities associated with an increased risk of surgical site infection may benefit from reinforcement of grade 2 ventral hernias with biologic scaffolds rather than synthetic repair materials. However, given the high cost of biologic scaffolds (Table 44.1) and the insufficient evidence that biologic scaffolds confer clinical benefit over synthetic reinforcement materials for the repair of clean, uncontaminated hernia defects [30], it is difficult to justify routine use of biologic scaffolds for grade 1 or grade 2 ventral hernias. Grade 3 (contaminated) ventral hernias are contaminated or potentially contaminated surgical sites, including surgical sites in proximity to a stoma or a violation of the gastrointestinal tract, or with a prior history of infection. Grade 4 (infected) ventral hernias are surgical sites with active infection, infected foreign body, or septic dehiscence. Based on level A and B evidence, the VHWG contraindicates the use of synthetic reinforcement materials and instead advocates the use of biologic scaffold reinforcement for grade 3 and 4 ventral hernias. Twelve-month interim results of the RICH trial demonstrate safe, definitive, single-stage reconstruction using Strattice™ Reconstructive Tissue Matrix for 80% of studied contaminated and infected ventral incisional hernias, further reinforcing this VHWG recommendation [31]. It should be noted, however, that a recent warning issued by the FDA to the study sponsors cautions against the as-yet unapproved use of Strattice™ Reconstructive Tissue Matrix for the reinforcement of contaminated or infected soft tissue repair sites. [32]. Level B evidence supports the reduction of bioburden prior to reinforcement material placement and definitive repair of infected defects [29, 33]. A delayed approach to repair should be considered in the setting of gross, uncontrolled contamination of the surgical site.

Prophylaxis for Parastomal Hernias

Parastomal hernias, or incisional hernias at the site of a stoma, are a frequent and highly morbid complication of stoma formation. The incidence of parastomal hernia is as high as 48% [34], and as many as 30% of parastomal hernias require surgical intervention for pain, bowel obstruction, or fistulation [35]. Recurrence rates for surgical repair of parastomal hernias range between 30 and 76% [36]. Attention has therefore been focused on parastomal hernia prevention. Strong evidence supports the prophylactic reinforcement of stomas with prosthetic mesh to significantly reduce the incidence of parastomal herniation [37–40]. Prophylactic reinforcement of stomal sites using biologic or composite reinforcement materials at the time of stoma creation is associated with a 77% relative risk reduction in the incidence of parastomal herniation compared to conventional stoma formation [36]. Given concern for adhesion, erosion, fistulation, and mesh infection with synthetic material reinforcement in close proximity to the bowel, biologic scaffolds have been favored for both parastomal hernia prophylaxis and repair. However, given similar rates of recurrence and complications associated with the use of both synthetic and biologic scaffolds for parastomal hernia repair, some surgeons argue that insufficient evidence exists to justify the preferred use of expensive biologic scaffolds [41].

Bridging Abdominal Wall Defects

Reinforcement of soft tissue defects with repair material without primary closure of the fascial layer, otherwise referred to as the bridging of soft tissue defects, is strongly discouraged in ventral hernia repair. Bridging ventral incisional hernias with biologic scaffolds without reducing the size and the overdue tension of the fascial defect has been associated with an 80% rate of hernia recurrence [42, 43]. Abdominal wall component separation to approximate the fascial edges of the defect for primary closure with material reinforcement of the repair is an acceptable alternative with more favorable recurrence rates (0–20%) compared to bridging defects with repair material [42, 44, 45].

It should be emphasized that characterization studies and clinical trials evaluating the comparative effectiveness of available biologic scaffolds in ventral hernia repair are limited. Further comparative investigation is warranted to inform surgeon selection of appropriate biologic scaffold materials for different clinical circumstances.

References

1. Millennium Research Group. US markets for soft tissue repair devices 2006. Toronto, ON: Millennium Research Group, Inc.; 2006.
2. Burger JW, Luijendijk RW, Hop WC, Halm JA, Verdaasdonk EG, Jeekel J. Long-term follow-up of a randomized controlled trial of suture versus mesh repair of incisional hernia. Ann Surg. 2004;240(4):578–83.
3. Luijendijk RW, Hop WC, van den Tol MP, de Lange DC, Braaksma MM, IJzermans JN, Boelhouwer RU, de Vries BC, Salu MK, Wereldsma JC, Bruijninckx CM, Jeekel J. A comparison of suture repair with mesh repair for incisional hernia. N Engl J Med. 2000;343(6):393–8.
4. Millennium Research Group. US markets for soft tissue repair devices 2010. Toronto, ON: Millennium Research Group, Inc.; 2010.
5. Harth KC, Broome AM, Jacobs MR, Blatnik JA, Zeinali F, Bajaksouzian S, Rosen MJ. Bacterial clearance of biologic grafts used in hernia repair: an experimental study. Surg Endosc. 2011;25(7):2224–9.
6. Kim H, Bruen K, Vargo D. Acellular dermal matrix in the management of high-risk abdominal wall defects. Am J Surg. 2006;192(6):705–9.
7. Patton Jr JH, Berry S, Kralovich KA. Use of human acellular dermal matrix in complex and contaminated abdominal wall reconstructions. Am J Surg. 2007;193(3):360–3.
8. Maurice SM, Skeete DA. Use of human acellular dermal matrix for abdominal wall reconstructions. Am J Surg. 2009;197(1):35–42.
9. International Consensus. Acellular matrices for the treatment of wounds. An expert working group review. London: Wounds International; 2010.
10. Cornwell KG, Landsman A, James KS. Extracellular matrix biomaterials for soft tissue repair. Clin Podiatr Med Surg. 2009;26(4):507–23.
11. Badylak SF, Freytes DO, Gilbert TW. Extracellular matrix as a biological scaffold material: structure and function. Acta Biomater. 2009;5(1):1–13.
12. Gouk SS, Lim TM, Teoh SH, Sun WQ. Alterations of human acellular tissue matrix by gamma irradiation: histology, biomechanical property, stability, *in vitro* cell repopulation, and remodeling. J Biomed Mater Res B Appl Biomater. 2008;84(1): 205–17.
13. Freytes DO, Tullius RS, Valentin JE, Stewart-Akers AM, Badylak SF. Hydrated versus lyophilized forms of porcine extracellular matrix derived from the urinary bladder. J Biomed Mater Res A. 2008;87(4):862–72.
14. Badylak SF, Valentin JE, Ravindra AK, McCabe GP, Stewart-Akers AM. Macrophage phenotype as a determinant of biologic scaffold remodeling. Tissue Eng Part A. 2008;14(11):1835–42.

15. Klinge U, Si ZY, Zheng H, Schumpelick V, Bhardwaj RS, Klosterhalfen B. Abnormal collagen I to III distribution in the skin of patients with incisional hernia. Eur Surg Res. 2000;32(1):43–8.
16. Liang HC, Chang Y, Hsu CK, Lee MH, Sung HW. Effects of crosslinking degree of an acellular biologic tissue on its tissue regeneration pattern. Biomaterials. 2004;25(17): 3541–52.
17. Cavallo JA, Deeken CR, Melman L, Jenkins ED, Frisella MM, Matthews BD. Biomechanical properties of the porcine abdominal wall repaired with crosslinked versus non-crosslinked porcine dermis in a porcine model of ventral hernia repair. Hernia Repair 2011. San Francisco, CA: American Hernia Society; 2011.
18. Melman L, Jenkins ED, Hamilton NA, Bender LC, Brodt MD, Deeken CR, Greco SC, Frisella MM, Matthews BD. Early biocompatibility of crosslinked and non-crosslinked biologic meshes in a porcine model of ventral hernia repair. Hernia. 2011;15(2): 157–64.
19. Deeken CR, Melman L, Jenkins ED, Greco SC, Frisella MM, Matthews BD. Histologic and biomechanical evaluation of crosslinked and non-crosslinked biologic meshes in a porcine model of ventral incisional hernia repair. J Am Coll Surg. 2011;212(5): 880–8.
20. Wake MC, Patrick Jr CW, Mikos AG. Pore morphology effects on the fibrovascular tissue growth in porous polymer substrates. Cell Transplant. 1994;3(4):339–43.
21. Bezuidenhout D, Davies N, Zilla P. Effect of well defined dodecahedral porosity on inflammation and angiogenesis. ASAIO J. 2002;48(5):465–71.
22. Matthews BD, Pratt BL, Pollinger HS, Backus CL, Kercher KW, Sing RF, Heniford BT. Assessment of adhesion formation to intra-abdominal polypropylene mesh and polytetrafluoroethylene mesh. J Surg Res. 2003;114(2):126–32.
23. Otterburn D, Losken A. The use of porcine acellular dermal material for TRAM flap donor-site closure. Plast Reconstr Surg. 2009;123(2):74e–6.
24. Jenkins ED, Melman L, Deeken CR, Greco SC, Frisella MM, Matthews BD. Evaluation of fenestrated and non-fenestrated biologic grafts in a porcine model of mature ventral incisional hernia repair. Hernia. 2010;14(6):599–610.
25. Jenkins ED, Melman L, Deeken CR, Greco SC, Frisella MM, Matthews BD. Biomechanical and histologic evaluation of fenestrated and nonfenestrated biologic mesh in a porcine model of ventral hernia repair. J Am Coll Surg. 2011;212(3): 327–39.
26. Deeken CR, Eliason BJ, Pichert MD, Grant SA, Frisella MM, Matthews BD. Characterization of the physicomechanical, thermal, and degradation properties of biologic scaffold materials utilized for hernia repair applications. Hernia Repair 2011. San Francisco, CA: American Hernia Society; 2011.
27. Deeken CR, Abdo MS, Frisella MM, Matthews BD. Physicomechanical evaluation of absorbable and nonabsorbable barrier composite meshes for laparoscopic ventral hernia repair. Surg Endosc. 2010;25(5):1451–552.
28. Deeken CR, Abdo M, Frisella M, Matthews BD. Physicomechanical evaluation of polypropylene, polyester, and polytetrafluoroethylene meshes for inguinal hernia repair. J Am Coll Surg. 2011;212(1):68–79.

29. Ventral Hernia Working Group, Breuing K, Butler CE, Ferzoco S, Franz M, Hultman CS, Kilbridge JF, Rosen M, Silverman RP, Vargo D. Incisional ventral hernias: review of the literature and recommendations regarding the grading and technique of repair. Surgery. 2010;148(3):544–58.
30. Bachman S, Ramshaw B. Prosthetic material in ventral hernia repair: how do I choose? Surg Clin North Am. 2008;88(1):101–12. ix.
31. Awad S, Baumann D, Bellows C, DeNoto G, Franz M, Helton S, Hultman S, Itani K, Kavic S, Rosen M, Steeb G, Vargo D (2010) Prospective multicenter clinical study of single-stage repair of infected or contaminated abdominal incisional hernias using Strattice™ reconstructive tissue matrix. In: 2010 Clinical Congress of the American College of Surgeons, Washington, DC, 5 October 2010
32. U.S. Food and Drug Administration, U.S. Department of Health and Human Services (2011) Inspections, compliance, enforcement and criminal investigations: LifeCell Corporation enforcement action warning letter, 2011 May 5. www.fda.gov/ICECI/EnforcementActions/WarningLetters/ucm254916.htm.
33. Mangram AJ, Horan TC, Pearson ML, Silver LC, Jarvis WR. Guideline for prevention of surgical site infection, 1999. Hospital Infection Control Practices Advisory Committee. Infect Control Hosp Epidemiol. 1999;20(4):250–78.
34. Carne PW, Robertson GM, Frizelle FA. Parastomal Herni. Br J Surg. 2003;90(7):784–93.
35. Janes A, Cengiz Y, Israelsson LA. Randomized clinical trial of the use of a prosthetic mesh to prevent parastomal hernia. Br J Surg. 2004;91(3):280–2.
36. Wijeyekoon SP, Gurusamy K, El-Gendy K, Chan CL. Prevention of parastomal herniation with biologic/composite prosthetic mesh: a systematic review and meta-analysis of randomized controlled trials. J Am Coll Surg. 2010;211(5):637–45.
37. Serra-Aracil X, Bombardo-Junca J, Moreno-Matias J, Darnell A, Mora-Lopez L, Alcantara-Moral M, Ayguavives-Garnica I, Navarro-Soto S. Randomized, controlled, prospective trial of the use of a mesh to prevent parastomal hernia. Ann Surg. 2009;249(4):583–7.
38. Janes A, Cengiz Y, Israelsson LA. Preventing parastomal hernia with a prosthetic mesh: a 5-year follow-up of a randomized study. World J Surg. 2009;33(1):118–21.
39. Hammond TM, Huang A, Prosser K, Frye JN, Williams NS. Parastomal hernia prevention using a novel collagen implant: a randomised controlled phase 1 study. Hernia. 2008;12(5):475–81.
40. Tam KW, Wei PL, Kuo LJ, Wu CH. Systematic review of the use of a mesh to prevent parastomal hernia. World J Surg. 2010;34(11):2723–9.
41. Slater NJ, Hansson BME, Buyne OR, Hendriks T, Bleichrodt RP. Repair of parastomal hernias with biologic grafts: a systematic review. J Gastrointest Surg. 2011;15(7):1252–8.
42. Jin J, Rosen MJ, Blatnik J, McGee MF, Williams CP, Marks J, Ponsky J. Use of acellular dermal matrix for complicated ventral hernia repair: does technique affect outcomes? J Am Coll Surg. 2007;205(5):654–60.
43. Candage R, Jones K, Luchette FA, Sinacore JM, Vandevender D, Reed 2nd RL. Use of human acellular dermal matrix for hernia repair: friend or foe? Surgery. 2008;144(4):703–11.

44. Kolker AR, Brown DJ, Redstone JS, Scarpinato VM, Wallack MK. Multilayer reconstruction of abdominal wall defects with acellular dermal allograft (AlloDerm) and component separation. Ann Plast Surg. 2005;55(1):36–42.
45. Byrnes MC, Irwin E, Carlson D, Campeau A, Gipson JC, Beal A, Croston JK. Repair of high-risk incisional hernias and traumatic abdominal wall defects with porcine mesh. Am Surg. 2011;77(2):144–50.

Part IX
Other Hernias

45. Parastomal Hernia Repair: Latest Updates

Chee-Chee H. Stucky and Kristi L. Harold

Creation of an ostomy is a widely performed surgical procedure. Enterostomies and colostomies are frequently formed as temporary or permanent fecal diversions in the setting of inflammatory bowel disease, carcinoma, trauma, or incontinence. Ileal conduits are also common urinary diversion stomas formed for the treatment of urogenital diseases including carcinoma and urinary incontinence. All of these stoma variations have the potential for hernia development through the fascial defect created in the abdominal wall at the time of formation. In fact, parastomal hernias are considered the most common late complication of stoma formation and typically occur within the first 2 years following creation [1–3]. The risk of occurrence also increases with time [4, 5].

The incidence of parastomal hernias ranges between 30 and 50%; however, with increasing use of computed tomography imaging, detection of asymptomatic parastomal hernias is increasing [2, 6, 7]. Comorbidities predisposing patients to poor fascial integrity and increased intra-abdominal pressure are the main risk factors associated with parastomal hernia formation. These include older age, obesity, emphysema (chronic cough), steroid use, malignancy, malnutrition, and wound infection [5, 8–10]. Groups have also suggested that the type of stoma influences the incidence of parastomal hernia with paracolostomy hernias thought to be more common than paraileostomy hernias due to larger fascial defects. Reports on this topic demonstrate mixed results [11].

The majority of patients (up to 70%) with parastomal hernias will not require surgical intervention [1]. Nonoperative management includes weight loss, abdominal binders, hernia support belts, and flexible, low-profile (or flangeless) pouching systems which may be more easily applied in the setting of the hernia [10, 12]. Surgical intervention is indicated when secondary complications arise such as obstruction, pain, bleeding, and

B.P. Jacob and B. Ramshaw (eds.), *The SAGES Manual of Hernia Repair*, DOI 10.1007/978-1-4614-4824-2_45,

poorly fitting stoma appliances resulting in skin breakdown secondary to leakage of urine or intestinal contents. Stomal prolapse is often confused with parastomal herniation; however, this situation is less likely to result in functional compromise and therefore should be distinguished from herniation [3]. Parastomal hernia repair techniques include open suture repair of the fascial defect, stoma relocation to the contralateral side of the abdominal wall, and, more recently, reinforcement of the fascia with mesh either in an open or laparoscopic fashion. This chapter reviews the various methods of parastomal hernia repair as well as describes the latest updates regarding these techniques.

Open Repair

The most definitive method in repairing parastomal hernias is reversal of the stoma. Unfortunately, this is not always a feasible option. Therefore, many other methods have been described with variable success. A simple and local option is primary fascial repair of the parastomal defect. While this approach is quick and easy to perform, the risk of hernia recurrence is quite high with reports ranging from 46 to 100% [13, 14].

Relocating the stoma to the contralateral side of the abdominal wall has been considered more successful than primary repair in terms of hernia recurrence. Studies have demonstrated recurrence rates of 30–50%; however, this technique by definition results in multiple sites for potential hernia formation including the original stoma defect, the new stoma defect, and the laparotomy incision used to relocate the stoma [14]. Therefore, this method is not considered an ideal option for treatment of parastomal hernias.

More definitive management of these hernias has been established with the use of prosthetic mesh reinforcement as a tension-free repair. This may be done with either an onlay, sublay, or intraperitoneal approach. The latter approach has been shown to have a low recurrence rate of approximately 11% likely due to adequate mesh overlap on the abdominal fascia [2]. However, this technique requires a laparotomy incision and thus introduces the risks of further herniation as well as potential surgical site infection and subsequent mesh contamination. The use of laparoscopy in parastomal hernia repair has gained acceptance as a means of minimizing both the incision size and the potential for surgical site contamination while still adequately exposing the hernia defect for sufficient mesh overlap.

Laparoscopic Repair

With the popularization of laparoscopic parastomal hernia repair, two techniques adapted from open intraperitoneal repairs are predominantly used. The first technique incorporates a procedure described by Sugarbaker et al. in 1985 [15, 16]. In this technique, the bowel is tunneled superficially and laterally above the mesh, thereby creating a flap valve to prevent further herniation. In the original description, the mesh was sutured to the fascial edges as an inlay, but today, this procedure is performed similarly to a ventral hernia repair where the mesh overlaps the fascial edges by several centimeters.

The keyhole technique is another method used to repair parastomal hernias [17–19]. The mesh has a "keyhole" shape or a slit cut into it allowing the mesh to be wrapped completely around the ostomy with the edges of the mesh then sutured to the abdominal wall. Although the concept of this technique is to reinforce the ostomy while covering the hernia defect, the recurrence rates can be unacceptably high. Therefore, we have directed our laparoscopic parastomal hernia repair practice to performing a modified Sugarbaker technique as described below.

Laparoscopic Technique

The patient is placed in a supine position, and general anesthesia is induced with both arms tucked at the sides. All patients are given a first generation cephalosporin (or appropriate substitute in the case of an allergy) within 1 h of incision. The abdomen, including the ostomy, is prepped and draped. A sterile Foley catheter is then inserted into the ostomy, and the balloon filled to assist with identification of the correct intestinal loop when lysing adhesions (Fig. 45.1). We use a Ioban drape (3M Company, St. Paul, MN, USA) to cover the abdomen and stoma as well as to mark the abdomen later when measuring for mesh size.

The peritoneal cavity is accessed using a Veress needle inserted in the left subcostal margin in the midclavicular line. Once adequate pneumoperitoneum (15 mmHg of carbon dioxide) is achieved, a 5-mm OPTIVIEW port is placed superolaterally on the side contralateral to the ostomy. Two additional 5-mm trocars are placed on this contralateral side: one laterally on the level of the ostomy and the other inferolaterally to the ostomy (Fig. 45.2). Adhesiolysis is then performed using sharp

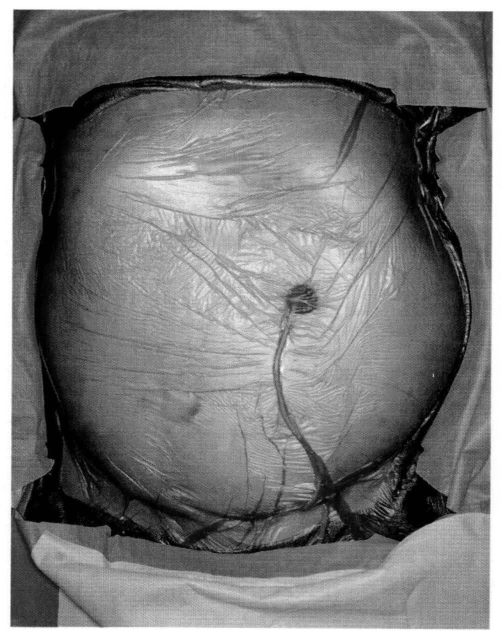

Fig. 45.1. A Foley balloon catheter in the ostomy to assist with localization of the correct intestinal loop when performing adhesiolysis.

dissection. At this stage, external manipulation of the Foley catheter placed in the stoma assists in identifying the ostomy intestinal loop (Fig. 45.3). Adhesiolysis is complete when the entire abdominal wall is visualized and the intestinal loop ending in the ostomy is circumferentially free of adhesions. At this time, spinal needles and an intra-abdominal ruler are used to measure the extent of the hernia defect, including any other coexisting ventral hernias. The defect is also measured and marked on the outside of the abdomen to ensure proper centering of the mesh (Fig. 45.4).

A sheet of GORE DUALMESH (W.L. Gore, Inc. Flagstaff, AZ), made from expanded polytetrafluoroethylene (ePTFE), is trimmed to a size allowing for 5 cm of overlap beyond the dimensions of the fascial defect. The mesh is marked for appropriate intra-abdominal orientation. A single 0-Gore-Tex suture is placed at the edge of the mesh on three of four sides. Two sutures are placed on the fourth side (either inferior or

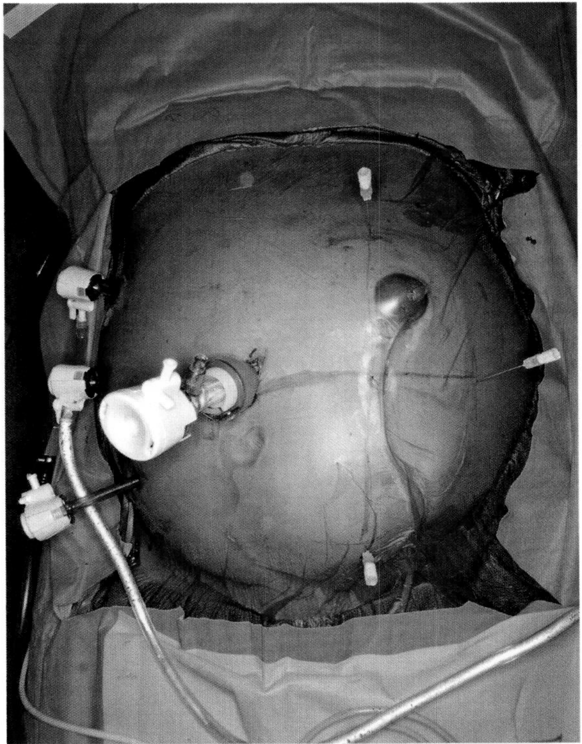

Fig. 45.2. Laparoscopic parastomal hernia port placement.

lateral edge) where the intestinal loop ending in the stoma will exit the created mesh flap valve (Fig. 45.4). The mesh is then rolled into a scroll to facilitate unfurling once introduced into the abdomen.

A 12-mm port is then introduced in a position which will later be covered by the mesh to prevent future trocar site herniation (Fig. 45.2). The scrolled-up mesh is inserted through this 12-mm port. The open jaws of a laparoscopic atraumatic bowel grasper are used to measure a 5-cm overlap from the edges of the fascial defect corresponding to the five points on the mesh where the Gore-Tex sutures were placed. These positions are aligned with the outside measurements and individually marked with spinal needles. A suture passer is used to transfer the Gore-

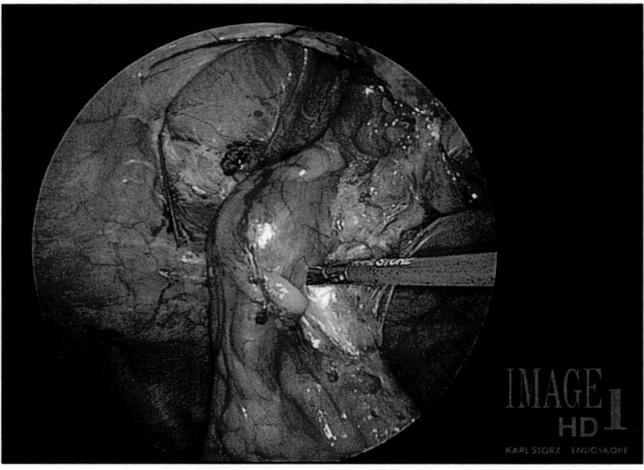

Fig. 45.3. Identification of intestinal loop containing ostomy and Foley catheter.

Tex sutures back through the fascia at these points. The mesh is then tacked circumferentially with spiral tacks except at the exit site of the stoma bowel loop (Fig. 45.5). Additional transfascial sutures are placed around the mesh every 4–5 cm circumferentially for fixation. All knots are tied in the subcutaneous tissue, and the port sites are closed after thorough evaluation of the final repair [20, 21].

Outcomes

Laparoscopic Versus Open Techniques

While long-term follow-up is not readily available specifically for laparoscopic parastomal hernia repair, its popularity over open repair stems from the same advantages of using laparoscopy in ventral or incisional hernia repairs [22]. These include decreased surgical site infection rate, decreased length of hospital stay, and earlier return to activities of daily living. Recurrence rates of incisional hernias have also been shown to be lower than in open repairs in many large studies [22, 23].

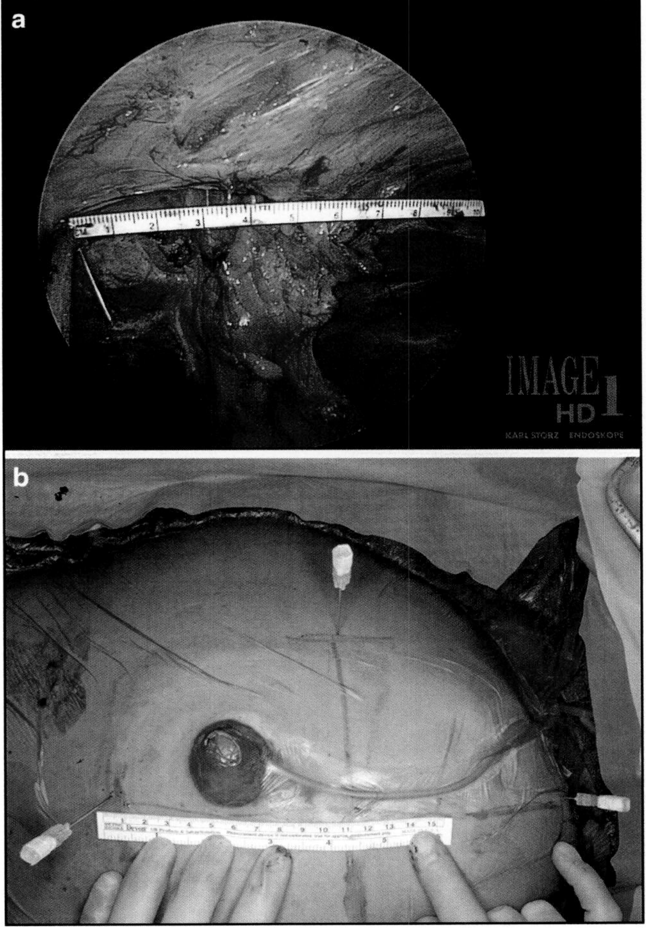

Fig. 45.4. (**a**) Intra-abdominal view of hernia defect marked by spinal needles. (**b**) Measurement of defect on outside of abdominal wall for appropriate mesh centering. (**c**) Gore-Tex sutures placed at five points along the mesh for parastomal hernia repair using the Sugarbaker technique.

In 2007, our institution reviewed 49 patients undergoing repair of symptomatic parastomal hernias [24]. Thirty patients underwent conventional open repair (total of 39 procedures), while 19 patients underwent successful laparoscopic repair. The postoperative follow-up

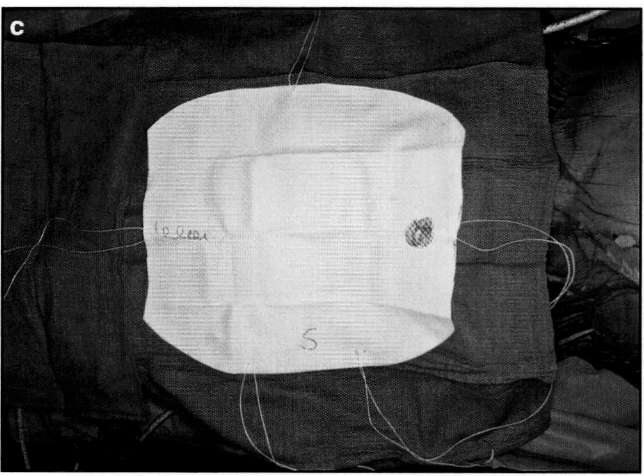

Fig. 45.4. (continued)

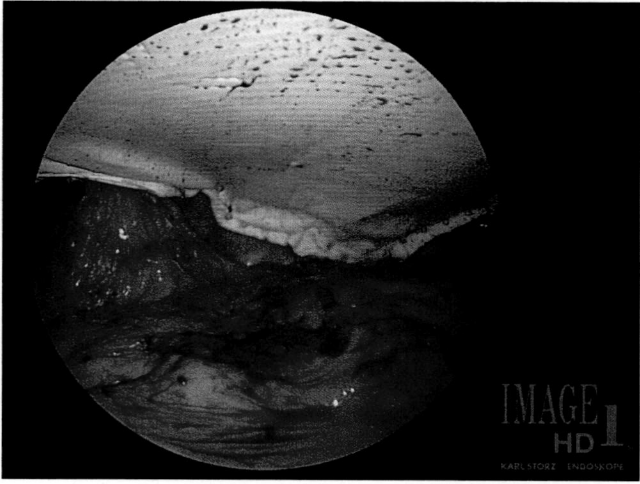

Fig. 45.5. Final orientation of the mesh with the loop of bowel containing the ostomy exiting at the flap valve.

was significantly shorter in the laparoscopic group (20 months vs. 65 months open repair, $p \leq 0.0001$), and, therefore, recurrence rates could not be appropriately compared. Complication rates were, however, equivalent, making laparoscopy a feasible approach at that time. Long-term follow-up is necessary to distinguish the major advantages of laparoscopic parastomal hernia repair.

Sugarbaker Versus Keyhole Techniques

Both the Sugarbaker and keyhole parastomal hernia repair techniques have been modified over the last several years. Despite improvements in the keyhole technique, current studies still demonstrate a recurrence rate of approximately 37–73% [25–27]. Our institution's series of 21 consecutive patients, all undergoing successful laparoscopic parastomal hernia repair with nonslit ePTFE mesh (Sugarbaker technique), demonstrated a 5% recurrence rate (1 patient) with a mean follow-up of 32 months (range = 1–63 months) [28]. This is similar to studies by Mancini et al. and Berger et al., both of which evaluated outcomes in 25 patients undergoing consecutive laparoscopic parastomal hernia repair at their individual institutions. These groups reported recurrence rates of 4% and 0%, respectively, while applying some variation of the Sugarbaker technique [16, 29].

Prosthetic Mesh

Initially, the main concerns with using prosthetic mesh in parastomal hernia repairs were exposure to and therefore potential erosion through the bowel wall as well as a source of adhesion development and intestinal obstruction. Polypropylene mesh has been particularly implicated in these complications, and therefore, using unprotected polypropylene mesh in the intraperitoneal laparoscopic repair has been essentially abandoned [30, 31].

Another common prosthetic mesh used in these repairs is ePTFE. This material has low bioavailability and therefore causes minimal adhesions and is less likely to become infected. The advantages to using ePTFE are offset by the lack of rigidity and poor memory making recurrence of the hernia possible despite adequate coverage of the defect. A study by Hansson et al. demonstrated a high recurrence rate with using ePTFE in the keyhole repair [27]. In these cases, shrinkage of the mesh at the site of the central hole, thereby making the hole larger, was the suggested cause of failure.

In light of the mesh-related complications, the focus of surgeons performing these repairs is now aimed toward identifying the ideal prosthetic mesh for this specific type of hernia. A recent study by Wara et al. reviewed results from 72 consecutive patients undergoing laparoscopic parastomal hernia repair (keyhole technique) with a bilayer mesh [32]. The polypropylene layer was placed on the parietal side, and the ePTFE later was placed toward the viscera. While this group reported substantial postoperative morbidity, including late mesh-related complications of abscesses and bowel fistulas requiring mesh removal, their recurrence rate of 3% was remarkably low for this technique [32]. In our repair, we also incorporate a dual-sided mesh composed entirely of ePTFE but with two different surfaces designed for host tissue incorporation on one textured side and minimal tissue attachment on the other smooth side. Our results, when evaluating both recurrence and overall complication rates, were similar to the Wara study but with fewer bowel injuries and therefore less abscess formation [28]. Therefore, standardization of a single mesh used in these cases may be less of an issue as surgeons become more experienced in the laparoscopic technique and the rate intra-abdominal complications decreases.

Parastomal Hernia Prevention

While the rate of parastomal hernia formation is quoted at 50%, many authors believe the actual rate is closer to 100%. Thus, prevention of hernia formation is ideal. Many groups have recently studied the effectiveness of placing a nonslit mesh prosthesis as a prophylactic reinforcement at the time of initial stoma creation. A prospective randomized trial performed by Jänes et al. compared the incidence of hernia development in 54 patients receiving either conventional colostomy formation without mesh reinforcement or UltraPro mesh placed in a sublay position at the time of colostomy formation [33]. With 5-year follow-up, their conclusions favored using mesh reinforcement citing a parastomal hernia incidence of 13% (vs. 81% with conventional colostomy, $p<0.001$). Their success was also supported by the fact that there were no mesh infections, no strictures, and no fistulas noted in either the mesh or conventional groups, making the use of prophylactic mesh reinforcement safe as well as effective. Two other randomized controlled trials with shorter follow-up have demonstrated similarly promising results [34, 35].

Given the substantial evidence supporting the use of prophylactic mesh reinforcement, some surgeons advocate this practice with every ostomy creation. Limitations to this becoming standard of care include persistent concerns of mesh complications and lack of evidence indicating an ideal prosthetic material. Regardless, these significantly decreased parastomal hernia incidences at the very least warrant consideration of using prophylactic mesh reinforcement when permanent ostomies are created.

Summary

The incidence of parastomal hernia formation is high ranging from 30 to 50%. The majority of these may be managed conservatively; however, indications for repair include pain, obstruction, bleeding, and poorly fitting stoma appliances resulting in poor quality of life. Repairs are typically performed either in an open fashion or laparoscopically. Modifications of two main techniques involving mesh reinforcement—the keyhole technique and the Sugarbaker technique—are typically used. Open repair involves the risks of incisional hernia development and presumably higher rates of wound infections. Laparoscopic repair may be more tedious and difficult to detect enterotomies at the time of adhesiolysis but minimizes the risk of incisional hernia while producing similar if not improved parastomal hernia recurrence rates. Prevention of parastomal hernia formation is ideal and may be attainable with the use of prophylactically placed mesh reinforcement at the time of ostomy creation.

References

1. Carne PW, Robertson GM, Frizelle FA. Parastomal hernia. Br J Surg. 2003;90: 784–93.
2. Israelsson LA. Parastomal hernias. Surg Clin North Am. 2008;88:113–25. ix.
3. Shellito PC. Complications of abdominal stoma surgery. Dis Colon Rectum. 1998;41: 1562–72.

4. Scarpa M, Barollo M, Keighley MRB. Ileostomy for constipation: long-term postoperative outcome. Colorectal Dis. 2005;7:224–7.
5. Mylonakis M, Scarpa M, Barollo M, et al. Life table analysis of stoma-related complications. Colorectal Dis. 2001;3:334–7.
6. Williams JG, Etherington R, Hayward MW, et al. Paraileostomy hernia: a clinical and radiological study. Br J Surg. 1990;77:1355–7.
7. Cingi A, Cakir T, Sever A, et al. Enterostomy site hernias: a clinical and computerized tomographic evaluation. Dis Colon Rectum. 2006;49:1559–63.
8. Duschesne JC, Wang YZ, Weintraub SL, et al. Stoma complications: a multivariate analysis. Am Surg. 2002;68:961–6.
9. Robertson I, Leung E, Hughes D, et al. Prospective analysis of stoma-related complications. Colorectal Dis. 2005;7:279–85.
10. Arumugam PJ, Bevan L, Macdonald AJ, et al. A prospective audit of stomas-analysis of risk factors and complications and their management. Colorectal Dis. 2003;5:49–52.
11. Shabbir J, Britton DC. Stoma complications: a literature review. Colorectal Dis. 2010;12:958–64.
12. Efron JE. Ostomies and stomal therapy. ASCRS. www.fascrs.org. Accessed 1 April 2011
13. Riansuwan W, Hull TL, Millan MM, et al. Surgery of recurrent parastomal hernia: direct repair or relocation? Colorectal Dis. 2010;12:681–6.
14. Rubin MS, Schoetz 2nd DJ, Mathews 2nd JB. Parastomal hernia. Is stoma relocation superior to fascial repair? Arch Surg. 1994;129:413–8.
15. Sugarbaker PH. Peritoneal approach to prosthetic mesh repair of paraostomy hernias. Ann Surg. 1985;201:344–6.
16. Mancini GJ, McClusky 3rd DA, Khaitan L, et al. Laparoscopic parastomal hernia repair using a nonslit mesh technique. Surg Endosc. 2007;21:1487–91.
17. Hofstetter WL, Vukasin P, Ortega AE, et al. New technique for mesh repair of paracolostomy hernias. Dis Colon Rectum. 1998;41:1054–5.
18. Bickel A, Shinkarevsky E, Eitan A. Laparoscopic repair of paracolostomy hernia. J Laparoendosc Adv Surg Tech A. 1999;9:353–5.
19. Gould JC, Ellison EC. Laparoscopic parastomal hernia repair. Surg Laparosc Endosc Percutan Tech. 2003;13:51–4.
20. Huguet KL, Harold KL. Laparoscopic parastomal hernia repair. Operat Tech Gen Surg. 2007;9:113–22.
21. Deol ZK, Shayani V. Laparoscopic parastomal hernia repair. Arch Surg. 2003;138: 203–5.
22. Heniford BT, Park A, Ramshaw BJ. Laparoscopic repair of ventral hernias: nine years' experience with 850 consecutive hernias. Ann Surg. 2003;238:391–9.
23. Novitsky YW, Paton LB, Heniford TB. Laparoscopic ventral hernia repair. Operat Tech Gen Surg. 2006;8:4–9.
24. McLemore EC, Harold KL, Efron JE, et al. Parastomal hernia: short-term outcome after laparoscopic and conventional repairs. Surg Innov. 2007;14:199–204.
25. Muysoms EE, Hauters PJ, VanNieuwenhove Y, et al. Laparoscopic repair of parastomal hernias: a multi-centre retrospective review and shift in technique. Acta Chir Belg. 2008;108:400–4.

26. Safadi B. Laparoscopic repair of parastomal hernias: early results. Surg Endosc. 2004;18:676–80.
27. Hansson BM, Bleichrodt RP, deHingh IH. Laparoscopic parastomal hernia repair using a keyhole technique results in a high recurrence rate. Surg Endosc. 2009;23: 1456–9.
28. Craft RO, Huguet KL, McLemore EC, Harold KL. Laparoscopic parastomal hernia repair. Hernia. 2008;12:137–40.
29. Berger D, Bientzle M. Laparoscopic repair of parastomal hernias: a single surgeon's experience in 66 patients. Dis Colon Rectum. 2007;50:1668–73.
30. Steele SR, Lee P, Martin JM, et al. Is parastomal hernia repair with polypropylene mesh safe? Am J Surg. 2003;185:436–40.
31. Morris-Stiff G, Hughes LE. The continuing challenge of parastomal hernia: failure of a novel polypropylene mesh repair. Ann R Coll Surg Engl. 1998;80:184–7.
32. Wara P, Andersen LM. Long-term follow-up of laparoscopic repair of parastomal hernia using a bilayer mesh with a slit. Surg Endosc. 2011;25:526–30.
33. Jänes A, Cengiz Y, Israelsson LA. Preventing parastomal hernia with a prosthetic mesh: a 5-year follow-up of a randomized study. World J Surg. 2009;33:118–21.
34. Serra-Aracil X, Bombardo-Junca J, Moreno-Matias J, et al. Randomized, controlled, prospective trial of the use of a mesh to prevent parastomal hernia. Ann Surg. 2009;249:583–7.
35. Wijeyekoon SP, Gurusamy K, El-Gendy K, et al. Prevention of parastomal herniation with biologic/composite prosthetic mesh: a systematic review and meta-analysis of randomized controlled trials. J Am Coll Surg. 2010;211:637–45.

46. Repair of Paraesophageal Hernia

Steven P. Bowers

Paraesophageal hiatal hernia (PEH) is one in which there is a fixed peritoneal sac above the diaphragm. This peritoneal sac is responsible for the unique spectrum of symptoms of PEH and also for the propensity for gastric volvulus and incarceration of viscera in the hernia sac. Although hiatal hernias are classified based on the anatomical location of the fundus of the stomach and the gastroesophageal junction, this classification has little bearing on the decision-making process of whether to repair a hiatal hernia. And for all hiatal hernias classified as types 1 through 4 that have a fixed hiatal sac, the technique of repair must include reduction of the peritoneal sac. This chapter will then focus on those aspects of paraesophageal hernia that directly impact surgical decision making.

Clinical Presentation

The paraesophageal hernia is more common in females, and its prevalence increases with age and obesity. Because of reconstitution of the angle of His above the diaphragm in many patients with PEH, the PEH is not uniformly associated with typical gastroesophageal reflux symptoms, and due to compression or angulation of the distal esophagus, dysphagia is a common symptom. Compression of the stomach at the hiatus is responsible for the most common symptoms of paraesophageal hernia, chest pain, and emesis and also for the development of erosions at the aspect of the stomach that is raked over the hiatus with respiration. Occult anemia and even acute hemorrhage can result from these lesions called Cameron's ulcers.

B.P. Jacob and B. Ramshaw (eds.), *The SAGES Manual of Hernia Repair*,
DOI 10.1007/978-1-4614-4824-2_46,

It is the natural history of PEH to gradually grow over time, ultimately culminating in the majority of the stomach lying in the mediastinum, potentially with omentum, colon, and even retroperitoneal structures. In order for the stomach to fit into the mediastinal peritoneal sac, it is obligated to be rotated in one of several patterns. Organo-axial volvulus denotes anterior rotation of the stomach along an axis made by the esophageal and pyloric attachments of the stomach and is surprisingly well tolerated from a symptom perspective. Mesentero-axial volvulus denotes either anterior or posterior rotation of the antrum cephalad about the axis made by the left gastric and short gastric vessels. It is this pattern of volvulus that is at highest risk for incarceration of the antrum at the hiatal opening, causing obstruction of the midstomach with or without compression of the blood supply to the upper stomach.

Acute obstruction due to gastric volvulus is a rare event and presents with a clinical scenario of retching without emesis, chest pain, and failure to pass a decompressive gastric tube (Borchardt's triad). Urgent repair for either acute hemorrhage or incarceration is reported in fewer than 5% of patients undergoing repair of PEH. There is a substantial amount of data to support nonoperative management of minimally symptomatic and uncomplicated paraesophageal hernia.

Patient Evaluation

Paraesophageal hernia is often found as a retrocardiac air bubble on chest radiograph or as an incidental finding on CT scan. Upper GI contrast study is used to assess the type and size of hiatal hernia and detect esophageal stricture or gastric volvulus and is helpful for preoperative planning. Upper endoscopy can be challenging in patients with gastric volvulus, but should be performed before PEH repair to exclude dysplastic Barrett's esophagus. Because many symptoms of paraesophageal hernia are not related to reflux, ambulatory pH testing is not an essential part of the preoperative evaluation. The esophageal stationary manometry catheter is unlikely to be passed successfully in PEH patients and has only a limited impact on operation even when correctly passed and interpreted. Gastric emptying study is also difficult to interpret in the setting of intrathoracic stomach and therefore has little to add in preoperative evaluation.

Surgical Technique

The author favors a laparoscopic transabdominal approach to repair of paraesophageal hernia due to the decreased morbidity of the approach. Visualization and esophageal mobilization are improved with laparoscopy compared to open operation, but population studies reveal open and transthoracic repair techniques are still prevalent in the United States. Gastropexy without excision of the sac or repair of the hiatus is an option to prevent complications of volvulus in frail and ill patients with symptomatic PEH.

Patient Positioning

The author favors operating with the patient in the split leg position, with the surgeon standing between the outstretched legs. A five-port approach is used, with port position similar to that of fundoplication.

Reduction of the Sac

The short gastric vessels are first divided with ultrasonic shears to expose the base of the left crus and fully mobilize the fundus of the stomach (Fig. 46.1). Using scissors with cautery, the leading edge of the peritoneum overlying the left pillar of the crus is incised from the base of the left crus in an anterior direction around the hiatus (Fig. 46.2). After dividing the hepatogastric ligament, the peritoneum at the leading edge of the right pillar of the crus is similarly divided from the base of the hiatus to the apex (Fig. 46.3). It is important to preserve the peritoneum of the crura to allow for more secure crural closure. A posterior window is dissected under direct visualization in the avascular retroesophageal space, and the hiatal contents are encircled with a rubber drain to allow retraction.

The sac is separated from the crural muscle and pleura and delivered into the abdomen. Once the sac is reduced into the abdomen, the Penrose drain enables esophageal retraction and ensures the vagus nerves are kept against the esophagus to avoid injury. The sac is excised from the attachments to the fundus—the right-sided sac contains the lesser curve mesentery of the stomach and cannot be fully excised. It is not uncommon

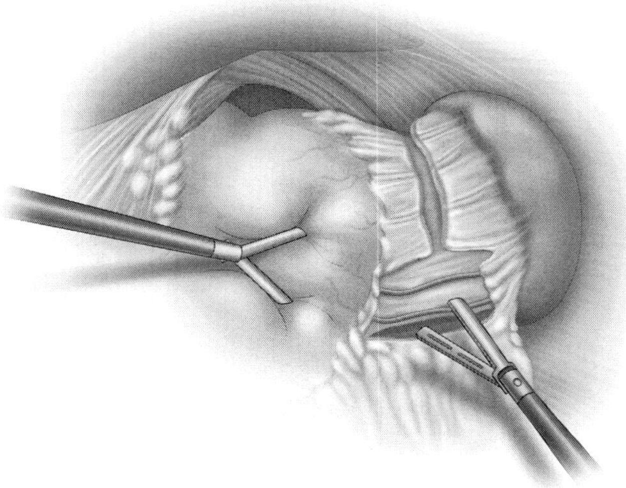

Fig. 46.1. The short gastric vessels are completely divided to expose the base of the left crus.

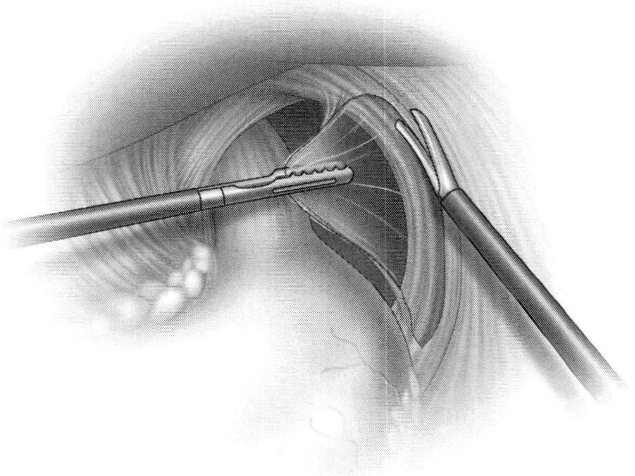

Fig. 46.2. The peritoneum overlying the left crus is incised from base to apex.

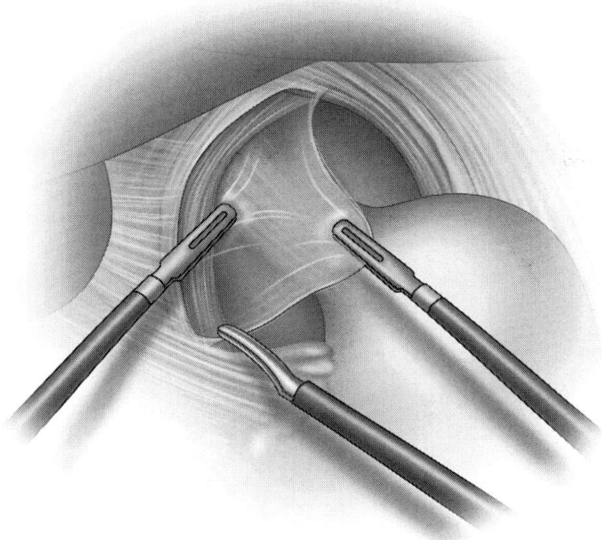

Fig. 46.3. The peritoneum overlying the right crus is incised and the sac is reduced.

to have a posterior lipoma of the sac, and this should be completely mobilized along with the sac to completely free the esophagus and fundus of the stomach from their posterior attachments.

Esophageal Mobilization

The mediastinal esophagus should be mobilized until the gastroesophageal junction remains comfortably in the abdomen without tension. The author prefers starting in the retroesophageal space and proceeding anteriorly, with dissection of both pleurae. Blunt dissection aided by the ultrasonic shears enables dissection to the level of the mid- to upper pericardium. The space anterior and left of the esophagus generally has the most difficult periesophageal adhesions, and this area is dissected last. Adequate esophageal mobilization is ensured when, after closure of the hiatus, there is greater than 3 cm of esophagus lying below the diaphragm without caudal traction on the drain. Endoscopy is recommended in cases of high mediastinal dissection, both to assess for esophageal injury and to definitively identify the location of the gastroesophageal junction (GEJ).

It is imperative, even when Collis gastroplasty is to be performed, to mobilize the esophagus such that GEJ lies comfortably below the diaphragm, as the fundoplication must include the GEJ. If the esophageal mobilization is restricted by tension on the vagus nerves, detachment of the vagal branches to the upper stomach, unilateral vagotomy, or transthoracic esophageal mobilization may be required to establish adequate esophageal length. If endoscopic assessment reveals inadequate esophageal length after mediastinal mobilization, the surgeon should consider Collis gastroplasty as an esophageal lengthening procedure.

Crural Closure

Crural closure should be performed such that the crura approximate the empty esophagus without constriction. A combination of interrupted simple and mattress sutures with cardiovascular pledgets is preferred by the author (Fig. 46.4). Because dysphagia may be decreased with some component of anterior crural closure, a consideration is given to place at least one anterior suture if more than three sutures are required for closure. The author decreases the pneumoperitoneum pressure when placing and securing the crural closures sutures.

Fundoplication

Although patients with PEH may not have GERD symptoms preoperatively, a third will complain of GERD or have endoscopic evidence of GERD following PEH repair without antireflux operation. It is therefore preferred to perform a fundoplication in all patients undergoing repair of paraesophageal hernia. Fundoplication increases the bulk of the gastroesophageal junction and may serve as a buttress preventing recurrence. Gastropexy of the fundoplication may further secure the stomach within the abdomen.

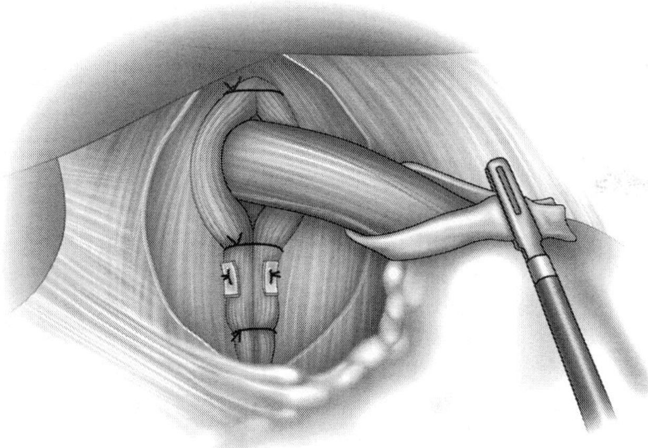

Fig. 46.4. Simple and mattress suture closure of the hiatus such that the crura approximate the empty esophagus.

An intraoperative assessment of the adequacy of the fundus of the stomach to comfortably create a Nissen fundoplication around an intraesophageal bougie is a crucial factor in helping decide what type of fundoplication is to be performed. If the fundus is thickened or fibrotic, a complete Nissen fundoplication may increase the risk of postoperative dysphagia. In this situation, a posterior hemifundoplication or anterior partial fundoplication should be considered.

Gastrostomy Tube

Selective use of percutaneous endoscopic gastrostomy (PEG) may be considered for patients in whom reduction of the hernia sac has been more difficult or required extensive manipulation of the stomach, those requiring urgent operation, or those in whom adjunctive measures were required for the short esophagus. The gastrostomy tube serves as an effective gastropexy technique. In patients in whom a Collis gastroplasty has been performed, a Witzel-type gastrostomy using a Foley catheter is performed to avoid dragging the PEG button across the Collis staple line.

Esophageal Lengthening

Authors reporting selective use of Collis gastroplasty report use of the technique in only 4–5% of patients undergoing hiatal hernia repair, although there are reports of less selective application of Collis gastroplasty in PEH patients. It has not been determined that use of Collis gastroplasty decreases the rate of reoperation for symptomatic recurrence. Long-term studies reveal that GERD-related outcomes are not as satisfactory in patients after Collis gastroplasty, because placing the fundoplication around the neoesophagus creates, at best, a slipped Nissen physiology. A highly selective use of the Collis gastroplasty is therefore encouraged.

When required, the author favors the stapled Collis gastroplasty to excise a triangular wedge of stomach at the angle of His, as this can increase the effective intra-abdominal length of esophagus by 2–3 cm. It is essential that the subsequent fundoplication includes the gastroesophageal junction to prevent an aperistaltic segment of neoesophagus above the fundoplication wrap and resultant two-compartment stomach physiology and dysphagia.

Mesh Repair of the Hiatal Defect

There is good evidence that both permanent and biological mesh reduce the short-term risk of radiological recurrence of PEH but that these benefits may be limited to the short term. It is clear that reoperation in the setting of prior hiatal mesh is more difficult and more morbid, and this should be factored into the decision to place hiatal mesh.

The use of biological or absorbable/nonpermanent mesh is recommended when concern for recurrence is especially high, as in patients undergoing an esophageal lengthening procedure and those with weak, thin or fibrotic crura, or large hiatal defects with crura approximated under tension. The optimal material and optimal technique of placement have not been determined, but, when mesh buttress of the hiatus is indicated, the author favors the technique used by Ohlschlager et al. in their pivotal randomized controlled trial. One technique to avoid due to the potential of mesh erosion into the esophagus is complete encircling of the esophagus with permanent macroporous synthetic mesh.

Obesity and Paraesophageal Hernia

In patients with class 2 obesity (BMI > 35) and paraesophageal hernia, it is optimal that the patient undergoes substantial weight loss prior to antireflux operation concomitant with PEH repair. The presence of fatty liver disease and visceral obesity significantly adds to the difficulty of PEH repair, and intra-abdominal pressure associated with obesity increases the risk of recurrent hiatal herniation, so a bariatric operation should be considered at the time of paraesophageal hernia repair.

Until longer term studies of patients undergoing sleeve gastrectomy at the time of PEH repair are reported, it is the author's opinion that the Roux-en-Y gastric bypass should be considered the standard operation for patients with morbid obesity and large hiatal hernia or paraesophageal hernia.

Suggested Reading

1. Allen MS, Trastek VF, Deschamps C, et al. Intrathoracic stomach. Presentation and results of operation. J Thorac Cardiovasc Surg. 1993;105(2):253–8 [discussion: 258–9].
2. Stylopoulos N, Gazelle GS, Rattner DW. Paraesophageal hernias: operation or observation? Ann Surg. 2002;236(4):492–500 [discussion: 492–500].
3. Edye M, Salky B, Posner A, Fierer A. Sac excision is essential to adequate laparoscopic repair of paraesophageal hernia. Surg Endosc. 1998;12(10):1259–63.
4. Frantzides CT, Madan AK, Carlson MA, Frantzides CT, Madan AK, Carlson MA, et al. A prospective, randomized trial of laparoscopic polytetrafluoroethylene (PTFE) patch repair vs. simple cruroplasty for large hiatal hernia. Arch Surg. 2002;137:649–52.
5. Oelschlager BK, Pellegrini CA, Hunter JG, et al. Biologic prosthesis to prevent recurrence after laparoscopic paraesophageal hernia repair: long-term follow-up from a multicenter, prospective, randomized trial. J Am Coll Surg. 2011;213(4):461–8.
6. Luketich JD, Nason KS, Christie NA, et al. Outcomes after a decade of laparoscopic giant paraesophageal hernia repair. J Thorac Cardiovasc Surg. 2010;139(2):395–404.
7. Parker M, Bowers SP, Bray JM, et al. Hiatal mesh is associated with major resection at revisional operation. Surg Endosc. 2010;24(12):3095–101.

47. Challenging Hernia Locations: Flank Hernias

Gregory F. Dakin and Michael L. Kendrick

Flank, or lumbar, hernias result from defects in the posterolateral abdominal wall. These are rare hernias, with several studies indicating as few as 300 cases reported in the literature. Flank hernias can be either acquired, usually from trauma or incisional, or congenital which generally occur in two anatomic locations: the inferior or superior lumbar triangles. Lumbar hernias are challenging to repair, principally because the boundaries of the defect are bony (iliac crest or 12th rib), thus making mesh fixation difficult. Given the rare nature of these defects, there is no consensus on technique of repair, nor are there significant prospective trials. Minimally invasive techniques have been applied since 1996 [1] to these challenging defects. This chapter will review flank hernias and discuss several technical considerations in performing laparoscopic repair.

History

The first publication on lumbar hernias was by Garangeot in 1731, though Barbette is credited with suggesting the existence of these hernias in 1672 [2, 3]. The first surgical repair of a lumbar hernia was by Ravaton in 1750 [2], performed for an incarcerated hernia in a pregnant patient. Petit is credited with describing the anatomic boundaries of the inferior lumbar triangle in 1783, while nearly a century later in 1866, Grynfeltt described the separate superior lumbar triangle [3]. Lesshaft also described the superior triangle in 1870; thus, this space is often referred to as the "triangle of Grynfeltt-Lesshaft." Early reports suggested that hernias of the inferior triangle were most common, but studies published

B.P. Jacob and B. Ramshaw (eds.), *The SAGES Manual of Hernia Repair*, DOI 10.1007/978-1-4614-4824-2_47,

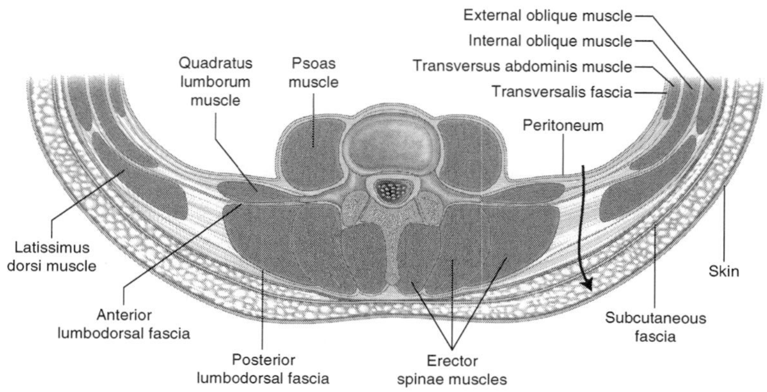

Fig. 47.1. Cross-sectional view of the abdominal musculature.

after 1920 indicated the superior triangle is the more common site of herniation. A posttraumatic hernia was first described by Selby in 1906, and post-incisional hernias were described in 1939 by Kelton [2, 3].

Anatomy

The lumbar region is defined anatomically as the area of the abdominal wall lateral to the midclavicular line between the ribs superiorly and the iliac crests inferiorly, extending posteriorly to the back. More precisely, the surgical anatomy of the lumbar portion of the abdominal wall is located between the lower edge of the 12th rib superiorly, the iliac crest inferiorly, the external oblique muscle laterally, and the erector spinae muscle medially [4]. A cross-sectional view of the abdomen in this area is useful to delineate the layers of the abdominal wall (from external to internal) (Fig. 47.1): (1) skin; (2) superficial fascia (membranous and fatty); (3) superficial muscle layer composed of external oblique anterolaterally and latissimus dorsi posterolaterally; (4) thoracolumbar (lumbodorsal) fascia, which is the union of all investing fasciae, covering muscles and their aponeuroses; (5) middle muscle layer, composed of the sacrospinalis muscle, internal oblique, and serratus posterior inferior muscles; (6) deep muscle layer, including the quadratus lumborum and psoas muscle; (7) transversalis fascia; (8)

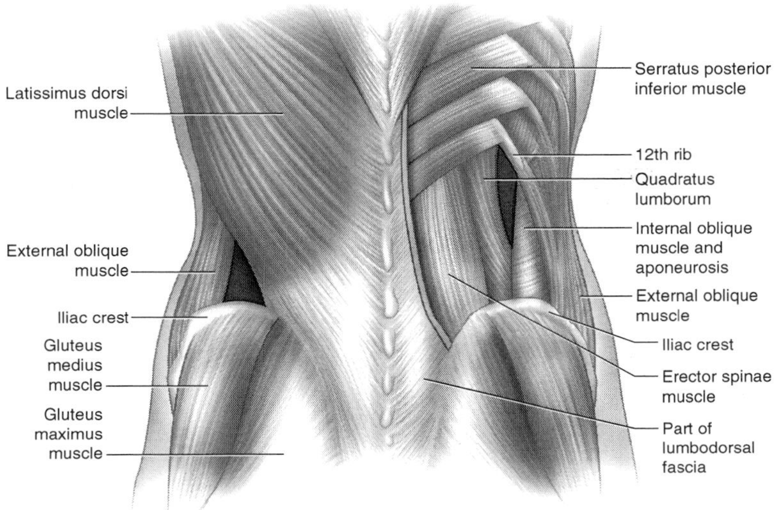

Fig. 47.2. View of boundaries of inferior and superior lumbar triangles.

preperitoneal fat; and (9) peritoneum [2, 3]. Knowledge of these layers is important for any surgical repair, especially when performing an extraperitoneal approach.

Most hernias in the lumbar region occur in two discrete areas of the flank, either the superior or inferior lumbar triangle. There are occasionally more diffuse hernias that extend beyond the boundaries of these two spaces. Such diffuse hernias are larger and generally the result of either surgical incisions or significant trauma such as automobile accidents. Diffuse hernias will often extend beyond the anatomic boundaries of the flank region to include portions of the rectus muscles anteriorly [2].

The inferior lumbar (Petit's) triangle is smaller than the superior triangle and is bounded by the iliac crest inferiorly (which forms the base of the triangle), the external oblique laterally, and the latissimus dorsi medially (Fig. 47.2). The roof of the triangle is the superficial fascia, and the floor is the internal oblique muscle. Authors speculate on certain factors that may predispose to hernias in this area, including alterations in the origin of the external oblique muscle and a more medial latissimus, leading to a wider triangle base [2, 3]. Unlike the superior triangle, there are no nerves or blood vessels penetrating through this area to weaken the floor and potentially lead to herniation [2].

Table 47.1. Classification of lumbar hernias.

I. Congenital
II. Acquired
a. Primary
b. Secondary
i. Post-incisional
ii. Traumatic
iii. Post-infectious

The superior (Grynfeltt-Lesshaft) triangle is bounded anteriorly by the posterior border of the internal oblique muscle, posteriorly by the anterior border of the sacrospinalis muscle, and the 12th rib and serratus posterior inferior muscle superiorly, which forms the base of this inverted triangular area [3] (Fig. 47.2). The roof is formed by the external oblique and latissimus, while the floor is formed by the transversalis fascia. There are several areas of natural weakness in the superior triangle, including beneath the rib where the transversalis fascia is not covered by the external oblique and the point of penetration of the 12th dorsal intercostal neurovascular pedicle [2]. Factors that may influence herniation in the superior triangle include the size of the triangle, the length and angulation of the 12th rib, and the size of quadratus lumborum and serratus posterior muscles. Authors speculate that a tall thin person with sharply angulated 12th ribs will have a smaller superior triangle space and thus be less likely to form hernias than a shorter, obese person with more horizontal ribs and a larger triangle [2].

Etiology

Lumbar hernias may be congenital or acquired (Table 47.1), with approximate incidences of 20% and 80%, respectively. Congenitally acquired lumbar hernias are reported rarely in the literature and can be due to neuropraxia, nerve entrapment, or abdominal masses [3]. Up to 67% of congenital lumbar hernias are associated with other anomalies, including diaphragmatic hernia, ureteropelvic junction obstruction, hydrocephalus, renal agenesis, meningomyelocele, high anorectal malformations, and undescended testis [3, 5–7].

Acquired hernias account for approximately 80% of lumbar hernias [8] overall and are classified as primary (spontaneous) or secondary if there is a causative factor. Primary acquired lumbar hernias represent

55% of acquired hernias and can be associated with several predisposing factors, such as excessive weight loss, advanced age, or pulmonary disease [8]. Secondary acquired hernias are caused by trauma, surgery, or infection (lumbar abscess). Lumbar hernias have been reported after a variety of surgical procedures, including nephrectomy, aortic aneurysm repair, iliac bone-graft harvest, and myocutaneous flap harvest [9–12].

Diagnosis

Lumbar hernias can present with a variety of manifestations, largely dependent on the hernia contents. Lumbar hernias containing colon, spleen, and liver have all been reported [3]. A hernia sac may also be absent, as in the case of a protrusion of extraperitoneal fat. Symptoms can include back pain, abdominal discomfort, and a flank mass. Pain can also be attributed to direct nerve compression. Many lumbar hernias, however, are asymptomatic. It is important to consider a wide differential diagnosis and exclude other common processes, such as flank lipomas, hematomas from trauma, abscesses, or kidney tumors [2]. CT scan has become the imaging modality of choice to confirm the diagnosis [13] (Fig. 47.3). The natural history of lumbar hernias is not rigorously delineated, due to their rare nature, though authors believe that, like other hernias, they tend to grow over time [2, 14]. Lumbar hernias have been reported to have a 25% risk of incarceration and an 8% risk of strangulation, making surgical repair a reasonable option [15].

Surgical Technique

Before embarking on minimally invasive lumbar hernia repair, it is important to consider the size and character of the defect. Diffuse, large defects or defects that result from muscular atrophy (pseudohernia) may be best approached with an open technique that will allow approximation of the muscular layers to provide an adequate functional and cosmetic result. However, smaller defects (<15 cm) can be repaired effectively with either retroperitoneal or transabdominal laparoscopic techniques. Regardless of the approach, difficulties with repair remain achieving adequate mesh overlap and fixation, owning to the fixed bony boundaries of these hernia defects.

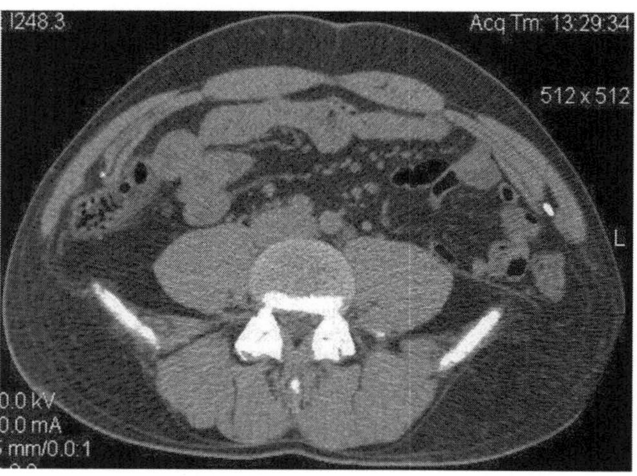

Fig. 47.3. CT scan showing lumbar hernia.

Laparoscopic Transabdominal Repair

The patient is placed in a semi-lateral decubitus position with a 45° elevation of the side ipsilateral to the hernia, which allows the patient to be rotated either fully flat or to a full lateral position to optimize visualization. Access to the abdomen is gained via the umbilicus, and a 10-mm port is placed. 5-mm ports are then placed in the midline above and below the umbilicus, with the exact position being determined by the location and size of the hernia defect. If necessary, an additional 5-mm port can be placed more laterally to facilitate dissection. The hernia contents are reduced, and any adhesions to the sac are divided. Frequently, adequate exposure of the defect will require mobilization of the colon and abdominal viscera medially. The psoas muscle is fully exposed with this maneuver and represents a useful anatomical landmark. Inferiorly, the dissection extends to Cooper's ligament. For superior defects, the dissection will extend to the diaphragm above the costal margin. Care is taken to identify and preserve retroperitoneal anatomical structures such as the ureter and vasculature, as well as the lateral femoral cutaneous nerve at the anterior superior iliac spine to avoid injury.

Once the defect is exposed, it can be measured and the appropriate mesh selected. Any mesh with an adhesion barrier designed for intra-abdominal use is an acceptable option (polypropylene, polyester, polytetrafluoroethylene). The use of mesh with an adhesion barrier obviates the need to repair the peritoneal flaps over the mesh after its placement. The mesh should be sized to provide a wide overlap of the hernia defect (at least 4–5 cm, with some authors recommending up to 10 cm [14]).

A key component to the repair is adequate mesh fixation, which can be difficult due to the bony boundaries of these hernias. Most authors utilize standard transfascial suture fixation [14, 16, 17], while some have reported using only laparoscopic tacking devices [1, 18]. Posteromedial fixation is to the paraspinous muscles posterior to the psoas and can be accomplished with intracorporeally tied sutures or with full thickness sutures placed through small skin incisions just lateral to the spine. Superiorly, the mesh can be fixed external to the costal margin as long as there is adequate overlap up onto the diaphragm. Inferiorly and anteriorly, the mesh can be held in place with tacks and then additional sutures passed transfascially as in standard ventral hernia repair.

For inferior defects extending to the iliac crest, the mesh is fixed to Cooper's ligament in addition to transfascial sutures just superior to the iliopubic tract [14]. The mesh must be cut so that there is enough overlap of the psoas and iliac crest. Perhaps a more reliable method of fixation is anchoring the mesh directly into the iliac crest itself. One technique is to drill through the iliac crest via one of the laparoscopic incisions and then pass a suture through the hole in the bone and anchor the mesh, akin to standard transfascial suture fixation [16]. Alternatively, titanium suture-armed bone anchors (e.g., Mitek GII QuickAnchor, DePuy Mitek Inc, Raynham, MA, USA) can be drilled directly into the iliac crest via one of the 5-mm trocar sites, and then the sutures passed through the mesh and tied intracorporeally [19]. These bone anchors are routinely used in orthopedic surgery and carry a very low incidence of infection or adverse bone reaction.

Laparoscopic Extraperitoneal Repair

Totally, extraperitoneal approaches have also been described [20, 21]. The patient is again placed in a lateral decubitus position. An incision is made in the midaxillary line halfway between the 12th rib and the iliac crest. A muscle-splitting dissection is carried down to the peritoneum. This plane is either then dissected with blunt finger dissection or a balloon dissector until enough space is created to permit additional trocar placement superiorly and inferiorly. The hernia contents are reduced, and the dissection is carried posteriorly beyond the psoas and erector spinae muscles. A prosthetic mesh can then be positioned and anchored as previously described. In this setting, polypropylene mesh without an adhesion barrier can be used because the mesh is isolated from the abdominal cavity.

Results

Since the first description of minimally invasive flank hernia repair by Burick in 1996 [1], numerous techniques have been described. However, virtually all of the reports in the literature are small non-comparative case series, making it difficult to adequately assess the effectiveness of any one technique. The largest series to date is a retrospective review of 27 patients over a 4-year period that underwent laparoscopic flank hernia repair [14]. This group repaired defects with an average operating time of 144 min with no conversions to open surgery. The mean length of hospital stay was 3.1 days with no postoperative complications. At a mean follow-up of 3.6 months, they found no recurrences. Two reoperations occurred, one for an unrelated midline hernia and one for removal of a previously placed flank mesh. Three patients had chronic pain at the repair site; two of these responded to treatment by pain management specialists, and the third responded after removal of mesh that had been previously placed by an outside surgeon.

The only comparative study of lumbar hernia repair deserves mention. In 2005, Moreno-Egea [22] conducted a prospective nonrandomized study of 16 patients who underwent repair of secondary lumbar hernias. Nine patients underwent laparoscopic repair with an adhesion barrier-coated polyester mesh, and seven patients underwent open repair with a preperitoneally placed polypropylene mesh based on the surgeon's discretion. The laparoscopic group had statistically significantly shorter operative times, shorter hospital stay, lower analgesic consumption, and quicker return to normal activity than the open group. While there were no recurrences in the laparoscopic group with 1–4 years follow-up, there were three recurrences in the open group during this time period. There was no statistical difference in cost between the procedures. Though there are obvious limitations to this study (nonrandomized, small sample size, possible selection bias, and short duration of follow-up), this is some evidence that the laparoscopic approach is an attractive option for patients with these rare hernias.

Conclusions

Lumbar hernias are rare defects that present technical challenges to the surgeon because of the bony boundaries of the defects. Laparoscopic repair is an attractive option that has been shown to be successful in numerous small case reports and series. Whether one takes a transabdominal or preperitoneal approach, it is imperative to achieve adequate mesh overlap. Fixation of the mesh to strong muscle posteriorly and to ligamentous or bony boundaries inferiorly is necessary to minimize chances of recurrence. Thorough knowledge of the relevant anatomy is also important to minimize inadvertent injury to surrounding structures and chronic pain.

References

1. Burick AJ, Parascandola SA. Laparoscopic repair of a traumatic lumbar hernia: a case report. J Laparoendosc Surg. 1996;6(4):259–62.
2. Moreno-Egea A, Baena EG, Calle MC, et al. Controversies in the current management of lumbar hernias. Arch Surg. 2007;142(1):82–8.
3. Stamatiou D, Skandalakis JE, Skandalakis LJ, et al. Lumbar hernia: surgical anatomy, embryology, and technique of repair. Am Surg. 2009;75(3):202–7.
4. Skandalakis JE, Skandalakis PN, Skandalakis LJ. Surgical anatomy and technique. 2nd ed. New York, NY: Springer-Verlag; 2000.
5. Wakhlu A, Wakhlu AK. Congenital lumbar hernia. Pediatr Surg Int. 2000;16(1–2):146–8.
6. Pul M, Pul N, Gürses N. Congenital lumbar (Grynfelt-Lesshaft) hernia. Eur J Pediatr Surg. 1991;1(2):115–7.
7. Akçora B, Temiz A, Babayi it C. A different type of congenital lumbar hernia associated with the lumbocostovertebral syndrome. J Pediatr Surg. 2008;43(1):e21–3.
8. Burt BM, Afifi HY, Wantz GE, et al. Traumatic lumbar hernia: report of cases and comprehensive review of the literature. J Trauma. 2004;57(6):1361–70.
9. Bayazit Y, Arido an IA, Tansu Z, et al. Morbidity of flank incision in 100 renal donors. Int Urol Nephrol. 2001;32(4):709–11.
10. Salameh JR, Salloum EJ. Lumbar incisional hernias: diagnostic and management dilemma. JSLS. 2004;8(4):391–4.
11. Stevens KJ, Banuls M. Iliolumbar hernia following bone grafting. Eur Spine J. 1994;3(2):118–9.
12. Mickel TJ, Barton FE, Rohrich RJ, et al. Management and prevention of lumbar herniation following a latissimus dorsi flap. Plast Reconstr Surg. 1999;103(5): 1473–5.
13. Baker ME, Weinerth JL, Andriani RT, et al. Lumbar hernia: diagnosis by CT. AJR Am J Roentgenol. 1987;148(3):565–7.

14. Edwards C, Geiger T, Bartow K, et al. Laparoscopic transperitoneal repair of flank hernias: a retrospective review of 27 patients. Surg Endosc. 2009;23(12):2692–6.
15. Sakarya A, Aydede H, Erhan MY, et al. Laparoscopic repair of acquired lumbar hernia. Surg Endosc. 2003;17(9):1494.
16. Arca MJ, Heniford BT, Pokorny R, et al. Laparoscopic repair of lumbar hernias. J Am Coll Surg. 1998;187(2):147–52.
17. Yavuz N, Ersoy YE, Demirkesen O, et al. Laparoscopic incisional lumbar hernia repair. Hernia. 2009;13(3):281–6.
18. Gagner M, Milone L, Gumbs A, et al. Laparoscopic repair of left lumbar hernia after laparoscopic left nephrectomy. JSLS. 2010;14(3):405–9.
19. Ho VP, Dakin GF. Video. Laparoscopic lumbar hernia repair with bone anchor fixation. Surg Endosc. 2011;25(5):1665.
20. Habib E. Retroperitoneoscopic tension-free repair of lumbar hernia. Hernia. 2003;7(3):150–2.
21. Meinke AK. Totally extraperitoneal laparoendoscopic repair of lumbar hernia. Surg Endosc. 2003;17(5):734–7.
22. Moreno-Egea A, Torralba-Martinez JA, Morales G, et al. Open vs laparoscopic repair of secondary lumbar hernias: a prospective nonrandomized study. Surg Endosc. 2005;19(2):184–7.

48. Challenging Hernia Locations: Suprapubic and Subxiphoid

John R. Romanelli and Jose E. Espinel

Incisional hernias develop in 11–20 % of patients undergoing laparotomy. Laparoscopic repair of these hernias is associated with less recurrence, shorter hospital stay, improved cosmesis in some patients, and most importantly, a reduced risk of wound infection. The terms suprapubic and parapubic are often used interchangeably. They refer to abdominal wall defects that are located just above the symphysis pubis. They often result from low midline and Pfannenstiel incisions used primarily for gynecologic, colorectal, and urological procedures.

Incisional hernias of the subxiphoid area may occur after an upper midline laparotomy incision, a median sternotomy, a mediastinal drainage tube incision, or a laparoscopic procedure. Incidence of incisional hernia after a sternotomy is 1.0–4.2 %. The majority of subxiphoidal hernias are asymptomatic due to the underlying liver, which prevents herniation of intestinal content. Because of the relative common mesh contraction of the prosthetic, 5-cm coverage of the defect in all directions is recommended. This is a difficult task when the abdominal wall defect is close to bone and cartilage structures like the rib cage and xiphoid process.

We consider all defects within 5 cm of the pubis to be suprapubic in nature and use the repair described here as a technique. Similarly, we consider all defects within 5 cm of the xiphoid process to be subxiphoid, and again use the described technique. This ensures that there is adequate mesh overlap to help reduce the chance of recurrence.

B.P. Jacob and B. Ramshaw (eds.), *The SAGES Manual of Hernia Repair*,
DOI 10.1007/978-1-4614-4824-2_48,

History

Supravesical hernias were first described by Sir Astley Cooper in 1804 [1]. This description originally detailed hernias de novo located within the supravesical fossa, or between the middle umbilical ligament and lateral umbilical ligament or the edge of the rectus sheath. Much more commonly, these defects are incisional hernias that are the result of either a midline laparotomy, with the hernia representing the inferior pole of the incision, or Pfannenstiel incisions. The earliest case report of a postoperative suprapubic hernia was in 1945 by Gerbode [2]. The term parapubic hernia first appeared in the literature in 1990, with a report by Bendavid from the Shouldice clinic in Toronto [3]. In this report, he specifically called attention to hernias created by Pfannenstiel incisions, or lower midline laparotomies that extended down to the pubis.

The earliest mention of a hernia in the epigastrium came from Arnauld de Villeneuve in 1285, and the term epigastric hernia came from Leveille in 1812. These defects were again considered to be de novo defects, located in the upper midline between the xiphoid process and umbilicus. The term subxiphoid hernia refers to hernia defects located immediately adjacent to the xiphoid process and are typically incisional hernias. These often occur after median sternotomy or as a consequence of an incision for a mediastinal drainage tube after median sternotomy. The first report in the literature utilizing the term "subxiphoid hernia" and detailing a mesh repair of the said defect came in 1985 by Cohen and Starling [4].

Anatomy

Suprapubic hernias are generally located in the midline, just cephalad to the pubis symphysis (Fig. 48.1). The lateral borders of the defect tend to be the rectus sheath on either side, and the most superior border tends to be the healed inferior end of the incision. Hernias along the pubis that are located lateral to the midline tend to be either supravesical or direct inguinal hernias. Other anatomic structures of consequence that must be kept in consideration during repair include but are not limited to the bladder, Cooper's ligament, and the pubic arcuate ligament.

Subxiphoid hernias are also generally located in the midline, just caudad to the tip of the xiphoid process (Fig. 48.2). While generally located in the midline, these can be just lateral to the midline,

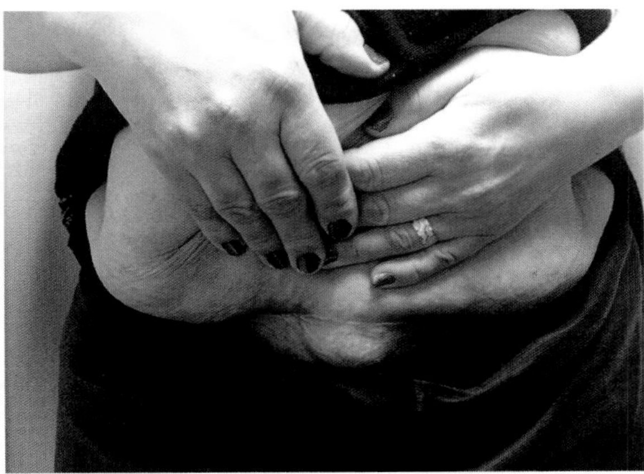

Fig. 48.1. Suprapubic hernia—external view (Courtesy of David B. Earle, M.D., F.A.C.S., with permission).

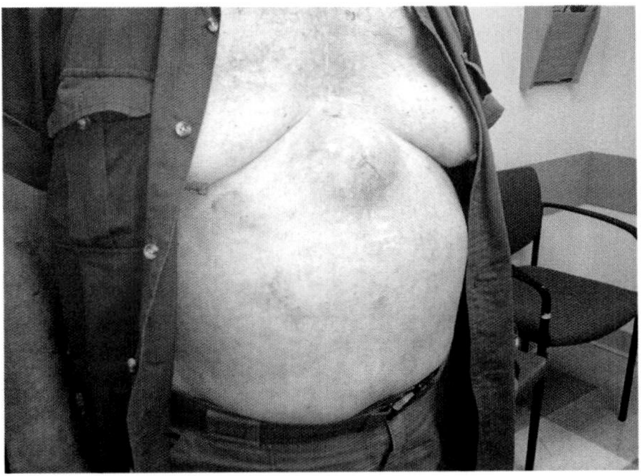

Fig. 48.2. Subxiphoid hernia—external view (Courtesy of David B. Earle, M.D., F.A.C.S., with permission).

especially if caused by an incision from a prior mediastinal drainage tube. These defects tend to be surrounded by intact rectus abdominis. Other anatomic structures of consequence that must be kept in consideration during repair include, but are not limited to, the 11th rib with the underlying intercostal nerve and artery, the inferior end of the pleural space, and the diaphragm.

Etiology

Most of suprapubic and subxiphoid hernias are acquired defects, typically the result of a prior surgical incision. Suprapubic hernias are most common after Pfannenstiel incisions but also occur after midline laparotomies performed for obstetric/gynecologic, colorectal, urologic, or other general surgical indications which require anterior access to the pelvic cavity. Subxiphoid hernias are rare de novo but also typically result from a prior surgical incision. Median sternotomies are the main culprit, in which the incision was carried down inferior to the xiphoid process. Incisions from mediastinal drainage tubes may also cause hernias. A more frequent recent occurrence has been a hernia resulting from a laparoscopic operation (such as that frequently made for a laparoscopic cholecystectomy), although these tend to be more inferiorly located, as the pneumoperitoneum tends to add distance from the xiphoid process. All of these defects share one property in common: close proximity to bony structures, which can hamper attempts at repair with sufficient mesh overlap.

Diagnosis

Both suprapubic and subxiphoid hernias present with typical symptoms of an incisional hernia: pain, a bulge at the location, and often the feeling of a loss of abdominal wall strength. The pain component may be a more common feature, due to the irritation of the adjacent periosteum from the hernia sac. While these defects, like all abdominal wall defects, may contain abdominal viscera; frequently, they *do not* due to the proximity of bony structures. In the case of suprapubic hernias, the bladder may be a component of the hernia or the structural defect itself. The falciform ligament may incarcerate into a subxiphoid defect, which can cause a painful bulge. Given the frequency with which abdominal complaints are diagnosed with the aid of imaging, CT scan of the abdomen may be performed to aid in the diagnosis; that said, history of prior incision and a physical examination consistent with a palpable defect, which protrudes upon increase of intra-abdominal pressure, may be sufficient to make the diagnosis. In the case of suprapubic hernias, physical examination may reveal a reducible mass over the groin area, often mistaken with an inguinal hernia. Closer examination demonstrates the defect adjacent to the pubic bone and not from the external inguinal ring.

Surgical Technique

Positioning and Preparation: Suprapubic

The patient undergoes general endotracheal intubation and is placed supine on the operating table. Both arms are tucked to the side of the patient when possible. A three-way Foley catheter is inserted to allow filling of the bladder intraoperatively and help identification of its borders during dissection.

Access, Port Placement, and Technique: Suprapubic

Access to the abdominal cavity is via a Veress needle, and an open technique (Hasson) or a closed technique is based on surgeon's experience. If a closed technique is chosen, an optical trocar is recommended. If the midline is to be avoided (e.g., due to the presence of a previous incision with anticipated adhesions), a left lateral subcostal incision off the tip of the 11th rib at the anterior axillary line is a safe place to insert the first trocar since the presence of preperitoneal fat and intra-abdominal adhesions in this location is rare. Two or three more trocars are placed under direct visualization. At least one of the trocars needs to be 12 mm in size to allow for the introduction of the prosthetic into the abdominal cavity.

The hernia contents are reduced, and adhesions are taken down sharply, when possible, with judicious use of ultrasonic dissection or electrocautery. The bladder is instilled with 250–400 cc of sterile water, often with the addition of blue dye, to aid in identification of an injury to the bladder during the dissection (Figs. 48.3 and 48.4). Then, a peritoneal flap is developed to be able to visualize the pubic bone, Cooper's ligament, inferior epigastric, and iliac vessels. This dissection resembles the one performed for a laparoscopic transabdominal (TAPP approach) inguinal hernia repair. The peritoneum is incised starting at the median umbilical fold using scissors (with or without cautery) in a horizontal pattern away from the midline. The length of the peritoneal flap should equal the size of the mesh that is going to be used. The hernia defect is measured intracorporeally by a variety of techniques, ranging from a thin plastic metric ruler to placing two spinal needles and using a piece of measured umbilical tape. The overlap of the hernia inferiorly is calculated to overlap 2 cm below the pubic bone. Once the hernia defect is measured, an appropriate-sized mesh should be selected

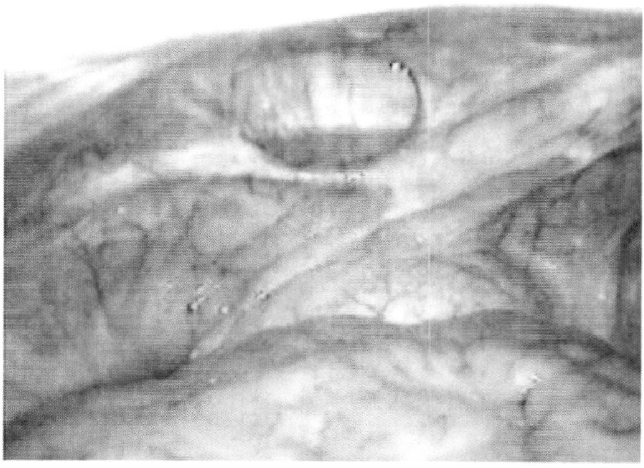

Fig. 48.3. Suprapubic hernia—internal view with bladder distention (Courtesy of David B. Earle, MD, FACS, with permission).

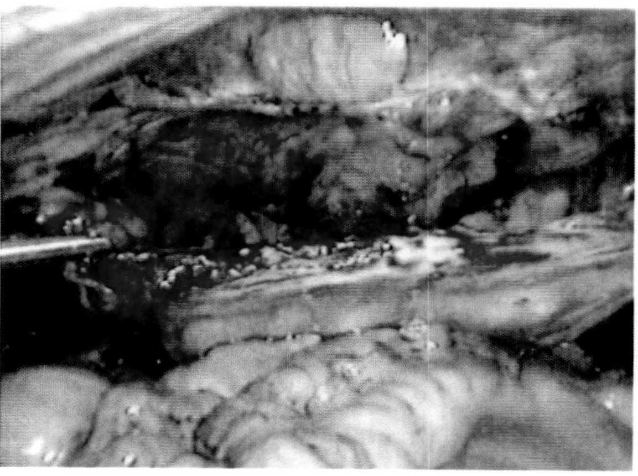

Fig. 48.4. Suprapubic hernia—internal view with bladder flap taken down (Courtesy of David B. Earle, MD, FACS, with permission).

that allows at least 4–5-cm overlap of the hernia defect in the cephalad and lateral dimensions. The choice of the prosthetic is up to the individual surgeon, and there is no clear data on the optimal prosthetic choice; polypropylene, polyester, PTFE, and biologic mesh have all been described for use in this indication.

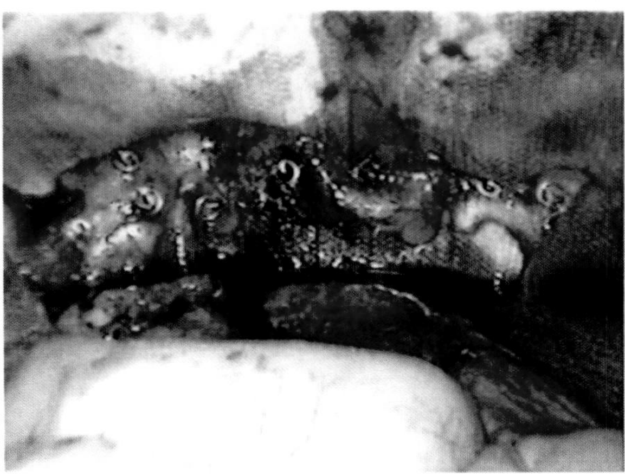

Fig. 48.5. Suprapubic hernia—internal view with mesh placed over Cooper's ligaments (indicated with asterisks) (Courtesy of David B. Earle, MD, FACS, with permission).

Pre-tied CV-0 PTFE sutures are placed in the midportion of the sides of the mesh to serve as initial transfascial fixation sutures. The mesh is placed intra-abdominally via the 12-mm trocar, and the sutures are retrieved with a suture passer on the preestablished skin sites. These sutures are pulled toward the abdominal wall, allowing the inferior portion of the mesh to be tacked to pubic bone and/or the pubic arcuate ligament medially and Cooper's ligament laterally (Fig. 48.5). All pre-tied sutures are retrieved from the abdominal cavity with the suture passer and tied extracorporeally via small stab incisions. Some authors advocate the use of additional transfascial sutures, which are placed every 5 cm circumferentially around the mesh. Careful attention must be given not to place these sutures below the iliopubic tract to avoid injury to the cutaneous nerves. Further fixation is achieved with helical tacks 1 cm apart, to prevent herniation of abdominal viscera above the mesh.

Positioning and Preparation: Subxiphoid

The patient undergoes general endotracheal intubation and is placed supine on the operating table. Both arms can be tucked to the side of the patient; however, when performing surgery below the umbilicus, the surgeons often need to stand above the umbilicus, thus necessitating the tucking of the arms. Similarly, for an operation such as a subxiphoid hernia repair, the surgeons need to stand below the umbilicus, and arm tucking is not necessary. No other special provisions are necessary to perform the repair.

Access, Port Placement, and Technique: Subxiphoid

After getting access to the abdominal cavity, adhesions are taken down from the anterior abdominal wall. Two other trocars are placed under direct visualization. The falciform ligament is dissected with an ultrasonic dissector or electrical diathermy. The subxiphoid hernia defect is measured intra-abdominally in a similar fashion to that described for the suprapubic hernia. The defect is measured in the longitudinal and transverse axis. Prosthetic material is chosen to the appropriate size required. It is important when deciding the mesh size to take into consideration any space between the edge of the defect and the xiphoid process itself. A 4–5-cm overlap of mesh in all directions should be taken into consideration when calculating the mesh size. Upon considering the superior overlap of the prosthetic, care must be taken not to reach the pericardium that lies directly behind and can be easily reached by a too extensive proximal dissection of the retroxiphoidal space. Further, allowing the mesh to lie freely over the liver generally comes without consequence and should be incorporated into the symmetry of the repair; in other words, given that the bony structures limit the size of the cephalad portion of the superior overlap, allowing the mesh to lie over the liver will account for this anatomically.

Pre-tied CV-0 PTFE sutures are placed on the mesh. The superior cardinal suture is placed toward the center of the mesh, which should be the first one to retrieve for easier manipulation of the mesh. Spiral tacks are placed over the costal margin, with care taken to avoid injury to the intercostal nerve and artery. When securing the mesh to the diaphragm, tacks are never used to avoid damage of the diaphragm, the pericardium, the pleural structures, or the heart. Intracorporeal stitches can be used to fix the mesh to the diaphragmatic peritoneal layer, if needed, or to the xiphoidal periosteum, allowing mesh overlap in a cephalad direction. A variety of tissue adhesives (glues) have also been used for this application. Additional transfascial sutures or tacks are placed, as described previously, up to the preference of the surgeon to allow for further fixation.

Results

Like most ventral hernias, the major concern is providing the patient with a durable repair that can minimize recurrence. Although data on these defects is admittedly scarce, recurrence rates in the studies referenced in this bibliography range from 5.5% to 10.0 % [5–7]. These rates are similar to many published series of laparoscopic ventral hernia repairs.

One recent study [5] details 33 hernias repairs relevant to this chapter: 18 suprapubic and 15 subxiphoidal. The mean operative time was 161.8 min. One patient suffered an enterotomy; this was repaired laparoscopically. There were seven minor complications in this series; recurrence was 7.7 % at a mean follow-up of 37 months.

Another study of 36 suprapubic repairs [6] performed with ePTFE prosthetics revealed similar results: a mean operative time of 178.7 min. Although the overall complication rate was higher (16.6 %), there were only two recurrences in this series, with a mean follow-up of 21 months. A change in the technique to mirror what is described in this chapter with tacking to Cooper's ligament and the pubis revealed no known recurrences in the last 27 cases, however.

Still another series [7] of ten subxiphoid poststernotomy hernia repairs produced similar data. Although the mean operative time was shorter (55 min), the minor complication rate (30 %) was higher, as was the recurrence rate (10 %). Given the small size of the series, however, it is difficult to understand the relevance of these data aside from the description of the technique utilized.

Complications beyond recurrence for these hernia repairs are also similar to other laparoscopic ventral hernia repairs, such as bleeding, enterotomy or injury to other viscera, infection, chronic pain, seroma, and conversion to open surgery. This chapter will not delve into individual discussion around these points. There are two unique complications, one for suprapubic hernias and one for subxiphoid hernias, which bear special mention.

Bladder injury during suprapubic hernia repair could be a potential complication. Distention of the bladder preoperatively, as described earlier, can aid in visualizing the bladder to avoid injury. The use of colored dye in the sterile water solution can also give a visual clue to an injury; this is especially helpful if the injury is too small to be found. When possible, the injury should be repaired laparoscopically with a two-layer technique using absorbable suture such as polyglycolic acid, with continuous drainage of the bladder with an indwelling catheter until a cystogram provides proof of healing (typically 7–10 days). If spillage was minimal, controlled, and there was no history of a urinary tract infection preoperatively, the procedure can be completed safely laparoscopically with concurrent prosthetic insertion, without additional risk of mesh infection.

In subxiphoid hernia repair, injury to the heart from the helical tacker could be a fatal complication, and it is incumbent on the surgeon to be aware of the cephalad limits of safety for utilizing the tacker. For this reason, we feel that the tacker should be used only as superiorly as the costal margin; the tacker can be used on the 11th rib, with attention placed on avoidance of injury to the intercostal artery and nerve. A recent report [8] details five cases, four of which were fatal, of cardiac injury from tacks during ventral hernia repair. Similarly, injury to the structures contained within the pleural space or pneumothorax can result if transfascial sutures or tacks are placed above the costal margin. Further complicating matters is that the distention of the abdominal cavity by pneumoperitoneum can make it less clear for surgeons where the cephalad border of the abdomen is located; we believe that the costal margin is an anatomic constant, and as such, should be used as the "safety" margin during subxiphoid hernia repairs.

Conclusion

The only laparoscopic approach for repair of suprapubic and subxiphoidal incisional hernias is very challenging for inexperienced surgeons. The anatomically complex location and the need to fixate the mesh to bone and ligaments provide unique anatomic challenges which may make the approach technically more difficult. Like most ventral hernia repairs, thorough knowledge of the anatomy will help the surgeon to avoid complications.

References

1. Cooper A. The anatomy and surgical treatment of inguinal and congenital hernia. London: Longman; 1804.
2. Gerbode F. Postoperative suprapubic hernia. Stanford Med Bull. 1945;3:190–3.
3. Bendavid R. Incisional parapubic hernias. Surgery. 1990;108(5):898–901.

4. Cohen MJ, Starling JR. Repair of subxiphoid incisional hernias with Marlex mesh after median sternotomy. Arch Surg. 1985;120(11):1270–1.
5. Ferrari G, Miranda A, Sansonna F, et al. Laparoscopic repair of incisional hernia located on the abdominal borders. A retrospective review. Surg Laparosc Endosc Percutan Tech. 2009;19(4):348–52.
6. Carbonell A, Kercher K, et al. The laparoscopic repair of suprapubic ventral hernias. Surg Endosc. 2005;19:174–7.
7. Landau O, Raziel A, Matz A, Kyzer S, Haruzi I. Laparoscopic repair of poststernotomy subxiphoid epigastric hernia. Surg Endosc. 2001;15:1313–4.
8. Frantzides C, Welle SN. Cardiac tamponade as a life-threatening injury during hernia repair. Surgery. 2012;152(1):133–5.

Suggested Reading

Conze J, Preschner A, Kisielinski K, Klinge U, Schumpelik V. Technical consideration for subxiphoidal incisional hernia repair. Hernia. 2005;9:84–7.

Hirasa T, Pickleman J, Shayani V. Laparoscopic repair of parapubic hernia. Arch Surg. 2001;136:1314–7.

Robin AP. “Epigastric Hernia”. In: Hernia, 4th ed. Philadelphia: Nyhus and Condon; 1995.

49. Hernias in the Pediatric Population

David M. Krpata and Todd A. Ponsky

Hernia repair, whether for inguinal or ventral hernias, offers different challenges in pediatrics than in the adult population. Of all hernia repairs performed by the pediatric surgeon, inguinal hernias are the most common. In addition to inguinal hernias, umbilical hernias and congenital abdominal wall defects comprise the great majority of hernias repaired in pediatrics. The pathophysiology, techniques, and controversies of these hernias will be discussed here.

Inguinal Hernias

Inguinal hernias in pediatrics are most commonly indirect inguinal hernias. The reported incidence of inguinal hernias in children is 0.8–4.4% [1], although the true incidence is difficult to establish and may be higher than this. Most commonly, these hernias are right sided with approximately 2/3 of unilateral inguinal hernias being right sided [2, 3]. Prematurity has been established as a significant risk factor of inguinal hernias, increasing the incidence up to 30% for premature infants [3].

The pathophysiology of the indirect inguinal hernia is based on the testicular descent and subsequent events that transpire, also explaining its dominance in young males. During embryologic development, the testes begin the process of dissention to the scrotum through hormonal signaling and shortening of the gubernaculum [4]. The processus vaginalis closes after the testis pass through, resulting in a completely intact peritoneum without communication into the internal ring (Fig. 49.1). Failure of this closure results in a patent processus vaginalis and puts patients at risk for developing an indirect

B.P. Jacob and B. Ramshaw (eds.), *The SAGES Manual of Hernia Repair*,
DOI 10.1007/978-1-4614-4824-2_49,

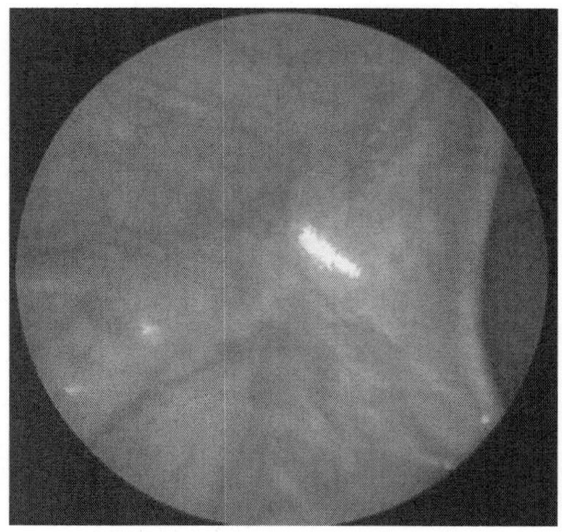

Fig. 49.1. Laparoscopic view of normal inguinal anatomy in a child.

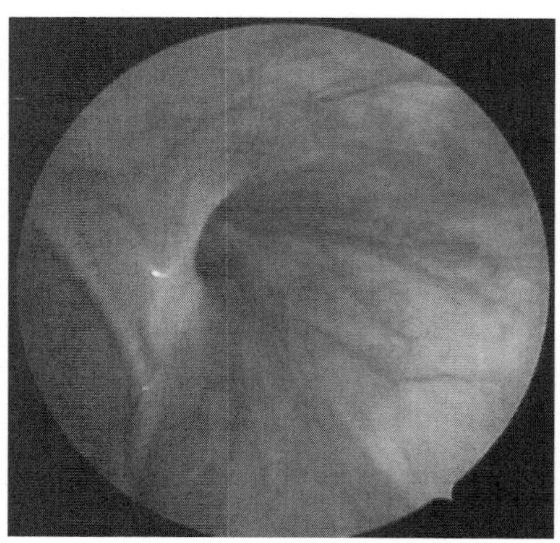

Fig. 49.2. Laparoscopic view of an indirect inguinal hernia in a child.

inguinal hernia (Fig. 49.2). This process is typically completed between 36 and 40 weeks gestational age, indicating why premature infants are at higher risk of developing an indirect inguinal hernia. Explaining the increased rate of right inguinal hernias is the fact that the left testis descends earlier than the right.

Diagnosis

The gold standard for diagnosis of inguinal hernias is a combination of physical examination, with presence of a groin bulge, coupled with a history reported by the parents of a bulging groin mass more prominent with activities causing increased intra-abdominal pressure, such as crying. These findings are certain to lead to surgical evaluation of the suspected groin and repair upon confirmation. The decision to operate can be more challenging when a parent gives a history of bulging in the groin, but the examiner cannot confirm the diagnosis on physical exam. To aid in confirming a diagnosis, the surgeon can suggest to the parents or guardian to photograph any bulging they notice and bring it in during subsequent visits.

The use of ultrasound offers an adjunct in the diagnosis of inguinal hernias. Initially studied for its role in evaluation of contralateral groin exploration, several studies have established ultrasonography as a highly accurate, inexpensive, and readily available technique for the diagnosis of patent processus vaginalis and indirect inguinal hernias [5–9].

Management

Undoubtedly, after diagnosis of an inguinal hernia in an infant or child, acute surgical therapy is necessary, although, unless incarcerated, it is not a surgical emergency. The timing of hernia repair in premies is challenging as the risks of anesthesia must be weighed against the risk of incarceration and possible strangulation. The incidence of incarceration has been described to be as high as 35% for infants under 12 months with a known hernia awaiting surgery [10]. Misra et al. reported an incidence of incarceration of 6% by limiting the wait for surgery to less than seven days [11]. In neonates, some advocate for repair of premature infants once they are ready for discharge from the neonatal unit. With such management, regular examination and hernia reduction should be performed to detect incarceration while in the NICU [12]. Others have shown a low risk (0%) of incarceration after discharge from the NICU followed by elective repair leaving the controversy of timing of inguinal hernia repair in premature infants still unclear [13]. Ultimately, the risks and benefits of repair must be weighed against the risks of anesthesia and potential respiratory complications in premies.

Surgical Techniques

Open Inguinal Hernia Repair

Open inguinal hernia repair in infants and children follows the same principles in anatomy and dissection as open inguinal hernia repair in adults. A 2- to 3-cm incision is made over the external ring. Dissection is carried down through Scarpa's fascia to the external oblique aponeurosis. Once encountered, the external oblique aponeurosis is completely exposed, and the external inguinal ring is identified. The external oblique aponeurosis is incised sharply. The incision is extended along the fibers of the external oblique aponeurosis to the external inguinal ring, to expose the inguinal canal.

In males, the spermatic cord and its structures including the testicular artery, the pampiniform venous plexus, the genital branch of the genitofemoral nerve, the vas deferens, the cremasteric muscle fibers, the cremasteric vessels, and the lymphatics are identified, mobilized, and isolated. The indirect inguinal hernia sac is identified and carefully dissected free from the spermatic cord down to the internal ring. After freeing the hernia sac, it is then divided between two hemostats, twisted 360 degrees and suture ligated with absorbable suture. The floor, transversalis fascia, of the inguinal canal should be inspected for direct hernias or any weakening. If either is found, a primary tissue repair should be performed to strengthen the floor of the inguinal canal. The external oblique aponeurosis is reapproximated followed by reapproximation of Scarpa's fascia. The skin is closed with subcuticular sutures.

Laparoscopic Inguinal Hernia Repair

With the advent of minimally invasive surgery, new approaches to old techniques have emerged. Several options for laparoscopic inguinal hernia repair exist, but the principle of high ligation of the hernia sac as in open repair persists.

The earliest experiences with a laparoscopic approach to inguinal hernia repair in children involve intracorporeal suturing of the peritoneal lining around the patent processus vaginalis, in a purse-string or Z-stitch fashion, resulting in hernia sac ligation [14–16]. The SEAL, subcutaneous endoscopically assisted ligation, technique employees a single umbilical port to visualize the extraperitoneal passing of a suture around the internal ring [17]. Our preferred method of laparoscopic involves hydrodissection around the internal ring with bupivacaine or saline

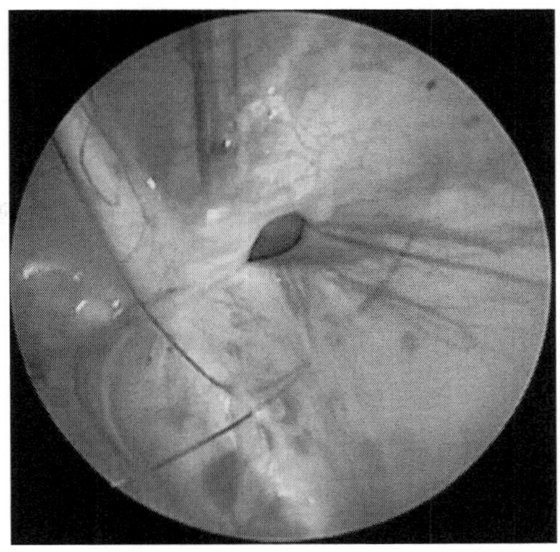

Fig. 49.3. The loop of polypropylene suture around the lateral portion of the internal ring after the needle is removed.

to elevate the peritoneum off of the cord structures. Following hydrodissection, an eighteen-gauge spinal needle is inserted into the preperitoneal space at the 12 O'clock position of the internal ring. The needle is then passed 180 degrees around the internal ring as it passes between the peritoneum and the cord structures. The needle then perforates through the peritoneum into the peritoneal space. At this point, a looped 3-0 polypropylene suture is passed through the needle (Fig. 49.3). This process is repeated along the medial side of the internal ring resulting in two loops of polypropylene within the peritoneal cavity. One loop is then used to snare the opposing polypropylene and is pulled through the incision (Fig. 49.4). We then interlock the loop of polypropylene with a looped nonabsorbable braided polyester suture and exchange one around the internal ring for the other by pulling the polypropylene back through the incision. The looped end of the suture is cut and tied. This results in double ligation of the hernia sac with the nonabsorbable braided polyester suture (Fig. 49.5).

Proponents of the laparoscopic hernia repair in infants and children site a potentially less pain and potentially less visible scar, but most importantly, potential reduced risk of trauma to cord structures, thus theoretically reducing the risk of infertility and testicular atrophy as well. While there is no evidence to support this, infertility following open inguinal hernia repair was reported to be as high as 40% in men who have had childhood bilateral inguinal herniorrhaphy [18].

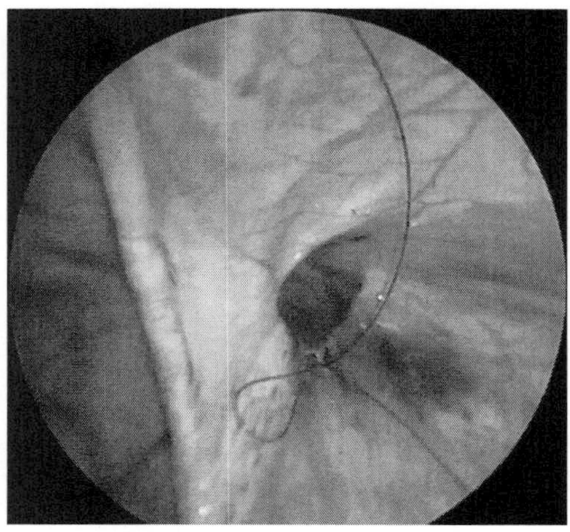

Fig. 49.4. Laparoscopic visualization of lateral polypropylene suture snaring the medial loop of polypropylene.

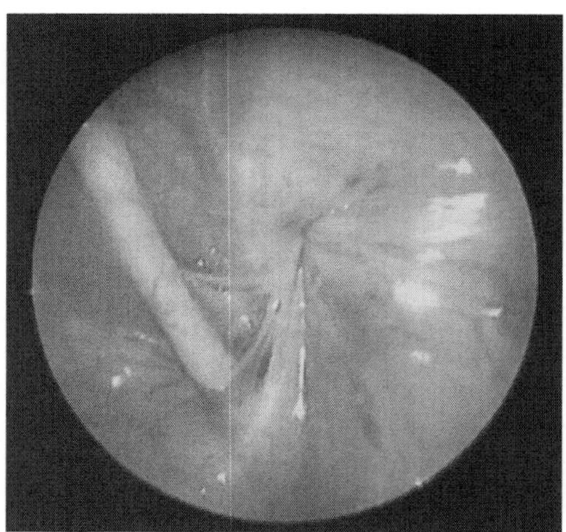

Fig. 49.5. A closed indirect inguinal hernia following laparoscopic repair.

The laparoscopic approach is also a nice option in recurrent hernias and incarcerated hernias. For recurrent hernias, the lap approach allows ligation of the hernia sac without entering into a reoperative field. For incarcerated hernias, the lap approach is helpful in assisting with reducing the bowel, assessing the viability of the incarcerated bowel, and allows for easy ligation of the sac despite an inflamed inguinal canal. An additional advantage to the laparoscopic repair is the direct visualization of the contralateral side.

Contralateral Groin Exploration

The issue of contralateral groin exploration has been a heavily debated topic over the years. There are two parts to the question of contralateral groin exploration in a child with a unilateral hernia; first, should you look for contralateral defects, and second, if you find one, should it be fixed? For years, prophylactic contralateral groin exploration was common practice during repair of a unilateral inguinal hernia. This practice fell out of favor in the 1990s due to concerns of unnecessary damage to the testicular artery and vas deferens causing testicular atrophy and infertility during groin explorations, as well as the additional risk of wound infection. A major advancement in contralateral groin exploration was the technique of transinguinal laparoscopic examination of the contralateral groin. This technique allows for direct visualization of the contralateral internal ring without having to make additional incisions and possibly reducing the risk of injury to the vas deferens and associated infertility seen with open exploration [19]. In the instance that a contralateral patent processus vaginalis or indirect hernia is found, that groin can then be repaired through an additional incision on the contralateral side. One of the advantages to performing laparoscopic inguinal hernia repair is that both groins are directly visualized through the umbilical port, and if a contralateral hernia is found, it too can be repaired with the same laparoscopic approach that was used for the original hernia.

Once a contralateral patent processus vaginalis is found, the second question arises; should it be repaired. Rowe et al. reported that 40% of patent processus vaginalis will close in the first few months and 60% will close by 2 years of age [20]. In a meta-analysis reviewing the risk of metachronous hernia in infants and children, Miltenburg et al. reviewed over 15,310 patients [21]. This group found that 7% of patients who presented for a unilateral inguinal hernia developed a contralateral hernia with 90% of these developing in the first 5 years following surgery. From these findings, they concluded that if a patent processus vaginalis is found, it should be repaired, and patients who do not undergo contralateral exploration should be followed up for 5 years.

Outcomes

The ultimate long-term outcome measure for inguinal hernia repair is recurrence. For open inguinal hernia repair in children, Ein et al., in the largest series of inguinal hernia repairs, reported a 1.2% recurrence rate in 6361 patients over a 35-year experience [3]. For laparoscopic repair, Montupet et al. recently reported a recurrence rate of 1.5% over a 15-year experience utilizing laparoscopic intracorporeal suture ligation of the hernia sac with a purse-string technique [22].

Adolescent Inguinal Hernia

The adolescent inguinal hernia is a challenging dilemma for pediatric and adult general surgeons alike. Whether mesh should be used in this population and at what age mesh is acceptable is debatable. From the perspective of a pediatric surgeon, adolescent inguinal hernias are often indirect and are believed to be a patent processus vaginalis instead of a muscle or floor defect as seen with most adult direct inguinal hernias and for this reason are typically treated with high ligation of the sac and not a mesh repair.

Umbilical Hernias

Congenital umbilical hernias are a common occurrence in infants and children. Their natural progression is such that most will close within this first 5 years of life, although one study has also reported the closure of congenital umbilical hernias until 14 years of age [23]. The incidence of umbilical hernias is higher in African American infants [23, 24]. The risk of incarceration with umbilical hernias is low, although there are several case reports in the literature describing this complication [25–29]. Spontaneous rupture of congenital umbilical hernias and evisceration has been described in the literature as well [30, 31].

Most surgeons will wait until 3–5 years of age before repairing an umbilical hernia. Indications for early repair of congenital umbilical hernias include pain, incarceration, and strangulation. Umbilical hernias are usually repaired through an infraumbilical incision through which the umbilical stalk is encircled. Once isolated, the umbilical stalk is incised leaving a hernia defect which is closed primarily with interrupted sutures. This practice of umbilical herniorrhaphy has been a relatively unchanged procedure throughout the years with few iterations except for in case of large umbilical defects requiring umbilicoplasty as well [32]. Minimally invasive closure of pediatric umbilical hernias using injectable dextranomer microspheres and hyaluronic acid has also been described, but long-term follow-up is still needed [33].

Congenital Abdominal Wall Defects

Gastroschisis and omphalocele, or exomphalos, are two congenital abdominal wall defects less frequently encountered than inguinal and umbilical hernias but are certainly of equal importance to the pediatric surgeon. Their presence provides many challenges to obstetricians, pediatricians, and pediatric surgeons alike. The incidence of gastroschisis is approximately 3 per 10,000 births and by some estimates is increasing [34]. Omphalocele has an incidence of about 2 per 10,000 births [35, 36]. The etiology and risk factors for their development are somewhat unclear, but gastroschisis is believed to be related more to environmental factors and less from genetic factors, whereas omphalocele is believed to be more genetic and less from environmental factors [37]. Classically, gastroschisis has been described as resulting from an ischemic insult during development that leads to impaired development of the abdominal wall [38].

Anatomically, there are several features that can be used to differentiate between gastroschisis and omphalocele. First, gastroschisis is always found off the midline from the umbilicus, most commonly to the right of midline. Additionally, there is evisceration of abdominal viscera without a protective sac to contain them. To the contrary, an omphalocele is a midline defect with herniated abdominal contents that are contained within a membranous sac consisting of peritoneum, Wharton's jelly, and amnion [39].

From a surgical standpoint, the management of these two abnormalities can be very difficult. Immediately after birth, neonates are evaluated and stabilized. Nasogastric tube decompression should be used for both abdominal wall defects. If a gastroschisis is present, the abdominal contents should be covered to reduce fluid losses from exposed bowel and broad-spectrum systemic antibiotics given. Once in the operating room, if possible, a gastroschisis should be primarily closed after inspecting for any associated bowel atresias. Some techniques to help reduce the abdominal contents included muscle relaxation, gastric

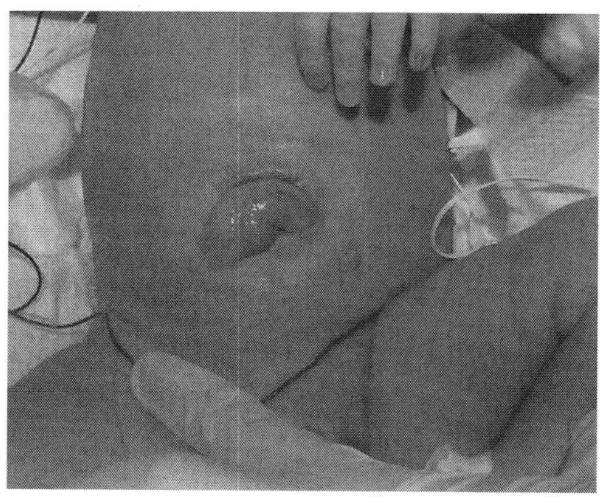

Fig. 49.6. Non-invasive closure of a gastroschisis.

decompression, and enlarging the defect before closing it. If reduction and primary closure are not possible, silo placement with serial reduction can be employed. This involves fixation of a silo to the fascia surrounding the defect followed by daily reduction of the silo contents back into the abdominal cavity allowing the abdominal wall to stretch over time and eventually lead to complete reduction. After complete reduction, closure of the defect in the operating room can be performed. An alternative technique for closure of a gastroschisis is a sutureless repair utilizing the umbilical cord as a natural patch to cover the defect [40, 41]. Utilizing general anesthesia or sedation, the bowel is decompressed and reduced. The umbilical cord is placed over the defect, typically in a coil fashion, and a 2×2 Tegaderm dressing (3M Health Care, MN) is fashioned over top to reinforce the closure (Fig. 49.6). This method offers a simple, safe, and cosmetically appealing option.

In the case of omphalocele, as long as the peritoneal covering is intact and the abdominal contents are not exposed to the environment, neonates can be managed nonemergently and evaluated for additional congenital defects. Such defects often associated with omphalocele include Beckwith-Wiedemann syndrome, Cantrell pentalogy, bladder or cloacal exstrophy, and chromosomal trisomies. After stabilization and preoperative assessment is complete, smaller omphaloceles are typically closed in the first few days of life. This typically involves excision of the sac, ligation of the umbilical vessels, and primary closure of the defect. In the case of giant omphaloceles in which the abdominal domain is not suitable for complete visceral reduction, several techniques can be employed. As with gastroschisis, silo reduction over days can be used. If the abdominal contents are not fixed to the omphalocele sac, the sac itself can be used as a silo, and sequential sac ligation can be performed. With this technique, as the viscera reduce, the sac is twisted and ligated daily with umbilical ties until fascial closure can be performed. An alternative, nonoperative approach involves treating the omphalocele sac with topical silver sulfadiazine, allowing epithelialization, and closing the defect weeks or months later [39, 42].

Following repair of a gastroschisis or omphalocele, close monitoring in the NICU should be utilized. It is important to monitor intra-abdominal pressure as abdominal compartment syndrome is a potential complication of being overly aggressive with reduction. Intra-abdominal pressures should remain below 20 mmHg. The inhospital mortality of neonates with gastroschisis is <5% [43], while outcomes for neonates with omphalocele tend to depend more on the associated chromosomal and structural abnormalities.

Summary

Pediatric inguinal hernia repair is a common procedure performed by pediatric surgeons. These hernias tend to be right sided and should be repaired soon after they are identified. Controversies, old and new, exist in their repair, including contralateral exploration and a newer debate over open versus laparoscopic repair. Umbilical hernias are very common but typically close on their own within the first 5 years of age. In congenital abdominal wall defects, the initial goal is stabilization and protection of the abdominal viscera. Once this goal is met, defects can be repaired primarily if the viscera are reducible and the fascia can be reapproximated. If the contents are not reducible, staged closure with progressive reduction of the viscera can be performed.

References

1. Bronsther B, Abrams MW, Elboim C. Inguinal hernias in children—A study of 1,000 cases and a review of the literature. J Am Med Womens Assoc. 1972;27:522–5. passim.
2. Manoharan S, Samarakkody U, Kulkarni M, Blakelock R, Brown S. Evidence-based change of practice in the management of unilateral inguinal hernia. J Pediatr Surg. 2005;40:1163–6.

3. Ein SH, Njere I, Ein A. Six thousand three hundred sixty-one pediatric inguinal hernias: a 35-year review. J Pediatr Surg. 2006;41:980–6.
4. Kubota Y, Temelcos C, Bathgate RA, et al. The role of insulin 3, testosterone, Mullerian inhibiting substance and relaxin in rat gubernacular growth. Mol Hum Reprod. 2002;8:900–5.
5. Chou TY, Chu CC, Diau GY, Wu CJ, Gueng MK. Inguinal hernia in children: US versus exploratory surgery and intraoperative contralateral laparoscopy. Radiology. 1996;201:385–8.
6. Toki A, Watanabe Y, Sasaki K, et al. Ultrasonographic diagnosis for potential contralateral inguinal hernia in children. J Pediatr Surg. 2003;38:224–6.
7. Erez I, Rathause V, Vacian I, et al. Preoperative ultrasound and intraoperative findings of inguinal hernias in children: a prospective study of 642 children. J Pediatr Surg. 2002;37:865–8.
8. Chen KC, Chu CC, Chou TY, Wu CJ. Ultrasonography for inguinal hernias in boys. J Pediatr Surg. 1998;33:1784–7.
9. Hata S, Takahashi Y, Nakamura T, Suzuki R, Kitada M, Shimano T. Preoperative sonographic evaluation is a useful method of detecting contralateral patent processus vaginalis in pediatric patients with unilateral inguinal hernia. J Pediatr Surg. 2004; 39:1396–9.
10. Stylianos S, Jacir NN, Harris BH. Incarceration of inguinal hernia in infants prior to elective repair. J Pediatr Surg. 1993;28:582–3.
11. Misra D, Hewitt G, Potts SR, Brown S, Boston VE. Inguinal herniotomy in young infants, with emphasis on premature neonates. J Pediatr Surg. 1994;29:1496–8.
12. Misra D. Inguinal hernias in premature babies: wait or operate? Acta Paediatr. 2001;90:370–1.
13. Lee SL, Gleason JM, Sydorak RM. A critical review of premature infants with inguinal hernias: optimal timing of repair, incarceration risk, and postoperative apnea. J Pediatr Surg. 2011;46:217–20.
14. Montupet P, Esposito C. Laparoscopic treatment of congenital inguinal hernia in children. J Pediatr Surg. 1999;34:420–3.
15. Shcheben'kov MV. The advantages of laparoscopic inguinal herniorrhaphy in children. Vestn Khir Im I I Grek. 1997;156:94–6.
16. Schier F. Laparoscopic herniorrhaphy in girls. J Pediatr Surg. 1998;33:1495–7.
17. Harrison MR, Lee H, Albanese CT, Farmer DL. Subcutaneous endoscopically assisted ligation (SEAL) of the internal ring for repair of inguinal hernias in children: a novel technique. J Pediatr Surg. 2005;40:1177–80.
18. Matsuda T, Muguruma K, Hiura Y, Okuno H, Shichiri Y, Yoshida O. Seminal tract obstruction caused by childhood inguinal herniorrhaphy: results of microsurgical reanastomosis. J Urol. 1998;159:837–40.
19. Miltenburg DM, Nuchtern JG, Jaksic T, Kozinetiz C, Brandt ML. Laparoscopic evaluation of the pediatric inguinal hernia–a meta-analysis. J Pediatr Surg. 1998; 33:874–9.
20. Rowe MI, Copelson LW, Clatworthy HW. The patent processus vaginalis and the inguinal hernia. J Pediatr Surg. 1969;4:102–7.

21. Miltenburg DM, Nuchtern JG, Jaksic T, Kozinetz CA, Brandt ML. Meta-analysis of the risk of metachronous hernia in infants and children. Am J Surg. 1997;174:741–4.
22. Montupet P, Esposito C. Fifteen years experience in laparoscopic inguinal hernia repair in pediatric patients. Results and considerations on a debated procedure. Surg Endosc. 2011;25:450–3.
23. Meier DE, OlaOlorun DA, Omodele RA, Nkor SK, Tarpley JL. Incidence of umbilical hernia in African children: redefinition of "normal" and reevaluation of indications for repair. World J Surg. 2001;25:645–8.
24. Hall DE, Roberts KB, Charney E. Umbilical hernia: what happens after age 5 years? J Pediatr. 1981;98:415–7.
25. Ameh EA, Chirdan LB, Nmadu PT, Yusufu LM. Complicated umbilical hernias in children. Pediatr Surg Int. 2003;19:280–2.
26. Brown RA, Numanoglu A, Rode H. Complicated umbilical hernia in childhood. S Afr J Surg. 2006;44:136–7.
27. Chatterjee H, Bhat SM. Incarcerated umbilical hernia in children. J Indian Med Assoc. 1986;84:238–9.
28. Hurlbut HJ, Moseley T. Incarcerated and strangulated umbilical hernia in infants and children. J Fla Med Assoc. 1966;53:504–6.
29. Chirdan LB, Uba AF, Kidmas AT. Incarcerated umbilical hernia in children. Eur J Pediatr Surg. 2006;16:45–8.
30. Weik J, Moores D. An unusual case of umbilical hernia rupture with evisceration. J Pediatr Surg. 2005;40:E33–5.
31. Durakbasa CU. Spontaneous rupture of an infantile umbilical hernia with intestinal evisceration. Pediatr Surg Int. 2006;22:567–9.
32. Ikeda H, Yamamoto H, Fujino J, et al. Umbilicoplasty for large protruding umbilicus accompanying umbilical hernia: a simple and effective technique. Pediatr Surg Int. 2004;20:105–7.
33. Feins NR, Dzakovic A, Papadakis K. Minimally invasive closure of pediatric umbilical hernias. J Pediatr Surg. 2008;43:127–30.
34. Alvarez SM, Burd RS. Increasing prevalence of gastroschisis repairs in the United States: 1996–2003. J Pediatr Surg. 2007;42:943–6.
35. Calzolari E, Bianchi F, Dolk H, Milan M. Omphalocele and gastroschisis in Europe: a survey of 3 million births 1980–1990. EUROCAT Working Group. Am J Med Genet. 1995;58:187–94.
36. Tan KH, Kilby MD, Whittle MJ, Beattie BR, Booth IW, Botting BJ. Congenital anterior abdominal wall defects in England and Wales 1987–93: retrospective analysis of OPCS data. BMJ. 1996;313:903–6.
37. Frolov P, Alali J, Klein MD. Clinical risk factors for gastroschisis and omphalocele in humans: a review of the literature. Pediatr Surg Int. 2010;26:1135–48.
38. Hoyme HE, Higginbottom MC, Jones KL. The vascular pathogenesis of gastroschisis: intrauterine interruption of the omphalomesenteric artery. J Pediatr. 1981;98:228–31.
39. Ledbetter DJ. Gastroschisis and omphalocele. Surg Clin North Am. 2006;86:249–60. vii.
40. Bianchi A, Dickson AP. Elective delayed reduction and no anesthesia: 'minimal intervention management' for gastroschisis. J Pediatr Surg. 1998;33:1338–40.

41. Sandler A, Lawrence J, Meehan J, Phearman L, Soper R. A "plastic" sutureless abdominal wall closure in gastroschisis. J Pediatr Surg. 2004;39:738–41.
42. Nuchtern JG, Baxter R, Hatch Jr EI. Nonoperative initial management versus silon chimney for treatment of giant omphalocele. J Pediatr Surg. 1995;30:771–6.
43. Lao OB, Larison C, Garrison MM, Waldhausen JH, Goldin AB. Outcomes in neonates with gastroschisis in U.S. children's hospitals. Am J Perinatol. 2010;27:97–101.

50. Spigelian Hernias: Diagnosis and Treatment

Marc Miserez and Marc H.F. Schreinemacher

A spigelian hernia is the protrusion of preperitoneal fat or a peritoneal sac, either containing an intraperitoneal organ or not, through a defect in the spigelian aponeurosis [1].

Anatomy and Pathophysiology

The spigelian aponeurosis is the aponeurosis of the transverse abdominal muscle limited laterally by the semilunar line and medially by the lateral edge of the rectus muscle [2] (Fig. 50.1). The semilunar line is the transition from the muscular to the aponeurotic part of the transverse abdominal muscle, extending from the ninth rib to the pubis. The line was first described in the seventeenth century by Adriaan van den Spieghel, a Flemish anatomist working at the University of Padua [3], and is also called the linea Spigeli. The first description of a hernia through the spigelian aponeurosis followed in 1764 by Joseph Klinkosch, another Flemish anatomist [4].

Ninety percent of all spigelian hernias occur in the transverse zone between the interspinal plane and the level of the umbilicus, the "spigelian belt" [1]. In this zone, the aponeurosis is at its widest, and the fibers of the transverse and internal oblique muscles run parallel, making them prone to separation [5, 6]. In addition, the intersection of the semilunar and arcuate line is especially weak, possibly related to a more muscular instead of aponeurotic part of the internal oblique muscle at that level [6]. Above the level of the umbilicus, the fibers of the transverse and internal oblique muscles cross at right angles, and even more cranial, the

B.P. Jacob and B. Ramshaw (eds.), *The SAGES Manual of Hernia Repair*, DOI 10.1007/978-1-4614-4824-2_50,

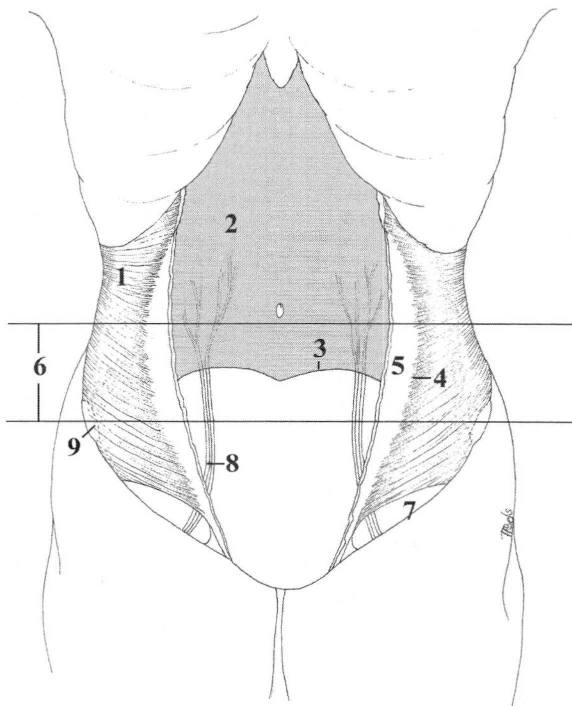

Fig. 50.1. Anatomy of the ventral abdominal wall. Schematic view of the ventral abdominal wall with the rectus muscle and external and internal oblique muscles removed. (1) transverse muscle, (2) posterior rectus sheath, (3) arcuate line (=semicircular line of Douglas), (4) semilunar line (=linea Spigeli), (5) spigelian aponeurosis, (6) spigelian belt, (7) medial of the epigastric vessels, (8) inferior epigastric vessels, (9) anterior superior iliac spine.

musculoaponeurotic transition lies behind the rectus muscles resulting in the absence of a spigelian aponeurosis [2].

A spigelian hernia most often penetrates the aponeuroses of the transverse and internal oblique muscles, while the aponeurosis of the external oblique muscle is generally thicker and stronger and therefore more resistant to herniation (Fig. 50.2). As a result, the hernia sac often expands in the space between the two oblique muscles thereby concealing the hernia and hindering correct diagnosis. The aponeurotic defect itself is often small (<2 cm in diameter) and has well-defined margins [2, 7]. The natural course is thought to be in line with other ventral abdominal

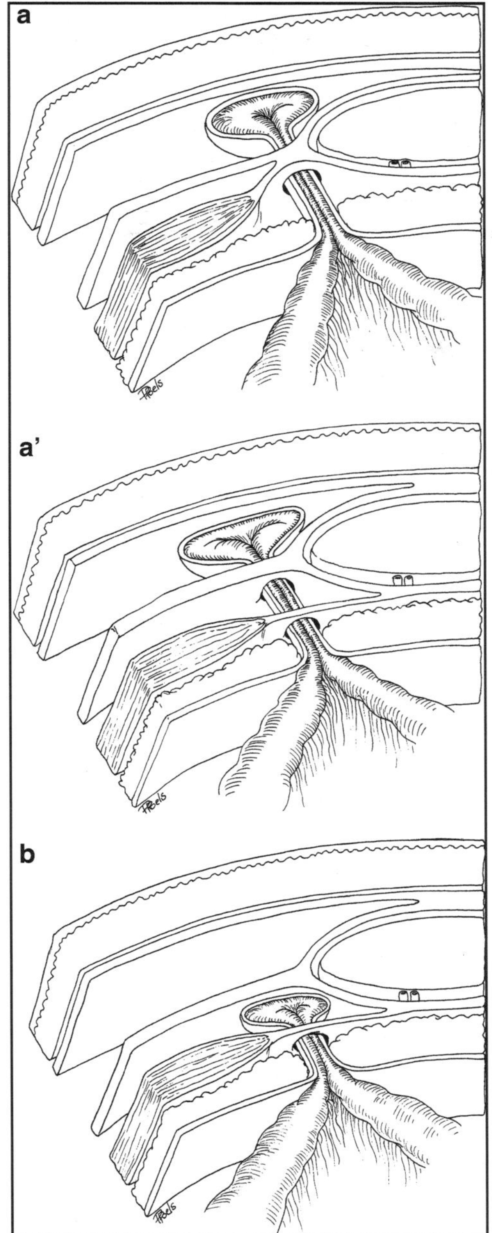

Fig. 50.2. A schematic transverse section of different spigelian hernias. Cranial to the arcuate line, the hernia most often penetrates the spigelian aponeurosis in conjunction with the internal oblique aponeurosis (**a** and **a**').

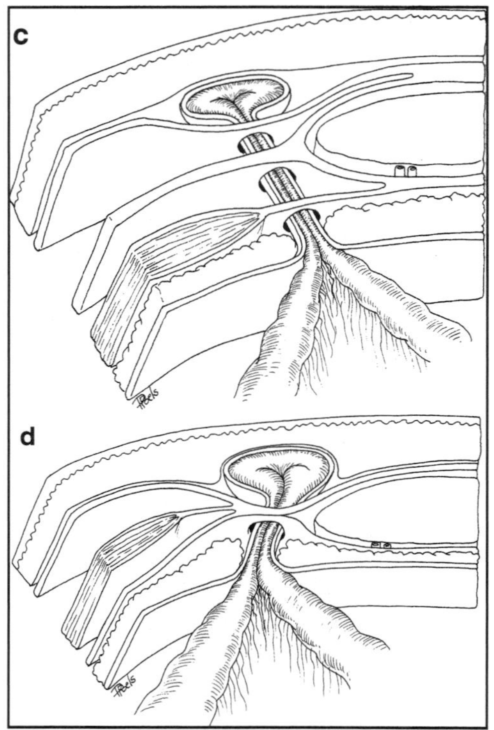

Fig. 50.2 Other possibilities are that the hernia only penetrates the spigelian aponeurosis (**b**), or even the external oblique aponeurosis (**c**). In addition, the occurrence of a spigelian hernia caudally from the arcuate line is shown (**d**). Seldom variants are the intravaginal hernia (**e**) and a spigelian hernia consisting only of preperitoneal fat (**f**).

hernias meaning that defects are expected to enlarge over time. Finally, the so-called low spigelian hernias can be found medial to the inferior epigastric vessels within Hesselbach's triangle. Because of this location, these hernias will be approached clinically as a direct inguinal hernia and treated accordingly [8].

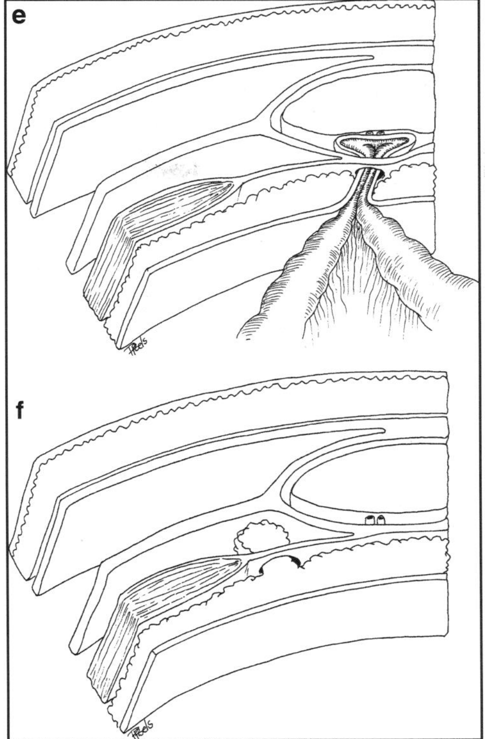

Fig. 50.2. (continued).

Etiology

Most spigelian hernias are considered to be acquired, although a congenital form is encountered in young children. In these children, an increased risk for cryptorchidism is observed leading to the suspicion of a congenital syndrome [9]. Based on a musculoaponeurotic defect etiology in acquired hernias, general risk factors for ventral abdominal hernias are considered to be of relevance for spigelian hernias as well.

Epidemiology

Spigelian hernias are relatively rare with a reported prevalence of 0.12–2% among all hernias [10–12]. Among all incarcerated hernias, about 1.5% are spigelian hernias [13]. Incarceration can be as high as 24%, and emergency procedures are performed in around 10% of patients presenting with a spigelian hernia [1, 14, 15]. The reason for this relatively high rate of incarceration might be related to the usual anatomy of the defect which is small and with well-defined margins. Most patients described in the literature are between 60 and 80 years old (excluding the congenital form), predominantly female (1.4:1 ratio), and exhibit hernias more often on the right side (1.2:1 ratio).

Diagnosis

Signs and Symptoms

Diagnosing a spigelian hernia may be straight forward in case of a painful, reducible mass at the lateral edge of the rectus muscles, justifying an operative repair. However, the diagnosis is generally challenging because of the low incidence, vague symptoms, and the often very subtle or even absent clinical signs. First of all, the most common symptom in case of a spigelian hernia is abdominal pain which can vary in type and severity, often related to the content of the hernia. The pain is often aggravated by maneuvers that increase abdominal pressure and relieved by rest [11].

Physical examination may show a palpable mass in the abdominal wall, but only about 60% of patients present with this finding [14, 15]. This is because of the common position of the hernia sac between the external and internal oblique muscles due to which the intact external oblique muscle conceals the hernia. Larson and Farley report in nonincarcerated hernias complaints of pain in 20%, intermittent mass in 35%, pain combined with intermittent mass in 27%, and 4% asymptomatic [14]. In case of incarceration, signs and symptoms are regarded to be more evident.

History taking and physical examination together confirm the diagnosis in 29–73% of patients [15]. The above mentioned aspects together with the relatively high incarceration rate justify a high suspicion for spigelian hernia in patients presenting with (vague or unusual) symptoms in the spigelian belt, in order not to delay diagnosis. Since pain can be musculotendinous or due to intraabdominal causes (e.g., diverticulitis and appendicitis), testing the abdominal wall with Valsalva maneuver provides more information [16, 17]. In addition, the finding of a palpable mass within the abdominal wall goes with a differential diagnosis including another type of ventral hernia, lipoma, hematoma, cyst, abscess, neoplasm, or ectopic testis [18].

Imaging: Ultrasound and Computed Tomography

One can conclude from the above that additional diagnostics are most often desirable in demonstrating a spigelian hernia and differentiating it from other pathology. In the literature, both ultrasound (US) and computed tomography (CT) have been used comparably to obtain the diagnosis [15].

US is an easy-to-perform, inexpensive, radiation-free, and noninvasive imaging modality. It is dynamic in nature allowing for real-time straining and relaxing of the abdominal muscles and has a sensitivity of 83–100% [14, 15]. However, the results of US are operator dependent and may be much less sensitive in case of obesity or when the operator is not instructed to search for a spigelian hernia [7, 18].

CT is another noninvasive imaging tool resulting in a sensitivity of 68–100% [14]. The addition of Valsalva maneuver and thin slices during CT examination significantly improves the sensitivity for ventral abdominal wall hernias [19]. An important benefit of CT is the detailed information about the whole ventral abdominal wall, the content of the hernia sac, and the possible intraperitoneal pathology (Fig. 50.3). However, an abdominal CT entails a relatively high radiation exposure with its associated risks, is more expensive, and may include the use of oral, rectal, and intravenous contrast.

Laparoscopy

In case imaging techniques result in equivocal results, but the patient's history and physical examination remains suspicious for a spigelian hernia, a diagnostic laparoscopy may ultimately be considered to confirm or exclude the diagnosis [16, 20]. Laparoscopy

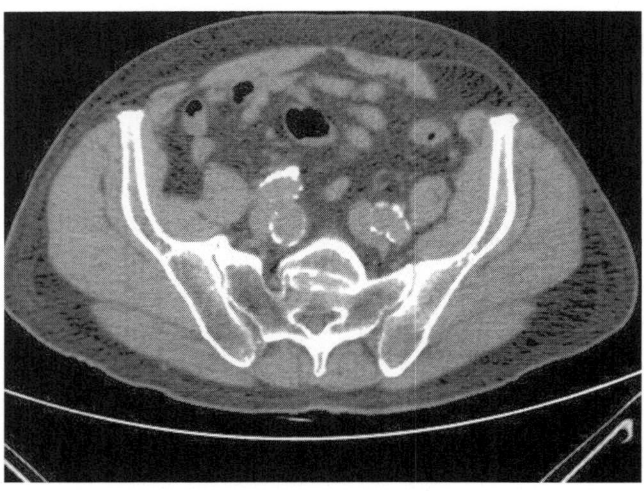

Fig. 50.3. CT scan with left-sided spigelian hernia with omentum in the hernia sac.

provides a direct inspection of the full ventral abdominal wall and possible hernias or other pathology. Furthermore, it provides an option for direct repair of the hernia. However, laparoscopy is an invasive procedure that may cause damage to intraperitoneal organs, and a hernia merely consisting of preperitoneal fat may be hard or even impossible to visualize in rare cases (Fig. 50.2, f). In case of the latter, a laparoscopic extraperitoneal (or open anterior) exploration may be required for diagnosis.

Proposed Diagnostic Process

Figure 50.4 depicts a proposed diagnostic flow chart for spigelian hernia in case of suggestive history and/or physical examination. We advocate that the repair of the hernia should be preceded by simple laparoscopy to confirm the diagnosis and location and the content of the hernia and to potentially identify any other abdominal (wall) pathology [14]. Repair of the defect(s) may then be performed consecutively or via an open approach if the surgeon is not familiar with endoscopic techniques (Fig. 50.5).

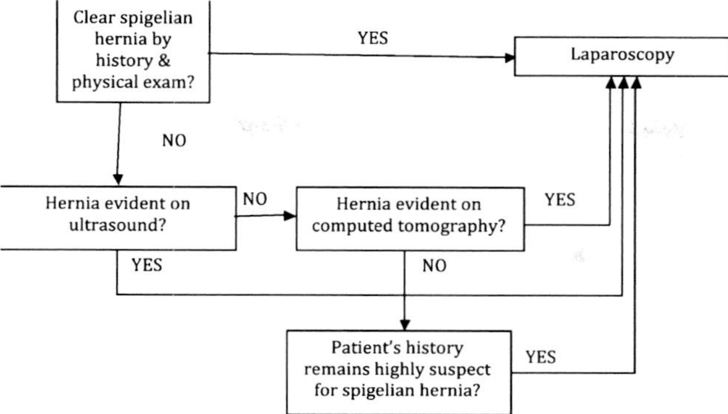

Fig. 50.4. Proposed diagnostic flow chart for spigelian hernia.

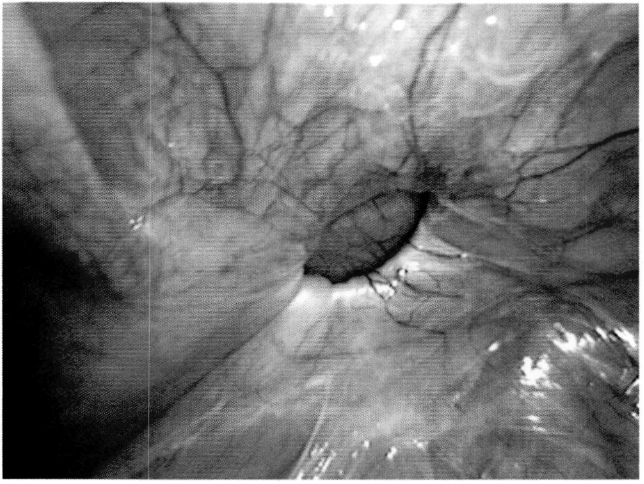

Fig. 50.5. Laparoscopic view of a left-sided spigelian hernia (same patient as in Fig. 50.3).

Treatment Options

In the treatment of spigelian hernias, two major questions exist. The first one concerns an open or laparoscopic mesh approach and the second whether a suture technique alone is still an option. Owing to the rarity of

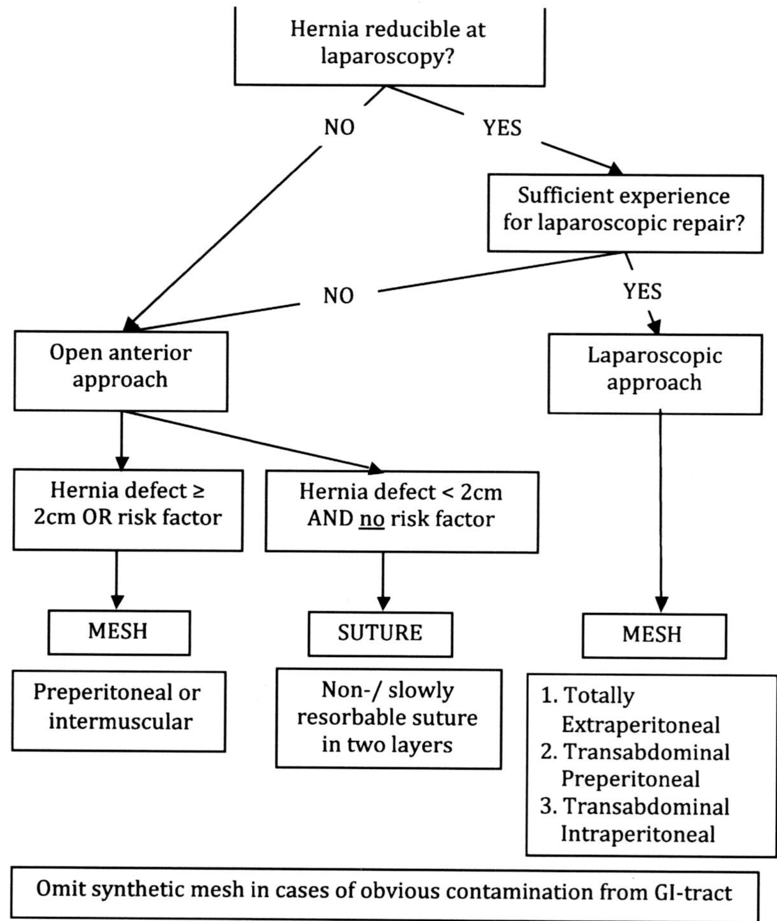

Fig. 50.6. Proposed surgical treatment flow chart for spigelian hernia.

spigelian hernias, only few studies and limited experience among surgeons are available. Nevertheless, we have formulated a proposal for the treatment of spigelian hernias based on best available evidence and our expert opinion (Fig. 50.6). Because of the increased risk for incarceration, it seems wise to advocate surgery also for asymptomatic spigelian hernias. However, this decision as well as the other treatment options described should be part of a shared decision process with an informed patient and family.

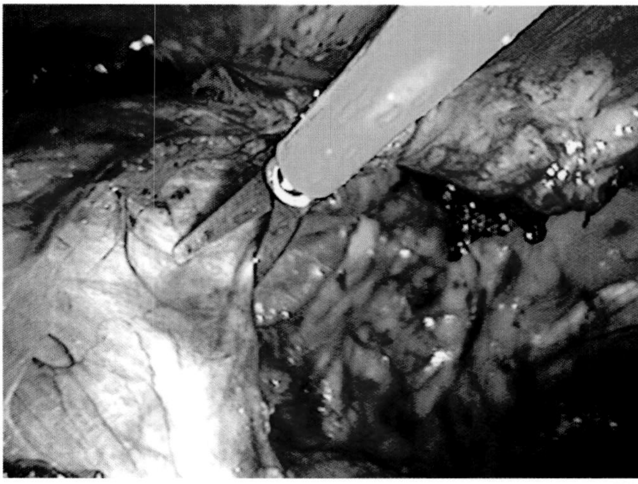

Fig. 50.7. Incision of the posterior rectus sheath laterally at the arcuate line in a totally extraperitoneal approach for laparoscopic repair of a left-sided spigelian hernia.

Open or Laparoscopic Mesh Placement

The laparoscopic repair of spigelian hernias is now well established [21, 22]. In 2002, the first and until now only randomized controlled trial on open and laparoscopic repair of spigelian hernias was published [23]. In this small trial, two groups of 11 patients with nonincarcerated hernias received a mesh either by open preperitoneal or laparoscopic repair (8 totally extraperitoneal, 3 intraperitoneal). There were no recurrences at a mean of 3.4-year follow-up, but length of stay and morbidity was significantly reduced in case of laparoscopy. The totally extraperitoneal approach was associated with the shortest hospital stay (5–9 h) and has been reported by others as well to be successful [24]. We therefore consider it the method of choice. However, in order to perform this procedure successfully, the surgeon must have sufficient experience with laparoscopic totally extraperitoneal inguinal hernia repair. The approach is identical, but it is advocated to incise the posterior rectus sheath laterally at the semicircular line of Douglas in order to have sufficient space laterally for placing a mesh with sufficient overlap (3–5 cm) (Fig. 50.7). We also propose the use of a 5-mm-angled endoscope with the three trocars in the midline (Fig. 50.8) so that the position of the

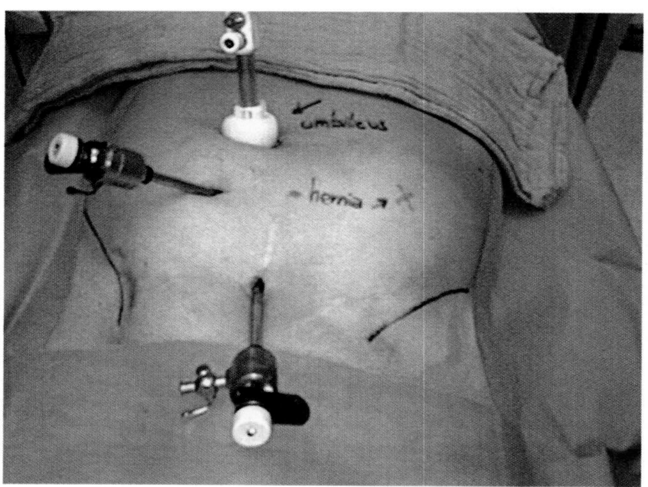

Fig. 50.8. Positioning of trocars in a totally extraperitoneal approach for laparoscopic repair of a left-sided spigelian hernia (same patient as in Fig. 50.3).

endoscope can be changed for obtaining the best view for dissection and placement of the mesh. Furthermore, the defect must generally be located well below the umbilicus in order to develop the preperitoneal plane adequately. As in laparoscopic inguinal hernia repair, also a transabdominal preperitoneal approach is possible [25, 26]. It offers a larger working space while mesh can still be placed preperitoneally after opening of the peritoneum. Otherwise, a laparoscopic intraperitoneal onlay mesh can be chosen [23, 27]. In these cases, as in laparoscopic incisional hernia repair, an adequate fixation of the intraperitoneal mesh is necessary. Although a laparoscopic technique might be especially useful in obese patients, the transabdominal approach may incur damage to the intestine, especially when adhesiolysis is required.

Opposed to the laparoscopic approach is the open mesh repair which was most dominant in the past century [15]. A transverse skin incision over the hernia, through the external oblique muscle is generally indicated. However, if the hernia cannot be palpated preoperatively and diagnosed laparoscopically or if there are multiple defects, a vertical skin incision will provide a good preperitoneal exposure [1, 2]. This incision can be extended easily craniocaudally and to the peritoneal cavity. Especially in case of an incarcerated or strangulated hernia, laparoscopic reduction of the hernia content may be difficult or even impossible

[28, 29]. Conversion to an open repair may then be necessary, and a partial bowel resection can be performed via the hernia defect or widened (umbilical) trocar site. In open surgery, a flat mesh can be placed preperitoneally or intermuscular. With sufficient overlap (3–5 cm), fixation of the mesh is probably unnecessary in a preperitoneal position. In the intermuscular positioning, the lateral edge of the rectus sheath should be opened for adequate expansion and overlap of the mesh behind the rectus muscle [30]. Also, the use of an intraperitoneal mesh or a mesh device by open approach has been described [31, 32].

Suture Technique

Following a landmark trial in 2000, tension-free mesh repair has become popularized since synthetic meshes reduced the recurrence rate of incisional hernias by about 50% [33]. In addition, the benefit of using mesh was not only found to be restricted to large hernia defects but also to defects ≤10 cm [2]. Another study also showed hernias with a diameter of 4 cm or more resulting in high recurrence rates after suture repair [34]. Schumacher et al. found recurrence rates after umbilical hernia repair with sutures to be 6% in defects up to 1 cm, 4% in defects up to 2 cm, 14% in defects up to 3 cm, 25% in defects up to 4 cm, and 54.4% in defects >4 cm [35].

Spigelian hernias are generally smaller than 4 cm, and about 90% are reported to be small (<2 cm in diameter). Suture repair concerns the closure of the hernia sac with an absorbable suture and the use of a running nonabsorbable or slowly absorbable monofilament suture to close the defect in two layers: first the deep layer (internal oblique and transversus muscle-spigelian aponeurosis) and then the external oblique aponeurosis [36–38]. Sutures are to be placed perpendicularly on the direction of the fibers. Also, laparoscopic suturing techniques have been described [15, 39].

Recent biological insights have shown multiple types of hernia to be related to a systemic collagen disorder [40–43]. What is more, most patients already display one or more risk factors for hernia development. Especially obesity is a major factor that shows high recurrence rates after ventral hernia repairs [44]. Since suture repair of spigelian hernias appears to have a lower recurrence rate compared to suture repair of inguinal and incisional hernias [1, 14], it seems a valuable option in case of small hernias (<2 cm in diameter) without any risk factors, such as obesity, smoking, heavy lifting, or known collagen disorders. However, we believe mesh repair can further reduce the risk for recurrence without increasing morbidity, such as postoperative (wound) complications, chronic pain, and adhesion formation, when placing the mesh extraperitoneally with minimal fixation, preferably by a totally extraperitoneal laparoscopic approach.

References

1. Spangen L. Spigelian hernia. World J Surg. 1989;13:573–80.
2. Skandalakis PN, Zoras O, Skandalakis JE, Mirilas P. Spigelian hernia: surgical anatomy, embryology, and technique of repair. Am Surg. 2006;72:42–8.
3. van den Spieghel A. Opera Quae Extant Omnia. Amsterdam: Johannes Blaeu; 1645.
4. Klinkosch JT. Programma Quo Divisionem Hernarium, Novumque Herniae Ventralis Specium Proponit. Rotterdam: Berman; 1764.
5. Spangen L. Spigelian hernia. Surg Clin N Am. 1984;64:351–66.
6. Read RC. Observations on the etiology of spigelian hernia. Ann Surg. 1960; 152:1004–9.
7. Salameh JR. Primary and unusual abdominal wall hernias. Surg Clin N Am. 2008; 88:45–60. viii.
8. Klimopoulos S, Kounoudes C, Validakis A, Galanis G. Low spigelian hernias: experience of 26 consecutive cases in 24 patients. Eur J Surg. 2001;167:631–3.
9. Raveenthiran V. Congenital Spigelian hernia with cryptorchidism: probably a new syndrome. Hernia. 2005;9:378–80.
10. Dabbas N, Adams K, Pearson K, Royle G. Frequency of abdominal wall hernias: is classical teaching out of date? J R Soc Med Sh Rep. 2011;2:5.
11. Patle NM, Tantia O, Sasmal PK, Khanna S, Sen B. Laparoscopic repair of spigelian hernia: our experience. J Laparoendosc Adv Surg Tech A. 2010;20:129–33.
12. Paajanen H, Ojala S, Virkkunen A. Incidence of occult inguinal and Spigelian hernias during laparoscopy of other reasons. Surgery. 2006;140:9–12.
13. Nieuwenhuizen J, van Ramshorst GH, Ten Brinke JG, de Wit T, van der Harst E, Hop WC, Jeekel J, Lange JF. The use of mesh in acute hernia: frequency and outcome in 99 cases. Hernia. 2011;15:297–300.
14. Larson DW, Farley DR. Spigelian hernias: repair and outcome for 81 patients. World J Surg. 2002;26:1277–81.
15. Bittner JG, Edwards MA, Shah MB, MacFadyen Jr BV, Mellinger JD. Mesh-free laparoscopic spigelian hernia repair. Am Surg. 2008;74:713–20.
16. Habib E, Elhadad A. Spigelian hernia long considered as diverticulitis: CT scan diagnosis and laparoscopic treatment. Computed tomography. Surg Endosc. 2003; 17:159.
17. Reid DR. Spigelian hernia simulating acute appendicitis. Br J Surg. 1949;36:433.
18. D'Hooge P, Van Der Bijl H, Miserez M. Update on Spigelian hernia: diagnosis and treatment by means of two cases. Acta Chir Belg. 2004;104:719–23.

19. Jaffe TA, O'Connell MJ, Harris JP, Paulson EK, Delong DM. MDCT of abdominal wall hernias: is there a role for Valsalva maneuver? Am J Roentgenol. 2005; 184:847–51.
20. Shenouda NF, Hyams BB, Rosenbloom MB. Evaluation of Spigelian hernia by CT. J Comput Assist Tomogr. 1990;14:777–8.
21. Carter JE, Mizes C. Laparoscopic diagnosis and repair of spigelian hernia: report of a case and technique. Am J Obstet Gynecol. 1992;167:77–8.
22. Skouras C, Purkayastha S, Jiao L, Tekkis P, Darzi A, Zacharakis E. Laparoscopic management of spigelian hernias. Surg Laparosc Endosc Percutan Tech. 2011; 21:76–81.
23. Moreno-Egea A, Carrasco L, Girela E, Martin JG, Aguayo JL, Canteras M. Open vs laparoscopic repair of spigelian hernia: a prospective randomized trial. Arch Surg. 2002;137:1266–8.
24. Tarnoff M, Rosen M, Brody F. Planned totally extraperitoneal laparoscopic Spigelian hernia repair. Surg Endosc. 2002;16:359.
25. Martell EG, Singh NN, Zagorski SM, Sawyer MA. Laparoscopic repair of a spigelian hernia: a case report and literature review. JSLS. 2004;8:269–74.
26. Palanivelu C, Viijaykumar M, Jani KV, Rajan PS, Maheshkumaar GS, Rajapandian S. Laparoscopic transabdominal preperitoneal repair of Spigelian hernia. JSLS. 2006; 10:193–8.
27. Saber AA, Elgamal MH, Rao AJ, Osmer RL, Itawi EA. Laparoscopic spigelian hernia repair: the scroll technique. Am Surg. 2008;74:108–12.
28. Subramanya MS, Chakraborty J, Memon B, Memon MA. Emergency intraperitoneal onlay mesh repair of incarcerated spigelian hernia. JSLS. 2010;14:275–8.
29. Yau KK, Siu WT, Chau CH, Yang GP, Li MK. A laparoscopic approach for incarcerated Spigelian hernia. J Laparoendosc Adv Surg Tech A. 2005;15:57–9.
30. Celdran A, Senaris J, Manas J, Frieyro O. The open mesh repair of Spigelian hernia. Am J Surg. 2007;193:111–3.
31. Malazgirt Z, Topgul K, Sokmen S, Ersin S, Turkcapar AG, Gok H, Gonullu N, Paksoy M, Ertem M. Spigelian hernias: a prospective analysis of baseline parameters and surgical outcome of 34 consecutive patients. Hernia. 2006;10:326–30.
32. Campanelli G, Pettinari D, Nicolosi FM, Avesani EC. Spigelian hernia. Hernia. 2005; 9:3–5.
33. Burger JW, Luijendijk RW, Hop WC, Halm JA, Verdaasdonk EG, Jeekel J. Long-term follow-up of a randomized controlled trial of suture versus mesh repair of incisional hernia. Ann Surg. 2004;240:578–83.
34. Hesselink VJ, Luijendijk RW, de Wilt JH, Heide R, Jeekel J. An evaluation of risk factors in incisional hernia recurrence. Surg Gynecol Obstet. 1993;176:228–34.
35. Schumacher OP, Peiper C, Lörken M, Schumpelick V. Long-term results after Spitzy's umbilical hernia repair. Chirurg. 2003;74:50–4.
36. Pélissier E, Ngo P. Traitement chirurgical des hernies de Spiegel. EMC (Elsevier Masson SAS, Paris), Techniques Chirurgicales—Appareil digestif, 40–151; 2010.

37. Bloemen A, van Dooren P, Huizinga BF, Hoofwijk AG. Randomized clinical trial comparing polypropylene or polydioxanone for midline abdominal wall closure. Br J Surg. 2011;98:633–9.
38. Van't Riet M, Steyerberg EW, Nellensteyn J, Bonjer HJ, Jeekel J. Meta-analysis of techniques for closure of midline abdominal incisions. Br J Surg. 2002;89:1350–6.
39. Ng WT, Kong CK, Kong KC. Facilitation of open Spigelian hernia repair by laparoscopic location of the hernial defect. Surg Endosc. 2004;18:561–2.
40. Klinge U, Junge K, Mertens PR. Herniosis: a biological approach. Hernia. 2004;8: 300–1.
41. Casanova AB, Trindade EN, Trindade MR. Collagen in the transversalis fascia of patients with indirect inguinal hernia: a case-control study. Am J Surg. 2009;198:1–5.
42. Asling B, Jirholt J, Hammond P, Knutsson M, Walentinsson A, Davidson G, Agreus L, Lehmann A, Lagerström-Fermer M. Collagen type III alpha I is a gastro-oesophageal reflux disease susceptibility gene and a male risk factor for hiatus hernia. Gut. 2009;58:1063–9.
43. Franz MG. The biology of hernia formation. Surg Clin N Am. 2008;88:1–15. vii.
44. Sauerland S, Korenkov M, Kleinen T, Arndt M, Paul A. Obesity is a risk factor for recurrence after incisional hernia repair. Hernia. 2004;8:42–6.

51. Hernia, Mesh, and Gynecology Procedures

Lauren Rascoff, Brian P. Jacob, and Charles Ascher-Walsh

Pelvic reconstructive surgeons, or urogynecologists, treat benign gynecologic conditions including pelvic organ prolapse and incontinence. Pelvic organ prolapse (POP) is the descent of the pelvic organs, including uterus, bladder, rectum, post-hysterectomy vaginal cuff, and small or large bowel, into the vaginal cavity. Stress urinary incontinence (SUI) is the involuntary leakage of urine on exertion, or while sneezing or laughing. These are common conditions—the lifetime risk of undergoing surgery for pelvic organ prolapse or incontinence, according to population-based studies, is 11–19% [1]. In addition, 6–29% of women who undergo surgical repair will need an additional surgery for recurrent prolapse or incontinence [2]. Risk factors for POP and SUI include parity, advanced age, and obesity, as well as chronic constipation [3]. Traditionally, prolapse was corrected using absorbable sutures. Given the high failure rates of these suture-only repairs and the success of mesh in general surgery, pelvic reconstructive surgeons began using synthetic mesh to augment prolapse repairs and treat stress urinary incontinence. Many studies have substantiated the efficacy and safety of mesh in abdominal surgery; however, the quantity and quality of research done concerning the use of mesh in gynecologic surgery is mixed. There is even less research concerning the safety in using mesh to repair a hernia concomitantly with gynecologic surgery. The question then becomes, if a patient has a symptomatic hernia and wants a repair at the same time as her prolapse repair, does placement of transvaginal mesh have any bearing on a hernia surgeon's decision to place mesh abdominally? Does it make a difference if the gynecologist opens the abdomen through the vagina during placement of the mesh? The main difficulty in answering these questions is that there are no studies on the topic. At this point in

B.P. Jacob and B. Ramshaw (eds.), *The SAGES Manual of Hernia Repair*,
DOI 10.1007/978-1-4614-4824-2_51,

time, more research needs to be done to fully address these issues. We will first give a detailed review of mesh in gynecologic surgery and then address these questions in more detail.

Grafts in Gynecologic Surgery

High failure rates with traditional surgeries for prolapse have led to the common use of grafts to repair pelvic floor defects and to treat stress incontinence. Pelvic floor defects are broadly characterized into three compartments—anterior (usually a cystocele), apical (usually uterine or vaginal cuff prolapse), or posterior (usually a rectocele). Pelvic floor defect repairs can be repaired either abdominally or vaginally. The most commonly performed abdominal surgery for apical pelvic floor defects that is loosely considered the gold standard for these types of defects is the sacrocolpopexy. This procedure, which can be done either laparoscopically—with or without robotic assistance—or via a laparotomy, involves the attachment of the top of the vagina or cervix (then called a sacrocervicopexy) to the promontorium of the sacrum. Because the vagina is not normally long enough to reach the sacrum, a graft is typically used to bridge the distance in this attachment. Although this procedure was originally done with permanent sutures or biologic grafts, currently, most pelvic surgeons opt for synthetic polypropylene mesh. Sacrocolpopexy has a reported success rate of 78–100% (no recurrent apical prolapse) and 58–100% (no recurrent prolapse in any compartment), as noted in a large review. Synthetic mesh erosion into the vagina, which is the most significant complication in many of the newer surgeries performed to treat prolapse, is reported to be 3.4%; however, rates vary by type of mesh, with polypropylene being 0.5% and non-expanded polytetrafluoroethylene being 5.5% [4]. There are two prospective, randomized trials comparing abdominal sacrocolpopexy with vaginal approaches to apical defects. One study followed 38 women in the abdominal group and 42 in the vaginal group for a mean of 2.5 years. Results showed a higher reoperation rate in the vaginal group for recurrent prolapse and incontinence. In this study, suture-only techniques were used to suspend the vaginal cuff to the sacrum [5]. Another prospective study comparing sacrocolpopexy with mesh to vaginal sacrospinous repair without mesh showed similar objective and subjective cure rates and concluded that both approaches are highly effective in the treatment of apical prolapse [6]. There is very little controversy regarding mesh in abdominal sacrocolpopexy given good prospective data and low erosion rates, especially when attaching the mesh to the cervix.

Grafts can be placed vaginally to treat anterior, apical, or posterior defects, and it is in this arena that the controversy arises. Traditionally, these defects were repaired with suture-only techniques. In the last 10 years, vaginal mesh kits have been made commercially available, which can repair any or all three of the compartments from the vaginal route. Transvaginal mesh kits have been developed to provide an efficient and minimally invasive approach to correct prolapse and as a response to high failure rates of traditional suture-only repairs. These kits are meant to be laid without tension and involve precut synthetic grafts with suspension of mesh arms either through sacrospinous ligaments, arcus tendineus fasciae pelvis, the obturator membrane, or iliococcygeus fascia. Transvaginal mesh kits were released into the market with very little data on their safety or efficacy. Success rates seem to be high according to the data that we have; for example, a meta-analysis showed high success rates for apical support—88% at 6.5–19.5 months; however, complication rates also seem to be high [7]. Two studies comparing traditional transvaginal repair for apical prolapse and polypropylene mesh kits showed a very high erosion rate—16% and 36% [8, 9]. A large review showed similar results—vaginal mesh kits had lower reoperation rates for prolapse recurrence but higher complication rates as a result of mesh erosion and fistula [10]. One prospective case series followed 110 patients for 3 months and found a recurrent prolapse rate of 4.7% and mesh erosion rate of 4.7% [11]. Similar data, although retrospective, looked at 120 patients at 13 months and found a 93% success rate and a mesh erosion rate, only in the anterior repair, of 3% [12]. Again, there are no long-term, large, prospective randomized trials looking at the safety and effectiveness of transvaginal mesh kits, and it is for this reason that we still have many unanswered questions regarding transvaginal mesh.

Graft material is also used to treat stress urinary incontinence, and midurethral slings are currently the gold standard operation. In one study, the objective cure rate after one midurethral sling placement (using polypropylene mesh) was 84.7% in a median 56-month follow-up [13]. Midurethral slings have been shown to be as effective as other surgical options for stress incontinence, such as retropubic colposuspension and bladder neck slings, but with shorter operative times and faster recovery; this was shown in a meta-analysis of 62 randomized trials [14]. In the same review, the perioperative complication rates did not differ among midurethral slings and more traditional surgeries. The only exception is bladder perforation; however, the clinical significance of this is low. Erosion rate after one midurethral sling has been reported at 0.4%, in one series of 241 women [15]. Given a number of well-conducted prospective studies and low erosion rates, mesh use for SUI is, on the whole, widely accepted.

Types of Grafts

In pelvic reconstructive surgery, the first grafts adopted were biologic. For example, autologous fascia lata slings for incontinence were popular and continue to be used. Other donor sites include abdominal wall fascia and vaginal skin. Autografts have also been used in sacrocolpopexy, but there are only two small case series looking at its use [16, 17]. The potential advantage of autologous materials over synthetic materials is the histologic similarity and low erosion rates. The main drawback, however, is the need to harvest the graft and potential complications at the donor site. Allografts, or cadaveric grafts, have been used in gynecologic surgery. One source of allograft material is derived from human dermis; it is a processed, acellular material that was used in repairing anterior and posterior defects, as well as treatment of stress incontinence [18]. Additionally, processed fascia lata has also been used for slings and for repair of anterior and posterior defects. The literature supports autografts over allografts in treatment of stress incontinence. In one study of 47 patients, 41.7% of allograft patients demonstrated SUI postoperatively compared with 0% of autograft patients [19]. Xenografts have also been used in reconstructive surgery, notably porcine and bovine grafts.

Synthetic grafts are currently the preferred material in gynecologic surgery. The properties of an ideal graft are as follows: (1) noncarcinogenic, (2) durable and able to withstand physical pressures, (3) chemically inert or have a predictable tissue response, (4) nontoxic to the host, (5) easily manufacturable and widely available, (6) resistant to infection, and (7) affordable [20]. Mesh is classified according to type, pore size, and filament number. Type I meshes are all polypropylene and are macroporous (pore size >75 μm) and monofilamentous. The advantage of type I mesh is their large interstices that allow passage of leukocytes and macrophages to fight infection. Type II meshes are microporous (<10 μm) and multifilamentous. Type III meshes are multifilamentous and can either have macroporous or microporous components. The disadvantage of type II and type III mesh is that multifilament mesh with small pore size allows the passage of small bacteria but not macrophages and leukocytes to fight off infection. Type IV mesh is a polypropylene sheet—monofilament and submicroporous—which is not used in pelvic surgery given its properties.

Polypropylene is popular among gynecologic surgeons for both abdominal and vaginal procedures because of its supposed inert behavior and ability to be reconfigured in different ways. It is becoming clear, however, that polypropylene is actually not inert. In one study, 100 vaginal mesh implants were explanted from patients secondary to complications and analyzed using histologic, microscopic, and chemical testing to determine degradation characteristics. The authors found that 75% of the multifilament and 33.3% of the monofilament polypropylene meshes were degraded. None of the polyethylene terephthalate (polyester) meshes were degraded even after being in the body for 3 years [21]. Additionally, this study found that low-weight meshes fared better than high-weight meshes, which is what gynecologists are currently using. This new data that polypropylene may not be as inert as gynecologists once thought is important and may shed light on erosion and infection rates.

Safety of Polypropylene Mesh

The Food and Drug Administration (FDA) has approved graft materials used in gynecologic surgery, since they are "equivalent" to existing materials already in use. However, this approval by the FDA does not speak to the graft safety or effectiveness. In 2008, the FDA put out a warning regarding mesh used in vaginal surgery for pelvic organ prolapse. The FDA received 1,000 reports from nine manufacturing companies regarding mesh complications. The warning did not specify the type of mesh used or the manufacturer. It did, however, indicate recommendations for physicians, which are as follows: (1) obtain specialized training for each mesh placement technique and be aware of its risks; (2) be vigilant for potential adverse events from the mesh, especially erosion and infection; (3) watch for complications associated with the tools used in transvaginal placement, especially bowel, bladder, and blood vessel perforations; (4) inform patients that implantation of surgical mesh is permanent, and that some complications associated with the implanted mesh may require additional surgery that may or may not correct the complication; (5) inform patients about the potential for serious complications and their effect on quality of life, including pain during sexual intercourse, scarring, and narrowing of the vaginal wall (in POP repair); and (6) provide patients with a written copy of the patient labeling from the surgical mesh manufacturer, if available [22].

On 13 July 2011, the FDA put out an additional warning regarding transvaginal mesh: "The FDA is issuing this update to inform you that serious complications associated with surgical mesh for transvaginal repair of POP are *not rare*. This is a change from what the FDA previously reported on 20 Oct 2008. Furthermore, it is not clear that transvaginal POP repair with mesh is more effective than traditional non-mesh repair in all patients with POP and it may expose patients to greater risk." As a result of this update and the numerous complications related to the use of mesh placed vaginally with these kits, a number of class action lawsuits have been created. Lawyers advertise in the media lumping together all types of treatments with synthetic mesh, making it more challenging to use these materials in any gynecologic surgery. Despite the new and increasing reports of mesh erosion, the FDA recommendations to the health care providers remain the same as the 2008 notice [23]. There are still many gynecologic surgeons who believe that its use enables better outcomes and continue to use it today.

Combined Hernia Repairs and Gynecologic Surgeries

When is it appropriate to do concomitant benign gynecologic surgeries and hernia repairs? Vaginal surgery does not preclude concomitant abdominal surgery. It is common practice for gynecologists to do both vaginal and abdominal procedures during the same case. Surgeons need to change gloves after completing the vaginal portion of a case and ensure a sterile setup abdominally. However, in light of the unknown long-term outcomes of placing mesh transvaginally, the question remains whether there is an increased infection and/or erosion rate of mesh placed during a hernia repair if it is done at the same time as a gynecologic procedure. What makes this question even more difficult is that there are no studies on the topic.

A look at surgical site classifications may give some insight into the vagina and the body's response to mesh. There is a widely accepted classification system for surgical sites, which was described 35 years ago by the National Academy of Sciences and the National Research Council [24]. The four categories are clean, clean-contaminated, contaminated, and dirty. Clean wounds are considered to be uninfected wounds in which a viscus was not entered. Clean-contaminated wounds are defined as an operative site where a viscus is entered under controlled conditions without significant bacterial contamination. Contaminated wounds are defined as procedures with spillage from a viscus, and dirty wounds include those that are infected or have existing perforated viscus. Vaginal surgery is considered to be a clean-contaminated operation. In a descriptive study done in 2001–2002, vaginal cultures were taken prior to the administration of antibiotics during a vaginal case and 30 and 90 min after the start of the case with the goal to see bacterial colony counts in the vagina [25]. The authors found that the highest total and anaerobic colony counts was at 30 min (52%), and it decreased to 41% at 90 min. Again, this was a descriptive pilot study, so statistical significance was not determined. However, this data may suggest either that the surgical scrub that is used is not killing off the bacteria or the preoperative antibiotics did not have time to affect vaginal colony counts. We also learn from this study that the clean-contaminated vagina cannot be fully sterilized.

We know that the vagina is colonized, so why doesn't all mesh become infected or erode? Many factors influence erosion, such as surface area of the mesh, pore size, infection, hematoma, elasticity of the mesh, and placement of the mesh. There are many techniques that may help to prevent infection or erosion of transvaginal mesh—a sheath around the mesh that is used for insertion, soaking the mesh in antibiotics prior to placing it, and routine parenteral antibiotics. In 1987, Gristina offered a conceptual way of understanding what happens to a foreign body as it is inserted into the body. He stated that there is a "race for the surface" of the mesh between host cells and bacteria, and if the host tissue wins, the material is less susceptible to bacterial colonization, subsequent infection, or erosion [26]. There are many factors involved in incorporation of foreign materials that we are still learning about.

In one study by Jacob BP et al., presented at the American Hernia Society 2012, designed to evaluate potential mesh contamination from insertion in a natural orifice, like the vaginal canal, polypropylene was used to culture both the unprepped and Betadine™-prepped vaginal canal in ten humans during a laparoscopic-assisted or robotic-assisted hysterectomy, and the results compared to a third culture from a prepped skin incision in the same patients [27]. The results are shown

Table 51.1. Mesh contamination microbiology results after polypropylene mesh insertion and removal in ten humans undergoing hysterectomy.

Unprepped vaginal canal	Betadine™-prepped vaginal canal	Betadine™-prepped skin incision
Lactobacilli	No growth	Coagulase-negative *Staphylococcus*
Coagulase-negative *Staphylococcus*		*Corynebacterium*
Corynebacterium		*Staphylococcus lugdunensis*
Streptococcus viridans		
Group B Strep		
Enterococcus		
Gardnerella vaginalis		

in Table 51.1. Impressively, there was no contamination on any of the mesh when inserted in a Betadine™-prepped vaginal canal, while there was contamination in three cases when the mesh was inserted through a prepped skin incision. The results suggest that a prepped vaginal canal is an acceptable and sterile environment for polypropylene mesh insertion.

What to do in a specific clinical scenario when a patient undergoing a gynecologic procedure has a symptomatic hernia requiring repair? As stated above, vaginal cases are clean-contaminated cases and therefore do not in and of themselves preclude simultaneous procedures. Additionally, if the transvaginal mesh were to erode or become infected, the disease state would be localized and will most likely not affect mesh placed abdominally. At this point in time, more research needs to be done in order to definitively answer this question.

References

1. Smith FJ, Holman CD, Moorin RE, Tsokos NS. Epidemiology of surgically managed pelvic organ prolapse and urinary incontinence. Obstet Gynecol. 1997;89(4):501.
2. Olsen AL, Smith VJ, Bergstrom JO, Colling JC, Clark AL. Epidemiology of surgically managed pelvic organ prolapse and urinary incontinence. Obstet Gynecol. 1997; 89(4):501.
3. Jelovsek JE, Maher C, Barber MD. Pelvic organ prolapse. Lancet. 2007; 369(9566): 1027.
4. Nygaard IE, McCreery R, Brubaker L, et al. Abdominal sacrocolpopexy: a comprehensive review. Obstet Gynecol. 2004;104:805.

5. Benson JT, Lucente V, McClellan E. Vaginal versus abdominal reconstructive surgery for the treatment of pelvic support defects. A prospective randomized study of long-term outcome evaluation. Am J Obstet Gynecol. 1996;175:1418–22.
6. Maher CF, Qatawneh AM, Dwyer PL, et al. Abdominal sacral colpopexy or vaginal sacrospinous colpopexy for vaginal vault prolapse: a prospective randomized study. Am J Obstet Gynecol. 2004;190:20–6.
7. Feiner B, Jelovsek JE, Maher C. Efficacy and safety of transvaginal mesh kits in the treatment of prolapse of the vaginal apex: a systematic review. BJOG. 2009;116:15.
8. Iglesia CB, Sokol AI, Sokol ER, Kudish BI, Gutman RE, Peterson JL, Shott S. Vaginal mesh for prolapse: a randomized controlled trial. Obstet Gynecol. 2010;116(2 Pt 1):293.
9. Lopes ED, Lemos NL, Carramão Sda S, Lunardelli JL, Ruano JM, Aoki T, Auge AP. Transvaginal polypropylene mesh versus sacrospinous ligament fixation for the treatment of uterine prolapse: 1-year follow-up of a randomized controlled trial. Int Urogynecol J Pelvic Floor Dysfunct. 2010;21(4):389.
10. Diwadker G, Barber M, Feiner B, Maher C, Jelovsek JE. Complication and reoperation rates after apical vaginal prolapse surgical repair. Obstet Gynecol. 2009;113(2): 367–73.
11. Fatton B, Amblard J, Debodinance P, et al. Transvaginal repair of genital prolapse: preliminary results of a new tension-free vaginal mesh (ProliftTM techniques)—a case series multicentric study. Int Urogynecol J Pelvic Floor Dysfunct. 2007;18:743–52.
12. Gauuder-Burmester A, Koutouzidou P, Rohne J, et al. Follow-up after polypropylene mesh repair of anterior and posterior compartments in patients with recurrent prolapse. Int Urogynecol J Pelvic Floor Dysfunct. 2007;18:1059–64.
13. Nilsson CG, Kuuva N, Falconer CA, et al. Long-term results of the tension-free vaginal tape (TVT) procedure for surgical treatment of female stress urinary incontinence. Int Urogynecol J. 2001;12 Suppl 2:S5–8.
14. Ogah J, Cody JD, Rogerson L. Minimally invasive synthetic suburethral sling operations for stress urinary incontinence. Cochrane Database Syst Rev 2009;(4): CD006375.
15. Abouassaly R, Steinberg JR, Lemieux M, Marois C, Gilchrist LI, Bourque JL, le Tu M, Corcos J. Complications of tension-free vaginal tape surgery: a multi-institutional review. BJU Int. 2004;94(1):110.
16. Culligan PJ, Murphy M, Blackwell L, Hammons G, Graham C, Heit MH. Long-term success of abdominal sacral colpopexy using synthetic mesh. Am J Obstet Gynecol. 2002;187(6):1473.
17. Brizzolara S, Pillai-Allen A. Risk of mesh erosion with sacral colpopexy and concurrent hysterectomy. Obstet Gynecol. 2003;102(2):306.
18. Crivellaro S, Smith JJ, Kocjancic E, et al. Transvaginal sling using acellular human dermal allograft: safety and efficacy in 253 patients. J Urol. 2004;172:1374–8.
19. McBride AW, Ellerkmann RM, Bent AE, Melick CF. Comparison of long-term outcomes of autologous fascia lata slings with Suspend Tutoplast fascia lata allograft slings for stress incontinence. Am J Obstet Gynecol. 2005;192:1677.
20. Bent A, Cundiff G, Swift S. Sutues and grafts in pelvic reconstructure surgery Ostergard's Urogynecology and Pelvic Floor Dysfunction. 6th ed. Pennsylvania: Lippincott Williams and Wilkns, 2008, p. 527.

21. Clave A, Yahi H, Hammou J, Montanaru S, Suzelei M, Gounon P, Clave H. Polypropylene as a reinforcement in pelvic surgery is not inert: a comparative analysis of 100 explants. Int Urogynecol J. 2010;21:261–70.
22. http://www.fda.gov/MedicalDevices/Safety/AlertsandNotices/PublicHealthNotifications/ucm061976.htm.
23. http://www.fda.gov/MedicalDevices/Safety/AlertsandNotices/ucm262435.htm.
24. Altemeier WA, Burke JF, Pruitt BA, Sandusky WR. Manual on control of infection in surgical patients. Philadelphia, PA: JB Lippincott; 1984.
25. Culligan P, Heit M, Blackwell L, Murphy M, Graham CA, Snyder J. Bacterial colony counts during vaginal surgery. Infect Dis Obstet Gynecol. 2003;11:161–5.
26. Gristina AG. Biomaterial-centered infection: microbial adhesion versus tissue integration. Science. 1987;237:1588–95.
27. Capes T, Krishan R, LaBombardi V, Pipia G, Ascher-Walsh C, Jacob B. The prepped vaginal canal may be a more sterile conduit for ventral hernia mesh insertion than a prepped laparoscopic skin incision: a prospective comparative study of mesh contamination for NOTES hernia repair. Accepted abstract and podium presentation at the AHS, New York, 2012.

Index

B.P. Jacob and B. Ramshaw (eds.), *The SAGES Manual of Hernia Repair*,
DOI 10.1007/978-1-4614-4824-2,

M

U

V